When this book was first published in 1993 it filled a real gap in the market. The need for a comprehensive, up-to-date text for the new student beginning health studies had been apparent for some time. Christine Brooker's *Human Structure and Function* satisfied these demands because it did not assume a background knowledge of general science. Instead, the principles of chemistry and physics were explained at appropriate points in the text while clear links between anatomy, physiology and the principles underpinning clinical practice were made throughout. Other strengths of the book could be identified in the key definitions which opened every chapter and the inclusion of a reference list with indicators for further reading for every topic. The book was generously and clearly illustrated throughout, with useful self-tests which students could use to monitor their own progress.

It gives me great pleasure to witness the publication of a second edition which retains all the original strengths of this now well-established text. *Human Structure and Function* has been thoroughly updated, ensuring that all the Nursing Practice Applications, Person-centred Studies and Special Focus sections are in line with current clinical practice. Moreover, these learning aids are now identified for the reader by a system of icons which effectively make the text even more user-friendly. The preface to this new edition provides the student with credible reasons for the need to master anatomy and physiology and the introduction provides a concise explanation of how to achieve maximum benefit from the text.

This second edition will continue to be widely appreciated by all those teaching the curricula on Project 2000 diploma courses and, with its attractive format, it will remain a firm favourite with students of nursing and the many other disciplines allied to health care.

Dinah Gould
Professor of Nursing
South Bank University
London

ACKNOWLEDGMENTS

With many thanks to Dinah Gould and Christine Hanks for reviewing the text; Ann Osborne at King's Lynn Health Service Library, The Queen Elizabeth Hospital; Janet Yeoman at the Resource Office, North West Anglia Health Promotion; Nicola Horton, Georgina Massy, Jill Northcott, Hannah Tudge and Cathryn Waters of Mosby International; Leander who helped to check the page proofs; and to my friends and colleagues for their help and support. Special thanks to my partner David who was his usual brilliant self with the computer 'stuff' and to our great chums – The Dalli who helped to preserve my mental health.

Disclaimer

This book should not be used as a prime source for prescribing and dispensing drugs. The publisher and author have undertaken reasonable endeavours to check dosage and nursing content for accuracy. We recommend that the reader should always check the manufacturer's product information for changes in dosage or administration before administering any medication.

Readers should also be aware that the publication of new research findings will continue to affect their evidence-based practice.

The people featured in the book are fictitious and are not based on any persons I have nursed or met while supervising students.

Nursing applications in clinical practice

Human Structure and Function

Second Edition

Christine Br̶o̶o̶k̶e̶r

BSc, RN, RM, RNT
formerly Senior Lecturer
in Nursing Studies
South Bank University
London

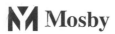 Mosby   London Philadelphia St Louis
Sydney Tokyo

Publisher:
Jill Northcott

Development Editor:
Gillian Harris

Project Manager:
Cathryn Waters

Index:
Nina Boyd

Production:
Hamish Adamson

Design:
Lara Last

Layout:
Gisli Thor

Illustration Manager:
Daniel Pyne

Cover Design:
Greg Smith

Illustration:
Evi Antoniou
John Cheung
Rob Dean
Diane Kinton
Debra Maizels
Jenni Miller
Amanda Williams
Debbie Woodward

First edition published by Mosby-Year Book Europe, Ltd, 1993

Reprinted 1996 by Times Mirror International Publishers Ltd.

Published by Mosby, an imprint of Mosby International Limited

Lynton House
7–12 Tavistock Square
London WC1H 9LB

Copyright © 1998 Mosby International Limited

ISBN 0 7234 2661 9

Printed by Printer Trento s.r.l., Trento, Italy
Text set in Sabon; captions set in Gill Sans

For full details of all Mosby titles please write to Mosby International Limited, Lynton House, 7–12 Tavistock Square, London WC1H 9LB, UK.

A CIP catalogue record for this book is available from the British Library.

CONTENTS

PREFACE

The major aims of *Human Structure and Function* are to provide students of nursing with the basic knowledge they need for the biology and physiology topics covered within Project 2000 diploma and nursing degree courses, and to form a firm base upon which to build the appropriate aspects of the branch programmes. The content and level of knowledge included in the book have been influenced by comments from students, lecturers, tutors and clinical nurses. This knowledge of human structure (anatomy) and function (physiology) is provided within the context of nursing practice applications.

The principal theme is that of structure and normal function, and the close relationship between structure and function is emphasized within the text. The information is provided within a logical framework. The eight sections cover the 'building' of a complete human organism from organic molecules through cells and tissues to the organs and functional systems which maintain homeostasis, the internal environment, functional areas of the body with overlap between sections as appropriate, basic genetics and an outline of developmental progress from embryo to older adult to provide an overview of the 'grand plan' which makes us unique and the significant physical events occurring during life.

The text is practice-based and, where appropriate, linked with relevant nursing research, health promotion initiatives and the pathophysiological changes which lead to disease states.

With assistance from learning aids incorporated throughout the text (see Introduction), students can use *Human Structure and Function* to:

- appreciate normal functioning of the body with its vital interactions that ensure homeostasis and health;

- understand how physiological dysfunction may lead to health deficiencies (illness);

- use their knowledge of body functioning during observation and assessment of people, clients and patients;

- apply this knowledge to appropriate areas of nursing practice with particular reference to current research into problems such as pain, incontinence or pressure sores; and

- integrate this knowledge with social and behavioural sciences in the promotion of health, prevention of ill-health, rehabilitation, and care relevant to the chosen branch programme.

No book or aid to learning is complete in itself. It succeeds only if it enables students to broaden and enhance their knowledge, and to apply this knowledge to daily nursing practice. As students prepare to pursue their chosen branch programme and beyond, *Human Structure and Function* will provide them with a firm knowledge of anatomy and physiology, founded in holism and health.

Christine Brooker

INTRODUCTION

To the Student

Why study structure and function?

Why is a detailed knowledge of human anatomy and physiology, and other basic biological sciences relevant to today's nurses? Apart from the fact that the roles and responsibilities of nurses are expanding in concert with our increasing knowledge of health issues and medical science, there are several reasons why these topics are of particular relevance to nurses and students of nursing:

- Health and health needs are better understood when there is an appreciation of the relevant biological sciences and an ability to integrate this knowledge with social and behavioural sciences.

- Breakdown in homeostasis can be more easily identified if normal functioning of physiological systems is clearly defined and there is an understanding of the biological factors that affect health.

- Physical care can be planned and implemented more effectively if the practitioner is familiar with relevant biological aspects of care. Knowledge of life sciences is considered, by students, to be important in physical care and in understanding reasons for a particular nursing action (Akinsanja, 1985).

- Outcomes of care can be more accurately predicted and evaluated by the practitioner who has a broad knowledge of body function.

- Knowledge of homeostatic processes is essential for an understanding of the implications for care should homeostasis fail.

- When nurses advise people about maintaining health and avoiding problems it is important that they have an understanding of normal body function.

- Study of body structure and function will ensure that the nurse has a complete picture of the person who requires their professional expertise. This enables the practitioner to respond with the appropriate nursing skills.

To help students relate the study of science to nursing practice, whenever basic scientific concepts are introduced they appear at a relevant point in the text and are presented in a way which is 'meaningful' for nursing students – rather than as a 'huge chunk' of scientific material which students may view as irrelevant to their preparation for practice.

Examples in the nursing literature support the view that the study of anatomy and physiology during a core/foundation course has relevance to nursing practice. Closs (1987), for example, concludes that education and research in biological sciences should aim to improve standards of practice in nursing.

Why emphasize healthy function?

A holistic approach to the study of nursing can be successful only if the structure and functioning of the human body is included and integrated with other areas of knowledge required for practice. Clark (1995) emphasizes that a knowledge of the biology of health and illness and of the biological aspects of nursing interventions is essential to holistic nursing practice.

Current nursing philosophy centres upon the whole person and emphasizes health and health maintenance through the integration of health promotion within practice. It is logical, therefore, to take a holistic view when learning about body structure and, more importantly, about the healthy functioning of its components. The holistic approach allows you to discover the close relationships between structure and function, and to appreciate the contribution that all body systems make towards homeostasis and health.

What is 'normal' function?

Body structures function as part of the integrated whole – no single organ or system can maintain homeostasis in isolation. At all levels – atoms, molecules, cells, tissues, organs, systems and the organism – there are interactions and essential relationships that affect the functioning of the whole person. A change in function in any major organ can affect the health of the individual. It is important, however, that we stress that 'normal' usually spans a range, e.g. core body temperature 36–37.6°C and that the range varies between individuals and changes under different conditions.

Physiological function and health can be summarized as:

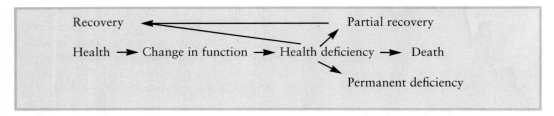

It is important that the image of a healthy person is retained during the study of body structure and function. As you pursue your nursing practice, you will find that most people within a community are not ill. They are normally functioning individuals who may become consumers of health care services at specific times, such as screening or during pregnancy. As illustrated in the health-illness continuum below, individuals become patients it they suffer health deficiencies (illness):

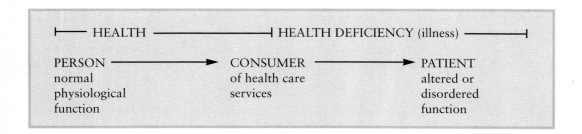

However, health is never static – it is a dynamic state which means different things to individual people and which may vary with their particular stage of life. The definition of 'health' for any individual, therefore, is never clear-cut.

The table below lists factors required for physiological health and those that alter the homeostatic balance.

Criteria for normal physiological function:	Factors associated with altered physiological function and homeostatic imbalance:
• genetic inheritance which programmes for normal function	• inheritance of genes which cause altered function
• normal chromosome complement	• chromosomal abnormality
• oxygen	• lack of oxygen or poor utilization of oxygen
• essential nutrients in the correct amounts	• malnutrition: incorrect nutrients, malabsorption and loss of nutrients
• water	• water imbalance
• ability to regulate pH and electrolyte levels and to remove waste	• electrolyte imbalance, and failure of excretory and homeostatic processes
• protection from hostile environmental factors, injury and disease	• lack of shelter, accidents, trauma, exposure to: toxic chemicals, radiation, contaminated water and food, pathogens (disease producing micro-organisms) and other stressors
• movement and stability	• immobility and instability of the body
• body temperature within normal range	• inability to maintain body temperature within normal range
• cell growth, replication and repair	• abnormal cell growth and division, e.g. malignant disease
• periods of inactivity and sleep	• lack of adequate rest and sleep (this varies with individuals)
• reproduction (not strictly essential for the individual but vital for the species)	

MAKING THIS BOOK WORK FOR YOU

A textbook can present a wealth of information; however, if that information is difficult to locate, to understand, and to apply to your daily activities as a nurse, then the textbook is of limited use. The learning aids featured in *Human Structure and Function* will enable you to locate and utilize the information so that it benefits you. These learning aids include the following:

Overview located at the beginning of every chapter, gives you a brief outline of topics covered in the chapter.

Learning Outcomes listed at the beginning of every chapter, tell you what you should know after reading the chapter. The learning outcomes provide a framework for learning and the means to plan and take responsibility for your learning.

Key Words also listed at the beginning of each chapter, define specific terms you will encounter throughout that chapter. The key words are presented in **boldface** when they appear within the text for the first time. Other important terms are defined when they are first used in the chapter.

Nursing Practice Applications, Healthier Living, Person/family-centred Studies, Special Focus and **Abnormal Function** topics scattered throughout the chapters, help you relate your knowledge of structure and normal function to health and the problems which may occur when function is disordered. The topics in each of the boxes can be identified by a distinctive icon (see above). This information also demonstrates the relevance of this knowledge to the daily practice of nursing.

Chapter Summary/Checklist located at the end of every chapter, enables you to review main topics and plan revision.

Self Test presented after the chapter summary, enables you to test your knowledge of the main topics covered in the chapter and alerts you to topics you may wish to review again.

Further Reading and **References** list additional sources of information to enhance your understanding of particular topics.

Useful Addresses located at the end of some chapters, includes those of organizations concerned with particular illnesses or disabilities discussed in the chapter. You can contact these organizations to obtain additional information about particular topics. It is also useful to be aware of these organizations when you practice as a nurse.

In addition to these features, a detailed **index,** numerous **cross-references,** and informative **illustrations** and **appendices** help guide you through *Human Structure and Function* to make the most of the information it presents. We hope you also will use your book to write important points in your own words (one of the best ways to check real understanding), and add related references and notes about how you used a particular topic during observation or practice situations.

REFERENCES

Akinsanja J (1985) Learning about life. *Sen Nurs* **2**(5): 24–25.
Clark M (1995) Guest Editorial. Nursing and the biological sciences. *J Adv Nurs* **22**(3): 405–406.
Closs J (1987) Biological science and nurses. *Sen Nurs* **7**(5): 45.

BEFORE YOU BEGIN

If you have not studied science subjects before, it might be helpful to read some basic texts prior to starting your exploration of human structure and function. A short list of appropriate books is provided but your tutors/lecturers will also offer advice and suggestions for your reading. If you have some knowledge of basic science, you may want to use these texts for a quick review:

Hinwood B (1993) *A Textbook of Science for the Health Professions,* 2nd edn. London: Chapman & Hall.
Johnson K (1991) *Physics for You.* Cheltenham: Stanley Thornes (GCSE level).
Minett P, Wayne D, Rubenstein D (1989) *Human Form and Function.* London: Collins Educational.
Raffan J, Ratcliff B (1995) *Foundation Chemistry.* Cambridge: Cambridge University Press.
Rockett B, Sutton R (1996) *Chemistry for Biologists at Advanced Level.* London: John Murray (Publishers) Ltd. (Part 1 is GCSE level with parts 2 and 3 aimed at tertiary level courses).
Rose S, Sanderson C (1979) *The Chemistry of Life,* 2nd edn. Harmondsworth: Penguin Books.

Outline of Living Material and Organization of the Body

Overview

- *Basic biochemistry – structure of major organic molecules.*
- *Chemical reactions.*
- *Cells – structure, transport, controls, division, nucleic acids, protein synthesis, differentiation.*
- *Abnormalities of cell growth.*
- *Tissues – overview of the main types.*
- *Organs, body cavities, functional systems.*
- *Anatomical terms, body planes.*

Learning Outcomes

After studying Chapter 1 you should be able to:

- Outline the structure of the major organic molecules and their roles in the body.
- Describe chemical reactions in the body, e.g. synthesis, decomposition, exchange and reversible reactions.
- Describe an 'idealized' cell.
- Describe the plasma membrane.
- Describe the main cellular organelles and their function.
- Explain how substances are transported across the plasma membrane.
- Outline ways in which cell function is controlled.
- Describe mitosis and state how it differs from meiosis.
- Define the terms 'chromosome' and 'gene'.
- Explain the structure and role of nucleic acids in protein synthesis.
- Define 'cellular differentiation'.
- Describe the common abnormalities of cell growth.
- Discuss the factors that predispose cells to neoplastic changes.
- Describe ways of reducing the risk of malignancy and of detecting cancers at an early stage.
- Outline how cells communicate with each other.
- Define 'tissue' and state the major types found in the body.
- State the types of structure found in organs.
- Name the body cavities.
- Outline the role of the functional systems.
- Define the common anatomical terms used to describe body directions.
- Describe the anatomical position of the body.
- Describe body planes.

Key Words

Active site – part of a protein molecule which is shaped exactly to fit and react with other molecules (substrates).

Adenosine triphosphate (ATP) – a chemical which provides the energy for vital cellular activities.

Key Words cont.

Atom – the smallest stable part of an element that can exist and display the properties of that element.

Chemical reactions – the energy-consuming and energy-releasing processes that change the structure of molecules as chemical bonds are formed, broken or changed. In the body they may be synthesis (anabolic or building up), decomposition (catabolic or breaking down) or involve the exchange of molecules. Many reactions important in biological systems are able to move in either direction and are said to be reversible.

Chromosomes – thread-like structures containing the genetic information (DNA). Present in the cell nucleus.

Deoxyribonucleic acid (DNA) – a nucleic acid found in the cell nucleus, it has a complex helical structure which carries the genetic code.

Differentiation – the changes that occur in cells and tissues as they develop the ability to perform specialized functions.

Diffusion – the process by which gas or liquid molecules of different densities/concentrations mix when brought into contact with one another.

Diploid – (2n) used to describe a cell that has a full set of paired chromosomes (46 arranged in 23 pairs), seen in all cells except the gametes.

Element – one of the unique substances (matter) that comprise all living and non living things, e.g. oxygen, potassium, zinc, carbon.

Gametes – the haploid (n) reproductive cells; ova and spermatozoa.

Genes – hereditary factors present on the chromosomes; consisting of DNA, they code for inherited characteristics or the precise replication of proteins.

Haploid – (n) used to describe a cell that has a half set of chromosomes (23 unpaired chromosomes), seen in the gametes following meiosis.

Hydrophilic – 'water-loving'; molecules that attract water and other polar substances.

Hydrophobic – 'water-fearing'; molecules that react with nonpolar substances.

Meiosis – a type of nuclear division that produces gametes. These special cells (ova and spermatozoa) are haploid.

Mitosis – a type of nuclear division in somatic (body) cells that results in the production of identical daughter cells with the same number of chromosomes as the original cell.

Molecule – two or more atoms joined together by a chemical bond, e.g. water.

Nonpolar – molecules with electrical balance.

Organelles – small structures within the cell, e.g. mitochondria, that perform specific functions.

Organic molecules – chemical molecules, e.g. glucose, that contain carbon and hydrogen in their structure. The large molecules of living systems are organic and include lipids, proteins, carbohydrates and nucleic acids.

Osmosis – the passage of a solvent (always water in a living system) from a dilute solution to a more concentrated one through a selectively permeable membrane.

Polar – molecules without electrical balance.

Ribonucleic acid (RNA) – a nucleic acid found in the cell nucleus and in ribosomes, vital in the process of protein synthesis.

Substrate – a chemical acted upon by an enzyme.

Transcription – the process by which genetic information is transferred from DNA to RNA, the first stage in the synthesis of proteins.

Translation – the process by which proteins are synthesized in the ribosomes from amino acids.

Introduction

Chapter 1 charts the 'building' of a complete human organism from **organic molecules** through cells and tissues to the organs and functional systems that maintain the body in a stable state (homeostasis).

The body is comprised of many billions of cells. These fundamental structural units form the great variety of tissues, organs and systems that perform the highly specialized biochemical processes required to maintain homeostasis. Biochemical processes are carried out by the smaller subcellular structures or **organelles** found in individual cells (see pages 14–16). The specific functions performed by a cell are determined by the type and numbers of these organelles. Continuity of the species depends on cells and the genetic material found in the nucleus. At fertilization the spermatozoon and oocyte (ovum) unite to form the zygote, a single cell which by cell division and differentiation eventually give rise to all the cells of the body. **Differentiation** is the term used to describe the changes that occur in cells and tissues as they develop the ability to perform specialized functions. This is an incredible process when you consider the diversity of cells produced in this way, e.g. excitable nerve cells, secretory cells of the digestive tract or structural bone cells. The study of cells is called cytology.

Generally, cells have an outer plasma membrane surrounding a gel-like fluid containing several organelles, and a nucleus containing the genetic material. The ingredients of these complex cellular components include water, organic molecules (see below) and electrolytes (see Chapter 2).

Basic Biochemistry

Before looking at the make-up and workings of body cells it would be helpful to take the time to cover some basic biochemical topics. For any study of cell structure and function it is necessary to have a basic understanding of the structure and roles of some organic molecules, and the types of **chemical reactions** occurring in cells. If you have not studied these areas before, this part will provide you with some basic facts, but if you are already familiar with the topics you can use it to revise and check your knowledge.

All living and nonliving things are formed from different combinations of unique substances (matter) called **elements**, e.g. oxygen, carbon, hydrogen and nitrogen. Each element is designated a letter code that is used as a type of shorthand, e.g. O = oxygen, C = carbon, H = hydrogen, N = nitrogen. The smallest stable part of an element that can exist and display the properties of that element is called an **atom**, but an atom generally combines with other atoms. By combining, the atoms form more complex chemicals called **molecules**, e.g. two atoms of oxygen form a molecule. When the atoms forming a molecule are from different elements the resultant substance is called a compound, e.g. water, which is formed from hydrogen and oxygen. Further coverage of basic chemistry including atoms, molecules, electrolytes and the chemical bonds holding atoms and molecules together is included in Chapter 2, which you should read in conjunction with this chapter.

Organic molecules

Organic molecules are those which contain carbon and hydrogen atoms in their structure. These molecules, which are often very large (macromolecules) as well as complex, include the raw materials from which cells are built and the chemicals needed for cell function, e.g. proteins, carbohydrates and lipids (fats). This huge variety of very different molecules is made possible by the chemical properties of carbon, which is able to join (or bond) with four other atoms to form many different structural arrangements – in much the same way that children build different structures with the same set of interlocking plastic shapes. This part of the chapter will deal with proteins (including enzymes), carbohydrates, lipids and **adenosine triphosphate** (ATP), but the nucleic acids are covered within the context of protein synthesis (see pages 21–22).

Proteins

Proteins (see Chapters 2 and 13) are complex macromolecules containing atoms of carbon, nitrogen, hydrogen and oxygen, and sometimes those of sulphur or phosphorus. They are vitally important and perform many diverse roles in the body, and range from the structural keratin of skin, nails and hair to the functional protein haemoglobin, found in erythrocytes, which transports oxygen around the body (*Table 1.1*).

All proteins are built from individual 'building blocks' called amino acids (see *Table 1.2*). Proteins are long chains formed from the combination of 20 or so amino acids joined together in different sequences and numbers. Some

Table 1.1 Types and roles of proteins in the body			
Type of protein	**Globular**	**Fibrous**	
General role	**Functional**	**Movement**	**Structural**
Detailed role with examples	Regulation and control – enzymes that catalyze chemical reactions, e.g. carbonic anhydrase, and hormones that regulate body processes, e.g. thyroid hormones. Protection and defence – components of the immune system, e.g. antibodies and complement. Transport – the protein haemoglobin transports oxygen. Plasma proteins transport other substances. Energy – protein can be used to supply energy. pH maintenance – proteins in the blood act as buffers, which limit pH changes.	Contraction – actin and myosin are contractile proteins found in muscle.	Structural support in tissues, e.g. collagen in connective tissue and keratin in skin, nails and hair.

Table 1.1 Types and roles of proteins in the body.

amino acids are indispensable (essential) and must be taken in the diet, but others are termed dispensable (non essential) because they can be synthesized in the body. The exact sequence and number of amino acids is vital to the production of the correct protein. For example, if just one amino acid (valine instead of glutamic acid) is incorrect in one of the chains making up the haemoglobin molecule, the individual will have the inherited haemoglobinopathy (disease affecting haemoglobin) known as sickle-cell disease (see Chapter 9). Each amino acid has two functional chemical groups – a basic amino end (NH_2) and an acidic carboxyl end (COOH). In addition, each of the amino acids has a hydrogen atom and its own special arrangement of atoms known as the 'R' group – it is the distinctive 'R' group, bonded (joined) to a carbon atom that gives the amino acid its individual chemical characteristics (*Figure 1.1*). Depending upon their 'R' groups, amino acids will be acidic (donating hydrogen), basic (accepting hydrogen) or neutral (neither acidic or basic), and will demonstrate **hydrophilia** (attracting water), **hydrophobia** (repelling water) or mixed characteristics.

A protein may consist of many hundreds of amino acids linked together by peptide bonds (*Figure 1.1*). To form amino acid chains the amine end of one amino acid reacts with the carboxyl end of another in a dehydration synthesis reaction (see page 11) – a reaction in which a water molecule is released (condensation) to form a peptide bond. The reverse happens when the body uses the proteins we eat; here the processes of chemical digestion break the peptide bonds of the protein chain by adding water (hydrolysis).

A pair of two linked amino acids is called a dipeptide, a chain of three is a tripeptide and many together is a polypeptide (*Figure 1.1*). Once the number of amino acids in the chain exceeds 50 or so, the structure is called a protein.

Apart from the peptide bonds linking individual amino acids, the more complex twisted or folded proteins are maintained by hydrogen and covalent bonds (see Chapter 2). There are four levels of complexity seen in protein structure (*Figure 1.1*):

Primary structure: a simple polypeptide strand consisting of its core chain of linked amino acids is the least complex level. Primary structure proteins are unusual.

Secondary structure: either a spiral alpha helical structure or a beta pleated sheet formed from two or more simple strands.

Tertiary structure: the next level is formed as an already folded alpha helix or beta sheet becomes folded on itself to form a rounded molecule.

Quaternary structure: the most complex form, such as that shown by the haemoglobin molecule, which has four polypeptide chains interlinked to give the molecule the unique physical and chemical characteristics required to transport oxygen.

It is important to understand how vital a protein's structure is to its particular function – having an exact structure ensures that the **active sites**, which are parts of the molecule that are shaped exactly-to-fit and react with other molecules called **substrates**, are placed correctly.

In addition to this classification, proteins may be defined as being fibrous or globular. Fibrous proteins usually have a secondary structure and perform a structural or mechanical role, e.g. actin in muscle and collagen. Globular proteins e.g. enzymes and some hormones, have a tertiary or quaternary structure, and perform a functional role, Fibrous structural proteins are usually resistant to changes in the prevailing physical and chemical environment and are said to be stable. However, the complex structure of globular proteins renders them very susceptible to changes in their environment. Extremes of temperature and pH (acidity/alkalinity) will unravel (denaturate) the protein. This renders it unable to function because its active sites for reacting with other molecules are no longer in the right place for a match. Some proteins can regain their original structure if normal conditions are resumed, but you only have to consider the change that occurs when the albumin of egg white is cooked to get an idea of how heat can permanently affect the structure of proteins. A discussion about the effects of extremely high temperatures on body function can be found in Chapter 19.

Enzymes

Enzymes are proteins that act as biological catalysts (a catalyst is a substance that controls or speeds up the rate of

Table 1.2 Amino acids	
Indispensable/essential (must be taken in the diet)	Dispensable/non-essential (can be synthesized in the body)
Isoleucine	Alanine
Leucine	Arginine (semi-essential)
Lysine	Asparagine
Methionine	Aspartate (aspartic acid)
Phenylalanine	Cysteine
Threonine	Glutamate (glutamic acid)
Tryptophan	Glutamine
Valine	Glycine
	Proline
Note: during childhood, histidine is indispensable	Serine
	Tyrosine

Table 1.2 Amino acids.

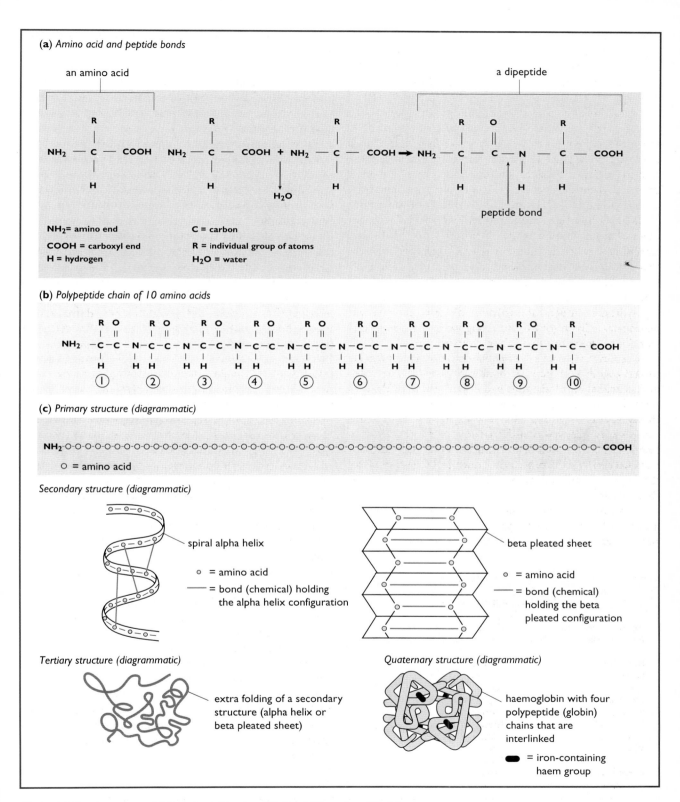

Figure 1.1 Protein structure. (**a**) An amino acid and peptide bond; (**b**) a polypeptide; (**c**) primary, secondary, tertiary and quaternary structures.

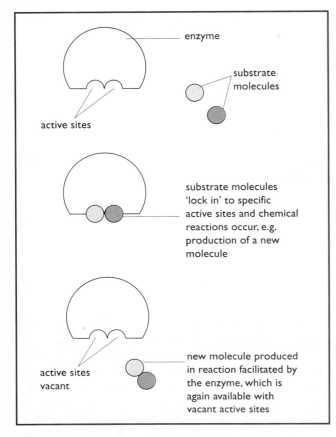

Figure 1.2 Enzyme active sites and substrate bonding.

active sites and the substrate is often likened to that of a key in a lock (suggested in 1890 by Fischer) – usually an exact fit is needed for the reaction to occur, but it is possible for a very similarly shaped molecule to attach to the active site just as a lock can sometimes be opened by another key. Certain drugs, e.g. the painkiller aspirin, can be used to modify biochemical reactions as they compete with the substrate by binding to the active sites of the enzyme.

Enzymes catalyze precise chemical processes and often their name will tell you what they do, e.g. proteases are involved in the breakdown of proteins and dehydrogenases remove hydrogen in oxidation reactions. Another guide to the recognition of enzymes and their role is the fact that many have the suffix 'ase' on the name of the substrate molecule, e.g. aminopeptidases act on the amino end of a peptide chain. Where enzymes have the potential to damage tissue they are usually released in an inactive form and are only activated when needed – this prevents the enzyme causing damage, e.g. some of the digestive enzymes. Occasionally, this goes wrong, such as in acute pancreatitis (inflammation of the pancreas), when the active pancreatic enzymes may start to digest the pancreas. Some enzymes need non-protein cofactors to function; for example, superoxide dismutase, which disarms harmful free radicals (see pages 16, 24, 25), needs copper and zinc. When the cofactors are organic molecules such as the B vitamins they are known as coenzymes.

Enzymes, like other protein molecules, only function properly within an environment where the physical and chemical characteristics are maintained within a limited normal range – this is why homeostatic mechanisms that maintain the internal environment are so vital. Both temperature and pH are important for enzyme function; for example, enzymes may be denatured by an abnormally high body temperature, and enzymes that normally function in an acid environment will not work in alkaline surroundings.

It only remains to stress just how important enzymes are in the control of many cellular activities and to remind you that further discussion about specific enzymes occurs throughout the book.

Carbohydrate

Carbohydrates (see Chapter 13) consist of carbon with hydrogen and oxygen in the same proportions as water (2:1) and include the simple sugars, the more complex starches and non-starch polysaccharides such as cellulose. Their major functions in the body are the supply and storage of energy, but other roles include forming part of both types of nucleic acid (*Table 1.3*).

a chemical reaction without itself being permanently altered) throughout the body. Many reactions in the body would be too slow to meet physiological needs without an enzyme, e.g. carbon dioxide transport needs the enzyme carbonic anhydrase to proceed rapidly enough to remove waste carbon dioxide from the tissues (Chapter 12). Enzymes are also discussed on page 11 as one of the factors affecting the rate of chemical reactions. The acceleration of reactions occurs because enzymes reduce the amount of energy required to get the process started – they reduce the activation energy. Just imagine that you are trying to get over a wall but cannot manage the leap needed to reach the top; but by standing on a box it is possible to reach the top. In this analogy the box acts as a catalyst by reducing the energy required.

Earlier we mentioned the importance of protein structure and the location of active sites. For an enzyme to work, its active sites must be in the right place so that substrate molecules can 'lock in' (*Figure 1.2*). The fit between the

Table 1.3 Types and roles of carbohydrates in the body		
Type of carbohydrate	Examples	Functions
Sugars (monosaccharides and disaccharides)	Glucose, galactose, fructose. Ribose Deoxyribose *Sucrose, lactose, maltose (disaccharides broken down to glucose for cell use)	Main energy source for cell use. Structural component of nucleic acids and adenosine triphosphate. Form glycoproteins found on the surface of the plasma membrane where they act as identification molecules.
Storage carbohydrates (polysaccharides)	Glycogen	Energy store in liver and muscles – reconverted to glucose when energy required.
	Plant starch	Converted to glucose for use as energy
Non-starch polysaccharides (NSP)	Cellulose	Adds bulk to faeces and reduces bowel transit times.

Table 1.3 Types and roles of carbohydrates in the body.

Monosaccharides and disaccharides

The basic unit forming the carbohydrates is the monosaccharide, or single simple sugar molecule, which usually has a closed ring structure (see *Figure 1.3*). Examples of monosaccharides are the sugars ribose and deoxyribose; these are both pentoses (5-carbon sugar) and are found in **ribonucleic acid** (RNA) and **deoxyribonucleic acid** (DNA). Other important monosaccharides are the hexoses (6-carbon sugars) glucose (the blood sugar that provides most cells with their fuel), galactose and fructose (fruit sugar). Usually galactose and fructose are converted into glucose before cellular use, but sometimes a baby inherits a condition where the enzymes required to convert galactose to glucose are missing, which results in galactosaemia (galactose in the blood). Without treatment the high levels of galactose would cause liver damage, failure to thrive and learning disabilities, but babies are managed successfully by excluding foods containing galactose from the diet and using specially formulated milks.

When two monosaccharides link together by dehydration synthesis (see page 11) they form a disaccharide joined by a glycosidic linkage (see *Figure 1.3*). Disaccharides of relevance to a study of cellular activity include:

- Sucrose (glucose + fructose), the 'sugar' you put in your tea.
- Lactose (glucose + galactose), milk sugar.
- Maltose (glucose + glucose), malt sugar.

The reverse happens when the body uses the disaccharides we eat. Here the processes of chemical digestion break the glycosidic linkage between the two sugar units by adding water (hydrolysis) to produce the simple sugar units for cell use.

Polysaccharides

The most complex carbohydrates or polysaccharides consist of long chains and branches of monosaccharide units joined by glycosidic linkages (see *Figure 1.3*). These large, non-sweet molecules include two storage carbohydrates formed from many glucose units – starch in plants and glycogen in animals. Glycogen is the form in which we store glucose reserves in the liver and skeletal muscle cells. When blood glucose levels fall we are able to convert liver glycogen into glucose, much as you use the contents of your cupboard or freezer to make a meal.

Again, the chemical processes of digestion eventually reduce most polysaccharides taken in the diet to their monosaccharide (glucose) subunits. However, the digestive process in humans is unable to break down some complex structural carbohydrates, e.g. cellulose, which provide faecal bulk as dietary fibre (non-starch polysaccharide).

Lipids

Lipids are a large and diverse group of molecules which include neutral fat, steroids, phospholipids, lipoproteins (see Chapter 10), prostaglandins, thromboxanes and leukotrienes, and many related molecules such as vitamins A, E and K (see Chapter 13). Lipids consist of carbon, hydrogen and oxygen, but in different proportions to carbohydrates (much less oxygen), and some contain phosphorus and nitrogen. They are insoluble in water (water and oil cannot mix), but they can be dissolved in organic solvents such as alcohol. Lipids are vitally important in the body – both structurally and functionally (see *Table 1.4*). Some lipids are discussed here, but others, such as lipoproteins and fat-soluble vitamins, are dealt with in later chapters.

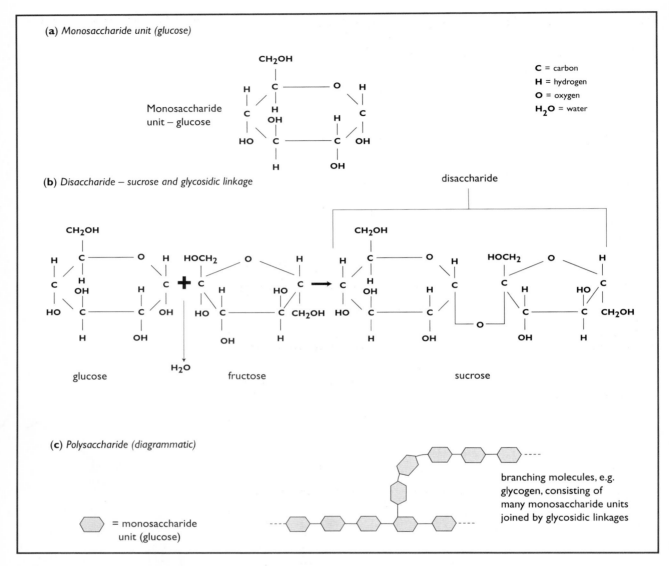

Figure 1.3 Carbohydrate structure. **(a)** Monosaccharide unit – glucose; **(b)** disaccharide (sucrose) showing glycosidic linkage; **(c)** polysaccharide.

Neutral fat

Most neutral fats in the body are triglycerides (also called triacylglycerols) and most dietary fat is also in this form. Triglycerides are formed from two distinct subunits: fatty acids and glycerol. As its name suggests, a triglyceride consists of three fatty acids (hydrocarbon chains) linked to a glycerol molecule (sugar with alcohol groups) by dehydration synthesis reactions (see page 11).

Variations in triglycerides depend on the fatty acids, which have different carbon–carbon bonds (single or double) and hydrocarbon chains of different lengths. Fats may be saturated; when all the carbon–carbon bonds (C–C) are single, these fats are usually solid at room temperature,

e.g. lard. Unsaturated fats, which are usually liquid at room temperature, may be monounsaturated (where one C–C bond is double, e.g. olive oil) or polyunsaturated (where two or more C–C bonds are double, e.g. sunflower oil).

The **nonpolar** (electrically balanced) neutral fats are used in the body to store energy, e.g. under the skin, where they also insulate and protect the deeper structures.

Steroids

Steroids (see Chapters 8 and 20) are lipid molecules having a common basic chemical structure comprising three 6-carbon rings and one 5-carbon ring (see *Figure 1.4*). The range of steroids in the body is wide and includes such

Table 1.4 Types of lipids and roles in the body	
Types of lipids, with examples	Outline of functions in the body
Neutral fats (triglycerides)	Energy store as fat deposits Insulation and protection
Steroids	
Cholesterol	Component of cell membranes and precursor of other steroid molecules
Sex hormones (testosterone, oestrogen and progesterone)	Control of reproductive function
Adrenal cortical hormones (corticosteroids such as cortisol and aldosterone)	Control metabolism of nutrients and electrolyte/water balance
Bile salts	Important for the digestion and absorption of fats
Vitamin D	Calcium homeostasis – bone growth and remodelling
Phospholipids	Component of the cell membrane – bilayer
Prostaglandins, thromboxanes and leukotrienes	Group of regulatory lipids concerned with blood clotting, inflammatory processes, reproduction and many other functions
Lipoproteins (high-density lipoproteins – HDLs and low density lipoproteins – LDLs)	Transport of fatty acids and cholesterol in the blood
Fat-soluble vitamins (Vitamin D, see above)	
Vitamin A	Visual functions, acts as antioxidant
Vitamin E	Acts as an antioxidant, in wound healing and possibly has a role in reproduction
Vitamin K	Blood clotting

Table 1.4 Types of lipids and roles in the body.

diverse molecules as cholesterol (a precursor of many other steroids), vitamin D, bile salts, sex hormones and those hormones secreted by the adrenal cortex (corticosteroids). Although all steroids have the same basic structure, their roles in the body could not be more different: cholesterol is a structural component of the plasma membrane as well as being the molecule from which other steroids are made; testosterone is the major male sex hormone; and vitamin D is concerned with calcium and phosphorus homeostasis (*Table 1.4*).

Phospholipids
Phospholipids are important in the formation of cell membranes. They are similar to triglycerides – with a basic glycerol molecule and two hydrocarbon chains, but this time a molecule containing phosphate groups and nitrogen replaces the third hydrocarbon (see *Figure 1.4*). An interesting point about phospholipids is that the phosphate end is **polar** (electrically unbalanced) and hydrophilic, whereas the fatty acid end is nonpolar and hydrophobic. This gives them the special properties required to form a bilayer, e.g. the plasma membrane (see page 13).

Prostaglandins, thromboxanes and leukotrienes
Prostaglandins, thromboxanes and leukotrienes are regulatory lipids derived from arachidonic acid (a fatty acid). This diverse group of lipids are important in blood clotting, the inflammatory process, reproduction and many other body functions (see Chapters 9, 19 and 20).

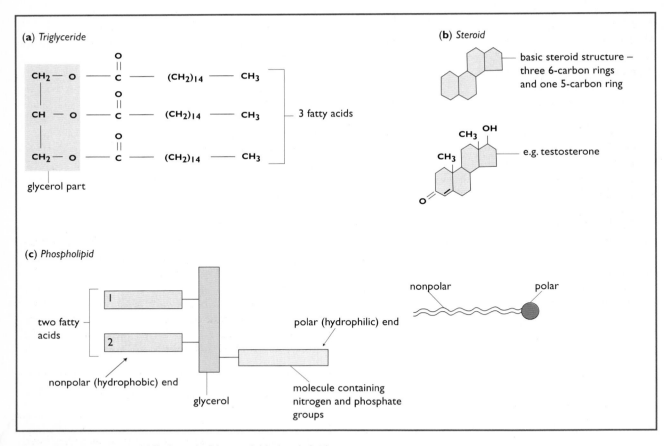

Figure 1.4 Lipid structure. (**a**) Triglyceride; (**b**) steroid; (**c**) phospholipid.

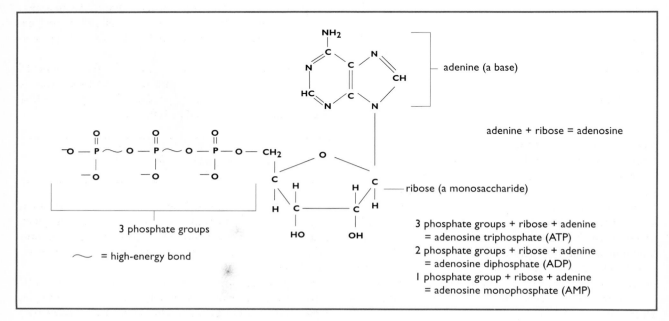

Figure 1.5 Adenosine triphosphate.

Adenosine triphosphate

All the organic molecules we have covered are important, but without the necessary energy they are merely interesting molecules – cells need energy in a usable form. Just as you cannot cook food until the gas supply is ignited to produce heat, cells cannot function without the means to convert the energy present in organic molecules. Cellular activities needed for homeostasis and health would be thwarted without adenosine triphosphate (ATP) the chemical that converts the energy obtained from organic molecules, such as glucose, into a form that the cells can use. ATP is formed from the base adenine, a ribose sugar and three phosphate groups (*Figure 1.5*).

The chemical energy is 'seized' from glucose breakdown and stored in the bonds between the phosphate groups, from where it is released, when needed, to power cellular processes such as moving molecules across cell membranes. The energy is released when the high-energy bond is broken by adding water (hydrolysis):

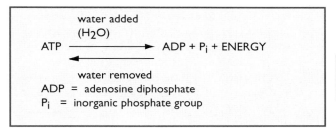

The balance between ATP production and breakdown to ADP must be maintained within a narrow range (much like paying into, and withdrawing money from, your current account) – too much ATP production would be wasteful of energy and not enough would stop vital cell processes. When ATP has been used to provide energy it is reformed to balance the energy account by virtue of the reaction being reversible (see page 12).

Chemical reactions

Chemical reactions are the energy-consuming (endergonic) or energy-releasing (exergonic) processes that change the structure of molecules as chemical bonds (see Chapter 2) are formed, broken or changed. Reactions take place between a number of reactants and result in product formation. The speed at which reactions take place is determined (within limits) by a variety of factors:

Concentration of the reactants: the chemical reaction is likely to proceed more quickly if there is a sufficient concentration of the reactants for them to meet (collide) and react.

Temperature: chemical reactions occur more rapidly as the temperature rises to the top of the normal range. This is because the reacting molecules 'whizz about' and collide more often. Reactions speed up when body temperature increases; conversely, when body temperature falls, chemical reactions slow down, such as in hypothermia (see Chapter 19). Obviously, temperature as a factor has some limitations in living systems – heating the body would damage biological molecules such as enzymes.

Enzymes: these are proteins that act as chemical catalysts (see pages 4, 6). They ensure that reactions that would be too slow at body temperature can proceed at an appropriate rate to maintain homeostasis.

Types of chemical reaction

The basic types of chemical reaction include: synthesis, decomposition and exchange (see below). In addition, some reactions can proceed in either direction, and are described as reversible.

Where a reaction between reactants results in a product which is larger and more complex it is called a synthesis reaction (see *Figure 1.6(a)*). A synthesis reaction, in its simplest form, can be symbolized by the following:

$$A + B \longrightarrow AB$$

In the body it is synthesis reactions that facilitate the 'building up' or anabolic processes by which the major organic molecules needed for tissue growth or repair are produced, e.g. proteins such as collagen being produced from amino acids (see pages 3, 4) to promote wound healing after surgery or injury. The topic of wound healing is given some prominence in Chapter 19.

Decomposition reactions are basically the opposite to those of synthesis – this time a large or complex molecule is broken down into simpler products [see *Figure 1.6(b)*]. Again it can be represented as follows:

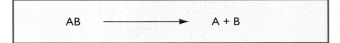

These 'breaking down' or catabolic processes of the body occur when large organic molecules such as polysaccharides are broken down to their constituent glucose subunits, e.g. during the chemical digestion of dietary starch (see page 7).

Chemical reactions where the reactants rearrange themselves are termed exchange or displacement reactions [see *Figure 1.6 (c)*]. Here part of one reactant combines with part of another to form different products. This pattern is seen in both synthesis and decomposition reactions. It can be represented by the following:

$$AB + CD \longrightarrow AD + CB$$

An example of an exchange reaction is the formation of a dipeptide from two amino acids. This involves the removal of a water molecule (a dehydration synthesis reac-

tion), but what makes it an exchange as well is the fact that part of the water molecule is formed from one amino acid and part from the other amino acid (see page 4).

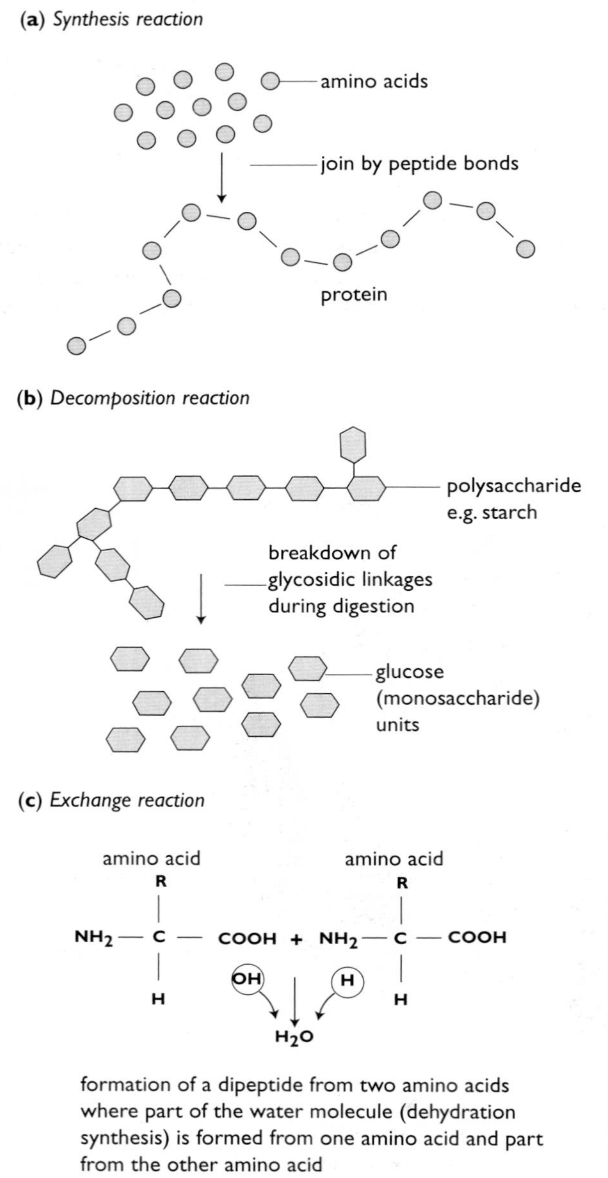

Reversible reactions
Chemical reactions that can proceed in either direction are said to be reversible. The reactants can form a product and the product can form the reactants:

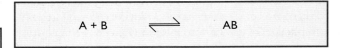

The two-directional arrows denote that the reaction is reversible and the length of the arrows relative to one another indicates the dominant direction of the reaction. In the example above the arrows are of equal length, which indicates that the reaction is in chemical equilibrium where the ratio of reactants used to product formed is constant. Should more reactants be added the reaction proceeds until the correct ratio between reactants and product is again achieved. An example in the body would be the multisystem homeostatic regulation of blood pH by maintaining the 20:1 ratio between hydrogen carbonate (bicarbonate) and carbonic acid (see Chapters 2 and 12). Maintenance of pH homeostasis is vital to cell function and ultimately life itself.

Cell Structure

Individual cells vary in form (related to function) and may have different lifespans. Generally, they all have an outer plasma membrane surrounding the cytoplasm, several organelles, and a nucleus containing the genetic material. Not all mature cells, however, retain a nucleus, e.g. erythrocytes (see Chapter 9). The structure of an idealized (showing most features) cell is shown in *Figure 1.10*, page 15. The functions of the various components are described below.

Cytoplasm
Cytoplasm is all the material within the cell outer boundary, but excluding that within the nuclear membrane. The cytoplasm consists of the viscous fluid part known as cytosol (a complex mixture of water, proteins, lipids, carbohydrates and electrolytes), the subcellular organelles (which perform functions within the cell) and inclusions related to particular cells, such as nutrients present in very active muscle cells.

(a) *Synthesis reaction*

amino acids

join by peptide bonds

protein

(b) *Decomposition reaction*

polysaccharide e.g. starch

breakdown of glycosidic linkages during digestion

glucose (monosaccharide) units

(c) *Exchange reaction*

amino acid

amino acid

$$NH_2 - C - COOH + NH_2 - C - COOH$$

R

H

OH

H

R

H

$$H_2O$$

formation of a dipeptide from two amino acids where part of the water molecule (dehydration synthesis) is formed from one amino acid and part from the other amino acid

Figure 1.6 Types of chemical reaction. **(a)** Synthesis reaction; **(b)** decomposition reaction; **(c)** exchange reaction.

Plasma membrane

The cell is surrounded by a complex protein/phospholipid structure known as the plasma membrane, which forms a boundary around individual cells, and separates intracellular and extracellular fluid. The fluid mosaic model proposed by Singer and Nicolson in 1972 is generally used to describe the semisolid phospholipid bilayer within which various protein molecules 'float' (*Figure 1.7*). The phospholipid bilayer (double layer) consists of match-like molecules that have polar heads facing outwards and nonpolar tails orientated towards the middle of the layer. The head parts, which contain phosphate groups, are hydrophilic and are in contact with the watery intracellular and extracellular fluids, whereas the tails are hydrophobic hydrocarbon molecules. One particular benefit of this highly specialized structure is that small membrane defects can be repaired.

Many other molecules contribute to the plasma membrane – cholesterol, which increases structural stability, and proteins, which may be within the bilayer (integral) or on either surface (peripheral). The many peripheral proteins, which are linked to carbohydrate molecules, are known as glycoproteins.

The integral proteins, some of which penetrate the entire bilayer, and peripheral proteins, are central to membrane function (see *Figure 1.8*). Integral proteins are involved with:

• Transport mechanisms moving substances in and out of the cell. They may form channels or act as carrier molecules.

Peripheral proteins including glycoproteins may be:

• Enzyme catalysts for a variety of biochemical reactions.
• Identity markers for cell recognition, such as the glycoprotein on the surface of erythrocytes that determines ABO blood groups (see Chapter 9).
• Receptors that respond to specific chemicals, e.g. hormones (see Chapter 8) or neurotransmitters (see Chapter 3) as part of intercellular communication (see pages 24, 25).
• Structural supports, through their ability to attach themselves to the structures of the cytoskeleton (see page 16).

In addition to the peripheral proteins and glycoproteins on the surface of the plasma membrane, there are other molecules containing carbohydrate, including glycolipids. All these surface molecules are important in providing the

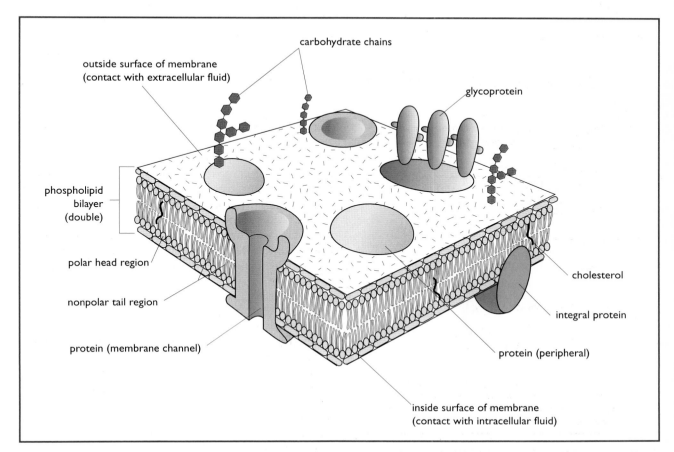

Figure 1.7 Plasma membrane (fluid mosaic model).

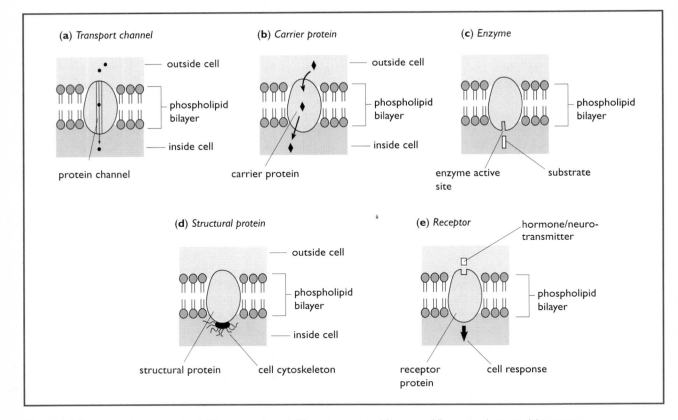

Figure 1.8 Plasma membrane proteins. (**a**) Transport channel; (**b**) carrier protein; (**c**) enzyme; (**d**) structural protein; (**e**) receptor.

markers that ensure cell recognition and in helping cells adhere together. Just imagine what might happen if the spermatozoon did not recognize the ovum or if the cells of the immune system were unable to discriminate between the body's own cells and pathogenic (disease-producing) bacteria.

The plasma membrane maintains cell integrity and determines which substances pass into or out of the cell by a variety of different processes, which are discussed later (see pages 17, 18).

Special features of the plasma membrane

Before leaving the plasma membrane we should consider the special structural adaptations that form tiny projections called microvilli and junctions between cells. Cell junctions come in three main forms – each designed to perform specific functions (*Figure 1.9*).

Microvilli

Microvilli are tiny structures that grow out from areas of open cell surface. They enhance the work of cells concerned with absorption, e.g. cells lining the small intestine, by increasing the surface area available for absorption.

Tight junction

As its name suggests, the tight junction is designed to prevent leaks from cells. A special arrangement of protein molecules stops the movement of molecules between cells.

Gap junction

A gap junction has small gaps that allow the movement of small water-soluble molecules between cells. Some exchange of nutrients, such as sugars, occurs, and in excitable cells, e.g. those of myocardium (heart muscle), the movement of ions (electrically charged atoms) between cells allows the smooth passage of the electrical impulse during muscle contraction.

Desmosome

Desmosomes are complex junctions that 'nail' cells together. In tissues such as the skin, which are subjected to considerable mechanical stress, it is the desmosomes that help to prevent structural damage.

Organelles

Inside the cell, situated within the cytoplasm, are several

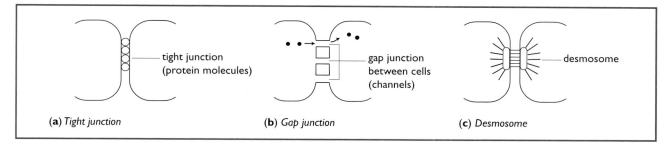

(a) Tight junction   (b) Gap junction   (c) Desmosome

Figure 1.9 Junctions between cells. (**a**) Tight junction; (**b**) gap junction; (**c**) desmosome.

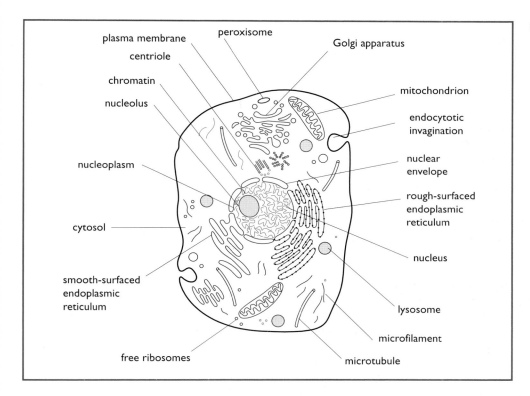

Figure 1.10 A cell (idealized).

smaller structures known generally as organelles; these perform a variety of metabolic functions. In addition to the plasma membrane around each cell, most organelles are surrounded by phospholipid bilayers that allow them to operate as discrete units within the cell.

Mitochondria
Mitochondria are the 'power stations' in the cell, the structures concerned with energy production from nutrients. The series of complex biochemical reactions known as the Krebs' (or citric acid) cycle (fuel molecules undergo changes in the presence of oxygen to produce energy, water and carbon dioxide) and oxidative phosphorylation (further reactions that generate large amounts of energy) occur in the mito-

chondria to produce energy in the form of ATP (see page 11). Cell function determines the number of mitochondria – greater numbers are present in liver and muscle cells, which are very active (they have a large energy requirement).

Endoplasmic reticulum (rough and smooth)
The endoplasmic reticulum (ER) consists of a network of membranes and channels inside the cell that are contiguous with the nuclear membrane. The ER is involved with the synthesis and movement of various substances, e.g. proteins and lipids. The rough ER is so called because of the presence of many ribosomes on its surface. Ribosomes have an important role in protein synthesis, which explains why many rough ER are found in secretory cells.

In contrast, the smooth ER has no ribosomes attached and has no role in protein synthesis. It is concerned with the synthesis and metabolism of lipids such as cholesterol and steroid hormones, and breaking down drugs in the liver.

Ribosomes

Ribosomes are very tiny organelles consisting of granules of protein and ribonucleic acid (RNA). RNA is the nucleic acid found in the ribosomes and nucleus, and is concerned with protein synthesis (see pages 22, 23). Ribosomes may be free in the cytoplasm or associated with the rough ER. Free ribosomes tend to be involved in the synthesis of proteins destined for intracellular use, whereas the ribosomes associated with the rough ER are concerned with membrane proteins and those that leave the cell.

Golgi apparatus

The Golgi apparatus is a network of membranous sacs in the cytoplasm situated close to the nucleus. These act as a modification area for cellular proteins produced by the rough ER – some proteins are converted to glycoproteins and some to lipoproteins (a lipid and protein) before use. The proteins are transported to their destinations in secretory vesicles (small sacs) which are 'nipped off' from the surface of the Golgi apparatus. The vesicles and their 'cargo' may end up as part of the plasma membrane, be used within the cell as lysosomes (see below) or be discharged from the cell surface by a process called exocytosis (see page 18). The Golgi apparatus is larger and more extensive in cells with major secretory functions, e.g. cells in the digestive tract.

Lysosomes

Within the cell are membranous vesicles, derived from the Golgi apparatus, containing lytic enzymes (capable of breaking down proteins, carbohydrates, etc). These sacs, known as lysosomes, are involved in the breakdown of substances or particles entering the cell by endocytosis (see page 18), such as bacteria, and in the 'salvage operations' initiated when cells are damaged. Lysosomes, as you would expect, are particularly numerous in phagocytes, a type of white blood cell (see Chapter 9) that engulfs bacteria before their destruction by the lysosomal lytic enzymes. Several inherited errors of metabolism are caused by a malfunction of lysosomal enzyme systems. This results in the build-up of unwanted substances and cell damage; for example, in Tay–Sachs lipid storage disease the nervous system is damaged and death occurs during infancy.

It is important to note that the membranous organelles; ER (and its contact with the nuclear membrane), Golgi apparatus, secretory vesicles and lysosomes together form a system of membranes within the cell known as the endomembrane system.

Peroxisomes

Peroxisomes are small membranous sacs containing oxidase enzymes. These potent enzymes use molecular oxygen in the detoxification of substances that can damage cells, such as alcohol. During these normal oxidative processes cells produce hydrogen peroxide and reactive chemicals called free radicals, which destroy important molecules such as nucleic acids and disrupt cell function. The peroxisomes can 'make safe' the free radicals and utilize the enzyme catalase to convert the excess hydrogen peroxide to water and oxygen. Cells with a major detoxification role, e.g. liver cells, have an abundance of peroxisomes. Free radicals are discussed later (see Healthier Living Box – Free radicals and antioxidants, page 25).

Cytoskeleton of supporting structures

Cells contain an internal network of supporting structures known collectively as the cytoskeleton. The network includes microfilaments, microtubules and intermediate filaments.

Microfilaments are protein strands that are concerned with maintaining cell shape, movement within cells and the process of cytokinesis occurring during cell division (see page 21). They are of particular importance in contractile cells such as skeletal muscle, where they are highly developed.

Support is also achieved by the presence of microtubules, which are tubes arranged in bundles. These help to support the cell organelles and maintain cell shape. Microtubules develop close to the nucleus in an area of cytoplasm known as the centrosome. Another important function of the microtubules is to form part of the centrioles (organelles that form the spindle during nuclear division). They also have a role in the intracellular movement of various organelles.

Intermediate filaments are durable proteins concerned with keeping cell shape and in the formation of desmosomes (see page 14), which hold cells together.

Motile structures – flagella and cilia

Certain cells have motile structures that project from their surface. They are formed from microtubules and include the microscopic hair-like cilia. The cilia are present on the cells that line the respiratory tract, where they move mucus and debris out of the lungs. The uterine (fallopian) tubes also have cilia that assist fertilization by moving the ovum along the tube. A much longer single version of a cilium is known as a flagellum; the only human cell to have a flagellum is the spermatozoon, where it forms the 'tail' that allows the spermatozoon considerable motility (see Chapter 20).

The nucleus

The nucleus is concerned with cellular control through the synthesis of proteins and cell division. With the exception of erythrocytes, all mature cells have at least one nucleus; some, such as skeletal muscle cells, are multi-nucleate (contain many nuclei). The nucleus contains chromatin, a thread-like substance containing proteins and the genetic material of the cell. Within the chromatin are the 46 **chromosomes**, which are made of DNA, a complex helical structure that carries the genetic code. Each tiny segment of DNA is known as a **gene**. Genes are responsible for the transmission of inherited characteristics and the precise replication of proteins. The nucleus is enclosed by a double membrane formed from two phospholipid bilayers. This nuclear membrane or envelope separates nucleoplasm from cytoplasm, but contains 'pores' that allow the selective transfer of substances by various mechanisms. You will remember that the ER is contiguous with the nuclear membrane. Also situated inside the nuclear membrane are the nucleoli, of which there are usually two; they contain both DNA and RNA and are involved in cell division.

Transport of Substances Across the Plasma Membrane

For all the complex cellular processes required for health, various organic and inorganic substances must be able to pass through the plasma membrane in both directions. These include glucose, amino acids, lipids, water, electrolytes, gases, urea (a waste product of protein metabolism produced by the liver and excreted by the kidneys; see Chapters 14 and 15), cellular secretions and sometimes large particles for destruction, such as bacteria. The plasma membrane is selectively permeable, i.e. the movement of some substances is enabled whereas the movement of others is restricted. The transport of substances may be **passive**, as in **osmosis**, or may be an active energy-requiring process where ATP is expended.

Passive transport processes
Osmosis

The method by which water moves in and out of the cell is known as osmosis. Water molecules pass from dilute to more concentrated solutions and eventually an equilibrium of concentration is achieved. It is an important mechanism in the maintenance of normal fluid balance within the body and is discussed more fully in Chapter 2. Osmosis is the passive process by which the cell moves water in or out through membrane pores without the use of energy.

Diffusion

Diffusion is the movement of molecules from areas of high molecular concentration to areas of low concentration (a sugar cube dissolving in a cup of tea) – it always needs a concentration gradient.

Nonpolar substances diffuse through the plasma membrane by dissolving in its lipid component. They include oxygen, waste such as carbon dioxide and urea, and fats. Small polar substances, such as sodium ions, can diffuse through protein channels (see *Figure 1.8*), but size is critical and usually the channel is designed to allow the passage of a specific molecule. Diffusion is a passive process that allows substances to move in either direction down concentration gradients, e.g. oxygen into the cell and waste carbon dioxide out of the cell.

Facilitated diffusion

Some larger molecules, that do not dissolve in lipids, can only diffuse through the plasma membrane by 'hitching a lift' from highly selective protein carrier molecules (see *Figure 1.8*). This process is known as **facilitated diffusion.** This is the process that allows glucose, the major fuel source of cells, to be transported rapidly into the cell without the use of precious energy. However, the number of specific protein carriers available at any one time will always determine the maximum speed at which glucose can enter the cells. A useful analogy is a revolving door into a supermarket – once all the spaces contain a person and trolley, the people still outside must wait for those progressing through the door to enter the store and vacate a spare place.

It is important to know that diffusion is a passive process and, whether simple or involving a carrier molecule, it requires the presence of a concentration gradient.

Filtration

Filtration is a passive process by which water and small molecules are transported from areas of high fluid pressure to areas of lower pressure – a pressure gradient not a concentration gradient. The process is driven by the hydrostatic (fluid) pressure exerted on the membrane that forces water and small molecules through the membrane pores. The process only works with molecules small enough to pass through the pores – large protein molecules or blood cells cannot move through a normal membrane, but they may get through if the membrane is inflamed. Filtration is an important process in the kidney during the formation of urine.

Active transport processes
Active transport

Active transport is a process requiring energy (in the form ATP) to enable carrier molecules to move substances:

- Against a concentration gradient.
- Where no gradient exists.
- Where the substance is unable to diffuse through the plasma membrane.

Substances transported in this way include amino acids, glucose (in some cells) and ions, e.g. sodium and potassium. The carrier molecules are specific and often the mechanisms involve the coupled movement of more than one molecule – one molecule may assist another going in the same direction or the substances may exchange or cross over, e.g. the sodium–potassium exchange pump, where sodium is pumped out of the cell and potassium is pumped in against their concentration gradients. This mechanism is important in maintaining the correct balance of ions and water between the intracellular and extracellular compartments (see Chapter 2). In addition, the excitable nerve and muscle cells depend on the sodium–potassium pump to create the electrochemical gradients needed for their activities (see Chapters 3 and 17).

It is important to note that all body cells have a resting membrane potential (voltage) where the inside of the membrane is electrically negative relative to the outside of the membrane. This results from the movement of charged ions (mainly sodium and potassium) across the plasma membrane to ensure that the negative and positive charges balance to give the cell and the extracellular fluid overall electrical neutrality.

Sodium and potassium also leak through the membrane by passive facilitated diffusion (sodium in and potassium out) in response to their concentration gradients. However, there is a bonus because the sodium helps other molecules, such as amino acids, into the cell prior to the sodium being pumped out again. This mechanism is important in the absorption of nutrients from the small intestine.

Special bulk transport processes

Special transport processes requiring ATP are used in the bulk transport of substances such as water.

Endocytosis

Endocytosis is a general term covering all the bulk transport processes that move material into the cell (*Figure 1.11*). Particles may be engulfed by the cell, as in phagocytosis of bacteria by phagocytic leucocytes (see Chapter 9). Another example is pinocytosis, where the plasma membrane surrounds a tiny drop of water and nutrients, which is then taken into the cell. In some cases of endocytosis special protein receptors on the plasma membrane ensure that only specific molecules, e.g. insulin, are taken into the cell. This is known as receptor-mediated endocytosis.

Exocytosis

When the material is moved out of the cell, the mechanism is called exocytosis (*Figure 1.11*). The material being moved out of the cell is transported in a vesicle that fuses with the plasma membrane prior to discharging its contents outside the cell. Exocytosis is involved when hormones (see Chapter 8) or neurotransmitters (see Chapters 3 and 6) are released or when mucus and saliva are discharged from cells.

Cell Replication

Cells replicate at different rates. Skin cells, blood cells and cells lining the digestive tract are continuously replaced and are classified as labile. Other cells, such as liver cells, are classified as stable. They replicate only until the organ reaches

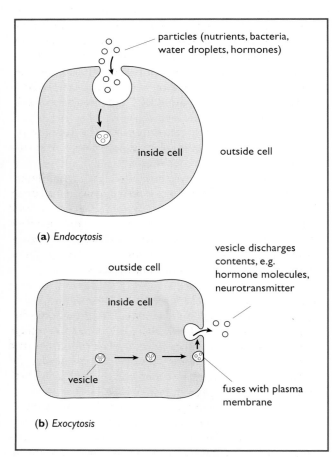

(a) *Endocytosis*

(b) *Exocytosis*

Figure 1.11 (a) Endocytosis; **(b)** exocytosis.

full size, but retain the ability to regenerate if the organ (e.g. the liver) is damaged. Permanent cells are not capable of replication after they mature; for example, cells of the central nervous system (neurones) cannot be repaired or replaced. The result of this can be seen after a stroke, where damage to the brain leads to a permanent loss of function, such as a weakness down one side of the body. It is sometimes possible, however, for a nerve fibre to regenerate if the nerve cell body of the neurone is intact (see Chapter 3). This is also true for cardiac and skeletal muscle cells, where damaged areas are replaced not by similar cells but by inelastic fibrous tissue during repair.

Cell division

Cells replicate through the division of existing cells. For cells to replicate, nuclear division must take place. The two types of nuclear division are **mitosis**, where identical daughter cells are produced, and **meiosis**. Meiosis is a more complex reduction division resulting in the production of **gametes**, the male and female reproductive cells (spermatozoa and ova), which have half the normal chromosome complement (**haploid**). This ensures that both parties each contribute half of the genetic material when the reproductive cells unite to form a zygote. The zygote then has the full complement of chromosomes (**diploid**):

Ovum   +   Spermatozoon   =   Zygote
(23 chromosomes) (23 chromosomes)   (46 chromosomes)

A more detailed explanation can be found in Chapter 20.

Mitosis is the process by which the somatic (non-gamete) cells of the body divide to produce new cells during periods of growth or as replacement for cells reaching the end of their lifespan. The events of somatic cell division, which include replication of the chromosomes, nuclear division and division of the cytoplasm, ensure that each new generation of cells contains the same genetic material.

The cell cycle

The cell cycle is the continuous process from one mitotic division to the next. The cycle includes all the processes necessary for nuclear and cell division. Very simply, the cell cycle can be divided into: interphase, during which DNA replicates; mitosis; and cytokinesis (cytoplasmic division) (see *Figure 1.12*). A knowledge of the cell cycle in 'normal' and malignant cells is used when planning radiotherapy for the treatment of some malignant diseases. During the cell cycle the cell is most susceptible to radiation, which disrupts DNA, during G_2 and mitosis. The dose and timing of radiation can be planned for maximum destruction of malignant cells while sparing 'normal' cells. Generally, cells that divide frequently, e.g. those lining the digestive tract, are most sensitive to radiation (they are said to be radiosensitive) – which explains why the side-effect of diarrhoea may be experienced during radiotherapy.

Another way to combat certain malignant conditions, e.g. leukaemia, is the use of cytotoxic (toxic to cells) drugs. Again, an exact knowledge of how cytotoxic substances work in relation to cell replication and the cell cycle is necessary. In this way, the team looking after the cancer patient can choose the correct cytotoxic drug for the specific malignancy and plan courses of treatment that offer maximum benefit with a minimum of distressing side-effects. The cytotoxic drugs used to treat malignant disease belong to many diverse groups, which act in a variety of ways to stop malignant cells dividing. They include:

- Vinca alkaloids derived from plants, e.g. vincristine, which stop the formation of microtubules needed for mitosis. They stop the cell cycle at metaphase.
- Alkylating agents such as mustine (used much less commonly), which is related to the mustard gas of World War I. These agents cause DNA damage and stop cells replicating.
- Antimetabolites, e.g. methotrexate, which inhibit the enzyme needed to make substances (purines and pyrimidines) needed for cell division.
- Cytotoxic antibiotics, e.g. doxorubicin, which inhibit the replication of DNA and work throughout the cell cycle.

Cytotoxic drugs, like radiotherapy, do not spare 'normal' cells and people taking these drugs can suffer from a variety of distressing side effects, such as nausea, hair loss and mouth ulcers, in addition to the more serious bone marrow depression and other toxic effects.

Interphase and DNA replication

Interphase is the stage during which all the day-to-day metabolic processes of cells occur. It is also the stage between two mitotic divisions when the cell grows and prepares the special structures and materials needed for division. The interphase can be subdivided into three stages: G_1, S and G_2 (see *Figure 1.12*).

The first part of interphase may last only hours in rapidly dividing cells, e.g. those of the digestive tract, but in others may take longer. The cell grows and proteins are synthesized. Close to the nucleus there are two centrioles lying at 90° to each other. These replicate during interphase and each resultant pair will move to the opposite poles of the cell to commence the formation of the mitotic spindle. The spindle is formed from protein strands which consist of microtubules. During the next stage the DNA in the chromatin replicates. This means that the two new cells that will result from mitosis will have identical genetic material. The triggers for DNA replication and cell division are not well understood, but it is probable that several factors are involved, e.g. cell volume/surface area ratio, which is known to determine the cell's ability to take in nutrients and excrete waste, and activation by proteins or the release of inhibition by other proteins. Normally cells are stopped from dividing too quickly by a process called contact inhibition (see page 28) that is initiated when cells are close enough to touch.

DNA is a complex chemical (see pages 21, 22). Each strand of DNA is built from subunits formed from nucleotides, each composed of a nitrogenous base, a sugar and a phosphate. It has two strands coiled into a double helix. During replication, the helical structure is uncoiled and the bonds between the two nucleotide strands are broken by enzymes (chemical catalysts) to produce two separated DNA strands. In an energy-requiring process, other enzymes cause two new nucleotide strands to be formed using the existing separate strands as a pattern or template (*Figure 1.13*). Once replication is complete, the double set of DNA joins with proteins to form new chromatin strands.

The last part of interphase involves the metabolic processes that provide the enzymes and energy needed for mitosis. Various factors such as chemicals, drugs and radiation may adversely affect this delicate process and prevent cell division. As already discussed, some of these are used therapeutically, to inhibit the growth and division of malignant cells, in the form of radiotherapy and cytotoxic drugs.

Mitosis

Mitosis is a continuous process, but is usually described as comprising four stages: prophase, metaphase, anaphase and telophase (*Figure 1.14*). The process of mitosis is usually, but not inevitably, followed by cytokinesis (see below). The whole process is completed within about 2 hours with some variation between different cell types.

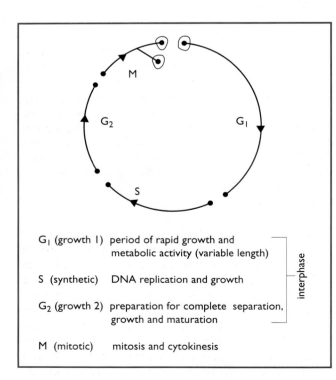

G₁ (growth 1) period of rapid growth and metabolic activity (variable length)

S (synthetic) DNA replication and growth

G₂ (growth 2) preparation for complete separation, growth and maturation

M (mitotic) mitosis and cytokinesis

Figure 1.12 The cell cycle.

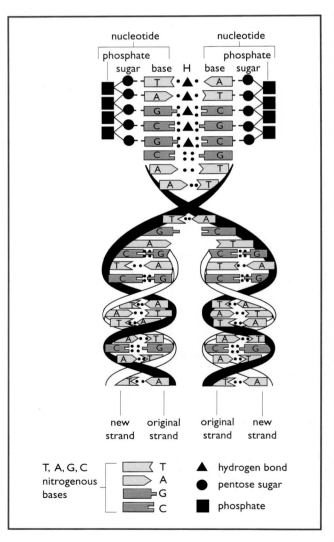

T, A, G, C nitrogenous bases — T, A, G, C

▲ hydrogen bond

● pentose sugar

■ phosphate

Figure 1.13 DNA replication.

Prophase [Figure 1.14(1a, 1b)]

Prophase commences with changes in the chromatin, which condenses and shortens to form visible chromosomes (there is a double set of chromosomes resulting from DNA replication during interphase). The double chromosomes are joined by the centromere. Each half of this double chromosome is known as a chromatid. The nucleoli start to breakdown and the nuclear membrane disappears. Each pair of centrioles moves to opposite poles of the cell where they commence the formation of the mitotic spindle which eventually reaches from one pair of centrioles to the other.

Metaphase [Figure 1.14(2)]

During metaphase, the double chromosomes move towards the middle of the cell so that their centromeres are arranged along the equator of the mitotic spindle.

Anaphase [Figure 1.14(3a, 3b)]

During anaphase the double chromosomes split at the centromere, each chromatid becoming a complete chromosome with its own centromere. The fibres of the mitotic spindle contract, causing one chromosome from each new pair to be pulled to the opposite pole of the cell.

Telophase [Figure 1.14(4)]

In telophase, the set of chromosomes at each pole uncoils to form the thread-like chromatin. Other changes include a reversal of the events occurring during prophase: the nuclear membrane reforms, the mitotic spindle disappears and the nucleoli reform.

Mitosis enables the body to grow and replace cells that sustain damage or reach the end of their allotted lifespan.

Cytokinesis

Cytokinesis (cytoplasmic division) is a separate process occurring after mitosis. The cleavage furrow that forms round the cell during late anaphase continues to progress inwards during telophase (*Figure 1.14(3b, 4)*). This continues until the original cell has been pinched into two 'daughter' cells, each with a nucleus containing identical genetic material.

Nuclear division is not always followed by cytokinesis. This results in some cells having more than one nucleus, such as may be seen in skeletal muscle. The two new cells, each of which is smaller than the original cell, now commence the cell cycle at interphase and a period of growth before their own division.

Nucleic Acids and Protein Synthesis

Nucleic acids

The two nucleic acids found in cells are DNA and RNA. They are organic macromolecules consisting of carbon, hydrogen, oxygen, nitrogen and phosphorus.

DNA consists of the pentose (5-carbon) sugar deoxyribose, phosphate groups and four nitrogenous bases: adenine (A), thymine (T), cytosine (C) and guanine (G). The nitrogenous bases are of two types: adenine and guanine are purines (double-ring structure) and cytosine and thymine are pyrimidines (single-ring structure). The three components:

- deoxyribose,
- phosphates, and
- nitrogenous bases,

form subunit, or nucleotides, which are arranged in a double helix with the two strands joined by hydrogen bonds. The bases are always paired A with T and C with G (*Figure 1.13*). These are known as complementary base pairs. DNA is the genetic material present within the nucleus which is replicated prior to cell division. Apart from its role in cell division, DNA acts as the master pattern for the precise synthesis of proteins. The term 'gene' is used to describe the tiny fragment of DNA that carries the information required to make a specific protein or subunit of a larger protein.

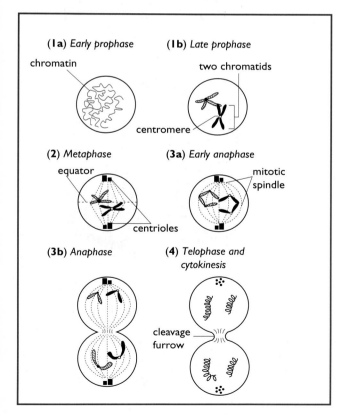

(1a) Early prophase
chromatin

(1b) Late prophase
two chromatids

centromere

(2) Metaphase
equator

(3a) Early anaphase
mitotic spindle

centrioles

(3b) Anaphase

(4) Telophase and cytokinesis

cleavage furrow

Figure 1.14 Stages of mitosis.

Table 1.5 Summary of DNA and RNA details.

Table 1.5 Summary of DNA and RNA details		
	DNA	**RNA**

Composition	Deoxyribose sugar
	Phosphate groups
	Nitrogenous bases:
	    adenine, thymine, guanine
	    and cytosine
		Ribose sugar
		Phosphate groups
		Nitrogenous bases:
		    adenine, uracil, guanine
		    and cytosine

Structure	Two nucleotide strands coiled into a double helix	Single nucleotide strand, which may be straight or folded
Sites	Nucleus	Nucleus, cytoplasm and ribosomes
Functions	Genetic material replicated in cell division acts as a pattern for protein synthesis	Undertakes the instructions needed for protein synthesis

RNA is found in the nucleus, cytoplasm and ribosomes. Although derived from DNA, it differs from DNA in several ways (*Table 1.5*). Its pentose sugar is ribose and its nitrogenous base sequence has the pyrimidine uracil (U) substituting for thymine. Structurally, it is a single strand that may be folded or straight. There are three types of RNA that perform specific roles during protein synthesis: messenger (mRNA), transfer (tRNA) and ribosomal (rRNA).

Protein Synthesis

All physiological functions are dependent upon the ability of the body to make proteins. A protein, remember, consists of many amino acids linked by peptide bonds to form polypeptide chains. We need to make many types of proteins: structural proteins, some hormones and the multitude of enzymes required for controlling biochemical reactions. The sequence of nitrogenous bases in the DNA molecule is in fact a genetic code (using the letters A, T, C and G), which is read and decoded by RNA. Three bases in the sequence form a triplet that codes for one amino acid in the new polypeptide chain, e.g. AAA codes for the amino acid phenylalanine. Several triplets arranged in a specific sequence in a gene will code for one complete polypeptide chain. The actual number of triplets needed will depend upon the length of the polypeptide chain to be made. Proteins are made by a complex process occurring in the nucleus, in the cytoplasm and inside the ribosomes. It has two distinct stages, **transcription** (the transfer of genetic information from DNA to RNA) and **translation** (the synthesis of proteins from amino acids within the ribosomes), and involves DNA and the three types of RNA. *Figure 1.15* illustrates the addition of the amino acid serine as part of a polypeptide chain.

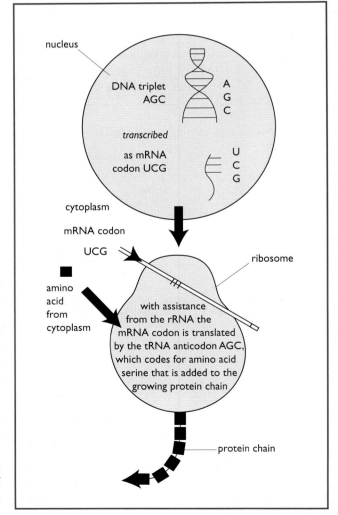

Figure 1.15 Transcription and translation.

Transcription

The first stage of transcription is to encode the DNA base sequence onto a molecule of mRNA. This base sequence is formed inside the nucleus by using one strand of the DNA as a pattern. The information from each DNA triplet is then carried as a codon of three complementary bases on the mRNA (remember – RNA has U instead of T). By this process the genetic code is transcribed. There is a total of 64 different codons as there are 64 different combinations of the four bases possible (*Table 1.6*). Each codon either codes for an amino acid, or switches on or turns off the process when the protein is complete (terminal codon). Most amino acids are coded for by more than one codon (remember there are only 20 amino acids and 64 codons). This complex code helps to minimize the effects of mutations or errors. Once transcription is complete the mRNA leaves the nucleus and migrates through the cytoplasm to the ribosomes ready for the next stage to start.

Translation

During this stage tRNA, with the help of rRNA, is able to translate the base sequence in the codon of the mRNA into the amino acid required to build the protein. It is the anti-codons (three bases) of tRNA that recognize the required amino acid, from the codon on the mRNA, and transfer this amino acid from the cytoplasm to the ribosome. Here the amino acid is added to the growing chain that will form the protein. The process of translation, which is summarized in *Figure 1.15*, occurs as the ribosome moves the mRNA strand along so that its coded message can be read sequentially. The exact mechanisms controlling protein synthesis are not fully understood but clearly the consequences of any small change in the process, such as the order of the bases, can have serious implications for the functioning of the individual. These changes, known as mutations, cause the production of abnormal proteins and result in genetic diseases. An example of a genetic disease involving an abnormal protein is sickle-cell disease (see page 4 and Chapter 9).

Table 1.6 RNA codons – the genetic code.

Table 1.6 RNA codons – the genetic code

1st position base	2nd position base				3rd position base
	U	C	A	G	
U	Phenylalanine	Serine	Tyrosine	Cysteine	U
	Phenylalanine	Serine	Tyrosine	Cysteine	C
	Leucine	Serine	Stop/terminate	Stop/terminate	A
	Leucine	Serine	Stop/terminate	Tryptophan	G
C	Leucine	Proline	Histidine	Arginine	U
	Leucine	Proline	Histidine	Arginine	C
	Leucine	Proline	Glutamine	Arginine	A
	Leucine	Proline	Glutamine	Arginine	G
A	Isoleucine	Threonine	Asparagine	Serine	U
	Isoleucine	Threonine	Asparagine	Serine	C
	Isoleucine	Threonine	Lysine	Arginine	A
	Methionine plus initiate	Threonine	Lysine	Arginine	G
G	Valine	Alanine	Aspartate (aspartic acid)	Glycine	U
	Valine	Alanine	Aspartate (aspartic acid)	Glycine	C
	Valine	Alanine	Glutamate (glutamic acid)	Glycine	A
	Valine	Alanine	Glutamate (glutamic acid)	Glycine	G

Codons code for an amino acid or they initiate or stop the process

Bases: U = uracil   C = cytosine   A = adenine   G = guanine

Cell Development

Cell differentiation

The body has many different types of cells, each with a characteristic structure and well-defined function. When you think about how life starts from only two cells, the ovum and spermatozoon, it becomes clear that some changes must occur in cells apart from the simple growth and division described in the cell cycle. The process by which a cell becomes more specialized structurally and functionally is known as differentiation. *Figure 1.16* illustrates the structural and hence functional changes that occur during erythrocyte maturation. A differentiated cell also loses the ability that embryronic cells have, to develop into other cell types. The fact that cells with identical genetic material can become so different suggests that gene expression and protein synthesis are subject to considerable control and regulation at a cellular level.

Cell ageing

Cells, like the complete organism they form, will eventually age (see Chapter 21). The exact cause of this decline is not fully understood. Theories put forward include: (i) a genetically determined failure of cellular repair mechanisms and replication as we simply run out of DNA, or inhibition of DNA synthesis by chemicals as we grow older. One explanation proposes that the progressive shortening of the DNA nucleotides (telomeres), which cover and protect the ends of the chromosomes, with each cell division, means that eventually the cells stop dividing. Telomeres are considered to be the 'biological clocks' that dictate the number of times an

individual cell may divide. (ii) Repeated injuries or 'wear and tear' to cells caused by toxins and chemicals, radiation, or lack of oxygen and nutrients over a period of many years. Some of these cellular insults result in the production of free radicals, which damage cells. (iii) A breakdown or change in the immunological responses which normally prevent cell damage by pathogenic microorganisms, malignant changes or the development of autoimmune conditions where the immune system 'attacks' tissues of the body. (iv) A reduction in endocrine gland activity and decline in pituitary hormones; for example, growth hormone plus decreased thymosine and melatonin may be implicated in ageing. (v) A lack of energy available for DNA maintenance and cell repair (disposable soma theory) – is also suggested as a factor in cell ageing. It is probable that many of these theories contribute to some degree to the process of cell ageing. It is well known that prolonged exposure to many of these factors can accelerate the cell changes that result in abnormal cell growth or premature ageing, such as the effects of excessive sunlight on skin – signs of ageing or skin cancers.

Cellular activity – communication and control

Cells do not exist in isolation – they must be able to 'send messages' out from their intracellular environment and to 'receive messages' from each other and chemicals in the extracellular environment.

Having looked at cell replication, protein synthesis and cell development, it would be helpful to outline some of the ways in which cell function is controlled before moving on to cells in association as tissues. Many

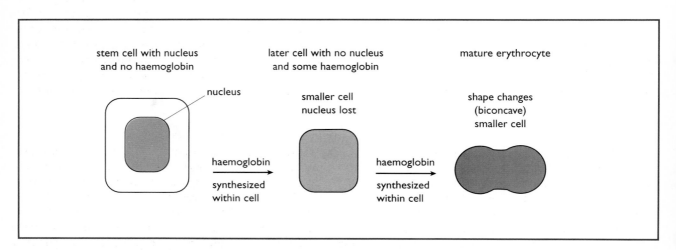

Figure 1.16 An example of differentiation – erythrocyte differentiation.

Healthier Living **Free radicals and antioxidants**

Free radicals, as we mentioned earlier, are extremely reactive chemicals (with unpaired electrons), produced during normal cellular processes. They are activated oxygen species, which include the superoxide ion (O_2^-) and the hydroxyl radical. Cells normally have the ability to deal with free radicals through complex antioxidant defence mechanisms. The defence strategies used against free radicals involve antioxidant enzyme systems that utilize trace element cofactors such as selenium, the antioxidant vitamins, e.g. vitamins C and E, and possibly beta carotene (vitamin A precursor). If free radicals accumulate the cell defences will be overwhelmed and damage will occur from oxidative stress (Kelly, 1994). There are several factors linked to an increased risk of oxidative stress, including smoking, alcohol misuse, build-up of metals such as iron, aluminium and lead in the body, and exposure to ultraviolet and ionizing radiation. Free radicals can cause great destruction within the cell by damaging nucleic acids, proteins and the lipids in cell membranes and lipoproteins. The cell damage and changes in lipid chemistry caused by free radicals may be implicated in the development of coronary heart disease, stroke and the cellular changes responsible for some cancers.

What can be done?

If all this sounds a bit gloomy, take heart — there are some common-sense measures that can be used as part of general health maintenance. It is important to stress, however, that current research findings regarding the protection afforded by the antioxidant vitamins C and E are persuasive rather than conclusive, and that increased intake is not recommended and high-dose supplements of these vitamins cannot be assumed to be safe (DoH, 1994).

- To ensure that the diet contains sufficient beta carotene, vitamins C and E, and trace elements such as selenium, zinc and manganese:

Increase the intake of fresh vegetables (dark green and orange) and fruit (yellow and orange).
Reduce the intake of saturated fats, replacing them with unsaturated fats.
Increase intake of whole cereals, nuts and seeds.
Include protein foods that also provide minerals.
- To avoid or minimize the factors linked to increases in oxidative stress: Stop or cut down on smoking.
Limit alcohol use.
Restrict exposure to ultraviolet radiation, e.g. sunlight.
Observe the safety protocols when dealing with ionizing radiation, e.g. using X-rays at work.
- To avoid a 'build-up' of metals such as lead use lead free petrol where possible, replacing old lead water pipes and lead-based paints; and not storing food or drinks in anything containing lead.

---

of the surface and integral molecules of the plasma membrane (see page 13) are involved with the communication necessary for cell regulation and ultimately, homeostasis. Some act as receptors that combine with specific signalling chemicals, such as hormones or neurotransmitters, known collectively as ligands. These ligands bind to the receptor and change cell proteins in various ways, thereby influencing function. These include:

- Activation and deactivation of membrane receptors which act as enzymes.
- Opening and closing the ion channels controlled by membrane proteins.
- Altering protein synthesis by affecting gene transcription.
- Initiating receptor-mediated endocytosis of regulatory molecules.

Many cell receptors (especially those involving ion channels or enzymes) act through regulatory intermediates called G proteins. The G protein-type receptors are often associated with other chemicals called second messengers. Important second messengers are cyclic adenosine monophosphate (cAMP), which is formed from ATP (see page 10) by the removal of two phosphate groups, and calcium. These two second messengers act as a link between the signalling chemical and the intracellular chemical reactions catalyzed by protein kinase enzymes. Second messengers are able to initiate intracellular processes by which many chemical reactions are catalyzed simultaneously (enzyme cascade amplification) and control the rate at which reactions occur. Calcium is the second messenger involved in muscle contraction (see Chapter 17).

Some cell receptors are situated within the cytoplasm or in the nucleus, which means that the ligand must first enter the cell to alter its function. Steroid hormones, which you will remember are lipids, are just such ligands. They dissolve in the lipid part of the plasma membrane and enter the cell where they bind to receptors, in the nucleus to alter gene transcription and protein synthesis.

Abnormalities of cell growth

As with any complex process the scope for error is ever present. Amazingly, protein synthesis, and growth and division in human cells, are, generally, accurate processes. When errors do occur they range from a failure of growth to a breakdown in control mechanisms that allows uncoordinated cell growth and division. This results in the development of tumours (mass of tissues), malignant or benign. Various cellular changes occur between the two

Nursing Practice Application *Ways in which drugs alter cell function*

Following the coverage of the surface and integral molecules of the plasma membrane (see page 13) and the ways in which cellular activity is controlled (see above), it is possible to apply this knowledge to a look at some of the ways in which drugs can be used to alter cell function. Drugs can alter cell function in a variety of ways by acting through the following targets: enzymes, receptors, ion channels and carrier molecules (Rang et al., 1995). Some of these principal sites for drug action are outlined in the following section:

(i) Enzymes. Enzymes, which normally catalyze cellular reactions, can be competitively inhibited by drugs, e.g. ibuprofen, a non-steroidal anti-inflammatory drug (NSAID), which reduces inflammation and pain by preventing the synthesis of prostaglandins (see page 9). Other drugs stop enzyme reactions by binding to the enzyme as false substrates (in place of its proper substrate) and producing an abnormal metabolite that disrupts a series of normal biochemical reactions. The drug methyldopa, now rarely used as an antihypertensive, acts as a false substrate. Another group of drugs require the action of a cellular enzyme to become activated; these are termed pro-drugs. Pro-drugs can be used to simplify administration and in some cases reduce toxicity as the active form is only produced after the action of liver enzymes, e.g. the cytotoxic drug cyclophosphamide.

(ii) Receptors (cytoplasmic or membrane). Cell receptors can be 'fooled' by drugs that are nearly the same shape as their normal ligand. The drug, which binds to the receptor and deceives the cell, can alter function in several ways. Some drugs are agonists, e.g. the analgesic morphine. These cause cells to act in exactly the same way as they would with the usual ligand, i.e. the expected cell response will occur. Some agonists alter cell function by opening membrane ion channels and allowing ions to enter the cell whereas others activate second messengers (e.g. cAMP) – systems to cause enzyme cascade amplification, which allows a widespread response. Lipid-soluble agonist drugs, such as corticosteroids, enter the cell and bind to cytoplasmic or nuclear receptors and eventually alter cell function by affecting gene activity and protein synthesis. Drugs that stop the cell ligand (the natural agonist) binding to the receptors are termed antagonists; for example, tamoxifen is used in the treatment of breast cancer because it stops the hormone oestrogen binding to its receptors. By stopping ligand binding, the drug prevents the normal cellular response, but please note that antagonists act by preventing a response rather than causing one, much as a parked car blocking your drive stops you driving your car into the garage, which is what normally happens. A further group of drugs act as partial agonists by being either agonists or antagonists, depending upon the prevailing physiological conditions. They tend to prevent the activation of a full cellular response.

(iii) Ion channels. Some membrane ion channels are not operated by ligands. These channels can be physically blocked by the binding of certain drugs that stop the movement of ions through the channel. This type of drug can alter function in excitable cells that depend upon ion movement and electrochemical gradients to produce the action potentials (see Chapter 3) required for the passage of nerve impulses – this can be demonstrated when local anaesthetics are used to block the transmission of pain impulses (see Chapter 4). Ion channel function can also be modulated by drugs which may increase or decrease the ability to open; for example, calcium antagonists such as nifedipine (a drug that dilates blood vessels) stop the entry of calcium ions into the cell and are used in the management of angina and hypertension.

(iv) Carrier proteins. Cell function can be altered if carrier proteins are prevented from transporting substances across the plasma membrane. Drugs may inhibit the carrier protein by binding to the carrier, thus preventing the normal transport of substances such as ions, amino acids and neurotransmitters. Drugs that act in this way include tricyclic antidepressants (see Chapter 6) such as clomipramine, which prevents the uptake of various neurotransmitters by nerve terminals, or loop diuretics such as frusemide (drugs that increase urine production – see Chapter 15), which prevent the movement of ions in the kidney tubules. Carrier protein function can also be affected by drugs that act as false substrates, e.g. amphetamine, which enters the cell to initiate the release of noradrenaline (a neurotransmitter) in the brain. Noradrenaline causes the heightened awareness, restlessness, appetite loss and insomnia associated with the use of amphetamines.

An understanding of how drugs work is obviously important if nurses, midwives and health visitors are to exercise their professional accountability in areas of practice that relate to the administration of medicines. The United Kingdom Central Council for Nursing, Midwifery and Health Visiting (UKCC) reiterates the importance of personal accountability for practice when they quote from the Code of Professional Conduct (1992a) in a later document dealing with the administration of medicines (UKCC, 1992b), which states that 'the practitioner will be satisfied that she or he has an understanding of substances used for therapeutic purposes' (UKCC, 1992b). Individual practitioners are recommended to update their drug knowledge by reading the manufacturer's most recent product information prior to administration and to obtain more general information from current drug reference books and the British National Formulary (BNF).

---

extremes of no growth (aplasia) and tumour formation (neoplasia), including: atrophy, hypertrophy, hyperplasia, metaplasia and dysplasia (*Figure 1.17*).

Aplasia

Aplasia means 'absence of growth' and applies to a situation where an organ or structure fails to develop during intrauterine life. This particular abnormality of cell growth affects paired structures: only one of the pair develops, e.g.

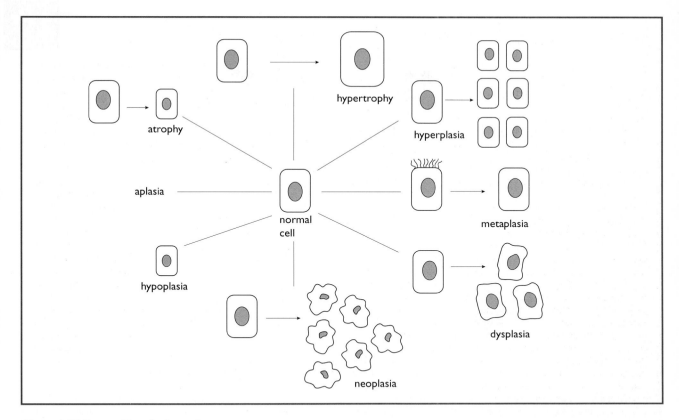

Figure 1.17 Abnormalities of cell growth.

kidney. A less severe form is hypoplasia, where organ development is incomplete, resulting in a smaller than normal structure with possible loss of function.

Atrophy
Atrophy is an acquired change occurring when a previously normal structure becomes wasted and smaller. Causes of atrophy include:
• Normal deterioration, e.g. during the climacteric (a period of time usually occurring between age 46 and 55 years, during which female reproductive function declines), when the ovaries atrophy.
• Abnormal deterioration, e.g. when a structure is starved of nutrients, its blood supply is impaired, it is subjected to constant pressure or after long-term disuse. This has particular relevance to nursing practice. People confined to bed because of illness or injury and those immobile for other reasons, e.g. severe arthritis, lose muscle mass (see Chapter 17).

Hypertrophy
With hypertrophy, individual cells increase in size, resulting in an overall enlargement of the organ. This may occur where use is increased, e.g. the leg muscles enlarge in a runner. It can happen as part of the compensation mech-

anisms by which the body tries to minimize the effects of declining function, e.g. enlargement of the myocardium (heart muscle) in heart failure (see Chapter 10).

Hyperplasia
An increase in actual cell numbers is known as hyperplasia. An example is the bone marrow hyperplasia that increases erythrocyte production in some types of anaemia or when an individual is living at high altitude (see Chapters 9 and 12).

Metaplasia
Metaplasia occurs when there is a change in cell type, usually with the cells becoming less specialized. This is a reversal of differentiation and may be seen in areas such as the cervix or gall bladder. It is caused by long-standing irritation or infection. If the cause is removed the cells return to normal. If the cause remains, further, more serious cell changes can occur, e.g. in the bronchial epithelium in smokers.

Dysplasia
Dysplasia is a change in the size and shape of the cells that form the covering and lining tissues of the body (the epithelia; see pages 30–31). It results from chronic irritation and

Special Focus **Cancer**

Predisposing factors

Geographical and environmental: e.g. breast cancer is uncommon in Japan, but common in Europe and North America, even in Japanese women living in these areas.

Genetic: certain cancers show an increased incidence within some families, e.g. colonic polyps.

Chronic physical irritation: e.g. bladder cancer may be associated with urinary calculi.

Chemicals: there are numerous examples of carcinogenic chemicals: those contained in cigarette smoke (lung cancer), asbestos (lung cancer and mesothelioma), aniline dyes (bladder cancer) and vinyl chloride (liver cancer and possibly lung and brain cancer). A link between alcohol misuse and head and neck cancers exists, but there is little public awareness (Buglass, 1995).

Infective agents: viruses are implicated as the causative agent in several animal and human cancers, e.g. the link between the herpes simplex virus (HSV2) and the papilloma virus (HPV) and some types of cervical cancer. Infection with the AIDS virus is also linked to a rare cancer affecting the skin (Kaposi's sarcoma).

Radiation: excess exposure to ultraviolet rays from sunlight causes skin cancers. Ionizing radiation causes an increased risk for cancer where environmental levels increase, e.g. following accidental leaks from nuclear plants.

Reducing the risks, including measures which may be realistic for individuals

Reduce tobacco smoking/chewing.

Modify diet: reduce fat and increase fibre. A high intake of a variety of fruit may be protective against some cancers (HEA, 1993). It is possible that beta-carotene, vitamin C and vitamin E all play a part in this protection (MAFF, 1995).

Limit alcohol consumption (see Chapter 14).

Avoid exposure to carcinogenic chemicals: in the workplace, follow safety procedures, e.g. wear protective clothing, and develop safer materials.

Practice safe sex: limit the number of partners, consider using a barrier method of contraception, e.g. cap or condom. Think carefully about long-term use of oral contraceptives or hormone replacement therapy (see Chapters 20 and 21).

Common cancers

Lung/bronchus, gastrointestinal tract (oesophagus, stomach, pancreas, bowel and rectum), breast (most common malignancy of women in Western industrial countries, DoH, 1993), ovary, cervix and uterus, prostate and bladder, skin, leukaemia.

NB Cancer causes nearly 25% of deaths in the countries of the UK.

Early detection – what you can do

Be aware of and report early warning signs, such as a change in a skin mole or blood in the urine.

Practice breast awareness or **testicular self-examination** (see Chapter 20).

Have routine screening tests – cervical smear tests, mammography (an X-ray of the breast). Monitoring of body fluids for cancer cells, e.g. urine for workers in some 'high risk' industries. Other screening tests that are not part of a national programme include faecal examination for occult blood (colorectal cancers) and ultrasound or CT scans to detect ovarian cancer (see Chapter 20).

commonly affects the skin, cervix and oesophagus. These serious changes can lead to the development of a malignant tumour. Interestingly, even at this stage spontaneous reversal to 'normal' can still occur if the chronic irritation ceases.

Neoplasia

Neoplasia, which means 'new growth', is characterized by very marked cellular changes. These include changes in DNA structure and abnormal, uncoordinated cell division that give rise to a tumour. Tumours are usually classified according to the type of tissue from which they develop. They may be benign or malignant:

- Benign localized tumours may cause problems from pressure or hormone production.
- Malignant tumours are invasive both locally and by

their ability to metastasize, that is spread to distant parts of the body through the blood or lymphatics (*Table 1.7*). Cancer is the lay term used to describe any malignant condition.

Tumour formation and defence

Tumour cells develop as various DNA mutations occur in cells exposed to some carcinogenic (cancer-causing) agent such as a virus or chemical. Normally cells stop dividing when they 'run out of room'; this is termed contact inhibition. This inhibition of continued cell division is apparently lost in cancer cells. Sometimes these changes result in a benign tumour, which may become malignant if an onco-gene (cancer gene) already present in body cells becomes

Table 1.7 Comparison of benign and malignant tumours		
	Benign	**Malignant**
Structure	Resembles its tissue of origin – well differentiated	May show any degree of differentiation; well to completely undifferentiated
Growth rate	Usually slow	Variable but usually rapid and uncoordinated; some malignant tumours are very slow growing
Enclosing capsule	Yes	No
Spread	No	Yes – locally by infiltration of tissues and by metastases that spread to other sites via blood, lymphatics, by 'seeding' along a natural channel and across body cavities
Effects	Pressure on a vital organ, e.g. brain. Production of hormones. Complications such as infection and bleeding. May become malignant.	Destroy vital organs. Cause weight loss and debility (cachexia) and eventual death in the absence of effective treatment. Some malignant tumours respond very well to treatment. (See also effects of benign tumours.)

Table 1.7 Comparison of benign and malignant tumours.

activated. Oncogenes are known to be present in around one in five cancers. At all stages the defence mechanisms of the body attempt to prevent the formation of cancer cells by the destruction of carcinogens by enzymes present in lysosomes and peroxisomes, and through the action of tumour suppressor genes (anti-oncogenes), which also code for the repair of damaged DNA and influence immunological cancer defences. Should this fail and a cell becomes malignant it can still be removed by specialized cells of the immune system. It is only in situations when these defences are completely overwhelmed that a malignant tumour develops. Malignant tumours occur most commonly in older people, which supports the genetic, repeated cell injury and immunological theories of cell ageing already described (see page 24). Tumours, in common with cell ageing, appear to have a multifactorial aetiology (cause).

Extracellular matrix

The gel-like extracellular matrix is the 'cement' secreted by cells to hold them together – much as the mortar holds the individual bricks of a wall. The composition of the extracellular matrix varies between different types of cells, but basically consists of:

- Water with salts and nutrients, which forms the interstitial fluid (see Chapter 2).
- Fibres of fibrous proteins, such as collagen and elastin.
- Polysaccharide molecules, e.g. hyaluronic acid, which link to other proteins to form proteoglycans.
- Cell adhesion proteins, e.g. fibronectin.

Apart from holding cells together, the extracellular matrix has other roles. A special sheet-like arrangement of extra-

cellular matrix, consisting of glycoproteins produced by epithelial cells, forms the basal lamina, which assists in cell migration, development and repair of damage, and acts as a filter that selectively allows molecules to diffuse between blood vessels and the cells. The basal lamina together with a reticular lamina of collagen and glycoproteins formed by connective cells forms the supportive basement membrane between the epithelial and connective tissues (see page 30).

Tissues

Cells in association form body tissues. The abilities of cells to migrate within the body and to become specialized by differentiation (see page 24) are central to tissue formation. A tissue consists of a number of cells and the extracellular matrix that binds them together. The cells that make up a tissue all have a similar structure and perform the same sort of functions in different parts of the body; for example, muscle tissue is concerned with contraction and movement regardless of its location. Tissues belong to one of four major types: epithelial, connective, muscle and nervous. The study of tissues is called histology. When laboratory techniques involve looking for abnormalities, such as the examination of biopsies (when tissue samples are examined), it is known as histopathology.

Tissue origin and classification

The early embryo has three basic tissues: ectoderm, mesoderm and endoderm (see Chapters 20 and 21). These are known as the primary germ layers. It is from these that the four groups of tissue (epithelium, connective, nervous and muscle) develop during embryonic life:

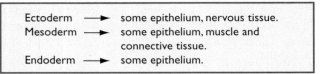

Ectoderm ──────▶ some epithelium, nervous tissue.
Mesoderm ──────▶ some epithelium, muscle and
                  connective tissue.
Endoderm ──────▶ some epithelium.

Epithelium is a covering and lining tissue, connective tissue is basically supportive but does much more, muscle tissue is concerned with movement, and nervous tissue is concerned with providing control and communication systems.

Epithelial tissues

Epithelial tissues cover the body, line body cavities and form glands. The cells of epithelial tissue are close together and usually lie on a basement membrane formed from the basal lamina and reticular lamina (see page 29). Some, however, do not have a basement membrane, e.g. liver sinusoids (see Chapter 14). There is little extracellular matrix between the cells. Each type of epithelium has developed to meet its basic function with further individual adaptations for special areas.

Simple epithelium

Epithelium may be simple, consisting of a single cell layer. These cells may be squamous, cuboidal or columnar. Squamous epithelium (*Figure 1.18*) is a single layer of flat cells found as a smooth lining in the heart and blood ves-sels (smooth tissue prevents blood clotting), in the lymph vessels, in the glomeruli of the kidney and in the alveoli of the lungs. The single layer of fragile cells allows easy transfer of substances; for example, by filtration in the glomeruli and by the diffusion of gases between blood capillaries and alveoli.

Cuboidal epithelium (*Figure 1.19*) is also a single layer, but here the cells are cube shaped. This tissue is found in the kidney tubules, where it is adapted for absorption, with many tiny projections called microvilli on its surface (see page 14), and secretion. Cuboidal epithelium is also found in small glands and their ducts.

Columnar epithelium (*Figure 1.20*) has cells which are tall. Many have microvilli, which increase the surface area available for absorption, and have goblet cells that produce mucus (see Chapters 12 and 13). Columnar epithelium is found in the gastrointestinal tract and gall bladder, again concerned with absorption and secretion. Some types found in the respiratory tract and uterine tubes have cilia (see page 16) upon their surfaces. The ciliated surface of these delicate, highly specialized cells helps move mucus or reproductive cells.

Stratified epithelium

Stratified epithelium consists of many cell layers. These cells may be squamous, cuboidal or columnar. In addition, there is the specialized transitional epithelium.

Stratified squamous epithelium (*Figure 1.21*) is composed of many layers of dividing columnar or cuboidal cells, which flatten as they move to the surface. They are protective and are found as skin in dry areas where the outer layer of cells are keratinized (keratin is a tough fibrous protein) and dead. In moist areas, which are subject to 'wear and tear', a non keratinized variety protects the mouth, oesophagus, pharynx, anus and vagina.

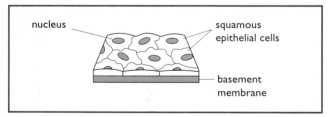

Figure 1.18 Squamous epithelium.

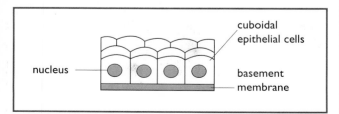

Figure 1.19 Cuboidal epithelium.

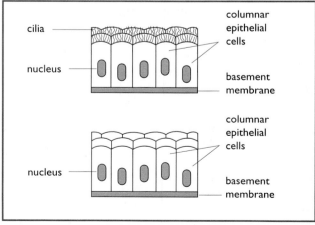

Figure 1.20 Columnar epithelium (above, ciliated; below, non-ciliated).

Transitional epithelium (*Figure 1.22*) is a type of epithelium found only in the urinary tract, where it lines the renal pelvis, ureter, bladder and urethra. Structurally it has cuboidal, columnar and dome-like surface cells that allow distension when the urinary structures fill with urine. Its surface cells are also able to withstand the effects of contact with urine.

Glands

Some epithelial tissues form specialized structures known as glands. These are groups of cells adapted to the production and secretion of various water-based secretions. Glands that secrete directly into the blood or lymph are known as endocrine glands and are ductless. With endocrine glands, secretions known as hormones are discharged directly into the extracellular spaces to enter the blood or lymph, e.g. the thyroid gland (see Chapter 8). Exocrine glands secrete their products into ducts. These secretions leave by a duct into a body cavity, or are discharged directly onto the surface skin, e.g. liver, mucous glands and sweat glands. Structurally, exocrine glands may have a simple or compound duct system with a tubular or alveolar secretory arrangement (*Figure 1.23*). The secretions may leave the gland by exocytosis (see page 18), cell rupture or partial disruption whereby the portion containing the secretion is 'nipped off'.

Connective tissues

There are a great variety of connective tissues. These range from loose connective tissue (adipose tissue), to supportive connective tissue (bone), to blood-forming tissue (haemopoietic bone marrow). Connective tissues are widespread throughout the body and are concerned with much more than just connection and support. Connective tissue around organs offers protection and insulation. In the form of fat it provides an energy source.

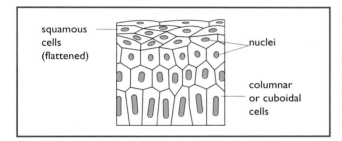

Figure 1.21 Stratified squamous epithelium.

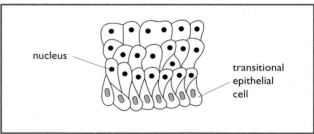

Figure 1.22 Transitional epithelium.

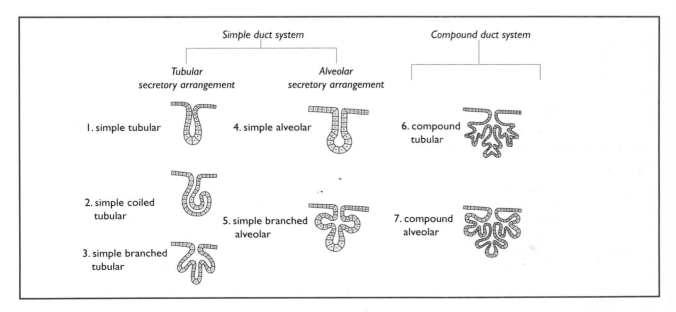

Figure 1.23 Types of exocrine glands.

It is also involved with body protection as reticular tissue and with transportation as blood.

The hallmark of connective tissue is cells surrounded by an extracellular matrix that may be rigid (bone), gel-like (areolar) or fluid (blood). Fibres are also present as a network within the matrix. These fibres are special fibrous proteins and take the form of collagen or elastin (elastic), or are reticular. The formation of a class of connective tissue is based on one of four types of primary cell: fibroblast, chondroblast, osteoblast or blood stem cell (haemocytoblast). The mature cells of the specific tissue develop from the primary cells. In addition, a variety of other cells may be involved, including fat cells, mast cells, (inflammatory response), leucocytes, plasma cells (immune response) and macrophages; the presence or otherwise of particular types of such cells depends on the nature of the connective tissue – for example, fat cells are found primarily in adipose connective tissue. The individual cells are discussed again in the relevant chapters, e.g. plasma cells (Chapter 19), but it might prove useful here to expand on the macrophage and its general importance in defence strategies. These large phagocytic cells are found fixed in certain organs and as freely mobile cells in other areas. As well as in connective tissues, they are seen in the liver as Kupffer cells (see Chapter 14), spleen, bone marrow and other lymphoid structures (see Chapter 11), and as microglial cells (see Chapter 3) in the brain. Macrophages are also part of the wider immune processes involving other cell types.

All the connective tissues discussed below are derived from a primitive embryonic tissue called mesenchyme, which itself develops from the mesoderm germ layer (see page 30). A mucous connective tissue found only in the embryo, called Wharton's jelly, supports the blood vessels in the umbilical cord.

Loose connective tissue

Areolar tissue (*Figure 1.24*) is a loose woven tissue with a semisolid matrix containing collagen, elastic and reticular fibres. The most prominent cells are fibroblasts, which are important in tissue repair. Also present are fat cells, mast cells and macrophages. Areolar tissue is found supporting vessels and nerves, around muscles, in glands and as the subcutaneous (under-the-skin) tissues. This open structure allows for considerable accumulation of water and salts. In certain pathological situations this leads to tissue swelling or oedema (see Chapter 10)

Adipose tissue (*Figure 1.25*) consists of many fat cells (adipocytes) in a basic areolar matrix. It is present in varying quantities, to some extent genetically determined, under the skin, around organs such as the kidneys, in the abdomen and between muscle fibres. Apart from support and insulation, it provides the body with a valuable source of fuel for energy. Adipose tissue accounts for around 15–22% of body weight in adults, with females having a greater percentage than males. A special type of adipose tissue called brown fat is widespread in newborn babies and persists into adult life within certain body sites such as in the axillae and around

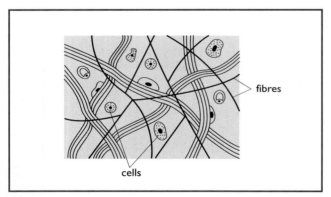

Figure 1.24 Areolar tissue.

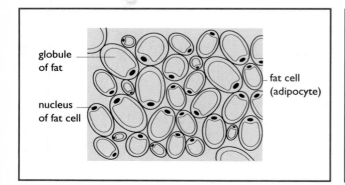

Figure 1.25 Adipose tissue.

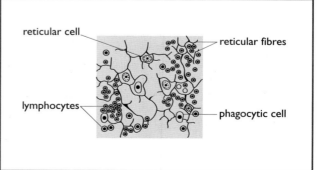

Figure 1.26 Reticular tissue.

the kidneys. Brown fat, which readily 'gives up' its energy as heat, is considered to be an important part of regulating body temperature in newborns.

Reticular tissue (*Figure 1.26*) consists of a network of reticular fibres. The matrix is loose and contains reticular cells (similar to fibroblasts), lymphocytes and phagocytic cells. It is found in the spleen, liver, lymph nodes and bone marrow, where it provides support and has a role in protecting the body.

Dense connective tissue

The two types of dense connective tissue are fibrous and elastic tissue. Fibrous tissue (*Figure 1.27*) has regular and irregular fibres. It is the tougher tissue, consisting of mainly collagen fibres and a few fibroblasts within a scanty matrix. It forms ligaments, tendons, and the covering for bones and organs such as the brain. This tissue is protective and assists with movement and stability by joining bones together and providing muscle attachments.

Elastic tissue (*Figure 1.28*), as its name suggests, is a tough tissue with the ability to stretch and recoil caused by the presence of elastic fibres within the matrix. It is an important component in structures required to distend and change shape: large arteries, epiglottis, vocal cords, trachea and the ear lobe.

Cartilage

Cartilage has a solid matrix containing chondrocytes (cartilage cells) and collagen fibres, which make the tissue firm and tough. The three types of cartilage – hyaline, white fibrocartilage and elastic yellow cartilage (*Figure 1.29*) – perform different functions.

Hyaline cartilage, a smooth, shiny tissue, forms the embryonic skeleton, covers the ends of long bones in joints and forms the cartilage of the nose, larynx, trachea, bronchi and the costal cartilages, which join the ribs to the sternum.

White fibrocartilage is a strong, flexible tissue able to absorb compressive forces. It is found as pads between the vertebrae (intervertebral discs) and the pubic bones of the pelvis (symphysis pubis), and as the semilunar cartilages of the knee joint.

Yellow elastic cartilage helps structures maintain their shape by its great flexibility. It is found in the pinna of the ear (see Chapter 7) and in the epiglottis (see Chapter 12).

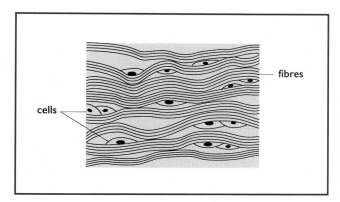

Figure 1.27 Fibrous tissue.

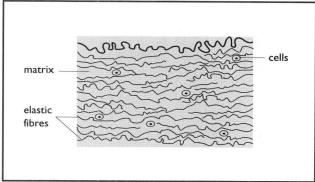

Figure 1.28 Elastic tissue.

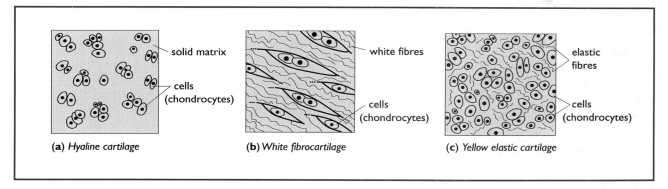

(a) *Hyaline cartilage* (b) *White fibrocartilage* (c) *Yellow elastic cartilage*

Figure 1.29 Cartilage.

Bone

There are two types of bone tissue, compact and cancellous (spongy), which are discussed in Chapter 16. The matrix in bone is hard because of its mineralization with calcium salts. The primary cells are osteoblasts, which differentiate to become osteocytes (bone cells).

Blood and blood-forming tissues

These tissues are discussed in detail in Chapter 9. Unusually for a connective tissue, blood has a fluid matrix. The haemocytoblasts (stem cells) in blood-forming tissues eventually give rise to all other blood cell types.

Membranes

Specialized secretory sheets of epithelial tissue with a connective tissue layer are called membranes. They cover organs, or line organs and body cavities. Here they provide support, reduce friction, provide nourishment and offer some protective functions. There are three types of epithelial membranes:

- Mucous membranes (mucosae): these are found in the respiratory, genitourinary and gastrointestinal tracts and produce a sticky viscous fluid called mucus.
- Serous membranes: these are double-layer membranes that line the major cavities of the body (parietal layer) and cover some organs (visceral layer). They form the peritoneum in the abdominal cavity, the pleura in the thoracic cavity and the pericardium around the heart (see Chapters 13, 12 and 10 respectively). Serous fluid produced between the two layers reduces friction during movement.
- Cutaneous membrane: this is found covering the body as the skin (see Chapter 19).

In addition to these membranes there is the synovial membrane found lining the cavity of freely movable joints (see Chapter 18). Synovial membrane is formed from modified connective tissue and secretes synovial fluid, which acts as a lubricant within the joint.

Nervous tissue

Nervous tissue can be classifed as neurones (excitable cells which transmit the nerve impulse) and the non-excitable neuroglia – cells that support, insulate and protect (see Chapter 3).

Muscle tissue

There are three types of muscle tissue: striated, which is voluntary (skeletal); non-striated, which is involuntary (smooth); and cardiac (heart) (see Chapters 10 and 17).

Individual muscle cells are generally referred to as muscle fibres.

Tissue repair

Physical or chemical injury to the body will initiate the inflammatory response and specific immune reactions within the tissues (see Chapter 19). The way in which healing occurs after tissue injury will depend on the type of tissue and the degree of damage involved. Repair can be either:

Regeneration: when the tissue is repaired by the proliferation of identical cells to those lost. New cells may be produced as existing cells divide, e.g. liver cells, or primitive stem cells such as blood cells differentiate. Regeneration occurs in relatively undifferentiated tissue, e.g. bone.

Replacement by fibrosis: here the repair is effected by the production of fibrous tissue (scar) in place of the damaged tissue. This occurs in differentiated tissues, e.g. cardiac muscle. In reality most healing occurs through a combination of both processes.

Highly specialized tissue, consisting of permanent cells, such as the nerve cells of the central nervous system and cardiac muscle, cannot regenerate. It is sometimes possible for a nerve fibre to regenerate if the nerve cell body is intact. Clearly any serious damage to these tissues will result in loss of functional ability, e.g. after a stroke (see Chapter 4) or heart attack (see Chapter 10). On the other hand, labile cells such as those in blood-forming tissues are continuously regenerated, and epithelial cells, e.g. those lining the gastrointestinal tract, continually wear away and regenerate to maintain tissue integrity. Between these two extremes are tissues made of stable cells, such as liver and bone, that can regenerate, but do so more slowly. Healing also depends on many other factors, such as tissue nutrition and oxygenation, presence of infection and age. Healing ability slows and becomes less efficient with increasing age. Tissue healing is addressed much more fully in Chapter 19, where it is applied to nursing practice in a discussion of wound care and healing.

Organs

Tissues grouping together eventually become discrete functional units called organs. These may be hollow, e.g. the stomach, or compact, e.g. the liver. Several types of tissue may be represented in one organ; for example, the stomach has an outer connective tissue and epithelium layer, middle muscle layer and a mucous membrane lining (epithelium). Compact organs consist of functional cells (parenchymal) supported by connective tissue and surrounded by a tough capsule.

Body Cavities

The body can be divided into cavities defined by the bony skeleton and muscles. The four main body cavities are the cranial, thoracic, abdominal and pelvic cavities. Many of the tissues and organs that constitute the functional systems of the body are grouped within these cavities, e.g. respiratory, digestive, nervous and reproductive systems (see pages 37, 38).

It is important to note that not all the structures or organs mentioned in the text are shown in the illustrations (*Figures 1.30–1.34*). Some are situated behind other structures and some are too small to be shown with any clarity.

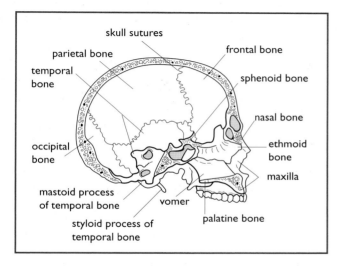

Figure 1.30 Cranial cavity (brain not shown).

The cranial cavity

The cranial cavity is formed by the bones of the cranium, which is the upper part of the skull. The bony box formed by the cranium surrounds and protects the brain. *Figure 1.30* shows the bones of the cranium (frontal, parietal-(2), temporal-(2), occipital, sphenoid and ethmoid) joined by fibrous joints called sutures. Also illustrated are some bones of the face (nasal, maxilla, palatine, vomer). See Chapter 18 for more details.

The thoracic cavity (thorax)

The cavity forming the upper portion of the trunk is known as the thoracic cavity (*Figure 1.31*). It is bounded by the structures of the root of the neck, ribs, costal cartilages, intercostal muscles, sternum, spine and diaphragm (the muscle dividing the thorax from the abdominal cavity). The thoracic cavity contains the trachea, two bronchi, two lungs, heart and great vessels, the oesophagus, nerves and lymphatics (see Chapters 10–13). The space between the lungs, occupied by the heart, is called the mediastinum.

The abdominal cavity

The large lower portion of the trunk is the abdominal cavity (see *Figure 1.32*). It is bounded by the spine, abdominal muscles (Chapter 18), lower ribs, diaphragm above and pelvic cavity below. Abdominal structures include the organs involved with digesting and absorb-

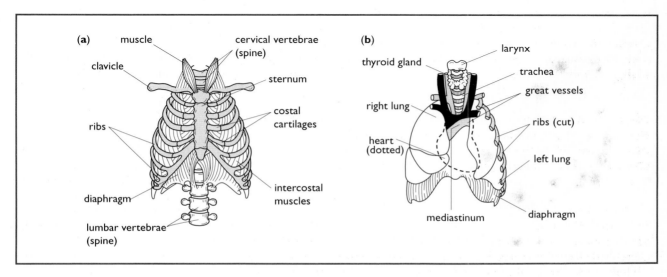

Figure 1.31 Thorax. (**a**) External structures; (**b**) internal structures.

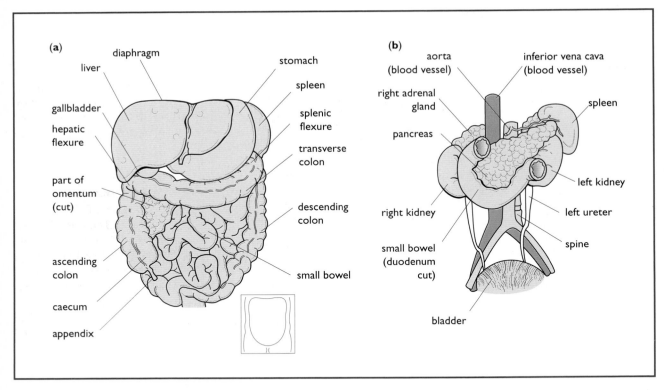

Figure 1.32 Abdominal cavity. (**a**) Anterior structures; (**b**) view with most of the organs of digestion removed.

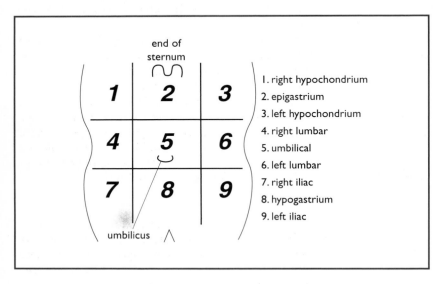

Figure 1.33 Regions of the abdomen.

1. right hypochondrium
2. epigastrium
3. left hypochondrium
4. right lumbar
5. umbilical
6. left lumbar
7. right iliac
8. hypogastrium
9. left iliac

ing nutrients, and the liver, kidneys and ureters, spleen, adrenal glands and associated blood vessels, nerves and lymphatics. *Figure 1.32(a)* shows the abdominal organs viewed from the front. The stomach, spleen, small bowel, caecum, appendix, colon, hepatic and splenic flexures, liver and gall bladder are shown. The omentum (a fold

of peritoneum) has been removed for clarity. *Figure 1.32(b)* illustrates the abdominal organs visible when most of the digestive organs have been removed.

The surface anatomy of the abdomen is divided into nine regions (*Figure 1.33*) – a useful tool when describing the location of the various organs or of pain.

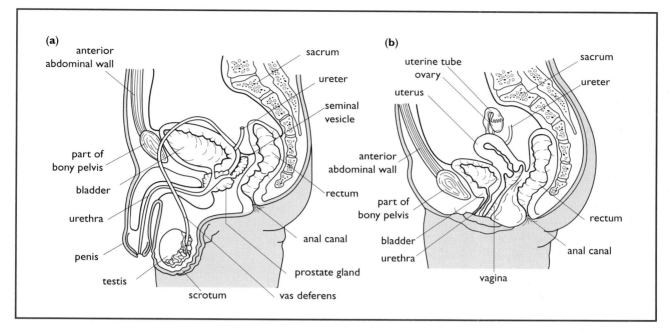

Figure 1.34 (a) Male and **(b)** female pelvis.

The pelvic cavity

The lowest portion of the trunk is the pelvic cavity (*Figure 1.34*). This is a continuation of the abdominal cavity. It is bounded by the bony pelvis, sacrum and muscles of the pelvic floor (Chapter 18), and contains openings for the urethra, vagina and anus. The pelvic cavity contains the female reproductive structures (ovaries, uterine tubes, uterus and vagina), some of the male reproductive structures (vas deferens, prostate gland and seminal vesicles, but not the penis, testes or scrotum), the lower ureters, bladder and urethra. Other pelvic organs are some coils of small bowel, the last part of the colon, the rectum and the anal canal.

Overview of Functional Systems

During your study of the functional systems, covered in Chapters 3–20, it is important to remember the vital interdependence between systems, and in certain situations the overlap of function. It is also useful to regard the functional systems of the body as the end point of an increasingly complex progression illustrated below:

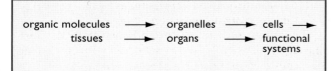

Regulation, control and communication

The nervous system (brain, spinal cord and peripheral nerves). Controls all other systems. Receives sensory information from sense organs. Initiates motor activity. Stores information as memory.

The special senses (eye, ear, olfactory epithelium, tongue and taste buds). Reception of sensory inputs as vision, hearing/balance, smell (olfaction) and taste (gustation).

The endocrine system and hormones (hypothalamus, pituitary, pineal, thyroid, parathyroids, thymus, pancreas, adrenals and gonads). Hormones, with nervous system, control all body functions, e.g. growth, reproduction, metabolism, stress responses, fluid balance, calcium and glucose homeostasis, immune responses, and other biological rhythms affecting mood and sleep.

Body transport systems

The blood (plasma, erythrocytes, leucocytes and platelets). Transportation of substances, e.g. gases, hormones and nutrients. Body defences and immune processes. Appropriate haemostasis to control blood loss following injury.

The cardiovascular system (heart and blood vessels). The heart pumps blood into a system of blood vessels and circulates blood through the lungs and around the body.

The lymphatic system (lymph, lymphatic vessels, lymph nodes and lymphoid tissues). Transportation of fats and return of tissue fluid to the circulation. Body defences and immune processes.

Obtaining and using raw material for metabolism and excreting waste

Respiratory system (nose, pharynx, larynx, trachea, bronchi, smaller bronchioles and lungs (tiny airways and alveoli). Air rich in oxygen moves into the lungs during inspiration; gaseous exchange occurs and air containing waste carbon dioxide leaves by expiration. Vital in the regulation of blood pH.

Digestive system (mouth, pharynx, oesophagus, stomach, small intestine, large intestine and accessory glands – salivary glands, pancreas and liver). Concerned with the ingestion of food, mastication, digestion, absorption and utilization of nutrients, and elimination of waste.

Liver and biliary tract (liver, gallbladder and bile ducts). The liver is concerned with metabolism of nutrients, synthesis of proteins and other molecules, detoxification of alcohol, drugs and modification of hormones, storage and bile production. Bile is stored in the gallbladder and transported in bile ducts.

Urinary system (kidneys, ureters, bladder and urethra). Production and excretion of urine vital in the maintenance of homeostasis: fluid and electrolyte balance, acid–base balance and the excretion of waste. Kidneys also stimulate haemopoietic bone marrow, control blood pressure and metabolize vitamin D.

Movement and stability

Locomotor system (bones, connective tissue, joints and skeletal muscles). Support, stability, movement, protection of organs, storage of minerals and haemopoiesis.

Defence and survival strategies

Integumentary system (skin and appendages). Protection, sensation, waterproofing, temperature regulation, storage, synthesis and excretion.

Immune system (blood cells, bone marrow, thymus gland, lymphoid tissues). Protects against infection, parasites and malignancy: inflammatory response, phagocytosis, immune response (humoral immunity and cell mediated immunity).

Ensuring continuity

Reproductive systems (male: testes, scrotum, duct system, glands and penis; female: ovaries, uterine tubes, uterus, vagina, vulva and breasts). Production of gametes, fertilization, nurture of developing embryo/fetus, parturition and lactation.

Anatomical Terminology

Anatomy is the study of body structures. A set of standard terms, accepted everywhere, is used to describe the position of body structures and their geographical relationships with each other. This ensures that the result will be both concise and understood.

The anatomical position and regional terms

The anatomical position of the body is used as a reference point when studying or describing the position of body structures. The person stands erect, faces forward, with arms at his/her side with palms uppermost (*Figure 1.35*). Each region of the body can be described using a specific term and many of these regional terms are illustrated in *Figure 1.35*.

Body planes

Body structures can be described in relation to three planes (imaginary lines) – median (midsagittal), coronal and transverse – which run through the body (*Figure 1.36*).

Directional terms

Directional terms are used to describe the position of structures relative to each other, e.g. the medial semilunar cartilage, which is often damaged while playing soccer, is on the inner side of the knee joint. The use of terms that have such a precise meaning can avoid mistakes because everyone is 'speaking the same language'.

- Superior – above.
- Inferior – below.
- Anterior (ventral) – in front.
- Posterior (dorsal) – at the back.

When describing the hands, the terms palmar and dorsal are used, with plantar and dorsal for the feet.

- Afferent – towards, e.g. sensory nerves going to the brain.
- Efferent – away from, e.g. motor nerves leaving the brain.
- Peripheral – at the edges of the body, e.g. fingers and toes.
- Lateral – away from the median line (middle), on the outer side.
- Medial – towards the median line, on the inner side.
- Distal – furthest away from a given point.

- Proximal – nearest the given point.
- Internal – towards the centre/inside of a cavity.
- External – towards the outside of a cavity.

- Deep – away from the surface of the body, e.g. deep veins.
- Superficial – near or on the surface of the body, e.g. superficial veins.

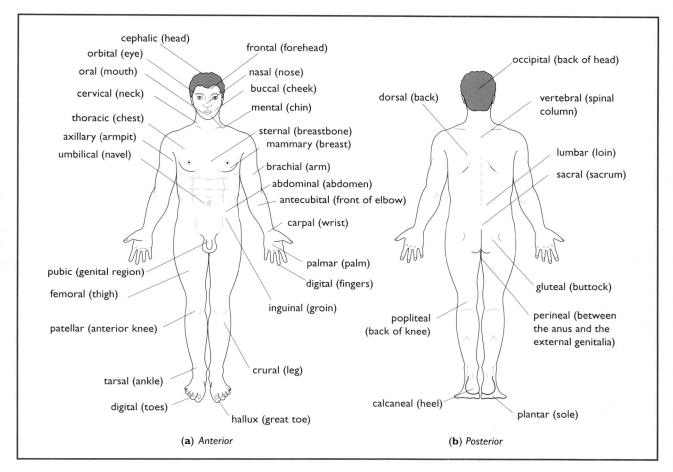

(a) Anterior

(b) Posterior

Figure 1.35 The anatomical position and regional terms.

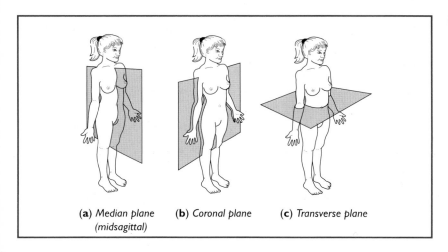

(a) Median plane (midsagittal)

(b) Coronal plane

(c) Transverse plane

Figure 1.36 Body planes.

Summary/Check List
••

Basic biochemistry – organic molecules (proteins, carbohydrates, lipids, ATP), chemical reactions.
Cell structure – cytoplasm, plasma membrane, organelles, cytoskeleton, motile structures, nucleus and related structures.
Transport across membranes – osmosis, diffusion, filtration, active transport, endocytosis, exocytosis.
Cell division – mitosis, meiosis, cell cycle (interphase, DNA replication, stages of mitosis and cytokinesis).
Protein synthesis and nucleic acids – nucleic acids (DNA and RNA), protein synthesis (transcription and translation).
Cell development – cell differentiation, cell ageing, Healthier living – free radicals and antioxidants. Cellular activity – communication and control. Nursing practice application –

ways in which drugs alter cell function. Abnormalities of cell growth. Tumours – benign, malignant, formation and defence. Special focus – cancer. Extracellular matrix.
Tissues – tissue origin (endoderm, ectoderm, mesoderm). Classification: epithelium (simple, stratified), glands (endocrine, exocrine); connective (loose, dense, cartilage, bone, blood); membranes; nervous (neurones, neuroglia); muscle (striated, smooth, cardiac). Tissue repair (regeneration, replacement, fibrosis).
Organs – hollow and compact.
Body cavities – cranium, thorax, abdomen, pelvis. Overview of functional systems.
Anatomical terminology – position, regional terms, planes, directional terms.

••

Self Test
••

1 What chemical features characterize an organic molecule, and why is it possible to have such a great variety of organic molecules?

2 Complete the following statements:
(a) Proteins are formed from 'building blocks' called
   _ _ _ _ _ _ _ _ _.
(b) The precise folded structure of proteins ensures that their _ _ _ _ _ _ _ _ _ _ _ are available for substrate binding.
(c) A protein may be _ _ _ _ _ _ _ _ _ by extremes of temperature or pH.
(d) Enzymes act as _ _ _ _ _ _ _ _ _ _ _ _ _ _ _ _ _ _ _.

3 Give one example of each of the following: a monosaccharide sugar, a disaccharide sugar and a polysaccharide.

4 Outline the diverse roles that lipids perform in the body.

5 What are the components of a triglyceride (triacylglycerol)?

6 How does ATP act as the 'energy currency' of the body?

7 Discuss the factors which influence the rate at which a chemical reaction proceeds.

8 The fundamental structural unit of the body is:
(a) an organelle
(b) an organ
(c) a cell
(d) a tissue.

9 Which of the following statements are true?
(a) The simple diffusion of substances across the plasma membrane is an active process.
(b) Osmosis is concerned with the movement of water across a selectively permeable membrane.
(c) Cells such as leucocytes are able to engulf (by phagocytosis) and destroy bacteria.
(d) Active transport processes using carrier molecules are able to move substances against a concentration gradient.

10 Which of the following is the correct sequence of events when somatic cells divide?
(a) Interphase, mitosis, DNA replication and cytokinesis.
(b) DNA replication, mitosis, interphase and cytokinesis.
(c) Interphase and DNA replication, mitosis and cytokinesis.
(d) Mitosis, interphase, DNA replication and cytokinesis.

11 Describe four ways in which DNA and RNA differ.

12 Explain the term 'differentiation'.

13 Which of the following statements about cancer are true?
(a) Malignant tumours often spread in the body through blood or lymph.
(b) Cancers cause about 40% of deaths in the UK.
(c) Infective agents are linked with some cancers.
(d) Prevention of cancer includes modifying diet and stopping smoking.

14 A relative asks why the damage after a stroke is permanent. What would you say?
15 Name the four basic tissues of the body. Give one example of each type.
16 Put the following directional terms in their correct pairs:
    (a) distal

    (b) afferent
    (c) lateral
    (d) superior
    (e) efferent
    (f) medial
    (g) inferior
    (h) proximal.

Answers

1   They contain carbon and hydrogen in their structure. The variety of organic molecules is possible because carbon is able to bond with four other atoms in several structural arrangements.
2   (a) amino acids;
    (b) active sites;
    (c) denatured;
    (d) biological catalysts.
3   See page 7.
4   See *Table 1.4*.
5   A glycerol molecule and three fatty acids.
6   See page 11.

7   Concentration of reactants, temperature and the presence of enzymes.
8   c.
9   b, c and d.
10 c.
11 See *Table 1.5*.
12 See page 24.
13 a, c and d.
14 See page 34.
15 Epithelium (squamous), connective (adipose), nervous (neurones) and muscle (striated).
16 a–h, b–e, c–f and d–g.

References

Buglass E (1995) Links between alcohol misuse and cancers of the head and neck. *Prof Nurs* **10**:(12)789–790.

Department of Health (DoH) (1993) *The Health of the Nation. Key Area Handbook. Cancers.* London: HMSO.

Department of Health (DoH). (1994) *Nutritional Aspects of Cardiovascular Disease.* Report on Health and Social Subjects, no. 46. Report of the Cardiovascular Review Group Committee on Medical Aspects of Food Policy. London: HMSO.

Health Education Authority (HEA) (1993) *Cancer: How to Reduce Your Risks.* London: Health Education Authority.

Kelly J (1994) Making sense of free radicals and their effects on the body. *Nurs Times* **90**:(18)34–36.

Ministry of Agriculture, Fisheries and Food (MAFF) (1995) *Manual of Nutrition*, 10th edn. London: HMSO.

Rang HP, Dale MM, Ritter JM (1995) *Pharmacology*, 3rd edn. Edinburgh: Churchill Livingstone.

Singer SJ, Nicolson GL (1972) The fluid mosaic model of the structure of cell membranes. *Science* **175**:720–731.

The United Kingdom Central Council for Nursing, Midwifery and Health Visiting (UKCC). (1992a) *Code of Professional Conduct for the Nurse, Midwife and Health Visitor*, 3rd edn. London: UKCC.

The United Kingdom Central Council for Nursing, Midwifery and Health Visiting (UKCC). (1992b) *Standards for the Administration of Medicines.* London: UKCC.

Further Reading

Alberts B, Bray D, Lewis J, Raff M, Roberts K, Watson JD (1988) *Molecular Biology of The Cell*, 2nd edn. New York: Garland Publishing.

Burkitt HG, Young B, Heath JW (1993) *Wheater's Functional Histology*, 3rd edn. Edinburgh: Churchill Livingstone.

National Heart Forum (1997) *At Least Five a Day: Strategies to Increase Vegetable and Fruit Consumption.* London: Stationery Office

Otto SE (1994) *Oncology Nursing*, 2nd edn. London: Mosby.

Rose S, Sanderson C. (1979) *The Chemistry of Life*, 2nd edn. Harmondsworth: Penguin Books.

Stryer L (1995) *Biochemistry*, 4th edn. New York: Freeman & Company.

Ward U (1995) Biological therapy in the treatment of cancer. *Br J Nurs* **4** (15):869–872, 889–891.

Watson JD, Crick FHC (1953) Molecular structure of nucleic acid. A structure for deoxyribose nucleic acid. *Nature* **171**:737–738.

The Internal Environment – Basic Concepts and Homeostasis

Overview

- *Homeostasis.*
- *Basic chemical concepts.*
- *Maintaining the internal environment.*
- *Fluid compartments, body fluids, electrolytes.*
- *Problems with water and electrolyte homeostasis, fluid replacement.*
- *Hydrogen ion concentration (pH) – control mechanisms, acid–base imbalance.*

Learning Outcomes

After studying Chapter 2 you should be able to:

- Define homeostasis.
- Describe negative and positive feedback control mechanisms.
- Discuss the general effects if homeostasis fails.
- Discuss basic chemical concepts: atom, element, molecule, compounds, ions and bonds.
- Discuss the importance of diffusion, osmosis and filtration in maintaining the internal environment.
- Describe the fluid compartments and body fluids.
- List the important electrolytes and their functions in the body.
- Outline the effects of electrolyte imbalance.
- Describe briefly how water balance is maintained.
- State how dehydration and fluid volume deficit might occur and describe their effects. Identify groups at particular risk and describe how fluid balance can be restored.
- Describe the concept of pH and its regulation.
- Outline the effects of a failure in acid–base homeostasis.

Key Words

Acid – a substance that combines with alkalis (bases) to form salts. It contains more hydrogen ions than hydroxyl ions, e.g. hydrochloric acid. Acids are hydrogen ion (proton) donors.

Alkali (base) – a substance that combines with acids to form salts. Contains more hydroxyl ions than hydrogen ions, e.g. sodium hydrogen carbonate (bicarbonate). Alkalis are hydrogen ion (proton) acceptors.

Atom – the smallest stable part of an element that can exist and display the properties of that element.

Autoregulation – 'self-regulation' by mechanisms occurring within the body. Usually applied to local changes to blood flow, or to other physical or chemical features that maintain

optimum conditions within an organ when internal or external environments change.

Base – see alkali.

Buffers – chemicals that limit changes in pH by donating or accepting hydrogen ions.

Electrolytes – ionic compounds that dissociate in water to form charged particles or ions. Able to conduct electricity.

Element – one of the unique substances (matter) that comprise all living and non-living things, e.g. oxygen, potassium, carbon.

Extracellular fluid – body fluid found outside the cells, e.g. blood, interstitial fluid.

Key Words cont.

Homeostasis – the maintenance of a stable but dynamic (within set parameters), physiological state by the autoregulatory processes of the body, e.g. temperature.
Inorganic compounds – compounds that generally contain no carbon or hydrogen in their chemical structure, e.g. sodium chloride.
Interstitial fluid (tissue fluid) – fluid surrounding the cells. Part of the extracellular fluid, it forms the fluid part of the extracellular matrix.
Intracellular fluid – fluid contained within the cell cytosol. Most body fluid is within the cells.
Ion – an atom with an electrical charge. There are two groups: cations, which have a positive charge, and anions, with a negative charge.

Molecule – two or more atoms joined together by chemical bonds, e.g. water.
Nonpolar – molecules with electrical balance, e.g. carbon dioxide.
Organic molecules – chemicals which contain carbon and hydrogen in their chemical structure, e.g. glucose. The large biological molecules found in 'living' systems are organic, e.g. proteins and carbohydrates.
Polar – molecules without electrical balance, e.g. water.
Solute – a substance that is dissolved in a solvent.
Solution – a liquid (solvent) containing a solid (solute) which has been dissolved in it.
Solvent – a liquid able to dissolve another substance.

Introduction

The chemical and physical internal environment of the body is determined by: the water content and its distribution within the fluid compartments (**intracellular** and **extracellular**), **electrolyte** levels, temperature, available nutrients, levels of waste and the pH of body fluids.

All cellular chemical reactions are dependent on the maintenance of these properties within a limited range. To this end, mechanisms operate in all body systems to maintain an optimum internal environment, thus ensuring that the complex interrelated functions of metabolism (all the biochemical processes occurring in the body) continue to occur. These mechanisms include:

- Oxygen (O_2) is taken in by the lungs and used to produce energy from fuel **molecules.**
- Nutrients and water are absorbed by the gastrointestinal tract as required.
- Waste carbon dioxide (CO_2) is excreted by the lungs. Retention of CO_2 affects blood pH.
- Hydrogen carbonates (bicarbonates), phosphates and proteins, which, acting as **buffers**, keep plasma pH within narrow limits. Buffers are chemicals which limit pH (acidity/alkalinity) changes (see pages 60, 61).
- The kidneys help to regulate water balance, pH and electrolyte levels by their ability to produce urine of variable composition in line with bodily needs.
- The skin is able to regulate temperature in several ways, e.g. by sweat glands. The amount of water lost through the skin helps to maintain water balance.

Homeostasis

Homeostasis is the maintenance of a stable but dynamic physiological state by **autoregulation** initiated from within the organism – a balance or equilibrium within set parameters. For example, the normal core body temperature is 36–37.6°C (at rest) and the temperature regulating mechanisms of the body are designed to keep it within this narrow range. Sometimes the mechanisms fail to maintain temperature homeostasis; for example, the heat regulating centre in the brain could be damaged by severe head injury, resulting in a dangerously high body temperature. Sometimes, however, an elevated temperature is adaptive, rather than loss of homeostasis – such as during infection, when higher temperatures help to destroy invading microorganisms and enhance healing (see Chapter 19).

While stressing that autoregulatory mechanisms work to maintain conditions within a normal range, it is worth mentioning that sometimes it is in your best interests to be able to exceed the normal value for a particular variable – if conditions change drastically, e.g. intense exercise, then the upper limit for 'everyday' situations can be reset. For example, when you run for a bus it is necessary for heart rate and blood pressure to increase so as to provide the muscles with enough oxygen-rich blood for contraction as you sprint for the last bus home.

For individual cells homeostasis provides a constant internal environment in which to function. For the person it means optimal functioning of all body systems, which is a good basis for health. The breakdown of homeostasis results in imbalance and possibly disease.

Homeostatic control mechanisms

A basic homeostatic mechanism has three components - (*Figure 2.1*): a receptor (usually nervous tissue), a control area and an effector. Communication between these three is neural by nerves (see Chapter 3) or by hormones released from endocrine structures (see Chapter 8).

The receptor samples the internal environment for changes and sends details to the control area. The control area determines the normal value for a particular chemical or physical variable; it interprets information received and then initiates a suitable response. The last part involves the effector structures, e.g. gland, muscle or blood vessel, which operate to either reverse the change (negative feedback control) or more unusually increase changes (positive feedback control).

Negative feedback controls

The majority of homeostatic mechanisms act by negative feedback, where the product of the process being monitored causes the process to slow or stop. In this way the specific variable being controlled returns to normal levels. This return to normal occurs from both low and high levels, e.g. low or high blood glucose returns to the normal level.

Physiological processes regulated by negative feedback operating through receptors, control areas and effectors include temperature control, rate and depth of respiration, water and electrolyte balance, and blood glucose (see *Figure 2.2*). As an example let us consider the three components involved in temperature control:

Receptors: thermoreceptors in the skin and body core, e.g. brain (hypothalamus), monitor temperature changes at the skin surface and in blood passing through the hypothalamus.

Control area: the thermoregulation centre (hypothalamic) receives this information via nerves and initiates responses that will return the temperature to normal.

Effectors: if body temperature is too low (e.g. when you get cold standing outside in winter), various structures in the skin (sweat glands, blood vessels) and skeletal muscles take measures to conserve or produce heat. Sweating ceases, blood vessels constrict (vasoconstriction) and muscles contract and relax to produce shivering. If temperature rises above normal (e.g. following vigorous exercise such as a game of squash) the measures taken to cause heat loss are sweat production and dilation of blood vessels (vasodilation). The negative feedback controls ensure that core body temperature returns to normal and homeostasis is maintained.

Positive feedback controls

Some (but very few) homeostatic mechanisms work through

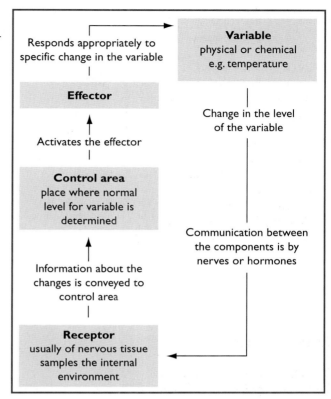

Figure 2.1 Homeostatic control – receptor, control area and effector.

positive feedback. Here an increase in the level of product from the process being monitored causes the process to be stimulated and the variable to move still further from the normal value (see *Figure 2.2*). These mechanisms usually involve reactions that occur infrequently, e.g. normal blood clotting (see Chapter 9) and the events of childbirth (see Chapter 20) – they are not everyday events that require constant regulation. Once these events start they accelerate and increase in intensity – as a giant snowball rolling down hill gets bigger and moves even faster.

A brief look at parturition (childbirth) can be used to illustrate a positive feedback control in a healthy individual. The events of labour are stimulated as the baby moves down the birth canal to exert pressure on the cervix. The pressure receptors in the cervix transmit impulses that cause hormone (oxytocin) release from the pituitary gland which in turn increases the rate and intensity of uterine muscle contractions. The increased contractions of the uterus push the baby down still further to exert more pressure on the cervix, which gradually dilates. Eventually the baby is born and the positive feedback causing the intense muscular contraction ceases. The positive feedback control of childbirth is a good example of both neural and hormonal communication between receptor, control centre and effector.

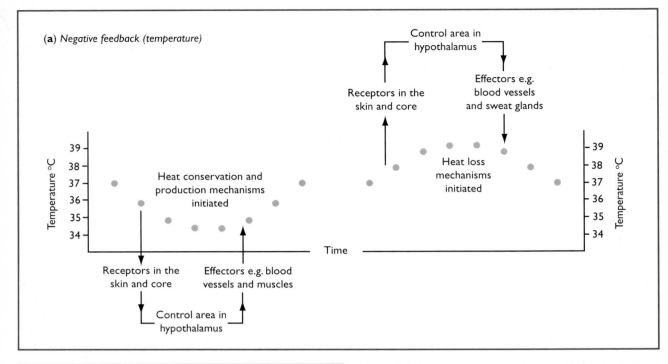

(a) *Negative feedback (temperature)*

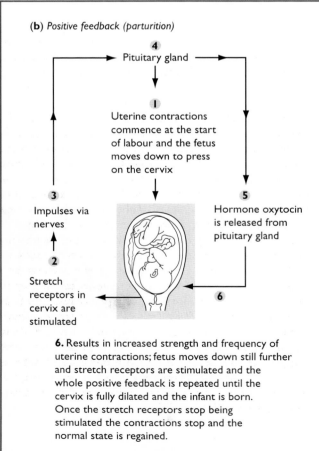

(b) *Positive feedback (parturition)*

4 Pituitary gland

1 Uterine contractions commence at the start of labour and the fetus moves down to press on the cervix

3 Impulses via nerves

5 Hormone oxytocin is released from pituitary gland

2

Stretch receptors in cervix are stimulated

6

6. Results in increased strength and frequency of uterine contractions; fetus moves down still further and stretch receptors are stimulated and the whole positive feedback is repeated until the cervix is fully dilated and the infant is born. Once the stretch receptors stop being stimulated the contractions stop and the normal state is regained.

Figure 2.2 Homeostatic control mechanisms. **(a)** Negative feedback (temperature); **(b)** positive feedback (parturition).

Abnormal Function **Problems with homeostasis**

Any imbalance in homeostasis will have implications for the individual's ability to function normally. For example, newborns have immature heat-regulating mechanisms which with other factors can mean that some babies have difficulty maintaining a normal temperature. At the other end of life, when cells and regulatory mechanisms are less efficient, there will be problems with homeostasis. Again this is illustrated by lack of temperature control. In older adults the thermoregulatory mechanisms cope less well with extremes of temperature (Herbert, 1986); this may result in hypothermia (temperature below normal; see Chapter 19).

Most health deficiencies are linked to a breakdown in negative feedback controls; for example, the loss of high carbon dioxide levels as a trigger for respiration in people with chronic lung disease causes carbon dioxide retention and problems with oxygenation. This and other problems caused by homeostatic imbalances as damaging positive feedback mechanisms spiral out of control, e.g. in shock (see Chapter 10) small blood vessels become permeable and fluid leaks from the blood to increase the degree of shock, are outlined with their practice implications in later chapters.

Basic Chemistry

It is appropriate here to explain some basic chemistry. You will find this helpful in understanding body processes and many practice applications. Only very basic facts have been included; these can form an introduction if science has not been studied before or as a revision of previous knowledge. You will find coverage of some **organic molecules** – proteins, carbohydrates, lipids and adenosine triphosphate in Chapter 1, where it is easier to appreciate their importance as cellular components and in the chemical reactions occurring in cells.

The composition of matter

All matter is made from substances known as **elements** (see *Table 2.1*). There are 92 elements that occur naturally, e.g. carbon, hydrogen, oxygen and iron. Individual elements consist of tiny particles called **atoms** which display the chemical and physical properties of that element.

Elements are identified by their chemical symbol, which is a shorthand code using one or two letters, e.g. hydrogen is H (its first letter) and sodium is Na, derived from the Latin name *natrium*.

Atoms

Atoms consist of smaller subatomic particles: protons (positive charge), neutrons (no charge) and electrons (negative charge). The protons and neutrons cluster together to form the nucleus around which the electrons orbit (just as some satellites orbit the Earth) (see *Figure 2.3*). The planetary model of atomic structure which we shall use describes electrons following fixed orbits within rings around the nucleus. A more recent orbital model, however, describes electron clouds moving without fixed orbits within electron shells (spaces) around the nucleus.

Atoms have equal numbers of positive protons and negative electrons, which means that overall the atom is neutral. Each element has a different number of subatomic particles within its atoms. This gives each element its unique properties: atomic number, mass number and atomic weight.

The atomic number

The atomic number is the number of protons within the nucleus, or the number of electrons in orbit; for example, hydrogen, with one of each, has the atomic number 1.

The mass number

The total mass of the protons and neutrons is the mass number. The electrons, which have an extremely small mass, are not significant within an atom. Rather confusingly, most elements have variable mass atoms (different number of neutrons) known as isotopes; these have the same atomic number but a different mass number, e.g. hydrogen atoms exist in three forms (hydrogen, deuterium and tritium).

Some elements produce 'heavy' isotopes which are unstable and radioactive. These are known as radioisotopes. They consist of unstable matter which emits radiation as the nucleus disintegrates. The radiation may be of several types – e.g. alpha (α), beta (β), gamma (γ). Each radioisotope has a half-life (the time taken for a radioactive isotope to decay to half its original activity). Radium has a long half-life of 1690 years, but others are much shorter, e.g. radioactive iodine at 8 days. Radioisotopes are widely used in diagnostic tests, e.g. certain scans, and in radiotherapy, where the radiation is used to treat cancers and some other conditions (see Chapter 1).

Table 2.1 Elements of physiological importance		
Element	**Symbol**	**Importance in the body**
Calcium	Ca	Forms structure of bone and teeth. Nerve impulse transmission, muscle contraction, and blood coagulation
Carbon	C	Present in all organic compounds, e.g. proteins, carbohydrates, lipids (fats)
Chlorine	Cl	As chloride an important negative ion (anion) in the extracellular fluid, maintenance of fluid compartments
Hydrogen	H	Concerned with body pH and as a constituent of organic compounds
Iodine	I	Required for the hormones of the thyroid gland
Iron	Fe	Constituent of haemoglobin, the oxygen-carrying pigment in the erythrocytes, and myoglobin in muscle
Magnesium	Mg	Found in bones and as a cofactor in many body reactions
Nitrogen	N	Constituent of proteins and nucleic acids
Oxygen	O	A constituent of many organic and inorganic compounds; needed for energy production
Phosphorus	P	As phosphates found in bone, teeth and nucleic acids
Potassium	K	An important positive ion (cation) found mostly in the intracellular fluid; required for nerve and muscle function. Maintenance of fluid compartments
Sodium	Na	An important positive ion (cation) found mostly in the extracellular fluid; required for nerve and muscle function. Maintenance of fluid compartments
Sulphur	S	A constituent of proteins

In addition to these, the body needs other elements in extremely small amounts. These are known as trace elements and include:

Chromium Cr	Fluorine F	Selenium Se
Cobalt Co	Manganese Mn	Silicon Si
Copper Cu	Molybdenum Mo	Zinc Zn

Table 2.1 Elements of physiological importance.

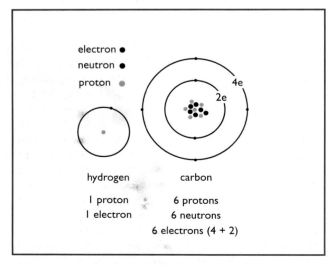

Figure 2.3 Atomic structure (diagrammatic – planetary model).

Atomic weight or mass

The atomic weight or mass is the weight (mass number) of an average atom of a particular element; it takes account of the different isotopes of that element. Hydrogen has an atomic weight of 1.008 (the average of its three isotopes), but for our purposes it is taken to be 1. The relative unit of weight used for measuring atoms and subatomic particles is the Dalton or atomic mass unit (amu). The weight of a neutron and a proton have each been designated as being 1 amu. An example to illustrate this is sodium, which with its 12 neutrons and 11 protons has a mass number of 23 and hence an atomic weight of 23. The weight of other elements can be compared with that of hydrogen, e.g. oxygen, with an atomic weight of 16, is 16 times heavier than hydrogen.

Combinations: molecules and compounds

In general, atoms cannot exist separately – they combine with other atoms. A molecule is formed when two or more atoms are chemically bonded together. These atoms may be from the same element, e.g. two atoms of oxygen form one molecule of the element oxygen (O_2). When atoms from different elements combine they form molecules of a compound, e.g. two atoms of hydrogen combine with one atom of oxygen to form one molecule of the compound water (H_2O).

A compound is a pure substance of which a molecule is the smallest unit that displays its individual properties. It is formed from the atoms of two or more elements, but has different characteristics from its constituent atoms, e.g. a molecule of the compound sodium chloride is formed from atoms of sodium and chlorine.

Compounds are formed by atoms with an outer shell (see page 47) electron number that makes them unstable (reactive), i.e. not full. Atoms without a full outer shell will become more stable by filling the shell. Conversely, when the outer electron shell is full or contains eight electrons the atom is very stable. These substances are described as being inert or unreactive, e.g. the gases helium, neon, argon, krypton and xenon.

Molecular weight

The molecular weight of a substance is the total atomic weights of its elements:

Water (H_2O)	
2 hydrogen (atomic weight 1) $2 \times 1 =$	2
1 oxygen (atomic weight 16) $16 \times 1 =$	16
molecular weight of water =	18
Glucose ($C_6H_{12}O_6$)	
6 carbon (atomic weight 12) $6 \times 12 =$	72
12 hydrogen (atomic weight 1) $12 \times 1 =$	12
6 oxygen (atomic weight 16) $6 \times 16 =$	96
molecular weight of glucose =	180

Molar concentration of solutions (molarity)

Molarity is very important and is used when expressing the concentration of substances in body fluids, e.g. glucose levels in the blood.

The unit of measure is the mole (mol), which is the atomic weight or molecular weight in grams (g) of a substance, e.g. 1 mol of glucose = 180 g of glucose. One mole of any substance will contain the same number of atoms or molecules: 6.02×10^{23} (known as Avogadro's number). This means that the numbers of particles in a solution is always known. The molar concentration of a **solution** (molarity) is measured by the number of moles of a substance present in 1 litre of the solution. It is part of the Systeme Internationale (SI) (see Appendix A: International System of Units), a system of measurement used for medical, scientific and technical purposes internationally.

A molar solution is one in which 1 mol of the substance is dissolved in enough **solvent** (a liquid which is able to dissolve another substance, usually water in the body) to produce 1 litre of solution. Chemical substances are usually in very low concentration in the body and for this reason we divide moles by 1000 to obtain the millimole (mmol). This is a much more appropriate unit when expressing the concentration of substances in the body fluids, e.g. serum calcium is 2.1–2.6 mmol/l. If an even smaller unit of measurement is needed, the millimole can be divided by 1000 to give the micromole (μmol). The SI system of measurement can be applied to any substance of known molecular weight (electrolytes and non-electrolytes), and it has replaced the milliequivalent for physiological purposes.

Chemical bonds

Earlier we considered the combination of two or more atoms to form molecules and compounds. Obviously some kind of bond must hold them together. This bond is formed by the energy reaction between the outer or valence shell electrons of the individual atoms as they seek to achieve stability. Chemical bonds can be of three types: ionic, covalent (**polar** or **nonpolar**) and hydrogen bonds.

Ionic bonds

One way in which atoms can bond together is through ionic bonds. The reactive electrons in the outer shells move between the reacting atoms. This results in one atom shedding one or more electrons (electron donor) and becoming a positively charged particle or **ion** (cation), and the other atom gaining one or more electrons (electron acceptor) and becoming a negatively charged ion (anion). The attraction between the charged ions holds the two ions together to form an ionic bond. A good example of an ionic bond is the formation of sodium chloride (NaCl): sodium atoms give up electrons to become the positive cation (Na^+) and chlorine atoms receive electrons to form the negative anion (Cl^-) (see *Figure 2.4*). Again this illustrates an attempt by atoms to fill their outer electron shells. When water is not present these compounds usually form crystals, e.g. common salt (sodium chloride). Many ionic compounds belong to the group of chemicals called salts, formed when an **acid** (substance which contains more hydrogen ions than hydroxyl ions, and therefore donates hydrogen ions) and an **alkali** (or **base**; substance which contains more

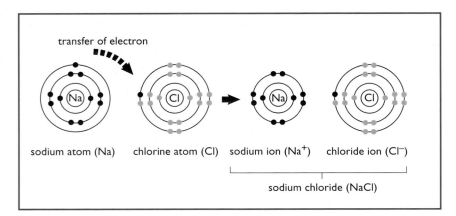

Figure 2.4 Ionic bond.

sodium atom (Na)   chlorine atom (Cl)   sodium ion (Na⁺)   chloride ion (Cl⁻)

sodium chloride (NaCl)

Figure 2.5 Covalent bonds (a) Single; (b) double; (c) triple.

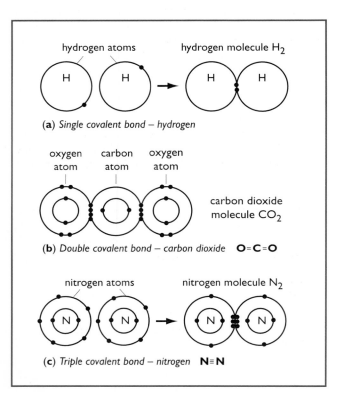

hydrogen atoms   hydrogen molecule H_2

(a) *Single covalent bond – hydrogen*

oxygen   carbon   oxygen
atom   atom   atom

carbon dioxide molecule CO_2

(b) *Double covalent bond – carbon dioxide*   **O=C=O**

nitrogen atoms   nitrogen molecule N_2

(c) *Triple covalent bond – nitrogen*   **N≡N**

hydroxyl ions than hydrogen ions, and therefore accepts hydrogen ions) combine, e.g. hydrochloric acid (HCl) and sodium hydroxide (NaOH).

acid + alkali = salt + water

$HCl + NaOH = NaCl + H_2O$

$\dfrac{\text{hydrochloric}}{\text{acid}} + \dfrac{\text{sodium}}{\text{hydroxide}} = \dfrac{\text{sodium} +}{\text{chloride}}$ water

Proteins, acids and bases are also ionic substances. When ionic compounds dissolve in water they dissociate or ionize into their ions, in which form they are known as electrolytes. The many electrolytes within the body are considered later in this chapter and in other chapters where appropriate.

Covalent bonds

In a covalent bond, the electrons are shared between the atoms, rather than the loss and gain situation of ionic bonds (*Figure 2.5*). In this way atoms can achieve partial stability. Covalent bonds may be single where the atoms share an electron pair, such as in the formation of a molecule of hydrogen (H_2) or methane (CH_4), in which one carbon atom (with four electrons in the outer shell) shares four electron pairs with four atoms of hydrogen (with one electron each). The ability of carbon to form single covalent bonds with hydrogen and other atoms such as nitrogen and oxygen is important in the formation of organic macromolecules required by the body (see Chapter 1). Other covalent bonds may be double, where two pairs of electrons are shared between two atoms, e.g. when carbon bonds with two atoms of oxygen to form carbon dioxide (CO_2), or triple, where three pairs of electrons are shared, e.g. a molecule of nitrogen (N_2).

Where the electrons are shared equally, as in the molecules already discussed, the substances are electrically balanced and are described as being nonpolar, e.g. carbon dioxide. If some atoms are 'greedier' than others and electrons are not shared equally the substance formed is electrically unbalanced (e.g. water) and is said to be polar. This property of some molecules to be polar or nonpolar, you will remember, is vital to the structure of biological membrane bilayers (see Chapter 1).

Hydrogen bond
A hydrogen bond is a weak bond found between polar water molecules and in certain complex biological molecules, such as proteins and nucleic acids (e.g. DNA; see

Figure 1.13). The hydrogen atoms involved in the bond are already bonded covalently to other atoms, e.g. oxygen or nitrogen. Hydrogen bonds help to maintain the three-dimensional structure vital to the functioning of biological molecules such as enzymes.

Maintaining the Internal Environment – Diffusion, Osmosis and Filtration

A further account of diffusion, osmosis and filtration is now appropriate, although they were discussed in Chapter 1 in terms of transport across plasma membranes. This further coverage will serve to illustrate the role of these three processes in maintaining fluid compartments and the concentration of substances within body fluids.

Diffusion
Diffusion involves the movement of substances from an area of high concentration to an area of lower concentration, i.e. down a concentration gradient. An everyday example of diffusion would be an air freshener: when used

Table 2.2 Chemical bonds – a comparison

Type of chemical bond	Distribution of electrical charge	Examples
Ionic – no electron sharing; there is complete electron transfer	Positively and negatively charged ions (cations and anions) exist separately	Sodium chloride Na^+ Cl^-
Covalent (a) nonpolar – electrons are shared equally	Electrical charge is balanced (even distribution) between the atoms	Methane 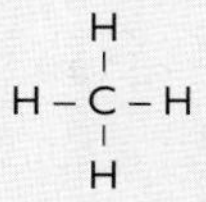 / Carbon dioxide O=C=O / H–C–H
(b) polar – electrons are shared unequally	One end of the molecule is slightly negative compared with the other end which is slightly positive	Water 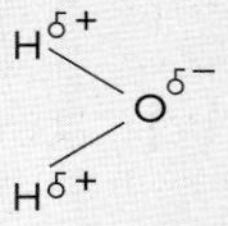
Hydrogen – the bond is formed by the weak attraction between the negatively and positively charged ends of polar molecules	Electrical charge is distributed in polar molecules by virtue of its polar covalent bonds	Two molecules of water 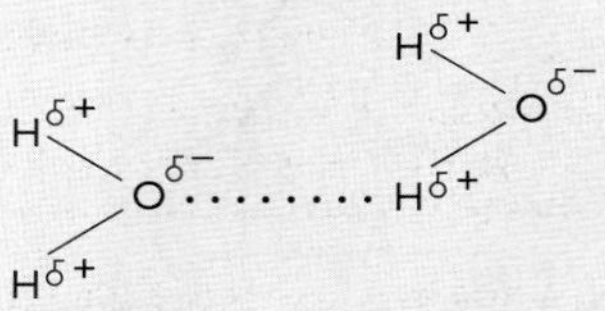

Table 2.2 Chemical bonds – a comparison.

in one part of a room it takes some time for you to smell the spray in another part of the room as the spray molecules need to diffuse through the air. In the body the movement of substances takes place either across a selectively permeable plasma membrane, which allows certain particles to pass through but holds back other larger particles, or down a concentration gradient within cells (*Figure 2.6*). Diffusion is passive and does not use energy (ATP). The kinetic energy which powers diffusion is produced by the constant collision of molecules as they move randomly in solution. In a closed system the end result of diffusion would be the concentration on both sides of the membrane being equal, i.e. in equilibrium.

For the body, diffusion is important in the movement of oxygen, carbon dioxide, fats, some hormones, electrolytes such as sodium, and the waste product urea. Particles pass through the membrane by either dissolving in the lipid part of the bilayer or using protein channel pores. Nonpolar substances such as carbon dioxide diffuse through the lipid part of the plasma membrane, but small polar substances and ions such as sodium use specific protein channels (sodium ions can only use a sodium channel). Some channel pores are permanently open, but others are operated by specific signalling chemicals known as ligands (see Chapter 1) or by electrical changes.

A more complex type of diffusion, known as facilitated diffusion, makes use of highly selective protein carrier molecules situated in the membrane. Facilitated diffusion is used by large, lipid-insoluble molecules such as glucose (which cannot dissolve in lipids or utilize protein channels), which uses such a carrier molecule to gain rapid entry into cells.

Osmosis

For physiological purposes the process of osmosis is the movement (diffusion) of water, which you will remember is a highly polar molecule, through a selectively permeable membrane. Pores in the membrane allow the movement of water molecules in either direction. Water will move when there is a difference in concentration on either side of the membrane. The direction of movement will be from high water to low water concentration, i.e. the water moves from a weak solution to a stronger, more concentrated solution. Most people will remember the experiment from school: a container of sucrose solution with a selectively permeable membrane at its base is placed in a beaker of water; after a while it becomes obvious that water has moved into the container as a rise in the level of the sucrose solution is observed (*Figure 2.7*).

The force required to oppose the movement of water by osmosis is known as the osmotic pressure; this increases with the concentration difference either side of the membrane. The total concentration of dissolved osmotically significant **solute** particles in a **solution** (the liquid/solvent in which the solute has been dissolved) is termed its osmolarity. Osmolarity is measured in osmoles/litre (osmol/l) or milliosmoles/litre (mosmol/l) of the solution (cf. osmolality, which is osmoles/kilogram of solution). This tells us about a solution's osmotic properties, including osmotic pressure, which depends upon the actual number of particles.

It is important to note that osmolarity and molarity are the same for undissociated non–electrolyte substances, but when substances dissociate into ions each ion has exactly the same osmotic action as an undissociated molecule. A 1-mol solution of sodium chloride which dissociates into sodium and chloride ions will contain 2 osmol.

The movement of water in and out of cells is influenced by the tonicity of the solutions to which they are exposed. Solution tonicity describes its power to alter cell shape, which depends on the osmotic concentration of nonpen-

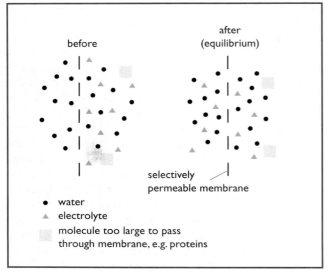

Figure 2.6 Diffusion in the body.

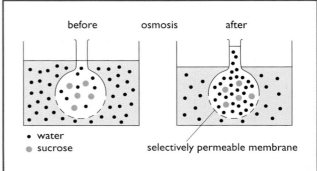

Figure 2.7 Osmosis.

etrating solutes, e.g. proteins (remember osmolarity is total solute concentration), in the solution compared with that of body fluids. Tonicity is implicated in the mechanisms involved in fluid and electrolyte imbalances and their management with fluid and electrolyte replacement (see pages 56–59). A solution with the same concentration as body fluids is called isotonic; cells placed in this solution show no water movement. A higher concentration solution is hypertonic (*Figure 2.8*); cells placed in it shrink (crenate) as water leaves the cells. A solution with a lower concentration is hypotonic; here the cells swell and burst as they draw in water from the solution.

Osmosis is vital in maintaining the correct water distribution within the fluid compartments. The movement of water stops when the opposing pressures on either side of the plasma membrane – osmotic and hydrostatic (see below) – are the same.

Filtration

The passive process of filtration provides another means by which the fluid compartments and the concentration of substances within body fluids is maintained; again there is a gradient difference either side of the membrane, but this time it is pressure rather than concentration. The pressure that forces water and small molecules through membrane pores is termed the hydrostatic (fluid) pressure. Fluids and small molecules leave the blood capillaries to supply cells with the raw materials for their metabolic processes in this way. Filtration is also an important process in the formation of urine. The hydrostatic pressure of the blood arriving at the nephron (functional unit of the kidney) causes water and other molecules to pass through into the tubule in the first stage of urine production. The composition of fluid (filtrate) in the kidney tubule is greatly modified by reabsorption and secretion before it becomes urine (see Chapter 15).

To summarize, it can be said that, when functioning properly in an integrated way, the three processes of diffusion, osmosis and filtration ensure that the state of the internal environment is always favourable to cellular processes.

Fluid Compartments and Body Fluids

In healthy young adults, water makes up approximately 50–63% of the body weight (see *Figure 2.9*). Different types of tissue contain different amounts of water; for example, muscle and bone have a higher water content than adipose tissue. Males, with their larger muscle mass, generally have a higher percentage of water than females, who have more adipose tissue. Newborns have a higher proportion of water (70–75%) which decreases to adult values during infancy and early childhood. Another difference with babies is that they have more water in the extracellular compartment; this increases the risk for fluid volume deficit (see pages 57, 58) (Heath, 1995). Obese individuals have a lower percentage of water because of their proportionally higher amount of adipose tissue. The proportion of water decreases in older people as part of normal ageing (45%). With the loss of muscle mass and an increase in adipose tissue, older adults have smaller water reserves, and because fluid homeostasis is less efficient they are at increased risk for dehydration (see pages 57, 58).

This water, with various non-electrolyte solutes, e.g. urea, and electrolytes such as sodium ions, is located within the intracellular and extracellular compartments of the body. In adults most of the water, about two-thirds, is within the cells as **intracellular fluid** (ICF). The remaining third is **extracellular fluid** (ECF). This consists of **interstitial fluid** (tissue fluid), which bathes the cells; plasma (fluid part of blood); and other types of ECF, including lymph, gastrointestinal juices and cerebrospinal fluid surrounding the brain and spinal cord. In health the overall water content of the body changes very little despite differences in fluid intake.

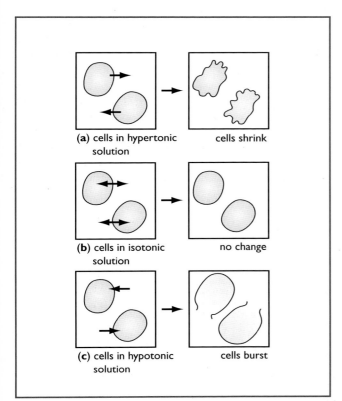

(a) cells in hypertonic solution — cells shrink

(b) cells in isotonic solution — no change

(c) cells in hypotonic solution — cells burst

Figure 2.8 Effects of tonicity on cells.

For example; a young adult male weighing 70 kg (11 stones) will have about 40 litres of water distributed around the fluid compartments, as shown in *Figure 2.10*. This can be summarized as:

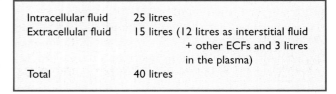

Intracellular fluid	25 litres
Extracellular fluid	15 litres (12 litres as interstitial fluid + other ECFs and 3 litres in the plasma)
Total	40 litres

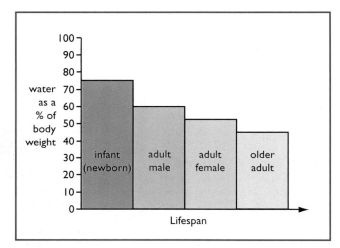

Figure 2.9 Water as a percentage of body weight in an infant (newborn), adult male, adult female and older adult.

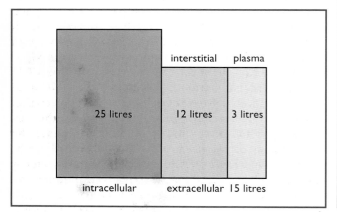

Figure 2.10 Fluid compartments.

Electrolyte composition of fluid compartments

Although we are considering water and electrolytes separately, it is important to stress that these two components of the ECF and ICF are inextricably linked; for example, water always moves after sodium – this means that the overall sodium concentration is maintained because if sodium is lost from the ECF the water content will be automatically adjusted. Each body fluid has its individual electrolyte composition. Some fluids are very different from each other; for example, intracellular and extracellular fluids are quite distinct. Others, such as the two extracellular fluids – interstitial fluid and plasma – exhibit similarities. They do, however, differ in one important respect: the protein content is higher in plasma (important in the production of osmotic pressure).

It is important to note that the positively and negatively charged ions (electrolytes) are balanced within a compartment to give an overall electrical neutrality. Remember, the non-electrolyte solutes do not have an electrical charge because chemical bonds prevent their dissociation in solution.

The electrolyte concentrations of ICF and ECF are set out below (*Figure 2.11*). Major anions and cations are those which predominate and the minor anions and cations are those which are present in small quantities only. This vital balance of electrolytes between the fluid compartments is maintained within the homeostatic range at the cellular level by selectively permeable membranes

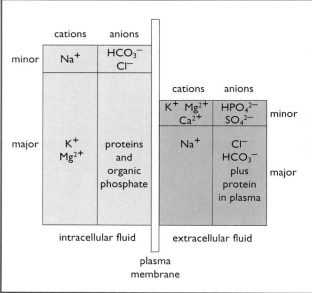

Figure 2.11 Comparison of the electrolyte composition of intracellular fluid (ICF) and extracellular fluid (ECF).

and active transport sodium–potassium pumps, and at the 'whole person' level by mechanisms which ensure that intake and excretion are matched, e.g. hormones such as aldosterone, glucocorticoids and parathyroid hormone, and the complex processes of the kidney (renal).

Intracellular fluid contains:
- Major anions – organic phosphates, proteins.
- Minor anions – hydrogen carbonate, chloride.
- Major cations – potassium, magnesium.
- Minor cations – sodium.

Extracellular fluid contains:
- Major anions – hydrogen carbonate and chloride in interstitial fluid, and these plus protein in plasma.
- Minor anions – hydrogen phosphate, sulphate and organic ions.
- Major cations – sodium.
- Minor cations – potassium, magnesium and calcium.

A common investigation used to assess health status is the measurement of the concentration of various ions in the serum (the fluid part of blood after the sample has clotted); this test monitors the serum electrolytes. The ions measured include: sodium, chloride, potassium, hydrogen carbonate (bicarbonate), calcium, magnesium and phosphates. Reference values for these are provided in *Table 2.3*. The results can give a guide to the functioning of many homeostatic mechanisms, e.g. renal excretion of potassium, which rises rapidly when the kidneys fail.

Table 2.3 Serum electrolytes – normal reference values

Electrolyte	Reference range (serum)	
Sodium (Na^+)	135–145	mmol/litre
Chloride (Cl^-)	95–105	mmol/litre
Potassium (K^+)	3.3–5.0	mmol/litre
Hydrogen carbonate (bicarbonate) (HCO_3^-)	22–28	mmol/litre
Calcium (Ca^{2+})	2.1–2.6	mmol/litre
Magnesium (Mg^{2+})	0.75–1.0	mmol/litre
Phosphate (PO_4^{2-})	0.8–1.4	mmol/litre

* Normal ranges may vary slightly on a local basis.

Table 2.3 Serum electrolytes – normal reference values.

Abnormal Function **Problems with electrolyte balance**

Problems with electrolyte concentrations can occur for many reasons and are often associated with problems of water (see pages 57, 58) and acid–base balance (see page 61). There may be loss of electrolytes such as sodium and water through excess sweating or burns; retention of electrolytes, e.g. potassium, when the kidneys fail; the intake of electrolytes may be excessive, e.g. the prolonged intake of magnesium indigestion medicines; or intake may be insufficient, e.g. magnesium in situations where protein-energy malnutrition exists. The causes and effects of some electrolyte imbalances are covered in *Table 2.4*, but readers requiring more detail are directed to Further Reading (Edwards *et al.*, 1995; Long *et al.*, 1995).

Water balance

Normally, the amount of water in the fluid compartments is determined by the amount: (i) taken in during eating and drinking; (ii) produced during metabolism; and (iii) leaving via the kidneys, skin, gastrointestinal tract and lungs:

IN	OUT
moist food	urine and faeces
fluids	sweat
metabolic processes	water vapour (via the lungs)

This is another example of a complex homeostatic mechanism involving the integration of many functional systems; for example, in hot weather, when sweating is excessive and water and electrolytes are lost through the skin, you pass urine less often – but note that to maintain health the adult kidneys must produce a minimum 500 ml of urine per day to excrete waste solutes. Overall control of this delicate balance is by the nervous and endocrine systems: through osmoreceptors in the hypothalamus which monitor the osmolarity of the ECF; hypothalamic thirst centres which alert you to the need to increase fluid intake when necessary; and the secretion of antidiuretic hormone (ADH), which affects the permeability of the renal tubules to water and hence the amount of water excreted in urine. When blood osmolarity is low, ADH is not released and excess water is excreted as urine. ADH secretion is also inhibited by atrial natriuretic peptides secreted by the heart (see Chapters 8, 10 and 15). As already discussed, the movement of water is intimately tied to that of sodium; together, these are important in maintaining normal blood pressure (see Chapters 10 and 15).

	Table 2.4 Problems with electrolyte balance		
Electrolyte	**Type of imbalance**	**Causes (selected)**	**Effects (selected)**
Sodium Na^+	Hyponatraemia (low sodium in the blood)	Failure to excrete water or excess intake. Sodium loss, e.g. vomiting, diarrhoea, sweating, burns etc. Diuretics. Aldosterone lack. Kidney disease. Excess ADH. Diabetes mellitus.	Cerebral oedema causing neurological problems, e.g. fits, coma. Hypovolaemic shock if present with water loss.
	Hypernatraemia (high sodium in the blood)	Water depletion, e.g. reduced intake in infants or older adults. Excessive sodium intake.	Cellular dehydration causing neurological problems, e.g. behaviour changes, dizziness and confusion. Muscle weakness. Thirst.
Chloride Cl^-	Hypochloraemia (low chlorides in the blood)	Vomiting - loss of hydrochloric acid from stomach. In association with low potassium levels. Prolonged use of alkali indigestion medicines.	Disruption of acid-base balance – metabolic alkalosis (hydrogen carbonate is retained)
	Hyperchloraemia (high chlorides in the blood)	Associated with high potassium levels. Where chlorides are retained or intakes are high.	– metabolic acidosis (hydrogen carbonate is lost) NB The concentrations of chlorides and hydrogen carbonates change relative to one another in order to maintain electrical neutrality.
Potassium K^+	Hypokalaemia (low potassium levels in the blood)	Loss in diarrhoea, vomiting and gastrointestinal drainage. Diuretics. Starvation. Excess loss in the urine, e.g. aldosteronism or Cushing's syndrome.	Muscle weakness. Life threatening cardiac arrhythmias. Alkalosis.
	Hyperkalaemia (high potassium levels in the blood)	Kidney failure. Excess intake in intravenous fluids or food. Tissue damage. Catabolic states. Acidosis. Aldosterone lack.	Muscle weakness. Life threatening cardiac arrhythmias (bradycardias).
Calcium Ca^{2+}	Hypocalcaemia (low calcium levels in the blood)	Vitamin D lack and impaired metabolism by the kidneys. Excess excretion of calcium by the kidneys. Alkalosis (calcium becomes unavailable).	Tingling of fingers & toes – carpopedal spasm. Tetany, convulsions.
	Hypercalcaemia (high calcium levels in the blood)	Hyperparathyroidism. Malignancy. Paget's disease. Excess vitamin D intake. Longterm immobilzation. Excess calcium intake and absorption.	Increased risk of fractures. Kidney stones. Cardiac arrhythmias and arrest. Nausea, vomiting, lethargy.
Magnesium Mg^{2+}	Hypomagnesaemia (low levels of magnesium in the blood)	Inadequate intake, e.g. with protein-energy malnutrition. Vomiting and diarrhoea. Excess loss in the urine, e.g. kidney disease and some drugs.	Neuromuscular problems – tremor and convulsions. Behavioural, e.g. agitation and confusion.
	Hypermagnesaemia (high levels of magnesium in the blood)	Acute and chronic kidney failure. Rarely due to excess intake of indigestion medicines containing magnesium.	General CNS effects and lethargy. Seen as part of uraemia.
Phosphates PO_4^{2-}	Hypophosphataemia (low levels of phosphates in the blood)	Alkalosis. Dialysis. Hyperparathyroidism. Parenteral nutrition. Reduced intake and absorption.	Muscular weakness and pain. Respiratory difficulties. Cardiac arrhythmias. Neurological problems, e.g. confusion, convulsions.
	Hyperphosphataemia (high levels of phosphates in the blood)	Acute and chronic kidney failure. Extensive tissue damage or necrosis.	Itching – pruritus. Disturbances of calcium homeostasis.

Hydrogen carbonates HCO_3^- (bicarbonate) – see pages 60, 61 and Chapters 8, 12, 13 & 15
NB Remember that a problem with one electrolyte will often affect the concentration levels of other electrolytes.

Table 2.4 Problems with electrolyte balance.

Abnormal Function **Problems with water balance**

Problems of water balance are divided into two basic types: those involving an equal movement of electrolytes, which are termed isotonic imbalances (osmolarity of the ECF may be unchanged); and osmolar imbalances, which involve a water loss or excess without an equal change in the electrolyte concentration (osmolarity of ECF will be affected).

Isotonic imbalances

When water and electrolytes are lost the person develops a fluid volume deficit. This situation can arise through vomiting, diarrhoea, sweating, drainage from the gastrointestinal tract and use of diuretic drugs (see Chapter 15). Further coverage of this important topic can be found in the Nursing Practice Application – People at risk for dehydration or fluid volume deficit, and the Patient-Centred Study – Natalie.

An increase in both water and electrolytes will cause a fluid volume excess. This may occur when intravenous fluids are infused too quickly, in people with cardiac and liver failure, and in those with excess secretion of hormones such as glucocorticoids and aldosterone. The results of fluid volume excess include the movement of fluid into the interstitial spaces to cause generalized tissue waterlogging (oedema) or pulmonary oedema where fluid enters the alveoli of the lungs.

Areas affected by generalized oedema look puffy and shiny, and form depressions (pits) when pressure is applied. Oedema often occurs in the dependent parts, such as the sacral area, feet and legs. The skin over an oedematous area has an increased risk for developing a pressure sore (see Chapter 19). The formation of oedema is discussed in Chapter 10.

Osmolar imbalances

Hyperosmolar fluid deficit or dehydration (water depletion) occurs when water intake is inadequate or excess fluid is lost from the body. Without a proportional loss of electrolytes, it is accompanied by a disturbance in electrolyte balance – especially sodium levels, which rise. Loss of water from the extracellular compartment increases the osmolarity of the ECF, which becomes hypertonic. Fluid then moves out of the cells in an effort to restore the osmotic equilibrium of the intracellular and extracellular fluids. The overall result will be cellular dehydration, which seriously disrupts cell function.

An increase in water without electrolytes results in a hypo-osmolar fluid excess (water intoxication). It can be caused by excessive water intake and from the inappropriate secretion of ADH, as may occur with some tumours. This time the extracellular fluid is diluted, its osmolarity decreases and, because it is hypotonic compared with the intracellular fluid, the movement of fluid is into the cells. Again cellular function will be adversely affected as cells swell with excess fluid (see Nursing Practice Application – Mental health problems and water intoxication).

Nursing Practice Application **Mental health problems and water intoxication**

Sometimes a person with severe mental health problems will have an abnormal desire to drink excessive amounts of water (psychogenic polydipsia), resulting in water intoxication. One of the most serious effects of the movement of water into the cells associated with hypo-osmolar fluid excess is swelling of brain cells (cerebral oedema), which can result in behavioural changes, altered consciousness, convulsions and even death. Health professionals need to be particularly alert for evidence of abnormal intake or its signs when caring for people at risk for water intoxication. The management of water intoxication may include: restricted fluids and intravenous infusion of hypertonic solutions of mannitol (a sugar) or saline, which causes water to leave the cells.

NB It is important to differentiate between psychogenic polydipsia and the excessive thirst experienced as an unwanted side-effect of lithium carbonate, a drug used to manage mental health problems such as manic-depressive (bipolar) disorders and depression.

Nursing Practice Application People at risk of dehydration or fluid volume deficit

Dehydration or fluid volume deficit occurs when the water (sometimes with electrolytes) lost over a period of time exceeds the water gained. Severe water loss can cause hypovolaemic shock due to reduced blood volume (see Chapter 10).

Causes of fluid imbalances and people at increased risk
Excess loss
Diarrhoea. Vomiting. Haemorrhage. Plasma loss from severe burns or scalds. Increased urinary output volume, such as diabetes mellitus and diabetes insipidus. Severe sweating. Diuretic drugs which increase urinary output volume.

Inadequate intake
Where suitable drinking water is unavail-

able. Physical factors such as unconsciousness. The inability of some people with severe learning disabilities to communicate their thirst and fluid needs. Psychological factors, e.g. a mental health problem such as severe depression, where the individual declines to take adequate fluids.

People at risk
Babies and young children are particularly vulnerable to water and electrolyte imbalances (see page 53). Diarrhoea is an important cause of dehydration in this group and is an especially important cause of ill health in developing countries.

Older adults have reduced water reserves, they may not respond to thirst and their kidneys are less efficient at conserving water by urine concentration. Frailty may mean that they do not

drink enough. Some may even restrict their intake because they fear urinary incontinence.

Others at risk include: people with jobs that involve heavy work in hot conditions, such as furnace workers; athletes and others who only replace water and not electrolytes after vigorous exercise; people exposed to high environmental temperatures, especially those on holiday in hot climates who may actually increase their fluid losses by mistakenly consuming alcoholic drinks to quench their thirst – alcohol increases fluid loss in the urine.

People whose homeostatic mechanisms are impaired by disordered body functions, e.g. people with diabetes mellitus who are passing large amounts of sugar in the urine (glycosuria) produce a greater volume of urine and lose fluid.

Person-Centred Study Natalie

Natalie, aged 2, is the second member of her family to have gastroenteritis; her brother has also been ill. She had been 'poorly' with diarrhoea and a fever for 24 hours when her worried father, who cares for the children alone, took Natalie to the health centre for some advice.

The doctor who saw Natalie decided that she did not need to go to hospital although she had lost both water and electrolytes through diarrhoea and sweating.

Initially the fluid lost by Natalie was from the ECF. When the negative fluid balance continued an osmotic movement of fluid from the ICF to the ECF occurred in an attempt to restore the osmolarity balance between the fluid compartments. Remember that this is only a shift of fluid from one compartment to another – there is still an overall reduction in body fluids. In Natalie's situation, where negative water balance is caused by diarrhoea, the electrolytes sodium and potassium would also be lost from the body. After asking Natalie's father about her condition and an examination of Natalie, the doctor noted the following effects of the negative water balance:

Dry, flushed skin: caused when fluid leaves the skin as ICF moves into the ECF. If fluid loss were to continue the skin

would eventually lose its elasticity (turgor) and the eyes would become sunken. NB Natalie may also feel hot and look flushed because her temperature is raised (see Chapter 19) in response to the infection causing her diarrhoea.

Dry mouth, sticky saliva, furred tongue: the salivary glands (see Chapter 13) produce less saliva in situations where the fluid volume of the body is reduced. The saliva that is produced tends to be sticky and viscous (thick). Without the normal cleansing action of saliva the mouth will feel dry and the tongue will be furred.

Thirst: Natalie will be thirsty. The loss of fluid from the ECF will initially increase its solute concentration (until fluid moves from the ICF). This increase in concentration stimulates the osmoreceptor cells in the thirst centre (see Chapter 4) situated in the hypothalamus. This and the dry mouth will increase the desire to drink, which eventually replaces fluid lost from the body.

Natalie is passing small amounts of **dark urine** – the dark urine is concentrated because it contains less water than normal. Homeostatic mechanisms concerned with fluid balance operate to conserve water within the body. The actual

mechanisms involved will depend on the type and severity of the imbalance – e.g. an increase in ADH secretion, from the posterior pituitary gland (see Chapter 8), in response to the reduction in plasma volume, or osmoreceptors within the brain respond to changes in the solute concentration of the ECF. This also initiates the release of ADH, which in turn increases kidney tubule permeability to water. This means that more water is reabsorbed rather than is excreted in the urine (see Chapter 15).

After discussion with Natalie's father, the doctor decided that, because Natalie was not vomiting and the imbalance was not severe, she could be rehydrated at home with oral fluids, and powders containing glucose and the electrolytes sodium and potassium. This treatment regimen replaces lost fluid and restores the electrolyte balance to normal. Although this soon restored Natalie to her normal self, her father was worried about protecting the family from future 'tummy upsets'. He decided to discuss his worries with the health visitor the next time he took Natalie for a routine assessment (see *Healthier Living – Food safety*).

Healthier Living **Food safety and basic hygiene**
....

When Natalie's father discussed his worries with the health visitor she listened to his fears and offered some suggestions regarding food safety and hygiene for his consideration. They included:
- Wash hands after using the toilet and before preparing or eating food.
- Select food which is fresh, in date and in good condition.
- Get frozen or chilled food home quickly.
- Store food at the correct temperature, e.g. 4°C or below in a refrigerator or freezer.
- Store food properly, e.g. keep raw and cooked foods separate.
- Defrost frozen poultry before cooking.
- Cook at temperatures high enough to kill food poisoning bacteria.
- Follow recommendations on cooking and 'stand time' for microwave ovens.
- Reheat food thoroughly and only once.
- Keep food preparation equipment and areas clean and dry, and have separate utensils for raw meat.
- Keep animals away from food and preparation areas and always wash your hands after handling animals.
- Avoid food containing raw egg and make sure that vulnerable groups such as young children only eat eggs that are completely cooked (yolk and white solid).
- Where possible do not prepare food if you have diarrhoea and vomiting or have a septic hand lesion. If this is not practical, cover hand lesions with coloured plasters or wear gloves.
- Keep kitchen clothes clean and dry.

Fluid replacement in dehydration and fluid volume deficit

Fluid replacement or rehydration can be achieved by:
- Oral fluids, if the fluid imbalance is not severe or when vomiting is not a problem (see Person-Centred Study – Natalie).
- Passing a tube into the gastrointestinal tract usually via the nose. This is used if the gastrointestinal tract is functioning (see Chapter 13) but when drinking is impossible, e.g. altered consciousness.
- Intravenous infusion, containing a combination of water and appropriate electrolytes used when the imbalance is severe (as with burns), or where the gastrointestinal tract is not absorbing fluid, such as after bowel surgery. Water and other substances in the infusion fluid are transported through the capillary walls into the interstitial fluid. From here some will enter the cells to restore the equilibrium between the extracellular and intracellular fluids.

- Fluid infused subcutaneously (under the skin). Challiner *et al.* (1994) propose that this route should be considered as an alternative to intravenous infusion in people unable to drink, and outline several advantages – nursing control, cheaper, fewer complications, vein damage avoided and more mobility allowed.

Nursing Practice Application **Monitoring and evaluating fluid replacement**
....

It is important that nurses are able to monitor and evaluate the adequacy of fluid replacement. The state of skin turgor, thirst and how the person feels are useful and simple assessments. A record of all intake and especially output in the form of a fluid balance chart is an important method of assessing hydration. Regular measurement of weight is a valuable guide to fluid loss or retention and urinary specific gravity may be used as a guide to urine concentration. When the imbalance is severe it may be necessary to use other criteria for assessing the volume of circulating fluid: blood pressure, pulse and central venous pressure (see Chapter 10). In addition, the results of blood tests (urea, electrolytes and packed cell volume) are used to assess the efficacy of nursing actions and treatment regimens.

Hydrogen Ion Concentration (Acid–Base Concentration)

The hydrogen ion concentration or pH is a method of expressing the acidity (concentration of hydrogen ions H$^+$) or alkalinity (concentration of hydroxyl ions OH$^-$) of a solution. pH is measured on a logarithmic scale of 0–14 (*Figure 2.12*); these figures represent the indices of the concentration, i.e. 10^0, 10^{-7}, 10^{-14}, and are easier to use than the actual number of hydrogen ions involved ($10^0 = 1$ mol/l, $10^{-7} = 0.0000001$ mol/l).

It is important to note that $10^0 = 1$ because the logarithm of 1 is 0.

A solution with a pH of 0 has the greatest concentration of hydrogen ions (10^0 or 1 mol/l) and the lowest concentration of hydroxyl ions. It is therefore acidic. pH 7 represents the point where hydrogen ions and hydroxyl ions are in the same concentration (10^{-7}); this solution is said to be neutral (neither acidic or alkaline), e.g. distilled water. At pH 14 (10^{-14}) the hydroxyl ions are at their greatest concentration and the hydrogen ions at their lowest. It is therefore alkaline or basic. A solution with a pH of less than 7 is acidic and one where the pH is greater than 7 is alkaline. As the hydrogen ion concentration decreases that of the hydroxyl ions increases and vice versa.

Since the pH scale is logarithmic, a change of one on the scale represents a tenfold change in the hydrogen ion concentration, e.g. a solution of pH 6 has ten times more hydrogen ions than one of pH 7. This is of particular importance when considering the pH of blood (normal range pH 7.35–7.45, i.e. slightly alkaline) as very small changes can affect the cell environment and function.

The pH of blood can also be expressed in nanomoles (see Appendix A) of hydrogen ions per litre (normal range 36–44 nmol/l); this is increasingly used in clinical situations.

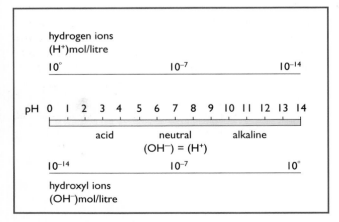

Figure 2.12 pH scale. Please note at 37^{0}C (body temperature) the neutral point is 6.8.

Regulation of pH

Acid–base balance in the body is maintained by several interdependent homeostatic mechanisms – chemical **buffer** systems in the ECF and ICF (see below), the respiratory centre and lungs, and the kidneys. The chemical buffers act immediately to regulate pH, respiratory regulation (through rate and depth of breathing) operates within minutes and the kidneys provide long-term regulation by processes occurring over many hours. These mechanisms ensure that the blood pH stays within the range 7.35–7.45 during health. This is vital for enzyme activity, which is dependent upon environmental pH, and for other functional proteins, such as haemoglobin, which require the correct pH range for optimal function. Some enzymes need a specific acid or alkaline environment – for example, the digestive enzymes which operate in the acid environment of the stomach stop working in the alkaline small intestine. *Table 2.5* details the pH ranges of some body fluids.

Table 2.5 pH range of some body fluids	
Fluid	**pH range**
Blood	7.35-7.45
Saliva	6.5-7.5
Gastric secretion	1.5-3.0
Pancreatic secretion	8.0-8.4
Urine	4.5-8.0

Table 2.5 pH range of some body fluids.

Buffers

Buffers are substances which limit pH change by their ability to accept hydrogen ions from acidic solutions and donate hydrogen ions to alkaline solutions. Buffers act as weak acids or alkalis, which is important because, unlike strong acids or alkalis, they only partially dissociate or ionize in solution and therefore have a much smaller effect on the pH of that solution. In this way it is possible for buffers to prevent large swings in pH which would otherwise inhibit cell function. The important buffer systems are:

The hydrogen carbonate (bicarbonate) system in the ECF (blood) and ICF

The hydrogen carbonate system consists of hydrogen carbonate (HCO_3^-) and carbonic acid (H_2CO_3) in a ratio of 20:1. The hydrogen carbonates, either sodium hydrogen carbonate (ECF) or potassium hydrogen carbonate (ICF), act as a weak alkali to 'mop up' excess hydrogen ions from a strong acid. They thus form more carbonic acid, which is a weak acid, and a neutral salt, leaving pH unaffected:

$$HCl + NaHCO_3 \rightarrow H_2CO_3 + NaCl$$

Hydrochloric acid (strong acid)	+	Sodium hydrogen carbonate (weak alkali)		Carbonic acid (weak acid)	+	Sodium chloride (salt)

The amount of hydrogen carbonate available in the blood for buffering pH is known as the alkaline reserve. It is regulated by the kidneys (see Chapter 15). Carbonic acid as a weak acid is able to donate hydrogen ions when the pH of a solution rises when a strong alkali is added:

$$NaOH + H_2CO_3 \rightarrow NaHCO_3 + H_2O$$

Sodium hydroxide (strong alkali)	+	Carbonic acid (weak acid)		Sodium hydrogen carbonate (weak alkali)	+ water

Carbonic acid is derived from cellular metabolism, and its level in the blood is regulated by the lungs (see Chapter 12). From our brief discussion of the functioning of this buffer system you can appreciate the importance of the three components (chemical buffers, respiratory and kidney mechanisms) of pH regulation working in a coordinated way.

Hydrogen phosphates in the ICF, kidney and blood

The hydrogen phosphate system consists of two sodium salts: sodium dihydrogen phosphate (NaH_2PO_4), which acts as a weak acid, and disodium hydrogen phosphate (Na_2HPO_4), which acts as a weak alkali.

NaOH (strong alkali)	+	NaH_2PO_4 (weak acid)	$\rightarrow$	Na_2HPO_4 (weak alkali)	+ H_2O water

HCl (strong acid)	+	Na_2HPO_4 (weak alkali)	$\rightarrow$	NaH_2PO_4 (weak acid)	+ NaCl (salt)

These two act like the hydrogen carbonate system by donating and accepting hydrogen ions.

Protein buffers

Intracellular proteins, such as haemoglobin, provide around 75% of the buffering capacity. They limit pH changes in the ICF and blood by their ability to ionize. Proteins, you will remember, are long chains of many amino acids joined together. One end of the chain has a carboxyl group (COOH) which acts as a weak acid and donates hydrogen ions:

$$R - COOH \rightleftharpoons R - COO^- + H^+$$
$$R = \text{different amino acid structures}$$

The other end has an amino group (NH_2) which acts as a weak alkali and accepts hydrogen ions:

$$R - NH_2 + H^+ \rightleftharpoons R - NH_3^+$$

When buffer systems are overwhelmed and other homeostatic mechanisms fail to cope, the pH of blood changes as the acid–base balance is disrupted. This may result in abnormalities, such as enzyme denaturation (see Chapter 1), which would seriously disturb normal physiological function. Acid–base imbalances, which are often associated with electrolyte or fluid imbalances, can be life threatening. Life is only possible within a blood pH range 7.0–7.8 (hydrogen ion concentration 16–100 nmol/litre) and people with a pH at the extremes of this range would be critically ill. The loss of homeostatic balance and disruption to pH occurs in two forms: (i) acidosis caused by a fall in pH; and (ii) alkalosis caused by a rise in pH. These opposites represent a shift beyond the values at either end of the normal range.

A fuller account of these departures from normal can be found in Chapters 8, 12, 13 and 15.

Summary/Check List

Homeostasis – control mechanisms, negative and positive feedback, breakdown in control.
Basic chemistry. Matter – elements, atoms, atomic number, mass number, atomic weight, isotopes, radioisotopes, half-life. Molecules and compounds – molecular weight, molar concentration and molarity. Chemical bonds – ionic (ions and electrolytes), covalent, hydrogen bond.
Diffusion – simple, facilitated.
Osmosis – osmotic pressure, osmolarity/osmolality, tonicity (isotonic, hypertonic and hypotonic solutions).
Filtration.
Fluid compartments and body fluids – intracellular fluid (ICF) and extracellular fluid (ECF). Electrolyte composition of fluid compartments – major anions and cations in ICF and

ECF. Problems with electrolyte balance. Water balance – water gain and loss. Problems with water balance. Nursing Practice Application – mental health problems and water intoxication. Nursing Practice Application – people at risk for dehydration or fluid volume deficit. Person-centred Study – Natalie. Healthier Living – food safety and basic hygiene. Fluid replacement in dehydration and fluid volume deficit. Nursing Practice Application – monitoring and evaluating fluid replacement.
Hydrogen ion concentration – the pH scale, regulation of pH, buffers (hydrogen carbonate system, hydrogen phosphates and proteins), outline of acid–base imbalances (acidosis and alkalosis).

Self Test

1   Which of the following statements about homeostasis are true?
    (a) It is the self-regulatory processes of the body which maintain the constancy of the internal environment.
    (b) All homeostatic mechanisms are controlled by negative feedback.
    (c) Homeostatic mechanisms only regulate the chemical concentration of body fluids.
    (d) A breakdown in homeostasis may lead to a health deficiency.
2   Describe the three components required for a homeostatic mechanism.
3   An atom with an electrical charge is called an:
    (a) isotope;
    (b) electron;
    (c) element;
    (d) ion.
4   What are the chemical symbols for the following elements? Sodium, calcium, potassium, iron, magnesium, chlorine, oxygen, hydrogen, nitrogen, carbon.
5   Describe the direction of water movement when cells are exposed to the following solutions of sodium chloride:
    (a) isotonic;
    (b) hypotonic;
    (c) hypertonic.

6   In a healthy newborn what percentage of their body weight will be water?
    (a) 45–50%;
    (b) 50–55%;
    (c) 60–65%;
    (d) 70–75%.
7   A man has 40 litres of body water. How much of this will be intracellular?
8   Which of the following statements are true?
    (a) Sodium is the major cation of the ECF.
    (b) Most potassium is intracellular.
    (c) Chloride, calcium and hydrogen carbonate are all anions.
    (d) Cations are ions with a positive charge.
9   Which groups are at increased risk for dehydration and fluid volume deficit?
10 How would you assess the efficacy of intravenous fluid replacement in a person with a fluid volume deficit?
11 Mark on the pH scale: neutral point, blood pH, acidic range, pH of gastric secretions, pH of urine, alkaline range.
12 Outline ways in which the body regulates acid–base balance.

Answers

1 a, d.
2 See page 45.
3 d.
4 Na, Ca, K, Fe, Mg, Cl, O, H, N, C.
5 (a) No movement; (b) from solution to cells; (c) from cells to solution.
6 d.
7 25 litres.
8 a, b, d.
9 See page 58.
10 See page 59.
11 See *Figure 2.12* and *Table 2.5*
12 Chemical buffers, respiratory system and kidneys.

References

Challiner YC, Jarrett D, Hayward MJ et al. (1994) A comparison of intravenous and subcutaneous hydration in elderly stroke patients. *Post-Grad Med J* **70**(821):195–197.

Heath HBM, Ed (1995) *Potter and Perry's Foundations in Nursing Theory and Practice*. London: Mosby.

Herbert R (1986) The biology of ageing: body temperature regulation. *Geriat Nurs Home Care* **6**(4):16–18.

Further Reading

Edwards CRW, Bouchier IAD, Haslett C *et al.,* Eds. (1995) *Davidson's Principles and Practice of Medicine*, 17th edn. Edinburgh: Churchill Livingstone.

Foss M (1988) Acid–base balance. *Prof Nurs* **3**(12):509, 511–513.

Herbert R (1986) The biology of ageing: maintenance of homeostasis. *Geriat Nurs Home Care* **6**(3):14–16.

Lewis M, Waller G (1980). *Thinking Chemistry*. Oxford: Oxford University Press. N.B. Provides coverage of basic chemical concepts.

Long BC, Phipps WJ and Cassmeyer VL, Eds, with Brooker CG, El-Gamel V, Gotecha P, UK Eds (1995) *Adult Nursing. A Nursing Process Approach*. London: Mosby.

McVicar A and Clancy J (1997) Principles of intravenous fluid replacement. *Prof Nurs* **12**(8) supplement S6–S9.

Miller JA (1989) Intravenous therapy in fluid and electrolyte imbalance. *Prof Nurs* **4**(5):237–241.

Robinson JR (1975) *Fundamentals of Acid–Base Regulation*, 5th edn. Oxford: Blackwell Scientific Publications.

Nervous Tissue and Basic Functions of the Nervous System

.....

Overview

- *Organization of nervous system.*
- *Nervous tissue.*
- *The nerve impulse.*
- *Reflex arc.*

Learning Outcomes

After studying Chapter 3 you should be able to:

- Outline the organization of the nervous system.
- Describe the structure of a neurone.
- Describe neuroglial cells and their functions.
- Describe the main types of sensory receptors.
- Explain the process of adaptation occurring in some sensory receptors.
- Discuss the transmission of nerve impulses.
- Describe a synapse and outline how it functions.
- Outline the variety and role of neurotransmitters.
- Describe factors influencing nerve transmission.
- Describe the reflex arc.

Key Words

Action potential – the change in electrical potential and charge across the cell membrane that occurs when a nerve conducts an impulse or when muscle fibres contract.

Autonomic nervous system (ANS) – the part of the nervous system controlling involuntary functions, e.g. heart rate, glandular secretion and smooth muscle contraction.

Axon – the long extension of a nerve cell that conducts impulses away from the nerve cell body.

Cell body (nerve cell body) – the part of the neurone containing the nucleus and other organelles.

Central nervous system (CNS) – the brain and spinal cord.

Dendrites – the branching processes of the nerve cell. They receive nerve impulses from other neurones and conduct them towards the nerve cell body.

Depolarization – a reduction in the difference in membrane charge where the resting membrane potential becomes less negative as it moves closer to 0 mV or becomes positive. This loss of polarity occurs during a stage of the action potential.

Electrochemical energy – energy that is produced by the electrical and concentration gradients that result from the movement of ions across an axon membrane.

Motor (efferent nerves) – convey impulses from the CNS to muscles and glands.

Myelin – the fatty material which covers some nerves. It insulates the nerve fibres and is analogous with the plastic cover around electrical wires.

Neuroglia – support cells of the nervous system.

Neurone – a nerve cell consisting of a cell body, an axon and dendrites.

Neurotransmitter – a chemical that facilitates the transmission of a nerve impulse across a junction, e.g. acetylcholine.

Key Words cont.

Peripheral nervous system (PNS) – the part of the nervous system outside the brain and spinal cord. The motor and sensory nerves carrying impulses between the CNS and the rest of the body.

Polarized – describes the resting state of the plasma membrane of an excitable cell (neurone or muscle fibre) in which there is no impulse transmission. The inside of the plasma membrane is electrically negative relative to the outside.

Potential difference – the voltage or potential energy in volts (V) or millivolts (mV) between two points, e.g. across a cell membrane.

Refractory period – the time for which a nerve or muscle fibre is unable to respond to a stimulus. It may be partial, when it may be overcome if the stimulus is sufficiently large, or absolute, when no response is possible.

Reflex – an instantaneous, involuntary (automatic) response to a stimulus (sensory input).

Repolarization – a stage of the action potential in which the membrane potential returns from a state of depolarization to its negative resting (polarized) potential. During repolarization there may be a short period of hyperpolarization when the membrane potential is briefly more negative than the resting level.

Resting potential – the difference in electrical charge (mV) between the inside and outside of the plasma membrane of an excitable cell in the resting state. Typically around –70mV for neurones, with the inside of the membrane negative relative to the outside.

Sensory (afferent nerves) – convey impulses to the CNS from organs, skin, joints and skeletal muscles.

Summation – the process by which the excitatory and inhibitory effects of stimuli arriving at a nerve cell body are added together, sorted and integrated.

Synapse – the gap between the axon of one neurone and the dendrites of another, or the gap between an axon and an effector cell. Transmission of the nerve impulse across the gap depends upon the release of a neurotransmitter.

Introduction and Basic Organization

The nervous system collaborates with the endocrine system (see Chapter 8) to control and regulate all body functions and maintain homeostasis (see Chapter 2). You will remember from our discussion in Chapter 1 that both **neurotransmitters** and hormones act as ligands (signalling chemicals) which bind to membrane receptors to influence cell function.

Communication within the body occurs by the two systems:

- The nervous system takes care of rapid communication between cells by the transmission of nerve impulses as **electrochemical energy** (see pages 71–73).
- In the endocrine system, in a slower process, hormones produced by the endocrine glands are transported in the blood or lymph to affect specific cell functions (see Chapter 8).

The nervous system receives sensory data from external and internal sources, handles the data and initiates an appropriate response. The ability to sort sensory input and determine the required action is called integration. The response – the motor output – results in glandular or muscular activity. For example, while strolling through a meadow you see a bull grazing (sensory input), realize the potential danger (integration) and remove yourself expeditiously from the

vicinity (motor output). Our understanding of the nervous system is increasing rapidly, but considerable research is still necessary before its functioning is fully understood.

The nervous system consists of several different parts, which contribute to the integrated working of the whole system. For convenience it can be divided structurally into:

- **Central nervous system** (CNS) – the brain and spinal cord. It is here that sensory input is received and processed before an appropriate motor output is produced.
- **Peripheral nervous system** (PNS) – the cranial nerves (12 pairs) and spinal nerves (31 pairs) linking the brain and spinal cord with the rest of the body.

The PNS is divided into two functional parts: the **sensory** division (**afferent nerves**), which carries sensory data to the CNS from receptors in the muscles, skin and joints (somatic) or from the organs (visceral); and the **motor** division (**efferent nerves**), which carries the motor output from the CNS. The motor division consists of the voluntary part of the PNS, which supplies skeletal muscle and can be controlled consciously, and the **autonomic nervous system** (ANS), which supplies involuntary muscle and glands and controls functions not normally under conscious control, e.g. heart rate and digestion. In turn, the ANS has two parts: the sympathetic ANS, which initiates the stress responses of the body, e.g. increased heart rate, and the parasympathetic ANS, which controls functions that are typically performed at rest, e.g. digestion.

To summarize:

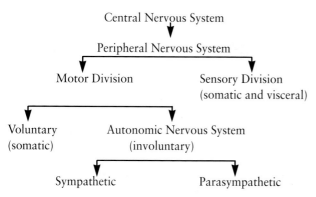

Nerve Tissue

Nerve tissue can be divided into:
- **Neurones** (excitable cells).
- **Neuroglia** (non-excitable cells).

Early development of nerve tissue

Neurones and neuroglia start their development from designated cells known as neuroepithelial cells, which are derived from the ectoderm of the neural tube (embryonic structure which gives rise to the CNS), about 4 weeks after conception. This very early start should alert you to just how important it is to have the optimal environment for healthy development already in place before conception and operative in the early weeks of pregnancy (see Chapter 4). The neuroepithelial cells are set on a fixed developmental path – they can only become nerve tissue. During several stages they increase in number and eventually differentiate into early excitable cells and neuroglia. These processes are not yet fully understood, but it is obviously extremely complex when you consider the many components required for the development of a functioning nervous system. Somehow the right nerve connections must be made as the now amitotic (remember in Chapter 1 we said that neurones could not divide) neurones (or neuroblasts) migrate to their correct locations and the development of different types of neurones, neuroglia, synapses and neurotransmitters must occur. There are various theories about how this happens:

- There appear to be chemical 'on/off switches' in the form of nerve growth factors and inhibitory chemicals released from developing nerve tissue.
- Growing **axons** use physical 'signposts' provided by older 'trail-blazing'neurones and neuroglial cells.
- Other chemicals may attract the growing axons to their destination.
- Special cell adhesion molecules (CAMs) cause the new axons to 'stick' properly when they arrive at their destination.
- Neurotransmitters appear to have a role in the differentiation processes.

Not all developing neurones make the right connections and many do not survive past the early developmental stages, as normal cell death occurs. What is important to realize is that although the nervous system continues to develop for several years after birth the total number of neurones present at birth is the most you will ever have.

Readers can find information about the development of specific areas of the nervous system in the relevant chapter, e.g. CNS in Chapter 4.

Neurones

Neurones (nerve cells) are the highly differentiated units of the nervous system (see *Figure 3.1*). They are very sensitive to changes in their environment and are easily damaged by exposure to microorganisms, chemicals, toxins and lack of oxygen. Permanent brain damage occurs when the brain is deprived of oxygen for several minutes, such as may occur during a cardiac arrest (see also Nursing Practice Application – Brains need oxygen).

As a result of their high degree of differentiation, neurones cannot replicate by mitosis (see Chapter 1), so damaged cells cannot be replaced. They compensate for this by being extremely long-lived. It is possible, however, to repair limited damage to neurones outside the CNS, provided that

Nursing Practice Application **Brains need oxygen**

Nervous tissue, with its high metabolic rate, needs a constant supply of oxygen and nutrients (glucose) to function normally. If the brain is deprived of oxygen the effects may include behavioural changes which range from confusion, restlessness and apprehension to alterations in consciousness. Nurses need to be alert to those people who are at risk for poor brain oxygenation, e.g. patients with chronic lung disease or after haemorrhage. Observing for changes indicative of poor brain oxygenation, ensuring that treatment such as oxygen therapy is administered safely and effectively, and monitoring for changes, e.g. respiratory rate and pulse oximetry, are vital nursing interventions (see Chapter 12).

the damage occurs some way from the **cell body** – a peripheral axon which is cut or compressed may regenerate and regain function.

There are several types of neurones (see below), but all are well adapted for the transmission of electrical impulses. A neurone consists of:

- A nerve cell body, which contains a nucleus, other organelles and Nissl granules (rough endoplasmic reticulum concerned with protein synthesis). There are no centrioles, which reflects the neurone's inability to divide by mitosis.
- A long process, or fibre (ranging from a few millimetres to 1 metre in length), called an axon, which transmits impulses away from the cell body. The axoplasm (cytoplasm) contains mitochondria and is enclosed by a membrane, the axolemma. The axon receives nutrients by the continuous movement of substances from the cell body. Axonal transport and axoplasmic flow carry organelles, enzymes and other substances from cell body to axon (anterograde), where they are used to maintain structural integrity and metabolic functions. Movement in the reverse direction, retrograde transport, occurs as organelles are returned to the cell body for destruction. Transport may be fast, intermediate or slow, and the mechanism suggested for the movement involves microtubules which act like a railway on which the substances and organelles are driven by contractile proteins.

  Unfortunately axonal transport can provide the means by which harmful agents such as viruses, e.g. rabies and herpes, gain access to the nerve cell body. Delieu and Keady (1996) describe the spread of the plaques and tangles associated with Alzheimer's disease as being by axonal transport mechanisms (see Chapter 4).
- Several short branching processes, called **dendrites**, which transmit nerve impulses towards the cell body.

(Readers requiring a revision of cell structure and organelles should have a quick look at Chapter 1.)

Some axons are covered with a white fatty material called **myelin**, which protects and insulates the fibre. Myelin insulates the axon and prevents leakage of the electrical charge generated by the nerve impulse. Myelination thus allows very rapid impulse transmission, of up to 120 m/s (see saltatory conduction, page 73).

Myelin is produced by specialized neuroglial cells, known as Schwann cells in the PNS and as oligodendrocytes within the CNS. These cells use their cell membrane to enclose the axon (see below); the layer they form around the axon is known as the neurilemma. In myelinated axons the neurilemma is wrapped around the axon several times, and forms the myelin sheath; in non-myelinated axons there is neurilemma but no myelin sheath. The mainly myelinated fibres form the 'white matter' of the CNS and the nerves of the PNS. The non-myelinated cell bodies form the 'grey matter' of the nervous system. Gaps in the myelin sheath, representing the boundaries between individual Schwann cells, occur at intervals along the myelinated axon and are known as the nodes of Ranvier. They assist in rapid transmission of the impulse.

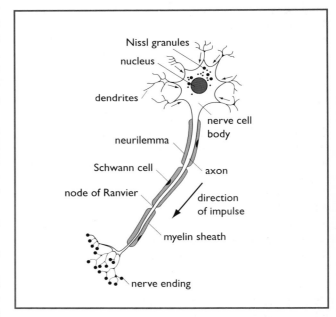

Figure 3.1 Neurone.

Nursing Practice Application **Myelination and motor development**

Nerve myelination commences during fetal life and continues into the teenage years, but it is during the all important first year of life that it proceeds at its most rapid rate. This express myelination is reflected in the amazing motor development milestones that the infant achieves during this period – from a newborn unable to lift its head to an infant who is able to stand, then walk. As myelination progresses the infant becomes mobile and acquires coordinated fine motor skills such as picking up small objects. The price, however, of such spectacular development is a vulnerability to factors that could delay or prevent normal development, e.g. infections affecting the CNS.

Family-Centred Study **Lisa, Darren, Carol and Tony**

Lisa is 35 and lives with Darren and their children (Carol 9 and Tony 5). Soon after Tony was born, Lisa experienced double vision and weakness in one arm. This soon cleared up and, being busy with the baby, she forgot all about it. All was well for about a year until weakness and tingling in her legs prompted Lisa to see her GP.

Following some tests, which included magnetic resonance imaging (MRI) and a lumbar puncture (LP), and many consultations at the hospital, Lisa and Darren were told that she probably had multiple sclerosis.

After four years Lisa is unable to walk and requires help with hygiene needs. Urinary incontinence (see Chapter 15) was a problem but intermittent self-catheterization has made life much easier for everyone. Preventing incontinence has also lessened the considerable risk for skin breakdown and pressure sore development (see Chapter 19).

Darren has learnt about skin care, moving/handling (see Chapter 18) and bladder management, and is able to care for Lisa when he is not working. Lisa's complete dependence puts a strain on their relationship and she worries that the children miss out on family outings. The family is well supported by Darren's parents, who live nearby, social services and the community nursing team, who provide specialist advice as required. Another help is the Multiple Sclerosis Society, who they contacted after the illness was diagnosed. They found that the chance to talk to people with similar problems helped them to develop more effective coping strategies as the disease progressed. They were able to talk about areas of anxiety such as sexuality and how best to help the children cope with Lisa's condition.

In many cases the condition progresses very slowly and there are periods of remission. However, the prognosis (outcome) for Lisa is poor and she has a high risk for developing pressure sores, urinary infection and pneumonia. Multiple sclerosis has a very variable presentation and outcome, which depend upon the neurones affected. The signs and symptoms are due to demyelination and hardened areas on the myelin sheath. There is no cure, but problems such as muscle spasm can be relieved with drugs, e.g. baclofen. Recently the use of beta interferon (immune chemical) has appeared to benefit some people – fewer 'flare ups' and some improvement. Some people have very little disability whilst others, like Lisa, become totally dependent. The severe form affects family relationships and causes financial problems, and presents health and social care professionals with an enormous challenge if quality of family life is to be maintained.

Neurones may be classified structurally on the number of processes they have – unipolar, bipolar or multipolar –or functionally, where neurones may be motor (carrying impulses from the CNS to the muscles or glands), sensory (carrying incoming sensory information to the CNS) or serve as connections in the CNS, when they are called interneurones.

Loss of myelin (demyelination) in previously myelinated fibres will result in serious impulse conduction problems. A common example of a demyelinating condition is multiple sclerosis, which affects 1 in 2000 of the population in the UK (Edwards *et al.*, 1995) – see the Family-Centred Study.

Supporting cells (non-excitable)

Supporting cells are known collectively as the neuroglia or glial cells. They are found in the CNS and PNS (where they are called Schwann cells), and they greatly outnumber the neurones (see *Figure 3.2*). Neuroglial cells can replicate and, if replication becomes disordered, may form tumours called gliomas. Glial cells include:

- Oligodendrocytes and Schwann cells, which produce myelin (see page 68). In addition, the phagocytic Schwann cells provide an important function in the PNS by clearing away cell detritus.
- Astrocytes (star-shaped cells in the CNS) support neurones and surround blood vessels in the CNS to form

an important component of the protective 'blood–brain barrier' (see Chapter 4).

- Microglial cells, also found in the CNS, are a type of macrophage; these phagocytic cells are active in areas of inflammation or damage (see Chapters 1, 9 and 19).
- Ependymal cells are found lining the fluid-filled cavities of the brain and spinal cord. Some cover the choroid plexuses (see Chapter 4), which secrete cerebrospinal fluid (CSF), and others have cilia (see Chapter 1) to circulate the CSF.

Nerve structure

The nerves of the PNS consist of many axons (nerve fibres) bound together to form a nerve (like the many tiny wires/fibres in a telephone cable) (see *Figure 3.3*).

Individual nerve fibres are surrounded by a delicate connective tissue, the endoneurium. Small bundles of nerve fibres are grouped together and enclosed in a sheath of connective tissue, the perineurium.

The entire nerve, which consists of many bundles of axons, is protected by an outer fibrous coat, the epineurium. Running between bundles of nerve fibres, and supported by connective tissue, are the blood (Chapter 10) and lymphatic (Chapter 11) vessels required by the nerve.

Nerves may be motor (efferent), sensory (afferent) or, more commonly, mixed (carrying both motor and sensory axons).

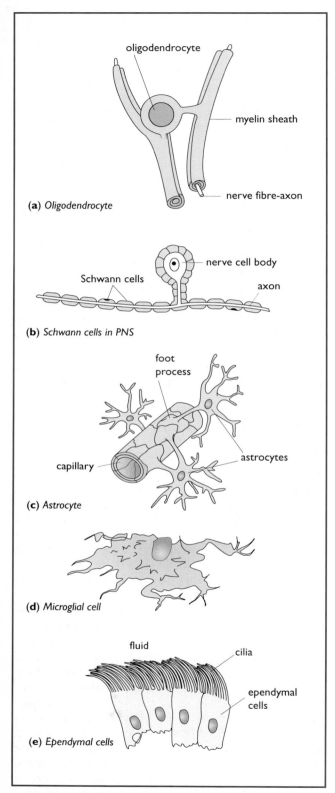

(a) Oligodendrocyte

(b) Schwann cells in PNS

(c) Astrocyte

(d) Microglial cell

(e) Ependymal cells

Figure 3.2 Types of neuroglia (supporting cells):. (a) oligodendrocyte, (b) Schwann cell, (c) astrocyte, (d) microglial cell, (e) ependymal cell.

Sensory receptors

Sensory receptors are specialized structures that monitor changes in the body's environment by reacting to external or internal stimuli. Receptors that respond to external stimuli are situated close to the body surface, e.g. in the skin or eye (exteroceptors), and those responding to internal stimuli can be found in 'deeper' structures, e.g. organs (visceroceptors), joints and muscles (proprioceptors). They range from a simple pressure receptor in the skin to very complex sense organs such as the eye (see Chapters 4 and 7).

The receptors send data through the sensory neurones to the CNS, where integration occurs at different levels; this means that not all the sensory input reaches our consciousness, but may be acted upon at a subconscious level, e.g. certain **reflexes**. Sometimes the perception of a sensation occurs without a stimulus, such as the hallucinations experienced by people with certain mental health problems. These can be very frightening even though they are entirely imagined.

The many types of receptors may be classified structurally or functionally as follows.

Structural classification

- Free dendritic nerve endings – found in the viscera, muscles, joints and skin, where they detect pain, touch and temperature.
- Encapsulated receptors (specialized nerve endings) – found in the skin, e.g. Meissner's corpuscles, which detect light pressure. Specialized receptors – Golgi organs in the tendons and muscle spindles in skeletal muscle monitor stretching and, together with receptors in the joints, provide information about position (proprioception).
- Non-nervous receptors – the specialized cells found in the sense organs, e.g. taste buds on the tongue.

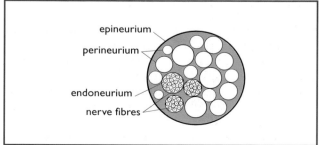

Figure 3.3 Nerve structure.

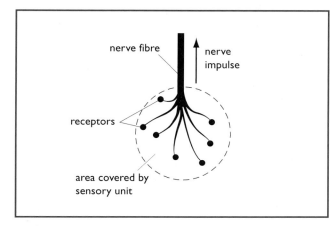

Figure 3.4 Sensory receptors and sensory unit.

Functional classification (by type of stimulus)

- Chemoreceptors can monitor changes in the chemical environment. They are concerned with taste and smell plus the vital monitoring of chemicals, e.g. carbon dioxide, in the blood.
- Mechanoreceptors are responsive to mechanical forces. They include pressure and touch receptors in the skin; proprioceptors, which monitor stretching, in muscles, joints and tendons, stretch receptors in the bladder, lung and gut; baroreceptors, which monitor pressure in blood vessels; and special receptors in the ear which respond to sound waves.
- Thermoreceptors situated in the skin and elsewhere respond to changes in temperature.
- Nociceptors (pain receptors) respond to many different stimuli, including intense pressure, extremes of temperature and the chemicals released during inflammation (see Chapter 19). All of these are harmful to tissue and cause pain (see Chapter 4).
- Photoreceptors are special receptors in the eye which respond to light energy.

Sensory receptors need a certain level of stimulation before they initiate a nerve impulse through the afferent fibres to the CNS; this is termed the threshold.

Some receptors modify their response when a stimulus is repeated continuously – after a while they stop responding to small constant stimuli and respond only to changes. This is termed adaptation and explains why, for instance, we are not aware of clothes touching our skin. Pain receptors, however, do not adapt, and continue to respond for as long as the potentially harmful stimulus is present.

Several sensory receptors channel their output into one afferent fibre; this is known as a sensory unit (*Figure 3.4*).

The Nerve Impulse

Transmission

Nerve impulses are transmitted by nerve fibres in the form of electrochemical energy – produced by the movement of ions across the axon membrane. The chemical composition of the body fluids is vital to nerve impulse transmission (see Chapter 2). It is the difference in ion concentration between the ICF and the ECF (which you will remember are both electrically neutral) that produces the electrical **potential difference** across the selectively permeable axon membrane.

The potential difference of –70 mV across the membrane is known as the **resting potential**. The negative sign indicates that the inside of the membrane is negative with respect to the outside. The resting potential is produced as ions leak through the axon membrane by passive facilitated diffusion – sodium (Na$^+$) leaks in slowly and potassium (K$^+$) leaks out more quickly in response to their concentration gradients. It is the positive potassium ions leaking out more quickly than positive sodium ions can replace them that causes the inside of the membrane to be electrically negative. At this stage there is no impulse transmission, most of the specific gated ion channels (see *Figure 3.5*) which will allow the rapid ion movement needed for impulse transmission are closed and the membrane is said

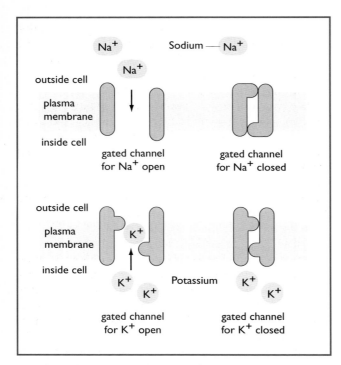

Figure 3.5 Gated ion channels (diagrammatic).

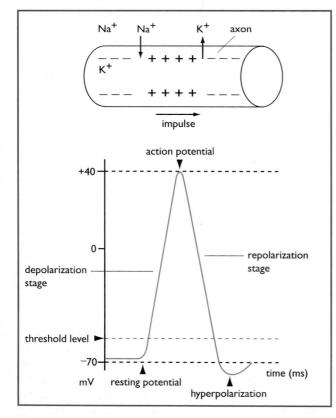

Figure 3.6 Transmission of the nerve impulse/action potential.

to be **polarized**. The resting potential is sustained by the active sodium–potassium pump which maintains the ion concentration gradients by pumping out more sodium than potassium into the axon.

For transmission of a nerve impulse to occur, a change in resting potential and membrane permeability (which ions the membrane will allow through) is needed. These changes occur when a stimulus reaches the axon. The rapid movement of ions through specific gated ion channels in the axon membrane causes a change in the potential difference, and this allows the nerve impulse to move along the axon. Some ion channels are operated chemically and some are voltage dependent. The change in potential difference is known as the **action potential**. As sodium and chloride (Cl$^-$) ions move rapidly across the membrane into the axon a potential difference of +40 mV is produced – a change of 110 mV.

The membrane is now depolarized – the inside is electrically positive with respect to the outside. The movement of sodium ions into the axon increases **depolarization**, which enhances membrane permeability with the opening of more sodium channels. The process of depolarization is now self-stimulating (positive feedback) and will occur sequentially along unmyelinated axons, allowing the propagation of the nerve impulse as the action potential regenerates in each segment of the axon (see page 73).

Sodium movement, which is all important, lasts for about 1 ms, but now at the height of the action potential (*Figure 3.6*) the sodium channels start to close and the membrane becomes more permeable to potassium ions, which move out of the axon as their specific channels open. As positive potassium ions move out of the axon (in response to its electrochemical gradient) the inside of the membrane becomes less positive and more negative, until the resting potential is restored.

After the passage of the impulse the membrane is repolarized – returned to the resting potential. During **repolarization** there is an increase in the negative potential as potassium ions continue to leave the axon (potassium channels take time to close), which results in a short period of hyperpolarization, a situation which reduces excitability and prevents the transmission of more impulses (*Figure 3.6*). The ion concentrations of the resting potential are soon restored by the active transport sodium–potassium exchange pump and diffusion (Chapters 1 and 2).

The ability to produce a resting membrane potential across their plasma membrane is a feature of all cells, but only the excitable cells – neurones and muscle cells (see Chapter 17) – can produce an action potential by reversibly altering the potential difference.

Some rather special features of the action potential merit further consideration. An action potential in a particular neurone is always of the same size and duration,

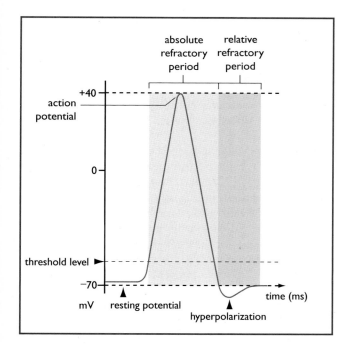

Figure 3.7 Absolute and relative refractory periods during an action potential.

regardless of the type and intensity of the stimulus. This is the all-or-none phenomenon – either a stimulus produces a full action potential or it produces nothing; there is no partial response to smaller stimuli. The intensity of the stimulus and the degree of membrane depolarization required for the passage of an impulse is called the threshold. During and following the production of an action potential the axon membrane is in a refractory state, when its threshold increases and its response to stimuli is altered. When an action potential is being generated the axon is in an absolute **refractory period**, which means that further stimuli, regardless of intensity, are incapable of producing another action potential. A relative refractory period, of around 5 ms follows the action potential, when only a very intense stimulus will cause a second action potential (*Figure 3.7*).

Propagation of the action potential

Earlier we mentioned that the nerve impulse is propagated along the axon as the action potential regenerates in each segment of unmyelinated axon. Depolarization occurring in a small segment is immediately followed by repolarization as gated ion channels open and close – first sodium and then potassium channels. The movement of ions inside and outside the axon set up local currents that cause depolarization and generation of an action potential in the next segment – the whole process is repeated

and the nerve impulse passes along the axon. Propagation of the impulse proceeds in one direction (away from the original stimulus) because the segment of axon which has just had an action potential will be in a refractory state and cannot respond while this persists.

The propagation of action potentials in myelinated nerves is much faster and can be explained by local currents operating between gaps (nodes of Ranvier) in the myelin sheath rather than from segment to segment (remember the myelin sheath insulates – so action potentials can only occur at gaps in the sheath). This is known as saltatory conduction, where impulses appear to leap from one node of Ranvier to the next.

Impulse transmission speed

The propagation of nerve impulses takes only a few milliseconds (ms); this is an important feature in a control system that relies upon rapid communication. Speed of transmission depends not only on whether the fibre is myelinated, but also on the diameter of the axon. Fibres can be divided into:

- The 'A' fibres (α, β, γ and δ, becoming progressively smaller and slower) are thick, heavily myelinated fibres capable of rapid transmission, e.g. motor and sensory fibres, some pain and thermal impulses.
- The 'B' fibres, or intermediate size fibres, which have some myelin and transmit more slowly, e.g. fibres in the autonomic nervous system.
- The 'C' fibres, which are thin and have no myelin sheath. The lack of myelin means that they transmit at the slowest rate, e.g. autonomic system and some types of pain.

Synapse

A **synapse** is a junction or gap between two neurones or between a neurone and an effector, such as a gland or muscle (see also neuromuscular junction, Chapter 17). The processes taking place at a synapse allow the nerve impulse to continue across the gap, a feature vital to the continuity and integration of the nervous system. The continuation of transmission can be achieved by electrical or chemical means.

Electrical synapse

In a few situations, where the gap between the cell membranes is extremely small and the electrical resistance (the resistance to flow of electrical charge) is low, it is possible for an impulse generated in the first neurone to cross the gap to the second neurone. This type of electrical synapse is uncommon, but examples exist in the brain, where they allow rapid transmission.

Chemical synapse

Most synapses are of the chemical type (*Figure 3.8*), where substances known as neurotransmitters, e.g. acetylcholine, are involved in the transmission of an impulse. A synapse consists of a presynaptic neurone, with a terminal knob containing vesicles (sacs) filled with the neurotransmitter, the synaptic cleft (gap) and a postsynaptic neurone, whose membrane contains receptor sites. These receptor sites are of different types; each type responds to a specific transmitter chemical, or to several.

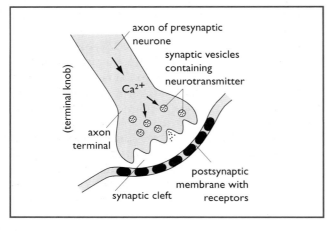

Figure 3.8 Synapse.

The complex events occurring at a chemical synapse can be summarized as:

- The action potential reaches the terminal knob of the axon.
- Gated calcium channels (voltage operated) in the membrane allow calcium ions (from the ECF) into the axon knob. It is important to note that the calcium ions are later pumped out.
- The influx of calcium causes the synaptic vesicles to fuse with the presynaptic membrane and release neurotransmitter into the cleft. It is generally accepted that neurotransmitter is released by exocytosis (see Chapter 1).
- Released neurotransmitter diffuses across the gap, which accounts for the small delay, and attaches to special receptor sites on the postsynaptic membrane.
- The neurotransmitter alters the potential difference of the postsynaptic membrane by opening channels that allow the movement of ions, or by using a series of reactions requiring a second messenger to cause a membrane response. The postsynaptic membrane potential may be excitatory, when sufficient impulses will produce the threshold depolarization required to generate an action potential in the axon distal to the synapse, or inhibitory, when hyperpolarization occurs and no action potential in the axon is possible (see pages 72–73).

Special Focus **Some drugs, chemicals and toxins acting at the synapse**

Drugs

Antagonist drugs such as atropine compete with acetylcholine at the postsynaptic receptor sites in parasympathetic neurones supplying the heart muscle, smooth muscle and exocrine glands, e.g. salivary glands. Atropine may be used to increase heart rate when an abnormally slow heart rate (bradycardia) has occurred following a myocardial infarction ('heart attack').

Pancuronium (synthetic curare) is a non-depolarizing blocking agent which competes with acetylcholine at the postsynaptic receptors, but it acts at neuromuscular junctions. It is used to relax skeletal muscle during surgery and sometimes in situations where ventilation is being provided by intermittent positive pressure respiration/ventilation (IPPR/V).

Anticholinesterase drugs such as neostigmine enhance synaptic transmission by inhibiting cholinesterase, resulting in the prolonged action of acetylcholine. It is used in the treatment of myasthenia gravis (see Chapter 17) and to reverse the effects of neuromuscular blocking agents.

Chemicals and Toxins

Organophosphorus pesticides produce their toxic effects by irreversibly inhibiting the action of cholinesterase at the synapse – they are known as anticholinesterases. People who have contact with these pesticides have bradycardia, vomiting and diarrhoea, and pulmonary oedema. These effects are reversed by the administration of cholinesterase reactivators which dislodge the enzyme from the receptor sites.

Toxins present in the venom of some snakes cause their paralytic effects by preventing the release of acetylcholine and by blocking the postsynaptic receptors.

The botulinum toxin is a neurotoxin produced by the food-poisoning bacterium *Clostridium botulinum*. It blocks the release of acetylcholine at the synapse – there is progressive paralysis which, without treatment, causes respiratory difficulties. The disease known as botulism is usually acquired from poorly preserved foods and has a high mortality rate.

The integration of synaptic transmission is a complex process involving hundreds of neurones. Some of these are excitatory and others inhibitory, and, as you would expect, not all are active at any one time.

The activity of many axon terminals, or the rapid production of impulses from a few, is required before the threshold is reached and the postsynaptic neurone can produce an action potential. This process, called **summation**, sorts, adds and integrates the effects of excitatory and inhibitory synapse activity on a temporal (when one or more axon terminals are producing rapid impulses) or spatial (when many axon terminals are active at the same time) basis.

The total process of synaptic transmission takes a few milliseconds and concludes with the destruction of the neurotransmitter by enzymes, e.g. cholinesterases destroy acetylcholine. This is necessary before the synapse can function again.

Neurotransmitters

Detailed consideration of specific neurotransmitters can be found in *Table 3.1* and in other chapters in Section 3. Neurotransmitters facilitate the passage of nerve impulses in all parts of the nervous system; they allow the vital connections between neurones, and between neurones, muscles and glands. Many different chemicals act as neurotransmitters, some of which are excitatory and others inhibitory. The major chemical groups of neurotransmitters are: monoamines; amino acids; and neuropeptides, a large group of substances acting as neurotransmitters.

Many neurones produce more than one neurotransmitter – this is termed co-transmission and is known to modify function. The release and activity of neurotransmitters is also subject to modulation by other chemical mediators, termed neuromodulators, which can inhibit or enhance neurotransmitter effects; for example, adrenaline and noradrenaline both inhibit acetylcholine. Modulation of neurotransmitter activity may be presynaptic or postsynaptic. There is considerable interest in chemical neuromodulators such as nitric oxide (NO), which, with other possible actions, appears to act like a neurotransmitter. There are differences, however: nitric oxide diffuses through membranes, synthesis occurs in neural and nonneural tissue, and it is not stored in vesicles. Nitric oxide is thought to be involved in areas such as learning, memory, nociception, gastric emptying and penile erection, and because it also acts as a free radical (see Chapter 1) it is implicated in the brain tissue damage seen in stroke. Readers requiring more details about nitric oxide and neuromodulation are directed to Rang *et al.*, (1995).

The list of neurotransmitters and neuromodulators is certainly not complete – more examples are being discovered as research continues.

Abnormal Function **Problems with nerve transmission**

Impulse transmission depends upon adequate stimuli, and the physical integrity of the neurone and functioning synapses.

Many drugs affect nerve transmission (see Special Focus box), including sedatives and local anaesthetics, e.g. lignocaine, which stops impulse transmission by blocking sodium channels, especially in fibres carrying pain impulses.

A nerve subjected to temporary pressure or extreme cold will not get enough blood and the consequent lack of oxygen reduces impulse transmission. When you get up after sitting on your leg, the 'pins and needles' you feel is caused by resumption of impulse transmission as the pressure on the nerve is released. Numbness of the fingers and toes on a winter's day is caused by the effect of cold on nerve function. Apart from pressure and cold, nerve impulse transmission may be disordered by factors which include:

- Trauma, where the nerve is subjected to prolonged compression, is crushed or severed.
- Bacterial toxins, such as those produced by the bacterium causing tetanus.
- The effects of viruses, e.g. herpes zoster (shingles) and human immunodeficiency virus (HIV) (see Chapter 19).

- Toxic metals, e.g. lead and mercury.
- Problems with neurotransmitters, e.g. lack of dopamine causes the condition of parkinsonism (see Chapter 4).
- Demyelination, with loss of impulse conduction, e.g. multiple sclerosis (see page 69). Neuropathies (nerve diseases) caused by lack of vitamin B_{12} and the Guillain–Barre syndrome are also caused by demyelination.
- Nutritional problems, e.g. lack of vitamin B causing peripheral neuropathy and spinal cord degeneration.
- Alcohol misuse.

Nursing Practice Application **Pressure on nerves**

Bandages, plaster casts, splints and crutches can cause pressure to be exerted on nerves (see also Chapter 5). Information for patients should reflect an awareness of this fact and should stress the importance of watching for altered nerve function caused by pressure, e.g. tingling 'pins and needles' or numbness, and reporting problems as soon as they are noticed. Tingling and numbness may also be caused by compression of blood vessels (see Chapter 17, Person-Centred Study – Dave).

Table 3.1 Neurotransmitters	
Neurotransmitter and production sites	**Action: excitatory (E) or inhibitory (I)**
(1) *Monoamines*	
Acetylcholine (classified by some authorities as a monoamine) – CNS: brain PNS: skeletal muscle neuromuscular junctions, some synapses of the autonomic nerves	Both (E) and (I) depending on site
Noradrenaline – CNS: brain PNS: some synapses of the autonomic nerves; adrenal medulla also secretes noradrenaline as one of its hormones	Both (E) and (I) depending on site and type of receptor
Dopamine – CNS: basal nuclei and extrapyramidal tracts PNS: sympathetic system	Mostly (E) but may be (I) in sympathetic system
5-hydroxytryptamine (5-HT) (serotonin) – CNS: brain and spinal cord	(I)
Histamine – CNS: brain. Also released as part of inflammatory response	Functions via a 'second messenger' system
(2) *Amino acids*	
Gamma-aminobutyric acid (GABA) – CNS: brain and spinal cord	(I)
Glycine – CNS: brain and spinal cord	(I)
Glutamate – CNS: brain and spinal cord	(E)
(3) *Neuropeptides*	
Enkephalin – CNS: brain and spinal cord; pituitary gland	(I) Acts as a natural opiate (painkiller)
Endorphins – see Enkephalin	
Somatostatin – CNS: brain; also secreted by the pancreas	(I) Also inhibits growth hormone release
Tachykinins, e.g. Substance P – CNS: brain PNS: sensory nerves carrying pain impulses	(E) Concerned with the transmission of pain and has an excitatory effect on nerves supplying the intestine. Also affects smooth muscle
(4) *Substances also considered to act as neurotransmitters / neuromodulators*	
Adenosine triphosphate (ATP) Neuropeptide Y (NPY) Prostaglandins Vasoactive intestinal peptide (VIP) Nitric oxide Cholecystokinin	
N.B. Remember that some neurotransmitters also function as hormones – the functional divisions are definitely blurred.	

Table 3.1. Neurotransmitters.

Healthier Living Keeping nerves 'in shape'

Throughout this book there are many reminders about just how important diet is in health maintenance. To stay healthy nerves need a balanced diet which includes the correct nutrients in the right amounts. Nerve impulse transmission depends on having the right levels of sodium, potassium and calcium in the body fluids, but these usually cause no problems unless fluid/electrolyte homeostasis is disturbed (see Chapter 2). Nerves need vitamins of the B group, especially folate and vitamin B_{12}, for myelination. Older adults, vegans

and others may have diets containing low levels of these vitamins (through lack of knowledge, financial constraints or choice). Those at risk for vitamin-B deficiencies need to increase their intake of meat, liver, eggs and dairy products, where acceptable, and fortified breakfast cereals or vitamin supplements. Those individuals unable to absorb vitamin B_{12} from the small bowel, e.g. those lacking the intrinsic factor (pernicious anaemia or after gastric surgery), will need regular intramuscular injections of the vitamin.

NB Folate deficiency and congenital abnormalities are discussed in Chapter 4.

Another way to keep nerves healthy is to keep alcohol intake within recommended limits. Excess alcohol is toxic to nerves and misuse may prevent vitamin-B absorption by causing gastritis (inflamed stomach lining does not produce intrinsic factor). Additionally, where alcohol is taken instead of food, the intake of vitamins B may be deficient.

The Reflex Arc

Reflexes are rapid involuntary motor responses to sensory inputs. They illustrate the integration of the fundamental concepts considered in this chapter – sensory receptors, neurones, nerve impulse transmission, synapses and effectors (*Figure 3.9*).

There are several types of reflex (see Chapters 5 and 6), but an example of a simple reflex action would be the events (reflex arc) initiated when you touch a needle. Sensory receptors in the skin send impulses through the sensory neurone (PNS) to the spinal cord (CNS), where synapses and an interneurone are used to transmit the impulse to the motor neurone (PNS) connected to the muscle (effector). Muscular contraction causes withdrawal of your finger from the needle.

There are situations where reflexes can be modified by voluntary control. For example, your parents have a very old and valuable dinner service. One mealtime you pick

up a very hot serving dish but, instead of dropping the dish (reflex), you hold on long enough to put it down safely. You modify the reflex because the dish is irreplaceable!

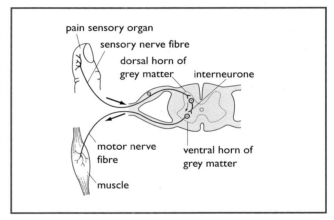

Figure 3.9 The reflex arc.

Summary/Check List

Introduction and basic organization – nervous system.
Nerve tissue – development. Neurones, Nursing Practice Application – brains need oxygen, cell body, axon, dendrites, myelination, Nursing Practice Application – myelination and motor development. Family-centred Study – Lisa, Darren, Carol and Tony. Supporting cells (neuroglia) – Schwann cells, oligodendrocytes, astrocytes, microglia, ependymal cells. Nerves – endoneurium, perineurium, epineurium. Sensory receptors – structural and functional classifications, adaptation, sensory unit. Nursing Practice Application – sensory overload.

Nerve impulse – transmission – resting potential, action potential, all-or-none phenomenon, thresholds, refractory periods, propagation of impulse, saltatory conduction, impulse transmission speed. Synapses – electrical, chemical, summation, Special Focus – some drugs, chemicals and toxins acting at the synapse. Neurotransmitters – monoamines, amino acids and neuropeptides. Neuromodulators. Problems with nerve transmission. Nursing Practice Application – pressure on nerves. Healthier Living – keeping nerves 'in shape'.
Reflex arc – basic components, example of simple reflex, voluntary modification.

Self Test

1 The brain and spinal cord are known collectively as the:
  (a) peripheral nervous system;
  (b) central nervous system;
  (c) voluntary nervous system;
  (d) autonomic nervous system.
2 Describe a typical neurone.
3 Which of the following statements are true?
  (a) neuroglial cells can replicate;
  (b) Schwann cells produce myelin in the CNS;
  (c) astrocytes are part of the 'blood–brain barrier';
  (d) myelin increases transmission speed.
4 Put the following sensory receptors with their correct function:
  (a) proprioceptor;
  (b) temperature;
  (c) photoreceptor;
  (d) chemical environment;
  (e) thermoreceptor;
  (f) pressure;
  (g) chemoreceptor;
  (h) light;
  (i) baroreceptor;
  (j) position sense.
5 Describe the events that cause an action potential.
6 What are the components of a chemical synapse?
7 Which of the following neurotransmitters is found at the neuromuscular junction in skeletal muscle?
  (a) dopamine;
  (b) noradrenaline;
  (c) acetylcholine;
  (d) γ-aminobutyric acid.
8 Which of the following statements about demyelinating conditions are true?
  (a) physical trauma causes loss of myelin;
  (b) multiple sclerosis is a common demyelinating condition;
  (c) poor absorption of vitamin B_{12} may lead to demyelination;
  (d) the effects of demyelination are always the same.

Answers

1 b.
2 See page 68.
3 a, c, d.
4 a–j, c–h, e–b, g–d and i–f.
5 See pages 71–73.
6 See page 74.
7 c.
8 b, c.

References

Delieu J, Keady J (1996) The biology of Alzheimer's disease. *Br J Nurs* 5(3):162–167.

Edwards CRW, Bouchier IAD, Haslett C *et al.* Eds (1995) *Davidson's Principles and Practice of Medicine*, 17th edn. Edinburgh: Churchill Livingstone.

Further Reading

Greenberg DA, Aminoff MJ, Simon RP (1993) *Clinical Neurology*, 2nd edn. Englewood Cliffs, NJ: Prentice-Hall.
Matthews GG (1991) *Cellular Physiology of Nerve and Muscle*. Oxford: Oxford Scientific Publications.

Rang HP, Dale MM, Ritter JM (1995) *Pharmacology*, 3rd edn. Edinburgh: Churchill Livingstone.

Useful Address

Multiple Sclerosis Society of
Great Britain and Northern Ireland
25 Effie Road
London SW6 1EE

The Central Nervous System

Overview

- *Central nervous system (CNS) – development, protection, blood supply.*
- *Brain, spinal cord.*
- *Sensory pathways, motor pathways.*

Learning Outcomes

After studying Chapter 4 you should be able to:

- Outline the development of the central nervous system.
- Describe the meninges and their function.
- Describe the ventricular system and the formation, circulation and functions of cerebrospinal fluid.
- Explain what is meant by the 'blood–brain barrier'.
- Explain how adequate blood supplies to the brain are maintained.
- Identify the main areas of the brain and their function.
- Describe the cerebral hemispheres.
- Discuss the functional areas of the cerebral cortex.
- Describe the location and role of the basal nuclei, thalamus, hypothalamus, epithalamus and pituitary gland.
- Discuss the internal capsule, pyramidal and extrapyramidal motor tracts.
- Discuss the effects of damage caused by cerebrovascular accident (CVA).
- Discuss the effects of extrapyramidal disorders such as parkinsonism.
- Identify the different areas of the brainstem and discuss their role in controlling vital functions.
- Describe the structure and function of the cerebellum.
- Describe the reticular formation and its role in consciousness and sleep.
- Discuss the nursing observations used to assess neurological status and describe how each is affected when intracranial pressure is raised.
- Describe the limbic system and its links with emotions.
- Outline the stages and types of memory and the learning process.
- Describe the structure of the spinal cord.
- Describe the major sensory and motor tracts in the spinal cord.
- Describe pain transmission and perception, and discuss methods of pain relief.
- Describe the effects of spinal injury and spinal shock.

Key Words

Basal nuclei – islands of grey matter situated deep within the white matter of the cerebral hemispheres.

Blood–brain barrier – the structural arrangement involving astrocytes that ensures that brain capillary walls are relatively impermeable. Generally prevents the passage of harmful substances from the blood to the brain.

Brainstem – collective name for the midbrain, pons varolii and the medulla oblongata.

Key Words cont.

Cerebellum – part of the hindbrain situated below the cerebrum and behind the pons varolii.

Cerebral cortex – the thin layer of grey matter which covers the white matter of the cerebral hemispheres.

Cerebrospinal fluid (CSF) – fluid found in the ventricles of the brain and between the membranes that cover the brain and spinal cord. It provides a protective cushion around these vital structures.

Cerebrum – the forebrain; divided into hemispheres, it forms the largest part of the brain.

Decussation – crossing over, i.e. of the motor nerves.

Meninges – three protective membranes (dura, arachnoid and pia maters) which cover the brain and spinal cord.

Spinal cord – the part of the central nervous system continuous with the medulla oblongata which runs inside the vertebral canal to the lumbar region.

Ventricles – cavities in the brain which contain CSF.

Introduction

The central nervous system (CNS) consists of the **brain** and **spinal cord** (*Figure 4.1*). It has been mentioned in Chapter 3, but now a more detailed approach will be taken. The CNS is the vital integration and communications network that controls and regulates every body function and every minute detail of our unique behaviour. As you would expect, the structure and functioning of the 'command centre' of the body are extremely complex.

Many areas are as yet poorly understood, but our knowledge of the structure and, more significantly, function continues to increase. This is especially so since the advent of advanced medical imaging technology, which has considerably increased access to the CNS.

Development of the CNS

Development of the brain and spinal cord has started by the third week of embryonic development. A neural plate formed from the embryonic tissue ectoderm (see Chapter 1) eventually gives rise to all the neural tissue. This plate grows and folds in on itself (invaginates) and eventually fuses to form the neural tube – the structure which, after many changes in shape, becomes the brain, spinal cord and **ventricles** (see *Figure 4.2*). The very early embryo has three primary brain vesicles: the prosencephalon (forebrain), mesencephalon (midbrain) and rhombencephalon (hindbrain). During embryonic development the forebrain becomes the telencephalon (endbrain), which grows rapidly to form the two cerebral hemispheres (responsible for higher functions) and the diencephalon (between brain), which in turn gives rise to the thalamus, hypothalamus and epithalamus. The midbrain becomes the adult midbrain.

The remaining adult brain structures are derived from the hindbrain, which divides into the metencephalon (afterbrain), to form the pons varolii and **cerebellum,** and the myelencephalon (spinal brain), which becomes the medulla oblongata (*Table 4.1*).

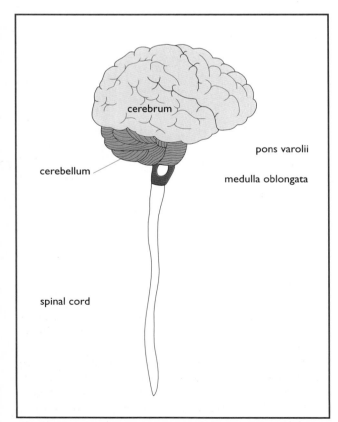

Figure 4.1 The central nervous system.

Special Focus **Discovering the brain – imaging techniques**

Computed tomography (CT scan): imaging technique that uses computer-linked X-ray equipment to provide cross-sectional views through various body planes. CT scans are used widely to investigate CNS structures.

Magnetic resonance imaging (MRI): a technique that utilizes the response of hydrogen nuclei within tissues when exposed to a strong magnetic field. Used to investigate function and to differentiate between different disease processes in soft tissues such as the brain. MRI is especially useful in the demonstration of CNS tumours, demyelination and other degenerative conditions. Recent innovations in MRI technology allow for three-dimensional images and the ability to link brain blood flow with activity.

Positron emission tomography (PET): an imaging technique that uses radioactive isotopes (very short half-life; see Chapter 2) to scan metabolically active tissues. The isotopes emit positrons (positively charged subatomic particles) which cause the emission of gamma radiation when they react with electrons in areas of high metabolic activity. Special equipment detects the gamma radiation in these tissues and records levels of activity. PET is used for research into brain function and for obtaining information about disease processes such as those occurring in Alzheimer's disease.

Ultrasonography (US): an imaging technique where high frequency sound waves are used to produce an image. Ultrasonography is not very useful for investigating the CNS because its surrounding bone is not penetrated by the sound waves. It does, however, have other applications, e.g. imaging in obstetrics and scanning other body structures.

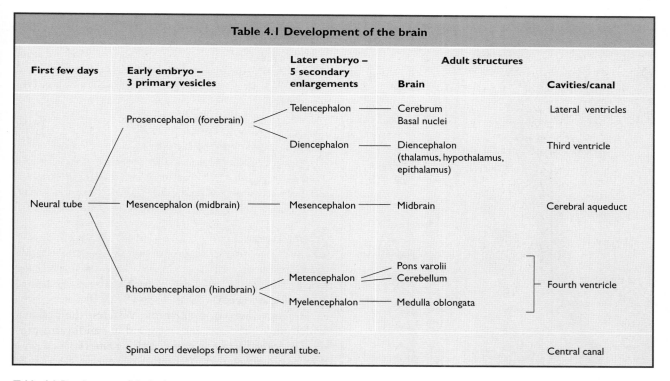

Table 4.1 Development of the brain.

CNS development also shows some gender differences – the male fetus is exposed to the male hormone testosterone, which appears to lead to variations in brain structure which may account for behavioural differences after birth.

During pregnancy the developing nervous system is vulnerable to any damage affecting formation and subsequent function. This is especially so in the early stages when several factors are associated with damage to the fetal nervous system, e.g. microorganisms, drugs and alcohol, lack of oxygen and lack of folate (folic acid) – a B vitamin (see Nursing Practice Application – Folate and CNS development).

After birth the CNS continues to develop; this development is especially important from birth to 4 years but continues until 13–15 years, when adult brain size is reached (1300–1500 g) and myelination is complete. The male brain is larger than that of the female, but brain size is proportional to body size.

Nursing Practice Application **Folate and CNS development**

Common developmental problems of the CNS, such as spina bifida (which may be associated with hydrocephaly; see page 85) and anencephaly, occur when the neural tube is developing. The figure for neural tube defects (NTDs) present at birth is 0.3/1000 in the UK. Some NTDs are associated with structural defects in the vertebral column, which can leave the delicate neural tissue exposed and unprotected. This can result in varying degrees of abnor-

mality. They may present no problems, cause disability or be incompatible with life.

NTDs have been linked to inadequate intakes of folate before conception and during the early weeks of pregnancy. The results of a study by Wald *et al.* (1991) confirmed that folate supplements should be taken by women planning to conceive and continued during early pregnancy if a previous pregnancy has been affected by a NTD. The same report also stated

that all women of childbearing age should have a diet containing adequate folate.

Health professionals, especially nurses, midwives and health visitors, can improve folate awareness amongst the public and hopefully reduce the risk of NTDs occurring. The Health Education Authority launched a major campaign, supported by literature (HEA, 1996), to encourage all women to increase their folate intake before conception and for the first 12 weeks of pregnancy.

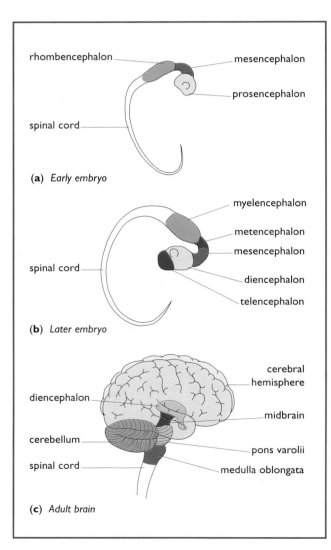

(a) *Early embryo*

(b) *Later embryo*

(c) *Adult brain*

Figure 4.2 Development of the brain – embryo to adult.

Protection for the CNS

The brain and spinal cord are well protected from external trauma and adverse internal changes by the skull bones and vertebrae, the **meninges**, ventricles and **cerebrospinal fluid** (CSF), the '**blood–brain barrier**' and an elaborate blood supply.

Skull and vertebrae
The brain is entirely enclosed by the skull and the spinal cord runs within the bones of the vertebral column (see Chapter 18), deep inside the body.

Meninges
The three meningeal membranes – the dura mater, the arachnoid mater and the pia mater – cover and enclose the brain and spinal cord. They are formed from connective tissue (*Figure 4.3*).

The outer meninges is the tough, fibrous dura mater, which lines the skull and vertebral column and forms double folds – the tentorium cerebelli and falx cerebri – which divide areas in the brain and enclose the venous sinuses which drain blood from the brain. The space between the dura mater and the skull/vertebrae is called the epidural space – injection of local anaesthetic drugs into this space in the lumbosacral region relieves pain. This route is often used during labour.

The middle meninges is the fragile, web-like arachnoid mater, which is separated from the dura mater by the subdural space. Beneath the arachnoid mater is the subarachnoid space, which is filled with cerebrospinal fluid. Bleeding into this space is known as subarachnoid haemorrhage and may result from the rupture of an aneurysm (an abnormal dilatation in the wall of an artery) or a cerebral bleed.

The inner meninges, or pia mater, is a fragile membrane containing many tiny blood vessels. It is in close contact with the brain and spinal cord, where it follows every contour.

Bacterial or viral inflammation of the meninges is known as meningitis – a serious condition characterized by 'flu-like' illness, headache, neck stiffness, pyrexia, vomiting and photophobia, and in some types a skin rash.

Ventricular system and cerebrospinal fluid

The ventricular system [see *Figure 4.4(a)*] of cavities within the brain consists of the two lateral ventricles, located in the **cerebrum**, which communicate with the third ventricle through the intraventricular foramina (a foramen is an opening). The third ventricle is situated between the two parts of the thalamus (see page 91); it is connected to the fourth ventricle by the cerebral aqueduct. The fourth ventricle, between the cerebellum and pons varolii (see *Figure 4.14*), is continuous with a central canal in the spinal cord.

Cerebrospinal fluid is produced by choroid plexuses – specialized capillaries derived from pia mater and covered by ependymal cells, which line the ventricles (a plexus is a network of blood vessels or nerves). The CSF is a crystal-clear, slightly alkaline fluid derived from blood plasma (Chapter 9). As much as 300–500 ml/day is produced, but only about 125–150 ml circulates within the system because it is continually being secreted and reabsorbed. It exerts a pressure of 1.33–4 kPa (10–30 mmHg), depending on body position. Its specific gravity is approximately 1.005, which is similar to that of the brain tissue. Specialized ependymal cells (see Chapter 3) with microvilli promote the circulation of CSF.

CSF consists of:
- Water.
- Proteins, e.g. globulins, albumin (total protein, at 100–400 mg/l, is lower than in plasma).
- Glucose 2.5–4.0 mmol/l; (a lower concentration than in plasma).
- Chloride, at 120–170 mmol/l, is higher than in plasma (other electrolytes differ – CSF has more sodium and less potassium and calcium than plasma).
- A few leucocytes.
- A small amount of waste, e.g. urea.

The CSF enters the subarachnoid space through foramina in the fourth ventricle and circulates around the brain and spinal cord with a small volume in the central canal. Reabsorption of CSF occurs through the arachnoid granulations – portions of arachnoid mater which project into the venous blood sinuses [see *Figure 4.4 (b)*]. The spinal cord ends at the level of the first/second lumbar vertebra (third in young children) and is secured to the vertebra by a modified portion of pia mater called the filum terminale (*Figure 4.3*). The fluid-filled space below the spinal cord, which contains the last spinal nerves (the cauda equina) (see *Figure 4.19*), provides a safe area for obtaining specimens of CSF by lumbar puncture.

Functions of CSF are:
- To provide a barrier/cushion between the brain and skull that acts as a shock absorber in the event of trauma.
- Involvement in brain metabolism by exchanging substances between brain and CSF.
- To support the CNS by providing the correct external pressure.

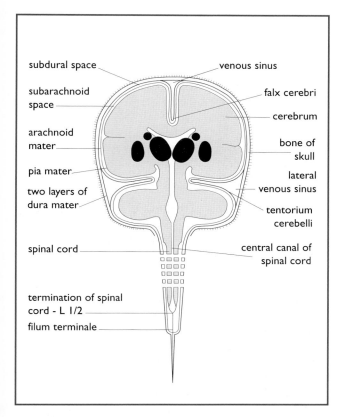

subdural space
venous sinus
subarachnoid space
falx cerebri
cerebrum
arachnoid mater
bone of skull
pia mater
two layers of dura mater
lateral venous sinus
tentorium cerebelli
spinal cord
central canal of spinal cord
termination of spinal cord - L 1/2
filum terminale

Figure 4.3 The meninges.

Nursing Practice Application **Lumbar puncture**

The diagnosis of conditions such as meningitis, multiple sclerosis and sub-arachnoid haemorrhage can be expedited by examining a specimen of CSF obtained by lumbar puncture. This involves the introduction of a hollow needle (with local anaesthesia) into the subarachnoid space between lumbar vertebrae 3 and 4 or 4 and 5; using these spaces ensures that the spinal cord is not damaged.

Lumbar puncture should not be under-taken when a person has raised intracra-nial pressure. Release of pressure during the puncture could cause the brainstem to be forced through the foramen magnum (see page 96) with serious results, including unconsciousness.

One nursing role is to ensure that the person understands what will happen, both during the lumbar puncture and after. The person is positioned either on their side with head flexed and knees drawn up towards the abdomen or strad-dling an upright chair – to open the spaces between the lumbar vertebrae. To prevent infection, sterile equipment is used and staff must adhere strictly to aseptic techniques. As well as obtaining specimens, the pressure of the CSF can be measured by attaching a manometer to the needle. Various drugs can be administered into the subarachnoid space (intrathecally) at the time of lumbar puncture – antimicrobials in meningitis, cytotoxic drugs in childhood leukaemias

and drugs to reduce muscle spasm, e.g. baclofen. Intrathecal administration can overcome the problem of getting the drug across the blood–brain barrier.

After lumbar puncture, the person should lie down for up to 24 hours with only one pillow and be advised to sit up only very gradually. This prevents headache caused by the loss of CSF and the reduction in its cushioning effect. Care planning should include: provision of adequate fluids to replace CSF volume, prescribed analgesia for headache or backache, reporting leg pain, which can indicate nerve damage, neurological observations where appropriate (see page 96) and checking the puncture site for CSF leakage.

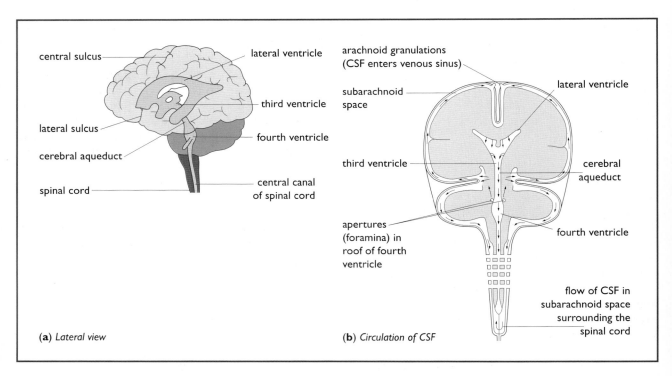

(a) *Lateral view*

(b) *Circulation of CSF*

Figure 4.4 Position of the ventricular system. (a) Lateral view (shown on intact brain); (b) circulation of cerebrospinal fluid (simplified).

Blood–brain barrier

In common with other parts of the body, the brain requires a stable internal environment for its proper functioning, but unlike other structures it is unable to tolerate even the smallest variation in the composition of its extracellular fluid. A special structural and functional arrangement of capillary endothelial (epithelium) cells forming tight junc-tions, a basal lamina and astrocytes (see Chapter 3) ensures that brain capillaries are relatively impermeable, and makes up the blood–brain barrier. This allows the pas-

---

Abnormal Function **Problems with CSF circulation and reabsorption**

....

Obstruction to the circulation of CSF or a failure to reabsorb causes hydrocephaly, or 'water on the brain', where excess CSF is present. This may be caused by problems with CNS development, such as neural tube defects, or may be secondary to infections and tumours. It

causes raised intracranial pressure and eventual damage to the ventricles and brain tissue. When hydrocephaly occurs in babies the bones of the skull, which are not fused, are pushed apart and the head circumference increases (skull structure in babies is discussed in Chapter 18). The

management of hydrocephaly involves the use of specialized shunts/valves, which drain excess CSF into the right side of the heart, a major vein or peritoneal cavity from where it enters the circulation.

---

sage of nutrients required by the neurones, but generally prevents the entry of substances which affect function and the loss of vital substances from the brain cells. There are, however, exceptions – lipid-soluble molecules such as fat, alcohol and drugs, e.g. anaesthetics, can cross the barrier and affect brain function. In babies and young children the barrier is less effective and allows the passage of substances such as the bile pigment bilirubin (see Chapter 14) and lead, which may damage the brain.

The relative impermeability of the blood–brain barrier can pose problems in treating brain disorders – drugs need to be able to diffuse through the barrier or cross by carrier transfer. Sometimes the disease process makes it easier, e.g. the inflammation of meningitis disrupts the barrier and allows systemically administered penicillin to cross. Drugs can also be given intrathecally (see Nursing Practice Application – Lumbar puncture).

Blood supply to the brain

It is essential that the brain receives sufficient oxygenated blood to maintain its complex metabolism (see Chapter 3). About 750–800 ml of blood circulates around the brain every minute, which means that the brain needs to receive approximately 15% of the cardiac output (the amount of blood leaving the heart in 1 min – approximately 5 litres at rest). This amount must be constant and any disruption in supply will rapidly cause changes in brain function; these range from the temporary unconsciousness of fainting (syncope) to the irreversible damage caused by longer disturbances, e.g. cardiac arrest.

To ensure the continuity of supply the brain has two pairs of major arteries (internal carotid arteries and vertebral arteries) feeding into a circular arrangement of arteries (circle of Willis) situated at the base of the brain (see Chapter 10). Branches from this circle maintain the blood supply to different areas of the brain; this means that a problem in one branch does not cut off supply to the whole brain.

Blood flow can be varied in response to changes in blood carbon dioxide and pH, and less so to oxygen levels, which

are continually monitored by the chemoreceptors; flow can also be diverted to active areas needing more oxygen. This is a good example of the ability of the brain to regulate its own homeostasis – autoregulation. Venous blood leaves the brain in blood plexuses and sinuses, which drain into the internal jugular vein and then into the superior vena cava, which carries blood to the right atrium of the heart (see Chapter 10).

The Brain

The brain is a semisolid (soft consistency between a fluid and a solid) organ that occupies the cranial cavity (*Figure 4.5*). It consists of the cerebrum (cerebral hemispheres and the **basal nuclei**), diencephalon (thalamus, hypothalamus and epithalamus), **brainstem** (midbrain, pons varolii, medulla oblongata and reticular formation) and cerebellum, which is part of the hindbrain.

Cerebrum

The cerebrum is the most highly developed and sophisticated part of the human brain. It consists of two cerebral hemispheres and the basal nuclei.

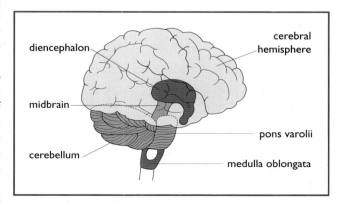

Figure 4.5 The brain.

Cerebral hemispheres

The cerebral hemispheres (*Figure 4.6*) are situated in the anterior and middle cranial fossae (depression in a bone) and form the bulk of the brain mass. The midsagittal or longitudinal fissure (split or cleft) divides the right and left hemispheres. They are also separated by a fold of dura mater, the falx cerebri, which dips down into the fissure to the level of the corpus callosum. The corpus callosum (see *Figure 4.11*) is the band of white matter connecting the two hemispheres deep within the brain. The nerve fibres in the corpus callosum are concerned with communication between the two hemispheres. On the outer surface of the cerebral hemispheres is a thin (about 3 mm thickness) layer of grey matter called the **cerebral cortex**. This cortex covers the white matter, which forms the major part of the hemispheres (although deep within the cortex there are isolated islands of grey matter – the basal nuclei; see *Figure 4.11*). The surface of the cerebral cortex has many folds and ridges. The raised parts of these convolutions are called gyri (singular, gyrus), which are separated by furrows – the sulci (singular, sulcus). Folding allows a much greater surface area of cerebral cortex to be contained within the skull.

Each hemisphere is divided into lobes: frontal, parietal, temporal and occipital, named after the bones of the skull that overlie them. Deep sulci separate each lobe: the central sulcus (sulcus of Rolando) between the frontal and parietal lobes, the lateral sulcus (sulcus of Sylvius) separates the frontal from the temporal lobe, and the parieto-occipital sulcus is found between the occipital and parietal lobes (*Figure 4.6*).

The gyri either side of the central sulcus are very important functionally: the precentral gyrus is the main motor area of the cortex and the postcentral gyrus is the main sensory area. The white matter lying under the nerve cells of the cortex consists of three types of myelinated nerve fibres which form large tracts:

- Commissures, which connect the two cerebral hemispheres, the most important being the corpus callosum.
- Association fibres, which allow communication between individual gyri and between the lobes of the same hemisphere.
- Projection fibres, which connect the cerebral cortex with other areas of the brain, sensory receptors (afferents) and effectors (efferents).

The internal capsule (see *Figure 4.11*) is an area between the thalamus and the basal nuclei. It is formed by projection fibres massing together as they pass through the restricted space. Motor fibres leaving the cortex and sensory fibres travelling to the cortex are particularly vulnerable to damage in this area from a stroke (cerebrovascular accident – CVA) (see page 91).

Functional areas of the cerebral cortex

The cerebral cortex is the 'thinking' or conscious part of the brain; it is where you process sensory inputs, communicate, understand, make decisions and regulate voluntary muscle action. It is responsible for intellect, memory, learning and sense of responsibility, and allows us to differentiate right from wrong (moral sense), i.e. the higher functions.

Knowledge of cortical function has increased tremendously with modern imaging techniques (see page 81) compared with the early 1900's, when Brodmann first proposed a map (with 52 areas) of the cortex. However, although we know a lot about cortical function, it should be remembered that functional areas overlap, and any description is bound to suffer from some degree of simplification (*Figure 4.7*).

Motor areas

The main motor area is the precentral primary motor area situated in the frontal lobes of both hemispheres just anterior to the central sulcus. The neurones in the motor cortex are the pyramidal Betz cells which control voluntary (skeletal) muscle contraction, e.g. deciding to flex your arm to pick up a glass. The fibres of the Betz cell bodies pass through the internal capsule to the medulla, where most cross over to the other side of the brain (**decussation**), with the result that the left motor cortex initiates voluntary movement on the right side of the body and vice versa (contralateral control).

The neurone from the cerebral cortex, known as the upper motor neurone, travels down the pyramidal or corticospinal tracts (see page 90) in the spinal cord to the appropriate level, where it synapses with the cell body of a second neurone, called the lower motor neurone (*Figure 4.8*). This second neurone, which arises in the spinal cord, carries the

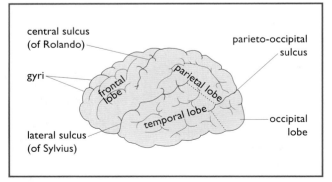

Figure 4.6 Cerebral hemispheres – gyri, sulci and lobes.

nerve impulse from the spinal cord to the neuromuscular junction in the voluntary muscle. One lower motor neurone supplies a number of muscle fibres known as a motor unit. Upper and lower motor neurones are discussed again on pages 100–101; more knowledge is helpful in understanding how neurone damage causes the different effects (paralysis and muscle atrophy) seen in nursing practice.

The body is represented upside-down on the motor cortex, with the toes being controlled from the medial part and the head from the lowest part by the temporal lobe. In *Figure 4.9* the size of some body areas has been distorted, so that the size represents the amount of innervation and hence the number of movements possible; for example, the tongue appears large because it has a large number of motor nerve fibres compared with areas such as the trunk.

Anterior to the precentral motor area is the premotor area (*Figure 4.7*), which exerts a general influence over the motor cortex and is responsible for motor skills requiring manual dexterity. These skills involve several muscle groups in a repeated series or pattern of movements, such as those needed to use a computer keyboard or tie a bow.

Within the premotor area of the dominant hemisphere (usually the left) is the motor speech area – Broca's area. The neurones here are responsible for the muscular movements needed for articulation. Broca's area is situated at the base of the frontal lobe just above the lateral sulcus. In right-handed individuals it is always found in the left hemisphere and in left-handed people it is usually on the left, but may be in the right hemisphere or shared – remember this when you try to make sense of the specific paralysis and speech problems experienced by people after a stroke.

Sensory areas
The main sensory area is the postcentral primary somatosensory cortex, which is situated immediately posterior to the central sulcus in the parietal lobes of both hemispheres. This area receives sensory input from receptors in the skin (temperature, pressure, light touch and pain) and the proprioceptors in voluntary skeletal muscles. It can localize sensation to particular areas of the body, with the sensory input from the right side of the body being received in the left hemisphere and vice versa. Decussation of some sensory fibres occurs in the spinal cord, with others crossing in the medulla. Sensory impulses are transmitted from receptor to sensory cortex through a three-neurone pathway; the first synapse is in the spinal cord or medulla and the second in the thalamus. Again, the parts of the body are represented upside-down on the sensory cortex, with highly sensitive areas drawn much larger than their real size on the sensory homunculus (see *Figure 4.9*); for example, the face and finger tips have many more sensory receptors than the trunk (demonstrated by the intense discomfort of burning your lips on hot food). The distribution of sensory receptors influences our ability to discriminate between two points of stimulation and discern their pattern (see *Figure 4.10*) – this is an important sensation for texture recognition.

The area immediately posterior to the postcentral primary somatosensory cortex is the somatosensory association area, which is concerned with our ability to remember objects and to identify them by touch; for example, with your eyes shut you can differentiate between a tennis ball and a golf ball placed one in each

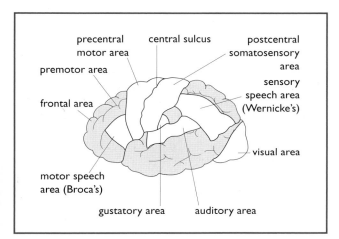

Figure 4.7 Functional areas of the cerebral cortex.

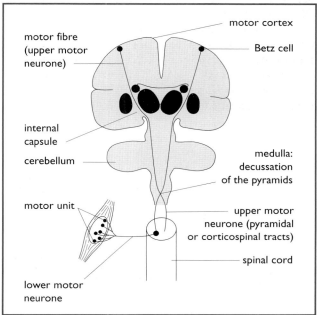

Figure 4.8 Upper and lower motor neurones.

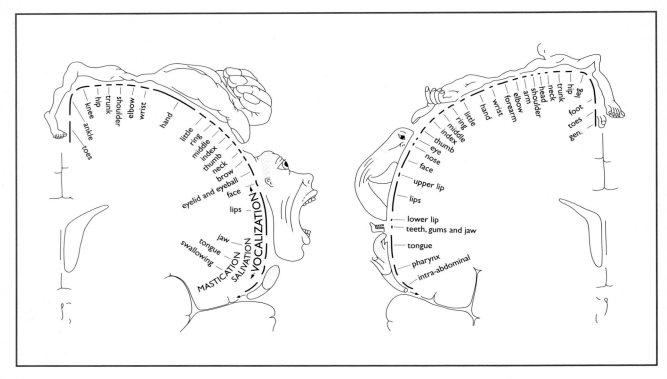

Figure 4.9 Representation of the motor and sensory areas (homunculus). (Adapted with permission of Macmillan Publishing Company from *The Cerebral Cortex of Man* by Wilder Penfield and Theodore Rassmussen. © 1950 Macmillan Publishing Company; copyright renewed © 1978 Theodore Rassmussen.)

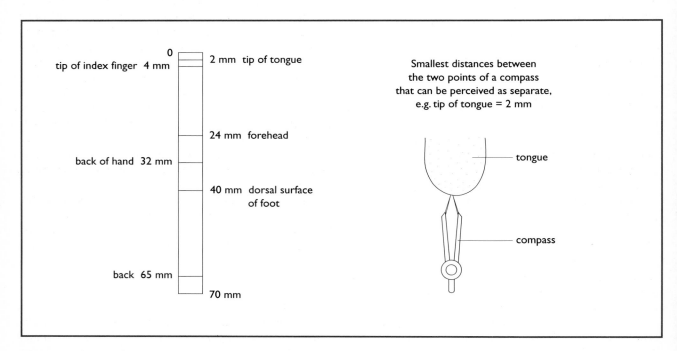

Figure 4.10 Two-point sensory discrimination.

hand. This ability requires the integration of information about different factors such as size, shape and texture. There are connections between this parietal area and the postcentral primary somatosensory cortex, which facilitates the integration of sensory input so that we can perceive specific sensations and know which area of the body is involved.

The sensory cortex has some highly specialized regions which receive sensory input from the sense organs. The sensory speech area, or Wernicke's area, is the part of the temporal lobe where the sounds of speech and visual impulses from written communications are received and understood. This area is situated with the motor speech area in the dominant left hemisphere in right-handed individuals and most left-handed individuals; connection between the two areas allows language to be both understood and articulated.

Affective (emotional) language areas are in the opposite hemispheres to Broca's and Wernicke's areas and put the 'feelings' element into communication; variations in voice intonation are enormous and can range from a gentle sympathetic tone when speaking to bereaved relatives to the sharp tone conveying displeasure.

Impulses from the retinae of the eyes are transmitted through the optic nerves for interpretation by the visual cortex, which is situated in the occipital lobes. Memories of previous experiences allow the recognition of familiar objects and people.

The auditory cortex (hearing) in the temporal lobes close to the lateral sulcus interprets impulses received through the vestibulocochlear (auditory) nerves from the cochlea of the inner ear.

Our ability to perceive taste is provided by the gustatory cortex in the parietal lobe. This receives impulses from the tongue via several different nerves.

The olfactory cortex (smell) is an area in the temporal lobes concerned with the sense of smell and the ability to differentiate odours. It receives impulses from the nose through the olfactory nerves. The functioning of this part of the brain is much more important in species that rely on smell for recognition than it is in humans.

Other cortical areas

Apart from motor and sensory aspects, the cerebral cortex is concerned with a variety of functions that affect our behaviour. The anterior part of the frontal lobe, known as the prefrontal cortex, controls areas such as personality, anticipation of events and their effects, intelligence and learning (cognition). This area of the human brain is more developed than in any other animal and accounts for characteristics which are probably unique to humans, such as moral sense. Characteristics controlled by the prefrontal cortex take time to mature and are greatly influenced by the environmental and social experiences of childhood.

Disorders arising in the prefrontal cortex can cause aggression or apathy. The person may lack concern about personal grooming, or may no longer conform to socially acceptable behaviour or think out the consequences of their actions. These changes can present great difficulties within the family, especially for those involved as informal carers. Nurses can provide support for the family through explanation and information regarding help available, and by listening to fears and feelings of anger or isolation.

Other cortical areas are involved with our ability to interpret events (interpretation areas): complex sensory inputs can be integrated so that you act quickly and appropriately. For example, a toddler pulls a bowl of tomato soup over his or her arm – the sensory input you receive includes hearing the child scream, seeing the red mark on the child's arm (and the stain spreading on the carpet) and, possibly, smelling the soup. You are probably unaware of these individual inputs as you pick up the child and run to the cold tap where immediate first aid with cold water will cool the area and reduce tissue damage.

Right versus left brain

Most functional areas are duplicated in both hemispheres but some, such as the speech areas, appear only on the dominant side of the brain – the left side in the majority of individuals. There seem to be functional differences between the hemispheres, with lateralization of some functions. For example, the dominant left hemisphere tends to control language, numeracy and processes requiring logic whereas the right hemisphere, in this instance, will control the creative, imaginative, intuitive and artistic aspects. Some left-handed individuals have cerebral hemisphere lateralization the opposite way round whereas others have a much more 'even-handed' situation with less lateralization – these people are often dextrous with either hand (ambidextrous).

There is communication between the two sides of the brain, with one side influencing the other. In this way a balance is created between 'sensible' behaviour and the more emotional side of our nature.

Basal nuclei

The basal nuclei are isolated areas of motor nerve cell bodies (grey matter) deep within the white matter of the cerebral hemispheres (see *Figure 4.11*). The basal nuclei are sometimes called the basal ganglia, which is not strictly correct as ganglia are structures of the PNS.

The basal nuclei consist of several masses of tissue (caudate nucleus, putamen and globus pallidus) situated close to the thalamus and internal capsule. When grouped together they are generally known as the corpus striatum (caudate, putamen) and the lentiform nucleus (putamen, globus pallidus), although there is controversy over this naming. Associated structures include the substantia nigra (midbrain), the subthalamic nuclei (diencephalon) and the amygdaloid nucleus, which is part of the limbic system (see page 98). The basal nuclei form part of the extrapyramidal (outside the pyramidal tracts) motor pathways and have connections with many areas of the brain, including the cerebral cortex, the thalamus and each other. Their exact functions are not well understood but they appear to be important in the initiation of slow and prolonged motor activities, such as arm swinging during walking, preventing inappropriate movements, posture and muscle tone. The basal nuclei allow us to do more than one activity at once and appear to play a part in how we remember the actions needed to perform a particular motor skill (see page 98).

Abnormal Function **Problems with basal nuclei function**

Functioning of the basal nuclei depends upon the release of the inhibitory neurotransmitter dopamine by the substantia nigra. When dopamine levels are reduced or response to dopamine is impaired, the basal nuclei no longer exert their inhibitory influences over motor activities. This leads to the development of the physical features of parkinsonism/Parkinson's disease. This is a common extrapyramidal condition that mainly affects older people. It is characterized by:

- Tremor, especially in the hands ('pill rolling').
- Hesitation in starting movements such as the initiation of walking – affected people shuffle and have difficulty stopping once they are moving.
- Rigidity, which causes a mask-like facial expression.

Drugs such as L-dopa (a precursor or forerunner of dopamine) are helpful in relieving the problems of parkinsonism, but may cease to be effective after prolonged use. Recent developments involving the transplantation of dopamine-producing fetal tissue into the brains of affected individuals have produced some encouraging results and the reduction of disability. There are, however, some very important ethical issues (the use of fetal tissue) and practical problems to be addressed before this technique becomes widely available. Parkinsonism has also been linked to the misuse of drugs (contaminated with methyl-phenyl-tetrahydropyridine – MPTP – which destroys neurones in the substantia nigra) by heroin addicts and exposure to herbicides, e.g. paraquat, which is similar to MPTP (Edwards et al., 1995).

Another example of an extrapyramidal disorder is Huntington's disease, a hereditary condition which appears during adult life (usually during the 30s and 40s). Destruction of the basal nuclei causes involuntary jerky movements of the facial muscles and limbs. Later it progresses to dementia as the cerebral cortex degenerates and eventual death. It is associated with normal dopamine levels with a lack of γ-aminobutyric acid (GABA, see Chapter 3) inhibition. Efforts to reduce the incidence of this tragic condition are currently centred around genetic screening and counselling services, but many couples have had their children before screening occurs.

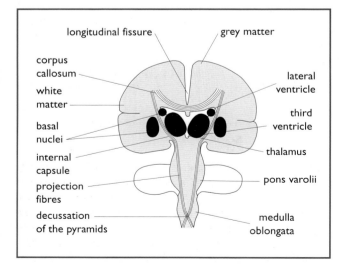

longitudinal fissure — grey matter

corpus callosum

white matter

basal nuclei

internal capsule

projection fibres

decussation of the pyramids

lateral ventricle

third ventricle

thalamus

pons varolii

medulla oblongata

Figure 4.11 Cerebrum – white matter, basal nuclei, internal capsule and thalamus.

Internal capsule

The internal capsule is the area between the basal nuclei and the thalamus; it is formed by the efferent and afferent projection fibres that connect the cerebral cortex to other parts of the brain, muscles and sensory receptors (*Figure 4.11*). The motor fibres that pass through the internal capsule form the pyramidal tracts (named for the pyramids in the medulla) or corticospinal tracts, which are the major motor pathways to the voluntary muscles. The motor activities controlled by these tracts are influenced (inhibited) by the extrapyramidal tracts, which pass outside the internal capsule.

It is important to note that the tremor and rigidity of Parkinson's disease can be explained by the loss of basal nuclei extrapyramidal inhibition, which allows the pyramidal influences to become exaggerated.

Special Focus Cerebrovascular accident (CVA)

CVA or stroke is a very common problem: according to Edwards et al., (1995), each year 2 people in every 1000 of the population will have an initial stroke. This pyramidal disorder, which usually affects older people, can cause considerable disability in the 70% of people surviving the initial event. The various types of stroke are a leading cause of death (third commonest) in developed countries and in 1991 caused around 12% of deaths in England (DoH, 1992). The disruption to cerebral blood supply and functioning may be due to cerebral infarction (tissue death), caused by thrombosis or embolism, or to haemorrhage. Temporary disruption to the blood supply can occur during a transient ischaemic attack (TIA), but here recovery occurs within hours. Increased incidence of stroke is associated with arterial disease and high blood

pressure. Frequently the damage occurs in the internal capsule and affects both the motor (UMN) and the sensory fibres. The resultant damage and physical presentation can vary considerably and obviously depend on the location, and the number and type of fibres affected. Nerve cell damage occurs as glutamate triggers the formation of free radicals such as nitric oxide and the influx of calcium ions, and later from swelling, which further reduces blood supply. The drug aspirin can be used after a stroke to 'mop up' free radicals in an effort to reduce cerebral damage (Kyriazis, 1994). Aspirin is also used to prevent further TIAs and stroke; however, a recent study (Algra and van Gijn, 1996) suggests that aspirin offers only modest protection and that a dose of 30 mg is enough to produce its maximal effect.

Common problems after stroke include: (i) changes in consciousness – may be deeply unconscious; (ii) hemiplegia (paralysis initially flaccid – muscles lack rigidity, decreased tone; becoming spastic – muscles are rigid, increased tone) or hemiparesis (weakness) on the side of the body opposite to the damage (remember motor fibres decussate in the medulla); (iii) vision problems – may include diplopia (double vision), visual field defects and blurring; (iv) communication difficulties if the speech areas in the dominant hemisphere are affected – the resultant speech problems include expressive (motor) dysphasia (unable to express oneself) or receptive (sensory) dysphasia (unable to understand what is being said); (v) emotional lability and associated depression; and (vi) varying degrees of sensory loss.

Nursing Practice Application Care priorities (initial and long-term) following a stroke

- Maintenance of the airway, especially if unconscious. Altered consciousness affects the cough reflex and increases the risk for inhalation of food, fluids or secretions (see Chapter 12).
- Neurological assessment (see page 96) to monitor changes, e.g. extension of the damaged area.
- Careful limb positioning will enhance eventual mobility by helping to prevent joint stiffness, foot drop and contractures.
- Frequent change of position to prevent pressure sore development (see Chapter 19). Remember that sensory loss may be present as well

as motor loss. Change of position and breathing exercises will help to prevent chest infections.
- Maintenance of nutrition and hydration – may have difficulty with swallowing or feeding (see Chapter 13).
- Early involvement of a multi-disciplinary team of health/social care professionals, e.g. nurse, physiotherapist, speech therapist, occupational therapist and social worker, in planning a realistic rehabilitation programme that involves the patient.
- Involvement of family/friends in rehabilitation, education, advice and support for informal carers.

- Increasing the awareness of the affected side, i.e. encouraging the person to 'remember' his or her affected limbs.
- Minimization of problems with visual fields by approaching person from the unaffected side.
- Provision of help with those activities that the individual is unable to manage, e.g. washing and dressing, but always encourage some independence.
- Encouragement in the use of specially adapted equipment, e.g. Velcro fastening on clothes and aids to mobility and continence.

Diencephalon

The diencephalon is the part of the forebrain that consists of the thalamus, hypothalamus and the epithalamus. It is situated between the cerebrum and the brainstem.

Thalamus

The thalamus comprises two masses of grey matter connected by a stalk or intermediate mass. It forms part of the third ventricle and with its many nuclei acts as a relay

station for incoming impulses (Figure 4.11). Some sensory neurones, you will remember, have their second synapse in the thalamus. The thalamus receives most of the sensory input from the sense organs, skin and viscera. It sorts this input and relays it via the internal capsule to the sensory cerebral cortex. The thalamus, which also receives impulses from the basal nuclei, hypothalamus and cerebellum, has a role in the functioning of the cerebral cortex, motor activity, strong emotions such as rage, and memory storage.

Hypothalamus

Positioned below the thalamus, the group of nerve cells known as the hypothalamus forms part of the third ventricle and lie close to the point where the optic nerves decussate (optic chiasma). Hypothalamic tissue forms a stalk from which the pituitary gland of the endocrine system (see Chapter 8) is suspended (*Figure 4.12*).

The hypothalamus is a vital component of homeostatic regulation; it contains very important nuclei that influence most body tissues in some way. It regulates the action of the autonomic nervous system (see Chapter 6), controlling involuntary functions such as heart rate, blood pressure and digestion. Body temperature is controlled by the hypothalamus, which acts as a thermostat – the temperature of blood passing through the hypothalamus activates heat loss or heat conservation mechanisms as appropriate (see Chapter 19). Appetite is regulated through the hunger and satiety centres in the hypothalamus, which control food intake; how useful it would be to have conscious control of these centres when trying to lose weight!

The hypothalamus is vital in the regulation of fluid balance and thirst; special cells called osmoreceptors respond to the osmolarity (see Chapter 2) of body fluids. When body fluid volume is reduced these cells activate hypothalamic nuclei which cause antidiuretic hormone (ADH) to be released from the posterior pituitary gland. This hormone controls water loss in the kidney and reduces urinary volume (see Chapter 15). Other cells in the thirst centre cause you to feel thirsty and drink more fluid. In this way, fluid balance is restored by reducing loss and increasing intake.

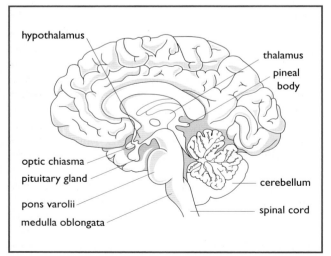

Figure 4.12 Section of the cerebrum showing hypothalamus, pituitary gland and pineal body.

Through connections with other brain areas the hypothalamus forms part of the limbic system (see page 98) concerned with the expression of emotions such as rage, fear, pleasure and those involved in certain biological drives and rhythms, such as sexual behaviour. Cells in the hypothalamus form pleasure and pain centres which appear to influence our behaviour to a limited extent. The hypothalamus also acts, with other brain parts, as a 'biological clock' to influence sleep–wake patterns, which are discussed on pages 94–96.

Earlier we mentioned that the pituitary gland is connected to the hypothalamus by a stalk, suggesting a close relationship between the two, which is the case. Substances produced in the hypothalamus affect the release of anterior pituitary hormones by acting as releasing or inhibiting factors. The other connection involves the two hormones released by the posterior pituitary (ADH and oxytocin) – these are actually produced by special hypothalamic nuclei. These links are discussed more fully in Chapter 8.

Epithalamus

The epithalamus, which lies superior and posterior to the thalamus, forms part of the third ventricle. It contains the hormone-secreting pineal body/gland, which can be considered part of the endocrine system (*Figure 4.12*). Its functions are not fully understood, but is known to produce melatonin (a hormone derived from an amino acid) cyclically during the diurnal/circadian (daily) cycle and the monoamine (chemical with one amine group) 5-hydroxytryptamine (5-HT), also derived from an amino acid.

Melatonin may inhibit the release of gonadotrophin-releasing hormone, which influences the onset of puberty and reproductive function. 5-HT, also known as serotonin, is found in cells lining the gastrointestinal tract, blood cells (platelets) and the brain. It is known to function as a neurotransmitter and is released when tissue damage occurs. A disturbance of 5-HT function is linked to conditions such as migraine, which may be treated with sumatriptan – a 5-HT agonist and depression/anxiety, which can be managed with 5-HT uptake inhibitors, e.g. fluoxetine.

The secretions of the pineal body are concerned with many biological functions and rhythms – various diurnal cycles such as sleep–wake patterns (see page 95), appetite, mood, sexual maturation and reproductive behaviour (see Chapters 8 and 20).

Brainstem

The brainstem is the lowest part of the brain and consists of the midbrain, pons varolii and medulla oblongata

(*Figure 4.13*). It basically consists of grey matter surrounded by white matter. This area of the brain controls the vital automatic functions, such as respiratory rate, contains the pathways which connect the cerebrum with the spinal cord and contains the nuclei of 10 of the 12 cranial nerves (see Chapter 5).

Midbrain

The midbrain is the part of the brainstem between the diencephalon and pons varolii, which surrounds the cerebral aqueduct (page 83) connecting the third and fourth ventricles. It contains several nuclei, including:

- Those of two cranial nerves (oculomotor and trochlear).
- Those associated with the basal nuclei and the extrapyramidal motor tracts, e.g. the substantia nigra (which contains the pigment melanin – the precursor for dopamine).
- The red nuclei involved with descending motor tracts.
- Nuclei involved with certain visual (two superior colliculi) and auditory (two inferior colliculi) reflex functions, e.g. turning your head towards a sudden sound. Together these four nuclei form the corpora quadrigemina.
- Pretectal nuclei involved with pupillary reaction to light.
- Those associated with the reticular formation.

The large descending and ascending nerve tracts form bulges in the midbrain known as the cerebral peduncles.

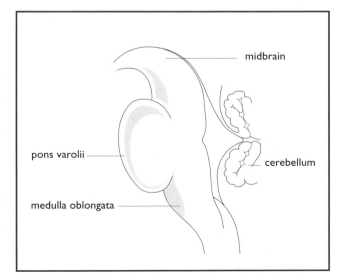

Figure 4.13 Brain stem.

Pons varolii

Situated between the midbrain and medulla, the pons varolii has fibres which form a bridge (pons) between the two hemispheres of the cerebellum and connect the brain and spinal cord. The pons forms part of the fourth ventricle. It contains the nuclei of several cranial nerves and the reticular formation, and its respiratory centre helps to control respiratory rhythm.

Medulla oblongata

The medulla oblongata is the lowest part of the brainstem (and therefore of the brain). It extends from the pons to become the spinal cord, which leaves the cranial cavity through an opening in the skull known as the foramen magnum. It is the site of decussation of the major motor nerves of the corticospinal tracts, which form enlargements in the medulla called pyramids (which give their name to the pyramidal motor pathways). It receives impulses from sensory receptors in the skin and skeletal muscles; some of these sensory fibres decussate in the medulla before being relayed on to the thalamus. The medulla, which has connections with the cerebellum, contains the nuclei of several cranial nerves and special nuclei concerned with maintaining body equilibrium.

Many vital autonomic reflex functions are controlled by centres in the medulla (with hypothalamic influences). Depth and rate of respiration is controlled by respiratory centres (see Chapter 12). Different parts of the respiratory centres respond to increased carbon dioxide levels and, less importantly, to reduced oxygen levels in the blood; gas levels are monitored by chemoreceptors. The medullary centres work with areas in the pons to control breathing rhythms.

The medulla has a cardiovascular centre which is divided into the cardiac centre and vasomotor centre (VMC). The cardiac centre controls the strength and rate of cardiac contraction through the autonomic nervous system (see Chapter 10). The vasomotor centre, which responds to signals from the baroreceptors, controls the diameter of the small peripheral arterioles (peripheral resistance) to regulate blood pressure. When the vessels constrict the blood pressure rises and vice versa (see Chapter 10).

The medulla also contains the centres which control reflexes such as sneezing, coughing, vomiting and swallowing.

Cerebellum

The cerebellum ('little brain') is situated in the posterior cranial fossa; it is located below the occipital lobe of the cerebrum and posterior to the pons and medulla (*Figure 4.14*). It has two hemispheres, connected by the vermis (worm-like structure), and consists of a cortex of grey matter covering the deeper white matter. The cerebellum communicates with the cerebral cortex and brainstem nuclei, e.g. red nuclei (see page 93), through three tracts called cerebellar peduncles. It also receives information from visual and vestibular pathways, and from proprioceptors in muscles and joints. These links allow the cerebellum to process sensory data and influence the voluntary motor activity required to maintain posture, balance and smooth coordinated motion. When the cerebral cortex signals a voluntary movement it also informs the cerebellum – much like the use of office memos or e-mail to let people know what is happening. The cerebellum checks that the intentions of the cerebral cortex are being carried out properly by comparing the instruction with what sensory inputs indicate is actually happening and makes minor adjustments as required. Unlike the cerebral cortex, the cerebellum has mostly ipsilateral (same-side) control – its fibres do not decussate. The functioning of the cerebellum is involuntary and we are not aware of its ability to correct and modify. When it becomes disordered, however, we can certainly appreciate the importance of healthy cerebellar functioning.

Functional Systems of the Brain and Higher Functions

These are areas of the brain which are described together because they perform a common function rather than have well-defined anatomical boundaries.

Reticular formation

The reticular formation is a functional system that consists of neurones, neural pathways and some isolated nuclei found throughout the brainstem (*Figure 4.15*). It has connections with the spinal cord, cerebellum, thalamus and hypothalamus. The reticular formation is important in the control of motor activity, some autonomic functions and the regulation of sensory inputs *en route* to the cerebral cortex. Through the reticular activating system (RAS) it is concerned with the state of cortical awareness and consciousness. Modification of sensory inputs prevents sensory overload (familiar inputs may be suppressed and unusual ones are allowed through); for example, living on a busy road you are unaware of the usual traffic noise, but you become aware of an isolated car travelling very fast. The RAS is normally inhibited by the hypothalamic and other sleep centres. In addition, RAS

Nursing Practice Application **Cerebellar dysfunction**

People with cerebellar dysfunction, caused by haemorrhage or tumour, require care that takes account of their clumsiness, vertigo, lack of balance increasing the risk of falls, inability to perform tasks requiring precise movements and staggering gait, which causes mobility problems. They may also have an intention tremor which occurs when they attempt to perform some task, such as lifting a cup. Communication problems occur in the form of dysarthria, characterized by slurred speech or scanning speech, where syllables become separated and have a 'sing song' quality.

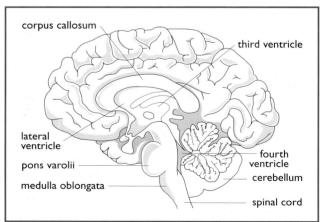

Figure 4.14 The cerebellum.

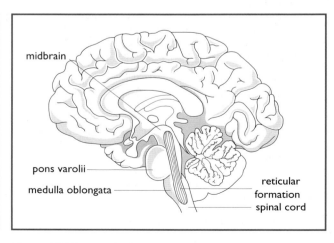

Figure 4.15 The reticular formation.

Special Focus **Sleep**

Sleep–wake cycles are controlled through the RAS, which keeps the cerebral cortex alert and awake, and sleep centres in the hypothalamus, which appear to control when sleep occurs. The hypothalamus contains the suprachiasmatic nucleus ('biological clock') and another nucleus which induces sleep. The process of sleep is more complex than this suggests and involves the whole brain in ways which remain unclear. Sleep–wake patterns usually follow a circadian biorhythm of around 24 hours, where sleep occurs during darkness and wakefulness during daylight hours. The amount of melatonin secretion by the pineal body, which is linked to dark–light cycles, affects the hypothalamic 'biological clock' through numerous receptors. Neurotransmitters such as 5-HT are also involved in sleep–wakefulness and levels of noradrenaline affects the type of sleep.

The actual amount of sleep required by individuals varies considerably, with some people needing only 4–5 hours whereas others 'feel deprived' if they do not sleep for 8–9 hours.

Modifications to the simple dark–light rhythm occur when routines are changed, such as shift working or travelling through time zones (jet lag). Anxiety and depression can disrupt sleep patterns (see box). Sedatives, tranquillizers and alcohol all affect the type and patterns of sleep. Other drugs may cause sleep disturbance; for example, diuretics cause the person to get up to pass urine and some, e.g. beta blockers and anti-ulcer medication, can cause vivid dreams and nightmares.

The functions of sleep are not fully understood, but all of us can remember that dreadful feeling that accompanies lack of sleep – such as staying up after a busy night duty. Sleep deprivation affects coping mechanisms, emotional stability, restorative properties, memory storage and our ability to perform skilled tasks.

One of the most common problems for people admitted to hospital is the disruption to their normal sleep–wake patterns. This is especially worrying when you consider that they are denied the restorative power of sleep during a period of increased physiological and psychological stress. In a study of 200 patients, Closs (1988) found that for most people sleep patterns changed after admission to hospital – 60% slept less

well, 27% slept the same and 11% slept better. The common reasons given for sleep disruption were pain, noise, environmental temperature and uncomfortable beds. In another study Southwell and Wistow (1995) found that 79% of patients on surgical wards reported one or more sleep disturbance compared with 49% on elderly care wards.

Stages and types of sleep

In adults a typical night's sleep consists of alternating cycles of non-rapid eye movement sleep (NREM), which has four stages (see below), and rapid eye movement sleep (REM). These types and stages are identified by different patterns of brain waves recorded by the EEG (see page 97).

NREM sleep occurs first:

Stage 1: (transition stage) relaxation and drifting into sleep, vital signs (blood pressure, temperature, respiration and heart rate) are still normal and we are easily roused.

Stage 2: more difficult to rouse.

Stage 3: sleep is deeper and muscles relaxed. Vital signs decline. Dreaming occurs at this stage.

Stage 4: the deepest level of sleep. Very difficult to rouse, often disorientated if woken. Vital signs at their lowest level. During this stage people may get out of bed or be incontinent of urine.

REM sleep occurs following a period of NREM sleep. It is characterized by a change in brain wave patterns, an increase in vital signs and inhibition of most muscles. Brain use of oxygen during REM exceeds the waking consumption. Vivid dreams occur during REM sleep.

In healthy adults the first period of REM sleep usually occurs after about 90 min, but subsequent NREM sleep periods become progressively shorter and the REM stages longer during a period of sleep. Each complete cycle lasts for about 90 min. The number of NREM/REM cycles is obviously related to the total time spent asleep.

Lifespan and changing sleep needs

Small babies are asleep for approximately 16 hours a day (however, their parents think it is much less!). They have many

sleep–wake cycles during the 24 hour period which take little account of day and night. Gradually they adapt to sleeping mainly at night and being awake during the day.

The amount of REM sleep gradually decreases during infancy and childhood and stabilizes at adult levels from about 10 years of age.

By the mid-teens most individuals have reached the average adult sleeping pattern of 7–8 hours.

Sleep patterns may change during mid-life, when a night's sleep may be broken by periods of wakefulness.

Older adults tend to have much lighter sleep with increasing periods of wakefulness, and the amount of NREM stage 4 sleep, which declines throughout life, may be very small or absent. The lack of sleep at night is usually compensated for by daytime naps. Older people appear to need more sleep and rest, and will often plan for a sleep after lunch.

These different sleep needs have obvious implications for the nurse, who somehow must try to provide the environment in which individuals can achieve adequate sleep. This is vitally important to enhance healing processes (see above and Chapter 19) and an individual's feeling of well-being, but very difficult to organize within a busy ward or where accommodation problems exist, such as a teenager sharing a bedroom with a grandparent.

Getting to sleep

Most people have a bedtime routine, which probably helps prepare for sleep, e.g. reading, having a milky drink and changing into nightclothes. There are many factors which prevent proper sleep, such as pain, a strange hospital bed, being with other people, the ward light, being too hot or cold, a full bladder, and the noise of other people and events. In one study, the two nursing actions which most helped people get back to sleep were found to be pain relief and a hot drink (Closs, 1988).

When individuals are still unable to sleep they might be prescribed a sedative drug, preferably for a limited period, as long-term use may lead to dependence and, paradoxically, to alteration in sleep patterns.

functioning is repressed by anaesthetics, drugs that reduce anxiety, sedatives, alcohol and severe trauma, which may result in unconsciousness.

The reticular formation is involved with other structures in the regulation of sleep–wake cycles. Sleep takes up about one third of our lives but its purpose and mechanisms are poorly understood (see Special Focus – Sleep). We do know, however, that the proper amount of sleep is important in maintaining health and for this reason it merits further discussion.

Nursing Practice Application Sleep disturbances and mental health problems

Sometimes a change in sleep patterns can indicate a mental health problem. People with anxiety or depression may find it difficult to get to sleep – initial insomnia.

Other types of depression cause early waking, where the person lies awake from the early hours. In some people an increase in sleeping time is associated with depression. The nurse should be alert to changing patterns and also consider the possibility that drug or alcohol intake is contributing to the changes.

Abnormal Function Problems causing alterations in level of consciousness

Although sleep represents an altered state of consciousness, it is not usually included in the causes of abnormal states of consciousness. Changes in consciousness result from impairment of brain functioning, causes of which include fainting (syncope), accidental or intentional overdose of drugs or alcohol, general anaesthesia, trauma, stroke and other brain disorders (see *Figure 4.16*, showing an intracranial haemorrhage), and homeostatic breakdown, e.g. reduced glucose in the blood.

Changes in the state of consciousness can be assessed using a standardized instrument, such as the Glasgow Coma Scale (Allan, 1984), which tests verbal response, motor response and eye opening. These criteria – with vital signs (blood pressure, pulse, temperature and respiration), pupil size, their reaction to light and limb movements – provide a comprehensive neurological assessment (see Person-Centred Study – Billie, see below).

Person-Centred Study Billie

Billie is admitted for observation after falling from his pony, Polly. He and some pals had been riding without hard hats and Billie was thrown to the ground. Billie hit his head and, according to his friends, was 'knocked out' for a few minutes.

Neurological assessment and/or observation is important after head injury. There is a risk that bleeding (haematoma formation) within the skull or brain swelling will cause an increase in intracranial pressure. Untreated, this raised intracranial pressure (RIP) may lead to further swelling, disruption to the blood supply, altered consciousness, brain damage and eventually death if the brainstem (with its vital centres) is forced down through the foramen magnum (herniation or coning).

During his hospital stay, Billie is observed carefully for any changes that might indicate increasing intracranial pressure. In an article concerning RIP,

Allan (1986) recommends the use of standardized assessment techniques, e.g. the Glasgow Coma Scale plus the other criteria mentioned above.

The changes indicative of raised intracranial pressure are:
Conscious level: becoming less responsive, using the criteria of eye opening, and verbal and motor response. Changes occur early.
Blood pressure: the systolic blood pressure increases (VMC involvement) as a late sign.
Pulse: the rate slows (cardiac centre involvement) as a late sign.
Respiration: changes in rate and depth (respiratory centre involvement).
Pupil size and reaction to light: if the brain is forced downwards it presses on the oculomotor nerve (third cranial nerve, see Chapter 5), which normally controls pupillary reflexes. If intracranial pressure is raised the pupils become unequal (dilate on affected side) and unresponsive to light; a fixed dilated pupil is an extremely grave prognostic sign.
Temperature: high body temperature may result from damage to the hypothalamic heat regulating centre.
Limb movement: spasticity or abnormal extension may occur as motor tracts and the brainstem are compressed. This is another poor prognostic sign.

Next morning the medical officer considers that Billie is fit for discharge – overnight all Billie's observations had been within normal limits and apart from the 'lump' on his head he feels well. When his parents arrive Billie goes home with a reminder about wearing his hard hat. The nurse advises Billie's parents about contacting their doctor if Billie has headache, vomiting, visual problems or drowsiness, and the need for a gradual return to energetic pastimes.

Brain wave patterns

The electrical activity of the many neurones in the brain can be recorded by using scalp electrodes and an electroencephalograph (*Figure 4.17*). The patterns of activity (brain waves) are represented visually as an electroencephalogram (EEG), which is a paper trace of the waves.

Brain wave patterns are very complex and unique to individuals; but there are four basic types:

- Alpha – low amplitude, slow waves associated with the relaxed awake state. Frequency 7–13 Hz.
- Beta – higher frequency (greater than 13 Hz) and less regular, they occur when we are awake and 'thinking' or concentrating.
- Theta – even more irregular, these are seen in children and the first stages of sleep. Frequency 4–6 Hz. Their presence in awake adults indicates abnormality.
- Delta – high amplitude waves recorded during deep sleep and where RAS activity is repressed. Frequency less than 4 Hz.

Brain wave patterns are useful in the diagnosis of many brain disorders, e.g. the epilepsies. These are characterized by abnormal electrical discharges in the brain that cause some alteration in consciousness, which may be accompanied by fits or seizures.

The EEG may be used in conjunction with other criteria to confirm 'brainstem death'. It is not routinely used in the UK (and several other countries), however, because some residual electrical activity may persist after brainstem death, and EEG measures cortical activity whereas tests for brain death are concerned with brainstem function (Allan, 1987).

Diagnosis of 'brainstem death' is of particular importance when decisions are to be made regarding the withdrawal of life-support systems (see Chapter 21), especially where organ donation is anticipated.

Healthier Living Protecting a child's head

Wearing a properly fitted protective helmet, of the most recent safety standard, can do much to protect a child from brain damage or death. Apart from Billie and his riding mishap, this head protection is vitally important when children ride bicycles on the road.

Proper head protection is one way of helping to achieve the 'Health of the Nation' target (DoH, 1992) of reducing the death rate for accidents in children under 15 by at least 33% by the year 2005. Nurses and health visitors working in schools and primary care are well placed to encourage the use of cycle helmets, reflective clothing and general road safety.

Provisional figures show a 10% fall in deaths from accidents in those under 15 (DoH 1997).

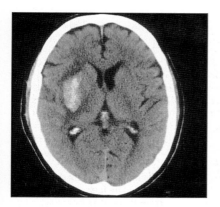

Figure 4.16 CT scan showing intracranial haemorrhage (pale area on left). (Simon Fraser/Science Photo Library. Reprinted with permission).

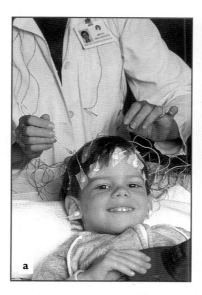

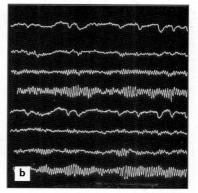

Figure 4.17 (a) Electroencephalograph electrodes in place (Larry Mulvehill/Science Photo Library. Reprinted with permission); (b) brain wave patterns (Science Photo Library. Reprinted with permission).

Limbic system

The limbic system is not a well-defined system, but rather a diffuse collection of nuclei and fibres in the cerebrum and diencephalon. These areas, which are part of the primitive brain, influence feelings and emotions. The 'limbic system' is really the link between the hippocampus and amygdaloid nucleus (involved in long-term memory), the thalamus, the hypothalamus (also concerned with emotions) and the cerebral cortex. Usually the cerebral cortex puts a 'brake' on our response to feelings and allows a socially acceptable response, but in some situations the primitive emotional brain wins and you give full vent to your feelings.

The olfactory system and its sensory inputs are important in the functioning of the primitive limbic system. We respond emotionally to odours that evoke memories; for example, the smell of fried onions and diesel may remind you of visiting a funfair.

Memory and learning

Memory is the ability to store past experiences which can be retrieved when required, much like saving data on a computer disk (*Figure 4.18*). To learn, we must have memory. As yet there is little information about the mechanisms involved in memory, but it would seem that we store facts in stages, that many areas of the brain are involved and processing depends on the hippocampus (area on the temporal lobe) and the amygdaloid nucleus. Our ability to learn new facts and store them in the memory decreases with age. Many older people have perfect recollection of memories of distant experiences but find they

have no recall of very recent events; for example, an older lady can tell you about food rationing during World War II but cannot recall whether she has had supper yet. In a small study, Dawe and Moore-Orr (1995) found that mild exercise programmes can improve memory and independence in people over 70 having long-term care.

Short-term memory, which involves important current matters (a working list), is temporary and limited. We can only remember around seven bits of data; you will recall what happens if you are trying to keep a telephone number in your head and someone tells you another fact – yes, the telephone number is lost! Some memory can be transferred to long-term storage, which is less limited and represents a permanent neuronal change. We can access these memories (like using a reference book) when required – apart from the bits you forget or suppress – but even the suppressed data can influence mental processes and behaviour. Several chemicals, e.g. glutamate and nitric oxide, are thought to play a part in the processes required for permanent memory storage.

Memory can involve facts such as the names of other students on your course or skills which involve a series of motor actions, e.g. applying a bandage. Fact memory relies heavily on associations – you may only remember fellow students who you particularly like or dislike. In contrast, the skill memory of bandaging will be re-activated whenever you pick up a bandage.

Our ability to store long-term memory and learn depends on factors which include:

- Being able to repeat new information – worth bearing in mind when teaching patients.
- Mood and state of arousal – we need to be interested

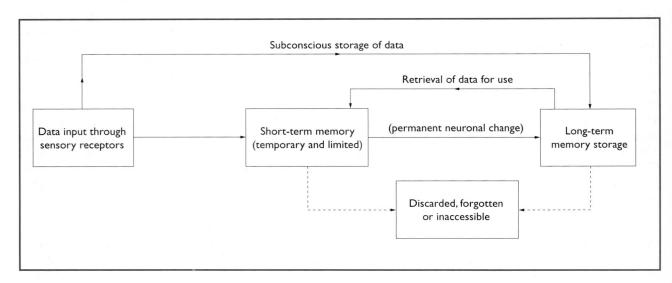

Figure 4.18 Memory – stages and storage.

and motivated; learning is impossible if you are distracted, e.g. not listening to a lecture if you are worried about getting a parking ticket.

• Tagging new facts on to those you already know makes

the process much simpler; for example, it is easier to learn how drugs work if you associate the new facts with those about cell membranes and transport.

Nursing Practice Application **Chaining – a strategy for people with learning disabilities**

Individuals with learning disabilities can be helped to learn skills such as dressing through chaining. This involves teaching tiny bits of the skill in sequence. It may be forward chaining, where the skill is learnt in the sequence that it normally occurs, with each step linking to the next; for example, a child learns the stages required to put on socks before those for trainers. Sometimes backwards chaining is used, with the skill being learnt by working backwards from the final step.

Abnormal Function **Problems with memory**

There are numerous reasons for memory problems, e.g. amnesia after head injury, but one of the most common is Alzheimer's disease. This is a degenerative brain condition that causes dementia (previously called senile dementia) and affects memory, learning and other higher functions. Alzheimer's disease is characterized by the formation of plaques and tangles in the brain, which may spread by axonal transport (see Delieu and Keady, 1996, Chapter 3), and with biochemical changes, including high levels of a specific protein. It runs in families (the likely gene has been identified) and is more common in people with Down syndrome. Alzheimer's disease usually occurs in older adults, but it can occur in mid-life. It is characterized by loss of short-term memory, an inability to learn new facts, confusion, disorientation and possible changes in personality. As you can imagine, this causes problems with everyday life for affected individuals and their families, who are often the only carers. Caring for and supporting people affected by Alzheimer's disease uses a 'big slice' of the health and social service budgets, both in the community and in hospital.

The Spinal Cord

The other part of the CNS is the spinal cord (see *Figure 4.19*). This is continuous with the medulla oblongata and runs inside the vertebral canal (surrounded by the vertebral column), down the length of the back to the level of the first or second lumbar vertebra (L1/L2) in adults, but in young children it may reach L3. The cord is about 2.5 cm thick and approximately 42 cm long in an adult male. The spinal cord is further protected by the three meningeal membranes and CSF (see pages 82–83). A modified portion of pia mater, the filum terminale, secures the end of the cord to the coccyx. Thirty-one pairs of spinal nerves (see Chapter 5) arise from the cord; these paired nerve roots enter and leave through apertures in the vertebrae (intervertebral foramina). At the level of L1/L2 the nerve roots fan out to form a structure resembling a horse's tail, the cauda equina.

Pathways in the spinal cord conduct sensory inputs to the brain and motor outputs from the brain. Various spinal reflexes occur within the spinal cord.

Structure of the spinal cord

The spinal cord consists of a butterfly-shaped area of grey matter, with a central canal, surrounded by white matter, neuroglia and blood vessels. The grey matter can be divided into:

• Two anterior (ventral) horns or motor horns – largest at the level where nerves for the limbs leave the cord. They contain the cell bodies of the lower motor neurones whose axons supply skeletal muscle.

• Two posterior (dorsal) horns or sensory horns. The cell bodies for the sensory nerves entering the dorsal horns of the spinal cord are in the dorsal/spinal ganglia which are outside the spinal cord. These sensory nerves may synapse in the cord at the level of entry or travel up the ascending tracts of the spinal cord to synapses higher up in the cord or in the brain. The dorsal horns also contain interneurones which link sensory and motor neurones (see simple reflex arc, Chapter 3).

• Lateral horns, present in the thoracic and lumbar regions of the cord, which contain autonomic motor neurones that innervate the viscera. They leave the spinal cord with the somatic motor neurones of the ventral horns.

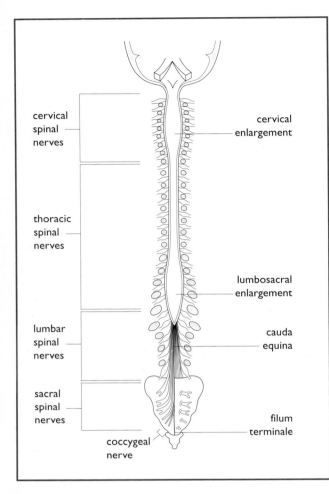

Figure 4.19 The spinal cord and spinal nerves.

The dorsal and ventral nerve roots entering and leaving the spinal cord fuse just outside the cord to become the mixed spinal nerve (*Figure 4.20*).

The white matter of the spinal cord consists of the ascending sensory tracts, carrying afferent impulses to the brain; descending motor tracts, carrying efferent impulses from the brain or from higher levels in the cord; and fibres, which connect one side of the cord with the other. The white matter is arranged into three columns, or funiculi, on each side of the cord: posterior, anterior and lateral. Many ascending and descending tracts are contained within each column. Generally, the tracts consist of two or three neurones that synapse. Most tracts decussate at some point and they are paired, one on the right side and one on the left side of the cord.

Motor pathways

The descending motor tracts are either pyramidal or extrapyramidal (see pages 86–87 and 90 and *Figures 4.8* and *4.21*).

Pyramidal tracts

The pyramidal or corticospinal tracts originate in the Betz (pyramidal) cells of the main motor area of the cerebral cortex. Their axons pass through the internal capsule and on to the medulla, where most decussate. This upper motor neurone (UMN) descends in the spinal cord tract to the appropriate level where it synapses with the lower

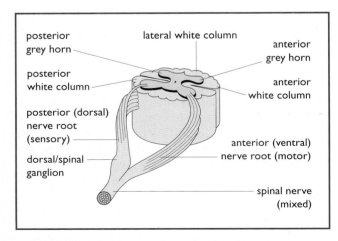

Figure 4.20 Section through the spinal cord showing structure and spinal nerve roots.

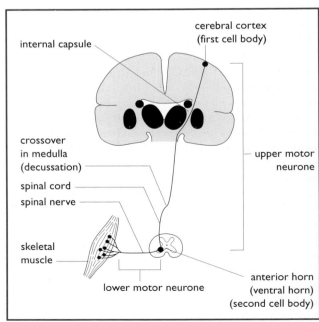

Figure 4.21 Motor pathways (pyramidal – two-neurone pathway).

Table 4.2 Comparison of UMN and LMN disorders

Site of problem	Type of paralysis	Muscle atrophy
Upper motor neurone, e.g. strokes	Spastic (increased tone), may be flaccid initially, affects one side of the body (hemiplegia)	No
Lower motor neurone, e.g. nerve trauma	Flaccid (decreased tone) affecting only the muscle groups innervated by that peripheral nerve	Yes

Damage to LMN may be accompanied by sensory disturbances such as an inability to detect temperature changes. This occurs because the peripheral nerves are usually mixed (both motor and sensory fibres).
NB   Reflexes are also affected, see Chapter 5.

Table 4.2 Comparison of UMN and LMN disorders.

motor neurone (LMN), also called the 'final common pathway', which leaves the cord by the ventral nerve root to innervate associated skeletal muscle fibres. The corticospinal tracts are concerned with voluntary movements.

At this point it is appropriate to consider the different effects of problems affecting the UMN and LMN; these are summarized in *Table 4.2*.

Extrapyramidal tracts
Extrapyramidal tracts include the tectospinal, rubrospinal, reticulospinal and vestibulospinal tracts (named for their origins – see below). They arise in subcortical areas and travel in the spinal cord columns to the anterior horn. Their activity is influenced by links with the cerebellum, basal nuclei and brainstem nuclei. The extrapyramidal tracts modify coarse voluntary movements and affect posture and coordination:

Tectospinal: fibres originate in an area of the midbrain known as the tectum, where they decussate. They travel in the anterior spinal cord column and control posture, balance and muscle coordination.

Rubrospinal: fibres originate in the red nucleus of the midbrain, where they decussate. They travel in the lateral columns of the cord and control muscle tone and posture.

Reticulospinal: fibres originate in the reticular formation; some decussate and others do not. They travel in the lateral and anterior columns to control muscle tone.

Vestibulospinal: fibres originate in the vestibular nuclei in the medulla; some decussate and others do not. They travel in the anterior and lateral columns to control muscle tone.

Sensory pathways
Sensory pathways carry various impulses from sensory receptors in the skin and proprioceptors in joints, muscles and tendons to the brain by a two-neurone or three-neurone system (*Figure 4.22*).

The pathways carry information about touch, pressure,

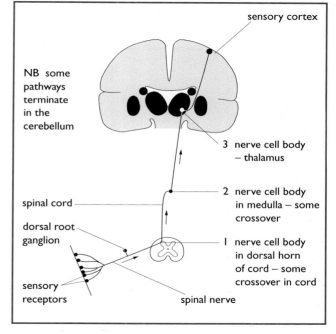

Figure 4.22 Sensory pathways (simplified two-neurone or three-neurone pathway).

temperature and pain to the sensory cortex, which in some instances can localize its site of origin. Information from the proprioceptors is carried to the cerebral cortex and to the cerebellum, where it is used to maintain posture and muscle tone. The major sensory pathways include: the fasciculi cuneatus and gracilis (a fasciculus is a small bundle), the anterior/lateral spinothalamic tract, and the anterior/posterior spinocerebellar tracts.

Fasciculi cuneatus and gracilis
The fasciculi cuneatus and gracilis carry touch and pressure impulses from skin receptors, and position sense from

proprioceptors, to the opposite side of the brain. First-order sensory neurones enter the cord and travel in the dorsal columns to synapse with second-order neurones in the nuclei cuneatus and gracilis in the medulla. The fibres decussate in the medulla before ascending to the thalamus, where they synapse with third-order neurones that carry the impulses to the sensory cortex.

Anterior/lateral spinothalamic tracts
The anterior/lateral spinothalamic tracts carry poorly localized pressure and touch impulses, plus impulses for temperature and pain (in A and C fibres), to the oppo-site side of the brain. They synapse and decussate in the cord before ascending in the anterior and lateral columns to the thalamus, where they synapse with third-order neurones that carry the impulses to the sensory cortex.

Anterior/posterior spinocerebellar tracts
The anterior/posterior spinocerebellar tracts carry pro-prioceptor and touch impulses to the cerebellum; some fibres decussate and others do not. They synapse in the spinal cord and the second-order neurones ascend in the lateral columns to terminate in the cerebellum.

Nursing Practice Application **Pain**

Pain transmission and perception involve the whole nervous system, but it seems logical to look at pain now, having covered the brain and sensory tracts.

The management of pain is one of the most important and challenging issues in nursing practice. Pain is subjective and individuals all feel and describe painful sensations differently. The biggest prob-lem is not being able to measure pain in units. Those working in health care must accept what the individual has to say about their pain and act upon this infor-mation in a positive way.

Over recent years the concept of 'pain meters' has been developed; these allow people to grade their painful sen-sations on a scale, e.g. 0 (no pain) to 10 (the worst pain possible). There are many ways of assessing and recording pain intensity, and Vandenbosch McCormick (1988) describes the use of 'pain flow sheets'. Schofield (1995) stresses the importance of pain assessment and doc-umentation using a pain assessment tool. Assessing pain in older adults, however, can present extra difficulties because age-related changes cause them to report pain differently, e.g. alterations in sensory per-ceptions (Closs, 1994).

Apart from what people say about pain, there is considerable information to be gained from their non-verbal commu-nication and physical appearance; for example, a person in pain may keep still, thrash around or become sweaty. Changes in vital signs, e.g. increasing pulse, may be detected in a person with pain.

Some of the many factors which influ-ence our response to pain include: (i) pain tolerance – people who are not easily bothered by pain are said to have high pain tolerance (we all feel pain at the same intensity of stimulus – threshold); (ii) cultural differences, such as adopting a 'stiff upper lip' attitude to pain; (iii) fac-tors which affect pain response, e.g. anx-iety and information. Hayward (1975) found that information regarding pain and its duration given before surgery reduced the need for painkillers after operation; (iv) the meaning of pain and past experi-ences, e.g. a man whose father died after a myocardial infarction will find his own response to chest pain influenced by this experience; and (v) Latham (1993) sug-gests that the presence of several coex-isting medical problems can amplify or confuse the picture of pain experienced and reported by older people.

Acute pain may have a physiological defence role and can be regarded in some situations as a warning that tissues are being damaged, e.g. acute inflammation. This is certainly not so for chronic pain, e.g. osteoarthritis (see Chapter 18), where joint damage has already occurred.

Physiology of transmission

Pain impulses are carried to the CNS by the 'A' delta and 'C' nerve fibres (see Chapter 3). The different fibres transmit different types of pain; for example, superficial somatic (skin, joints and mus-cles) pain uses 'A' delta fibres and deep somatic pain the 'C' fibres. Melzack and Wall (1965) proposed the gate control theory in which they suggested that a 'gate' operating at the spinal cord level can block pain impulses from reaching a conscious level unless the input of pain impulses is large. Gate control theory is very complex, but basically works by fibres from touch receptors inhibiting the fibres carrying pain impulses – the gate is shut. The descending spinal tracts are also involved. The gate control theory is important in our understanding of pain and we shall use it to explain other aspects of pain.

Various chemicals produced in the body are involved in the transmission and modulation of pain impulses. Many are neurotransmitters (see Chapter 3), e.g. substance P, which enhances pain trans-mission, the opiate-like substances enkephalin and endorphin, which act as natural analgesics by 'closing the gate', and the amino acid glutamate. Other chemi-cals involved are those produced by tissue damage and inflammation (see

THE CENTRAL NERVOUS SYSTEM ■ CHAPTER 4

Abnormal Function **Problems – spinal injury and spinal shock**

The pathological effects of spinal cord injury obviously depend on the extent of the damage and the level at which it occurs. Common causes of spinal cord transection are traffic, industrial and sporting accidents, but diseases such as spinal tumours and metastatic (spread from primary site) cancer can cause similar effects through cord compression.

Initially after cord injury there is spinal shock, which is characterized by loss of bowel and bladder control, paralysis (flaccid, becoming spastic) and loss of sensa-tion and reflexes below the level of damage, reduction in blood pressure, and problems with temperature control as sweating ceases below the damage level. If neurological function is still absent a few days after injury, it indicates that the cord damage and resultant disability is permanent.

Damage in the cervical region (see *Figure 4.19*) results in quadriplegia, which is paralysis of all four limbs, whereas damage in the thoracolumbar region results in paraplegia, where only the legs are affected. Various other effects include problems with sexual function and the enormous psychological and social prob-lems associated with a sudden and permanent disability.

Individuals with spinal injuries require nursing interventions that ensure correct limb positioning, prevent skin breakdown, deal with bladder and bowel function, assist the person to express his or her sexuality and help all concerned to cope with permanent disability.

Nursing Practice Application cont. **Pain**

Chapter 19) such as bradykinin, which stimulates pain receptors and intensifies pain, and histamine and prostaglandins (which fulfil many other roles in the body), which are involved in healing. 5-HT and nitric oxide also appear to have a role in pain transmission and perception.

Special types of pain
Referred pain
This is visceral pain felt in a different loca-tion from where it originates, e.g. cardiac pain felt in the left arm, neck and jaw. This occurs because pain fibres from the affected structure enter the spinal cord at the same level as somatic sensory fibres from the referred area and follow the same pathways. This is why visceral pain can be misinterpreted by the brain as being somatic in origin.

Phantom limb syndrome
Following amputation of a limb, the individual can still experience pain in the missing part. This happens because if the sensory nerves are stimulated anywhere along their length they continue to transmit pain impulses. Without the amputated limb to provide the touch fibre impulse transmission inhibition (gate theory) pain is experienced in the missing part as the brain localizes the pain incorrectly.

Chronic pain
As already discussed, chronic pain cannot be considered protective. Hanks and Hoskin (1986) state that chronic pain has no positive function. The perception of chronic pain, such as that caused by advanced malignancy, may also be influenced by the emotions of a person facing the prospect of death (Waugh, 1988). Another important aspect of chronic pain is that the cause cannot be cured (Hockley, 1988), but sensory stimulation may reduce its effects (Schofield, 1996).

Methods of pain relief
Just as pain perception is unique to the person, so is its relief equally individual. It is essential that assessment reflects a holistic approach to pain relief by con-sidering the physical, emotional, social and cultural aspects. The management of acute and chronic pain differs in several ways. For instance, relief of acute pain is usually only required for a limited dura-tion, e.g. postoperatively, but relief of chronic pain may be required for life. Closs (1996) found that although nurses had a good awareness of the negative effects of chronic pain, there were many misconceptions on the pharmacological treatment of pain.

NB Interventions such as joint replacement, discussed in Chapter 18, may reduce pain substantially.

Physical
(i) Basic comfort such as an extra pillow; (ii) massage to enhance relaxation and relieve pain by using large touch fibre transmission to 'shut the gate'; (iii) heat or cold, e.g. ice pack (care is needed to prevent skin damage); (iv) transcutaneous electrical nerve stimulation, which prob-ably works by stimulating the large fibres which inhibit the pain fibres (gate theory or the release of natural analgesic sub-stances; see Chapter 20); (v) radiation; (vi) surgical division of a nerve; (viii) acupunc-ture, which may well stimulate the release of the natural opiates.

Pharmacological
(i) Analgesic drugs, such as morphine, aspirin; (ii) drugs to lift mood, e.g. anti-depressants; (iii) nerve blocks and epidur-al analgesia.

Psychological
(i) Distraction and diversion, e.g. televi-sion; (ii) visualization techniques; (iii) relaxation and hypnosis; (iv) reducing anxiety and providing information; (v) therapeutic touch.

Various complementary therapies are used to relieve pain, and readers can find more information in a discussion of their use in stress management in Chapter 6.

Summary/Check List

Special focus – Discovering the brain.
Development of CNS – embryonic, factors causing damage, Nursing Practice Application – folate and CNS development, development during infancy and childhood.
Protection for the CNS – Skull and vertebrae. Meninges. Ventricular system and CSF – composition, circulation and functions of CSF, Nursing Practice Application – lumbar puncture, hydrocephaly. Blood–brain barrier. Blood supply.
The brain – cerebrum, cerebral hemispheres. Functional areas of cerebral cortex – motor areas, sensory areas, other cortical areas. Right brain versus left brain. Basal nuclei, parkinsonism, Huntington's disease. Internal capsule, Special Focus – CVA, Nursing Practice Application – stroke.

Diencephalon – thalamus, hypothalamus, epithalamus.
Brainstem – midbrain, pons varolii, medulla oblongata.
Cerebellum, Nursing Practice Application – cerebellar dysfunction. Reticular formation, Special Focus – sleep.
Alterations in consciousness, Person-centred Study – Billie.
Healthier Living – protecting a child's head. Brain wave patterns – fits, brainstem death. Limbic system. Memory and learning – Nursing Practice Application – chaining a strategy for people with learning disabilities, Alzheimer's disease.
Spinal cord – Structure (grey and white matter). Motor pathways – pyramidal, extrapyramidal tracts. Sensory pathways. Nursing Practice Application – pain. Spinal injury and spinal shock.

Self Test

1 During pregnancy, development of the CNS has commenced by the:
  (a) 3rd week;
  (b) 12th week;
  (c) 16th week;
  (d) 20th week.
2 Which of the following statements are true?
  (a) CSF is found between the dura and arachnoid mater.
  (b) The composition of CSF is similar to that of plasma.
  (c) The pia mater is the inner meningeal membrane.
  (d) The 'blood–brain barrier' prevents brain damage due to exposure to lead in young children.
3 Draw and label a diagram of the brain to show the cerebrum, brainstem and cerebellum.
4 Put the following in their correct pairs:
  (a) basal nuclei;
  (b) Broca's area;
  (c) extrapyramidal motor tracts;
  (d) internal capsule;
  (e) motor speech area;
  (f) occipital lobe;
  (g) pyramidal motor tracts;
  (h) visual cortex.
5 Describe briefly how the hypothalamus influences sleep patterns.
6 Why is the medulla oblongata so vital in maintaining homeostasis?
7 Which of the following indicate a rise in intracranial pressure?
  (a) Fall in blood pressure.
  (b) Decreasing verbal response.
  (c) Slowing pulse rate.
  (d) Pupils unresponsive to light.
  (e) Rise in blood pressure.
  (f) Rising pulse rate.
8 Which of the following statements are true?
  (a) The spinal cord terminates at the level of L1 or L2 in adults.
  (b) The grey matter of the cord surrounds the central white matter.
  (c) Sensory nerves entering the dorsal horn have their cell bodies outside the spinal cord.
  (d) Motor nerves leave the cord via the posterior horn.
9 Describe the route taken by a nerve impulse from the Betz cells in the motor cortex until it reaches the motor unit.
10 Quadriplegia will follow spinal cord transection in which region:
  (a) thoracic;
  (b) lumbar;
  (c) sacral;
  (d) cervical.

Answers

1 a.
2 b, c.
3 See pages 85, 86.
4 a–c, b–e, d–g and f–h.
5 See pages 92, 94-96.
6 See page 93.
7 b, c, d, e.
8 a, c.
9 See pages 100, 101.
10 d.

References

Algra A, van Gijn J. (1996) Aspirin at any dose above 30 mg offers only modest protection after cerebral ischaemia. *J Neurol Neurosurg Psychiat* **60**(2): 197–199.

Allan D (1984) Glasgow coma chart. *Nurs Mirror* **158**(23): 32–34.

Allan D (1986) Raised intracranial pressure. *Prof Nurs* **2**(3): 78–80.

Allan D (1987) Criteria for brain stem death. *Prof Nurs* **2**(11): 357–359.

Closs J (1988) Sleep in surgical wards. *Nurs Times,* **84**(22): 52.

Closs J (1994) Pain in elderly patients: a neglected phenomenon? *J Adv Nurs* **19**(6): 1072–1081.

Closs J (1996) Pain and elderly patients: a survey of nurses' knowledge and experiences. *J Adv Nurs* **23**(2): 237–242.

Dawe D, Moore-Orr R (1995) Low-intensity range-of-motion exercise: invaluable nursing care for elderly patients. *J Adv Nurs* **21**(4): 675–681.

Department of Health (DoH) (1992) *The Health of the Nation. A Summary of the Strategy for Health in England.* London: HMSO.

Department of Health (DoH) (1997) *Health of the Nation.* http://www.open.gov.uk/doh/dhhome.htm

Edwards CRW, Bouchier IAD, Haslett C, Chilvers ER, Eds (1995) *Davidson's Principles and Practice of Medicine,* 17th edn. Edinburgh: Churchill Livingstone.

Hanks GW, Hoskin PJ (1986) Pain control in advanced cancer: pharmacological methods. *J Roy Coll Phys* **20**(4): 276–281.

Hayward J (1975) *Information, a prescription against pain.* London: Royal College of Nursing.

Health Education Authority (HEA) (1996) *Folic Acid – What All Women Should Know.* London: Health Education Authority.

Hockley J (1988) Setting standards for pain control. *Prof Nurs* **3**(8): 310–313.

Kyriazis M (1994) Developments in the treatment of stroke patients. *Nurs Times* **90** (29): 30–32.

Latham J (1993) Treatment we can all believe in. Pain and its management in later life. *Prof Nurs* **8**(4): 212–220.

Melzack R, Wall PD (1965) Pain mechanisms: a new theory. *Science* **150**: 971–979.

Schofield P (1995) Using assessment tools to help patients in pain. *Prof Nurs* **10** (11): 703–706.

Schofield P (1996) Sensory delights. *Nurs Times,* **92**(5): 40.

Southwell MT, Wistow G (1995) Sleep in hospital at night: are patient's needs being met? *J Adv Nurs* **21**(6): 1101–1109.

Vandenbosch McCormick T (1988) How to use a pain flow sheet effectively. *Nursing 88* (USA) **18**(8): 50–51.

Wald N *et al.* (MRC Vitamin Study Research Group) (1991) Prevention of neural tube defects: results of the Medical Research Council Vitamin Study. *Lancet,* **ii**: 131–137.

Waugh L (1988) Psychological aspects of cancer pain. *Prof Nurs* **3**(12): 504–508.

Further Reading

Barasi S (1991) The physiology of pain. *Surg Nurs* **4**(5): 14–20.

Barker E (1994) Neuroscience Nursing. London: Mosby.

Clark AJ, Flowers J, Boots L, Shettar S (1995) Sleep disturbances in mid-life women. *J Adv Nurs* **22**(3): 562–568.

Jacques A (1992) Do you believe I'm in pain? Nurses' assessment of patient's pain. *Prof Nurs* **7**(4): 249–251.

McCaffery M, Beeb A (Latham J, Ball D, UK eds) (1994) *Pain: Clinical Manual for Nursing Practice.* London: Mosby.

Shapiro CM, Ed (1994) *The ABC of Sleep Disorders.* London: British Medical Journal Publications.

Wilson-Barnett J, Batehup L (1988) *Patient problems: A Research Base for Nursing Care.* London: Scutari Press.

Useful Addresses

Alzheimer's Disease Society
Gordon House, 10 Greencoat Place,
London SW1P 1PH

British Epilepsy Association
Anstey House, 40 Hanover Square,
Leeds LS3 1BE

Disabled Living Foundation
380–384 Harrow Road,
London W9 2HU

Headway – National Head Injuries Association
7 King Edward Court, King Edward Street,
Nottingham NG1 1EW

National Meningitis Trust
Fern House, Bath Road,
Stroud GL5 3TJ

Spinal Injuries Association
Newpoint House, 76 St James's Lane
London N10 3DF

The Peripheral Nervous System

Overview

- *Peripheral nervous system (PNS).*
- *Cranial nerves, spinal nerves, plexuses, peripheral nerves.*
- *Reflexes.*

Learning Outcomes

After studying Chapter 5 you should be able to:

- Describe the different divisions of the PNS.
- Describe the cranial nerves and their functions.
- Describe the structure and formation of the spinal nerves.
- Identify the nerve plexuses and the major peripheral nerves arising from them.
- Outline the different types of reflex and be aware of their significance in neurological assessment.

Key Words

Autonomic – meaning independent and self-governing, i.e. peripheral motor nerve fibres innervating involuntary muscle and glands. Form the autonomic (involuntary) nervous system.

Cranial nerves – 12 pairs of peripheral nerves which originate from the brain.

Ganglion – a collection of nerve cell bodies in the PNS.

Plexus – a network or mass of nerve fibres (or blood vessels).

Somatic – meaning 'of the body', i.e. peripheral motor nerve fibres which innervate voluntary muscles.

Spinal nerves – 31 pairs of peripheral nerves which originate from the spinal cord.

Introduction

The peripheral nervous system (PNS) consists of all the nervous system outside the brain and spinal cord. It is of vital importance in the reception and transfer of sensory data, which is relayed to the CNS by afferent (conducting inwards, towards the CNS) fibres, and in carrying motor impulses from the CNS, via efferent (conducting outwards, away from the CNS) fibres, to effectors such as muscles and glands. Rather like the cables connecting the central processing unit of a computer to its peripherals – messages in from the keyboard or modem convey information to the computer and messages out from the computer, e.g. to the printer – they give instructions for a specific action. Without this two-way contact with the outside world all the complex functions of the CNS would be useless – rather like having a good idea which you keep to yourself!

The Peripheral Nervous System

The PNS consists of the peripheral nerves, of which most have both motor and sensory fibres (or mixed nerves), ganglia and sensory receptors. The PNS has two types of ganglia: the dorsal root ganglia, which contain the cell bodies of the sensory nerves, and those which contain the cell bodies of **autonomic** motor neurones.

The peripheral nerves are either cranial or spinal, depending on whether they originate from the brain or spinal cord.

Early development of the PNS

PNS structures arise from two embryonic sources: **somatic** motor neurones from the neural tube, and sensory neurones and autonomic components from special neural crest cells (which detach themselves from the neural plate; see Chapter 4).

From around the fifth week of development the **spinal nerves** start to branch from the spinal cord and grow out to the limb buds and the trunk. The **cranial nerves** develop to supply the head and neck. During early embryonic development the body forms in segments or blocks. Motor and sensory nerve fibres grow out to innervate (supply nerves to) blocks of skeletal muscle and cutaneous spinal nerves innervate areas of skin known as dermatomes (see page 112). The overlap and size differences of adult dermatomes can be explained by the rotation that occurs during embryonic limb development and the varying growth rates in different parts of the body.

An outline of autonomic nervous system development can be found in Chapter 6.

Division of the PNS

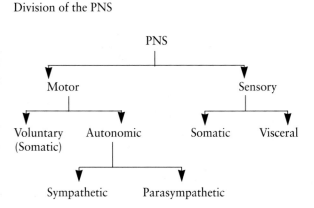

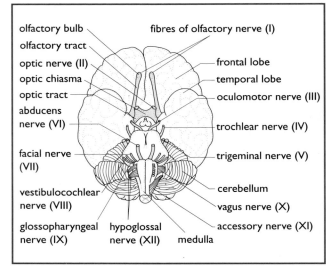

Figure 5.1 The origins of the cranial nerves.

Cranial Nerves

The term 'cranial nerves' is used for the 12 pairs of nerves that originate in the brain – pairs I and II from the forebrain and pairs III–XII from the brainstem (*Figure 5.1*). The nerves are identified by names and Roman numerals. Most are concerned with the innervation of the head, neck and associated structures, but the vagus nerves (X) extend to structures in the thorax and abdomen.

Olfactory nerves (I) (*Figure 5.2*)

These are sensory and are concerned with the sense of smell. They carry impulses from the epithelium of the nasal cavity to the olfactory cortex in the temporal lobe of the cerebral hemispheres.

Optic nerves (II) (*Figure 5.3*)

These are sensory and are concerned with sight. Impulses from the retina of the eye are conveyed to the visual cortex in the occipital lobe of the cerebral hemispheres. The optic nerves enter the cranial cavity and converge at the optic chiasma, where some fibres cross over. The optic tracts pass through the thalamus to terminate in the visual cortex. Some tracts terminate in midbrain nuclei, e.g. superior colliculi (nuclei controlling visual reflexes). Damage to the optic nerves may cause blindness, whereas partial damage to the optic tracts (Chapter 7) distal to the chiasma may cause visual field defects.

Oculomotor nerves (III)

These are mostly motor (somatic and parasympathetic), with some sensory (proprioception) fibres, and originate in the midbrain. The motor somatic fibres innervate four of the extrinsic (external) muscles that move the eyeball and the muscle that raises the upper eyelid. The parasympathetic fibres innervate the iris muscle, which constricts the pupil (see Chapter 4), and the ciliary muscle, which changes the shape of the lens.

You will remember from Chapter 4 the importance of checking pupil size and reaction to light in situations where changes to normal pupillary reflexes can indicate the extremely serious problem of raised intracranial pressure, e.g. after head injury. Other disorders of the oculomotor nerves cause problems with eyeball movement – squints (strabismus), eyelid drooping (ptosis), focusing difficulties and double vision (diplopia).

Trochlear nerves (IV)

These are mainly motor, arise in the midbrain and innervate one extrinsic muscle of the eyeball. They also convey some proprioceptor fibres from the extrinsic eyeball muscle.

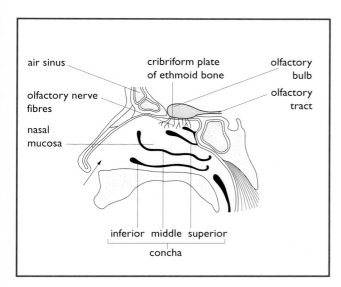

Figure 5.2 Olfactory nerves.

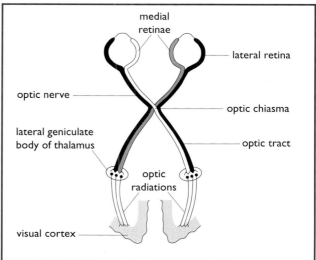

Figure 5.3 Optic nerves (visual pathways).

Trigeminal nerves (V) (*Figure 5.4*)

These are sensory and motor. The largest cranial nerve runs from the pons varolii to supply the head and face. Its sensory fibres have their cell bodies in the trigeminal **ganglion.** The trigeminal nerve has three divisions: (i) ophthalmic, which carries sensory information from the anterior scalp, forehead, cornea, lacrimal glands, upper eyelids, nose and nasal mucosa; (ii) maxillary, which carries sensory information from the lower eyelids, the upper gums, teeth and lip, and the cheeks; and (iii) mandibular, which carries sensory information from the lower gums, teeth and lip, chin, tongue and pinna of the ear. The mandibular division also contains motor fibres, which innervate the muscles involved in mastication (chewing). A branch also supplies the tensor tympani (a muscle of the middle ear). Proprioceptor fibres are also conveyed from the muscles of mastication.

A condition of generally unknown cause, called trigeminal neuralgia, results in agonizing pain felt in the face. McConaghy (1994) states that the pain has been described as the most excruciating known to man. The pain may be precipitated by simple stimuli, such as chewing and cold air. Treatment with drugs, e.g. carbamazepine, may be ineffective and more drastic methods may be needed. These include injecting alcohol into the nerve, thermocoagulation or dividing the trigeminal nerve. The virus that causes herpes zoster (shingles) can affect the trigeminal nerve, producing a face rash, and corneal ulceration with possible eye damage if the ophthalmic division is involved (see also page 113).

Abducens nerves (VI)

These are mainly motor and arise in the pons varolii. They innervate the remaining extrinsic muscle of the eyeball.

They also convey some proprioceptor fibres from the extrinsic eyeball muscle. Disorders cause strabismus.

Facial nerves (VII)

These are sensory, motor and parasympathetic (motor), and originate in the pons varolii. The sensory fibres carry impulses from the anterior part of the tongue (taste buds) to the cortex. The parasympathetic fibres supply the salivary glands, the lacrimal glands and the glands of the nasal mucosa. The motor component innervates facial muscles and controls facial expression – controlling the muscles needed to smile, frown or whistle. A branch also supplies the stapedius (muscle of the middle ear).

Disorders such as Bell's palsy cause paralysis of one side of the face, which leads to difficulty with eating and talking, loss of taste and an eye that waters constantly and will not close. Individuals with an affected eye are advised to protect it from dust etc., and to cover the eye with a pad during sleep. Luckily, spontaneous recovery usually occurs within a few weeks.

Vestibulocochlear/auditory nerves (VIII)

These are sensory and carry impulses from structures in the inner ear. The cochlear branch carries impulses from the organ of Corti (hearing) to the auditory cortex in the temporal lobe via midbrain nuclei, e.g. inferior colliculi (nuclei controlling auditory reflexes) and other relays. The vestibular branch carries impulses from the semicircular canals (balance) to the cerebellum. Damage can cause tinnitus (ringing/roaring noises in the ear), nerve deafness, balance problems, dizziness and nausea.

Glossopharyngeal nerves (IX)

These are motor, sensory and parasympathetic (motor), and originate in the medulla oblongata. The motor fibres serve the tongue and pharynx and are concerned with swallowing and the gag reflex. They convey proprioceptor fibres from the pharyngeal muscles. The sensory fibres transmit taste impulses from the back of the tongue to the cortex and general sensory impulses from the pharynx and the back part of tongue. They also transmit information from the carotid body (a chemoreceptor) vital for the control of respiration and the carotid sinus (a baroreceptor), which supplies data needed to regulate blood pressure. The parasympathetic fibres stimulate the secretion of saliva from the parotid glands.

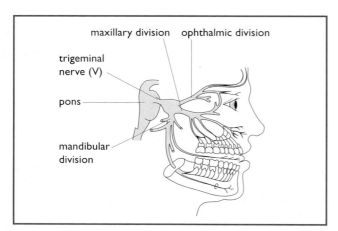

Figure 5.4 Trigeminal nerve.

Vagus nerves (X) (*Figure 5.5*)

These are parasympathetic (motor), motor and sensory. They originate in the medulla oblongata, extend down the neck to innervate the muscle and glands of the pharynx, larynx, trachea, lungs and heart, and pass into the abdomen to supply the viscera (organs). They convey proprioceptor fibres from the pharyngeal and laryngeal muscles. The sensory fibres transmit impulses to the brain from these structures and various chemoreceptors and baroreceptors. As you can imagine, the proper functioning of the vagus (X) nerve is vital to life and is discussed many times throughout the book.

Accessory nerves (XI)

These are mostly motor and originate in the medulla oblongata. They innervate the muscles of the pharynx, larynx, head, neck and shoulders, and carry proprioceptor fibres from these muscles. They control head movements and shrugging of the shoulders – a useful part of non-verbal communication.

Hypoglossal nerves (XII)

These are mostly motor and originate in the medulla oblongata. They provide motor fibres for fine tongue movements, which are required for moving food, swallowing and speaking, and carry proprioceptor fibres from these muscles.

Spinal Nerves

The 31 pairs of mixed nerves arising from the spinal cord provide the connections between the CNS and the neck, body and limbs (*Figure 5.6*). They are classified and named by the level at which they leave the spinal cord:

- 8 cervical (C1–C8).
- 12 thoracic (T1–T12).
- 5 lumbar (L1–L5).
- 5 sacral (S1–S5).
- 1 coccygeal (C_x0).

There are eight cervical nerves but only seven vertebrae; the first pair of cervical nerves exit between the skull and the first cervical vertebra, and the eighth pair exit below the last cervical vertebra. The other nerves are named for the vertebra immediately above their exit points. The nerve roots of the lumbar, sacral and coccygeal region extend into the vertebral canal as the cauda equina, before emerging from the vertebral column at the appropriate level.

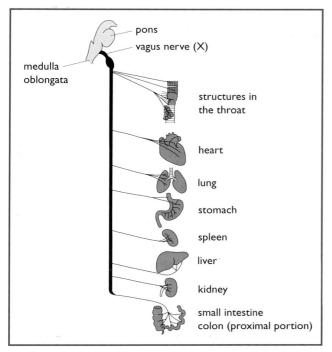

Figure 5.5 Vagus nerve.

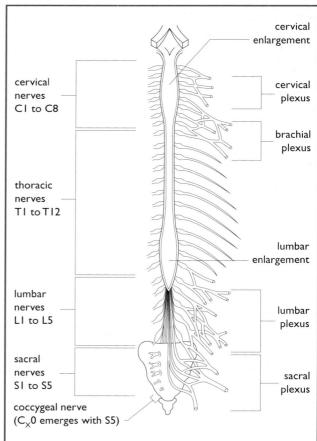

Figure 5.6 Spinal nerves (NB for clarity the coccygeal plexus is shown in Figure 5.12).

Each spinal nerve has two connections with the spinal cord (*Figure 5.7*). These are the ventral (motor) root, with its efferent fibres from the lower motor neurone (LMN), and the dorsal (sensory) root, with afferent fibres from the cell bodies in the dorsal root ganglion. These roots, covered with dura and arachnoid mater, fuse to form the mixed spinal nerve before emerging from the vertebral column by the intervertebral foramina.

Fibres of the autonomic system are associated with the ventral roots of the spinal nerves, sympathetic fibres in the thoracolumbar region and parasympathetic fibres in the sacral region (plus the cranial nerves, as discussed earlier).

After leaving the vertebral column each spinal nerve divides into:

- A thin dorsal ramus (branch) of mixed fibres, which innervates the skin and muscles of the posterior part of the head, neck and trunk.
- A thicker ventral ramus, also of mixed fibres, which innervates the anterolateral aspects of the trunk and limbs.
- The rami communicantes in the thoracic region, which form part of the sympathetic nervous system (see Chapter 6).

In the cervical, lumbar and sacral/coccygeal regions the ventral rami mass together to form the major **plexuses**. The thoracic spinal nerves do not form a plexus but their ventral rami form the intercostal nerves that supply the ribs, the intercostal muscles (respiratory muscles), and the skin and muscle of the thorax and abdominal wall.

Dermatomes

The cutaneous branches of a particular spinal nerve provide sensory innervation to an area or segment of skin known as a dermatome. From *Figure 5.8* it can be seen that each nerve supplies a horizontal strip of trunk at the approximate level of its exit point. The situation is rather more complex for the limbs and there is considerable overlap of dermatomes. Earlier, we mentioned that during embryonic development the body forms in segments, which are innervated by a corresponding cutaneous spinal nerve to form dermatomes, and that the overlap and size differences of adult dermatomes can be explained by embryonic developmental patterns. There is less overlap in the thoracic region than in the lower trunk, where dermatome boundaries are far from clear. In regions where considerable overlap exists a strip of skin may be innervated by two or more spinal nerves. It follows that malfunction of a single nerve in these regions may have only a limited adverse effect upon sensation.

Major plexuses

These are formed by the ventral rami of spinal nerves (except thoracic nerves T2–T12) which mass together at the side of the vertebral column before forming plexuses with branches that contain fibres from more than one nerve root. This adaptation serves to safeguard the nerve supply to individual parts of the body; for example, a muscle has fibres from more than one spinal nerve (a good example of 'not putting all your eggs in one basket').

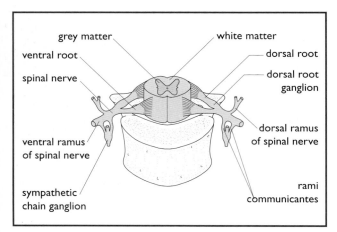

Figure 5.7 Formation of a spinal nerve.

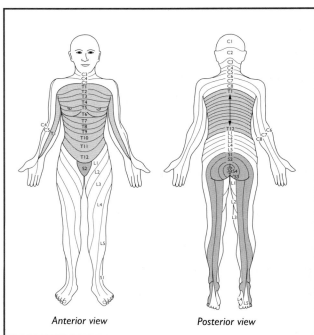

Figure 5.8 Sensory dermatomes.

The plexuses formed are the cervical, brachial, lumbar, sacral and coccygeal, which are mostly concerned with the innervation of the limbs. For most nursing purposes the identification of every individual nerve is not required and we will discuss only the major nerves of each plexus, where appropriate within the context of a nursing application. Readers requiring additional information should consult Further Reading – Williams *et al.* (1995).

Cervical plexus (*Figure 5.9*)

The cervical plexus is situated in the neck underneath the sternocleidomastoid muscle (see Chapter 18) and is formed by spinal nerves C1–C4. Its branches supply the back of the head, the neck and the diaphragm (respiratory muscle), which is innervated through an important branch called the phrenic nerve (see Nursing Practice Application – Hiccups). Damage to the phrenic nerve(s), e.g. by bronchial cancers or during chest surgery, leads to problems with breathing caused by paralysis of the diaphragm (part or whole).

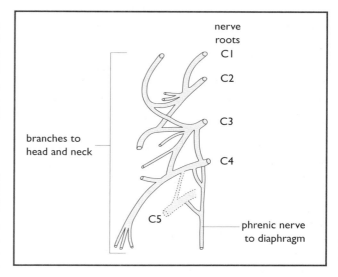

Figure 5.9 Cervical plexus.

Nursing Practice Application **Shingles (herpes zoster)**

The varicella zoster virus can remain dormant in a sensory nerve root ganglion long after a childhood infection with chickenpox. The virus may undergo reactivation in older adults and in those who are immunologically compromised in some way, e.g. by HIV infection or immunosuppressive drugs for cancer. The person complains of severe pain in the dermatomes innervated by the affected cutaneous spinal nerve or in the areas covered by a particular cranial nerve, e.g. trigeminal nerve (see page 110), and a few days later a rash appears in the affected area. Nurses who care for older adults or others at risk can encourage them to seek early medical advice as prompt treatment with antiviral drugs, e.g. acyclovir, can reduce the unpleasant effects of shingles, such as intractable neuralgia (pain along the distribution of a nerve), which can persist for many months. Other effects of shingles include abnormal sensation, sensory loss and occasionally motor root involvement with muscle wasting.

Nursing Practice Application **Hiccups**

Hiccups (diaphragm spasm), are caused by irritation of the phrenic nerve. This usually causes only minor inconvenience for a short while in a healthy person, but when it is associated with physiological dysfunction, such as uraemia (high levels of nitrogenous waste in the blood), it may result in considerable distress and discomfort. The person affected soon becomes exhausted, eating and drinking become difficult, and in some situations the hiccups may cause pain, e.g. when abdominal muscles are strained or where the person has had surgery. Nursing interventions should include: pain relief and rest, help with eating/drinking and the administration of prescribed medication to stop the hiccups, such as chlorpromazine.

Brachial plexus (*Figure 5.10*)

The brachial plexus is found in the neck and axilla, and is formed from the spinal nerves C5–C8 and T1. Nerves from this plexus innervate the skin and muscles of the shoulder and arm, and include the axillary, radial, ulnar and median nerves. When you hit your 'funny bone' it is the ulnar nerve that causes the pain and tingling. (See also Nursing Practice Application – Brachial plexus damage.)

Lumbar plexus (*Figure 5.11*)

The lumbar plexus is situated within the psoas muscle of the back (see Chapter 18). It is formed from the spinal nerves L1–L3 and part of L4. Nerves from this plexus innervate the psoas muscle, lower abdomen, hip, part of the genitalia, thighs and legs, and include the iliohypogastric, ilioinguinal, genitofemoral, lateral cutaneous nerve of the thigh, femoral and obturator nerves.

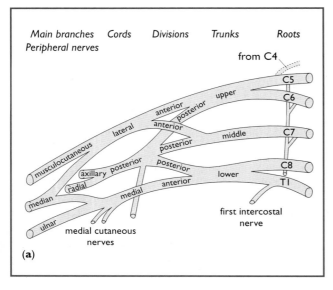

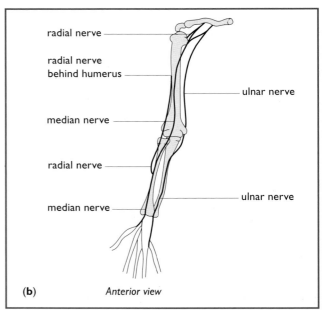

Figure 5.10 (a) Brachial plexus; **(b)** nerves of the arm (simplified).

Nursing Practice Application **Brachial plexus damage**

Damage to the brachial plexus occurs mainly through trauma that involves extreme abduction of the shoulder or forced separation of the shoulder and head. It can be associated with birth injuries, abnormal pressure or surgery.

Radial nerve compression leading to 'wrist drop' may be caused by the incorrect use of crutches, such as leaning with all the pressure in the axilla or having crutches that are too long. The nerve supply to the muscles which straighten or extend the wrist and fingers is interrupted, which results in bending or flexion of the fingers, hand and elbow. It is thus important to provide crutches of the correct size and teach patients about their use. Damage to the radial nerve may occur if a person's arms are not handled or positioned carefully, as might be the case if consciousness is altered, e.g. during a general anaesthetic. The radial nerve may also be affected by a condition known as 'Saturday night' palsy, which occurs if an inebriated person goes to sleep with his or her arm over a chair – they wake up with an arm that does not function properly as well as a 'hangover'.

Entrapment of the median nerve may occur at the wrist as it passes through the connective tissue carpal tunnel. This causes pain, numbness and tingling of the hand and fingers, and is known as carpal tunnel syndrome. Often caused by repetitive wrist movements, this common condition (incidence of 100 per 100 000) may be treated by avoiding particular wrist movements, splinting or surgery.

Sacral plexus (*Figure 5.12*)

Situated in the posterior part of pelvic cavity, the sacral plexus is formed from the spinal nerves L4/L5 (lumbosacral trunk) and S1–S3/S4. Nerves from this plexus innervate the pelvic floor, pelvic structures, buttock and leg, and include the sciatic (the largest nerve in the body), posterior cutaneous nerve of the thigh, pudendal, tibial and peroneal nerves (See Nursing Practice Application – Sciatic nerve and injections).

Coccygeal plexus (*Figure 5.12*)

The coccygeal plexus is formed from part of S4, S5 and the coccygeal spinal nerve C_x0. It innervates the pelvic floor and the skin over the coccyx.

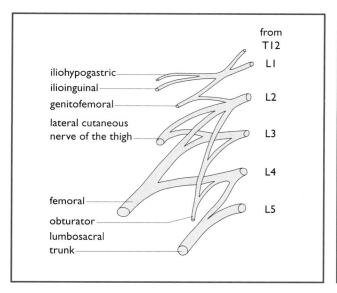

Figure 5.11 Lumbar plexus.

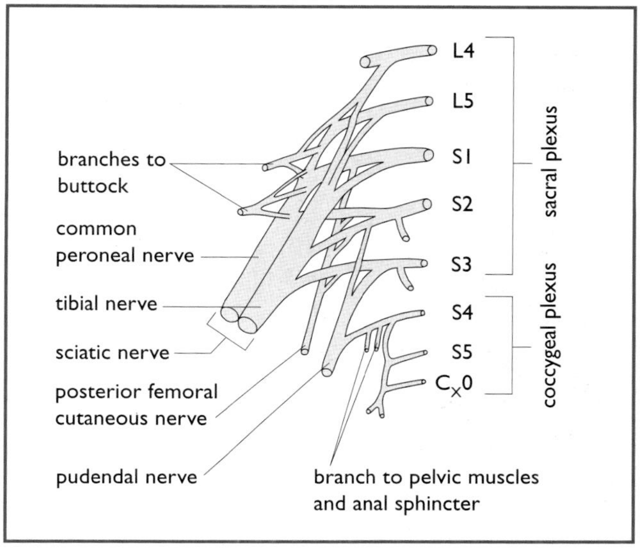

Figure 5.12 Sacral and coccygeal plexuses.

Nursing Practice Application **Sciatic nerve and injections**

In a review of basic texts, Beyea and Nicolls (1995) found that intramuscular (i.m.) injection procedures were not always research-based and showed evidence of outdated ideas, traditions and myths. The administration of medication by i.m. injection can be a hazardous procedure – especially for the sciatic nerve.

The position of the sciatic nerve has important implications for nursing practice. When using the buttock as a site for (i.m.) injections it must be remembered that the nerve passes through three quadrants of the buttock. This leaves only the outer upper quadrant as the area for injection, which reduces the risk of nerve damage (see *Figure 5.13*). Campbell (1995) reported that many hospitals do not include the buttock as a site for i.m. injections in their protocols because of the nearness of the sciatic nerve.

NB Back problems, e.g. prolapse of a lumbar intervertebral disc, can also damage the sciatic nerve (see Chapter 18).

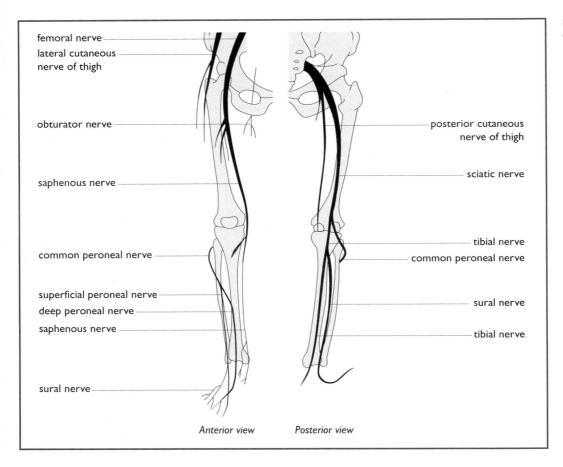

Figure 5.13 Nerves of the leg (simplified).

femoral nerve

lateral cutaneous nerve of thigh

obturator nerve

saphenous nerve

common peroneal nerve

superficial peroneal nerve

deep peroneal nerve

saphenous nerve

sural nerve

posterior cutaneous nerve of thigh

sciatic nerve

tibial nerve

common peroneal nerve

sural nerve

tibial nerve

Anterior view   *Posterior view*

Reflexes

Reflexes, you will remember from Chapter 3, are the mainly protective, rapid involuntary motor responses to sensory inputs. The components of a reflex arc are discussed in Chapter 3. Functionally, reflexes can be divided into:

- Those controlled by the autonomic nervous system (see Chapter 6), which initiate coughing, vomiting, secretion of saliva, maintenance of blood pressure etc., by acting upon involuntary muscle and glands. Many of these reflexes operate through the medulla oblongata.
- Those that involve the contraction of voluntary muscle, which may be innate (inborn) or the result of learned behaviour that allows the automatic performance of some complex activity. Many of these postural or protective reflexes operate through the spinal cord and are known as spinal reflexes. Most reflexes are excitatory – they cause muscle contraction. Usually they are accompanied by reflex inhibition of antagonist muscle groups – a process known as reciprocal inhibition. In certain situations there is also some brain involvement, which will influence and modify the spinal reflexes which helps to coordinate muscle contraction and maintain posture.

Spinal reflexes
Withdrawal or flexion reflexes

Withdrawal or flexion reflexes are important protective reflexes which allow you to respond to harmful or painful stimuli by removing the body part. They involve more than one synapse (polysynaptic) and interneurones connect the sensory and motor neurones involved in the reflex. Examples of withdrawal reflexes include: removing your hand when you prick it on brambles while picking blackberries and your foot if you stand on a sharp pebble on the beach (*Figure 5.14*). These reflexes also initiate relaxation of the opposing muscle groups (reciprocal inhibition) and sometimes contralateral (opposite) side extension (see crossed extensor reflex) so that posture and balance are maintained as you move from pain or danger.

Crossed extensor reflexes

Crossed extensor reflexes occur with withdrawal reflexes (*Figure 5.14*). For example, when you stand on a drawing pin there is ipsilateral withdrawal flexion of the affected leg accompanied by contralateral extension of the other leg. The crossed extensor reflex uses interneurones to cross the spinal cord, where it stimulates the motor neurones which innervate the leg extensor muscles on the opposite side of the body. This complex adaptive reflex keeps you upright – without the contralateral extensor reflex you would fall to the ground.

Plantar and abdominal reflexes (superficial reflexes)

The polysynaptic superficial reflexes can be demonstrated by stimulating the skin. The plantar reflex occurs as part of the withdrawal reflex in response to painful/dangerous stimulation of the foot. It can be tested by stroking the sole of the foot: normally, after infancy, the toes curl up towards the sole (plantar flexor); in infants, before standing and walking, the response is plantar extensor, where the toes extend and spread out. The change, at around 1 year, to the adult plantar flexor reflex occurs when corticospinal tract myelination is complete. Disorders affecting the corticospinal tracts (the upper motor neurone; UMN), such as a stroke, may cause the plantar response to be extensor; this sign of disordered function is known as a positive Babinski response/sign. The plantar response may be normal in disorders of the LMN but will be affected if the innervation to the relevant muscles is damaged.

The abdominal reflex can be demonstrated by stroking the skin of the abdomen. Normally the underlying muscles will contract, but the vigour of response varies in healthy individuals. The reflex is usually absent on one side if cor-ticospinal tracts disease is present, and damage to the lower thoracic spinal nerves will also prevent the reflex occurring.

Stretch reflexes (tendon stretch)

Stretch reflexes are concerned with muscle tone and posture. They depend on the stretching of muscle fibres which activates stretch receptors, called muscle spindles (specialized muscle cells), within the muscle. Stretch reflexes are simple monosynaptic (there is no interneurone) reflexes involving sensory afferent fibres from the muscle spindle. These synapse with an alpha LMN in the ventral horn of the spinal cord which stimulates the contraction of the stretched muscle fibres. Muscle spindles are also innervated by gamma motor fibres which increase their sensitivity to additional stretch. The gamma fibres are influenced by impulses from the brain, which further modifies the characteristics of the stretch reflex (see abnormal stretch reflexes below). As mentioned earlier, there is reciprocal inhibition of the antagonist muscle group that would oppose the movement.

The stretch reflexes can be tested where a tendon is stretched over a joint, e.g. the knee-jerk reflex (of the patellar tendon below the knee). When the patellar tendon is tapped sharply the quadriceps muscle of the thigh is stretched and contracts, causing the leg to jerk (see *Figure 5.15*).

Stretch reflexes are exaggerated where a disorder affects the UMN because the descending influences on the gamma fibres are modified by pathological changes such as those

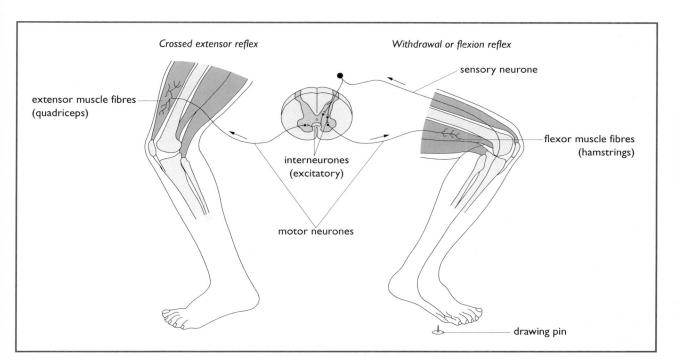

Figure 5.14 Withdrawal reflex and crossed extensor reflex.

caused by a stroke (see Chapter 4). The reflex is absent where the LMN of the reflex arc is affected by disease or injury. It will also be reduced or absent if the function of the muscle groups involved is disordered (see *Table 4.2*).

Golgi tendon organ reflexes

Tendon receptors known as Golgi tendon organs (see Chapter 3) reverse the contraction initiated by a stretch reflex if the tension in the muscle becomes too great. The Golgi tendon organs monitor the amount of tension occurring as the muscle contracts and can send inhibito-ry impulses through interneurones to the motor neurones and reduce the amount of muscle contraction. In certain situations the Golgi tendon organs have a protective role in preventing muscle damage as well as smoothing out the start and finish of muscle contraction and providing pro-prioceptive information for the brain.

Reflexes, then, are altered in various ways by disor-dered function of the nervous system (see also spinal shock, Chapter 4); testing reflexes may help to localize cer-tain disorders and is an important part of any neurologi-cal examination.

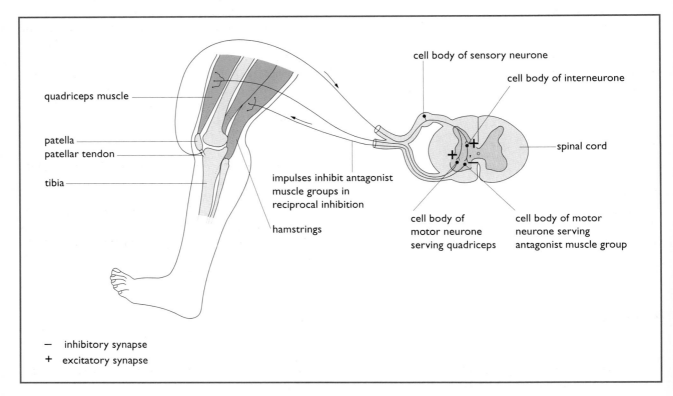

Figure 5.15 Knee-jerk reflex.

Summary/Check List

PNS introduction – early development, components, divisions.
Cranial nerves – function, disordered function.
Spinal nerves – cervical, thoracic, lumbar, sacral and coccygeal, structure and formation. Dermatomes. Nursing Practice Application – shingles. Major plexuses – cervical plexus, Nursing Practice Application – hiccups. Brachial plexus, Nursing Practice Application – brachial plexus damage. Lumbar plexus. Sacral plexus, Nursing Practice Application – sciatic nerve and injections. Coccygeal plexus.
Reflexes – autonomic reflexes, spinal reflexes – withdrawal/flexion, crossed extensor, plantar and abdominal, stretch, Golgi tendon organ.

Self Test

1 The PNS consists of the:
   (a) brain and peripheral nerves;
   (b) muscles and lower motor neurones;
   (c) sensory receptors, peripheral nerves and ganglia;
   (d) spinal cord and peripheral nerves.
2 Which of the following statements are true?
   (a) All cranial nerves arise from the brain stem.
   (b) There are twelve pairs of cranial nerves.
   (c) The vagus nerve innervates structures in the chest and abdomen.
   (d) The trigeminal is the largest cranial nerve.
3 Define: dorsal root, ventral root, mixed nerve, dorsal ramus and ventral ramus.
4 Correct the following statements:
   (a) There are seven cervical spinal nerves.
   (b) The thoracic spinal nerves form a plexus.
   (c) The phrenic nerve forms part of the brachial plexus.
   (d) The sciatic nerve runs through the outer upper quadrant of the buttock.
5 Lan-Ying is troubled by persistent hiccups and asks you to explain what is happening. What would you say to her?
6 One of your patients, who has been working very hard to 'master' his crutches, complains that he cannot straighten his elbow, wrist and fingers. What do you think has happened and what might have caused this to occur?
7 How do crossed extensor reflexes maintain balance and posture during a withdrawal reflex?

Answers

1 c.
2 b, c, d.
3 See page 112.
4 (a) Eight cervical nerves;
   (b) thoracic nerves do not form a plexus;
   (c) phrenic nerve is part of the cervical plexus;
   (d) the sciatic nerve does not run through the outer upper quadrant but is found in the other three quadrants.
5 See page 113.
6 He may have 'wrist drop' due to radial nerve compression in the axilla. This could be due to crutches that are too long or leaning with all the pressure in the axilla.
7 See pages 116, 117 and *Figure 5.14*.

References

Beyea SC, Nicoll LH (1995) Administration of medications via the intramuscular route: an integrative review of the literature and research-based protocol for the procedure. *App Nurs Res* **8**(1): 23–33.

Campbell J (1995) Injections. *Prof Nurs* **10**(7): 455–458.
McConaghy DJ. (1994). Trigeminal neuralgia: a personal review and nursing implications. *J Neurosci Nurs* **26**(2): 85–90.

Further Reading

Williams PL, Warwick R, Dyson M, Bannister LH *et al.* (1995) *Gray's Anatomy*, 38th edn. Edinburgh: Churchill Livingstone.

The Autonomic Nervous System

Overview

- *Autonomic nervous system (ANS).*
- *Sympathetic and parasympathetic divisions.*
- *Neurotransmitters.*
- *Homeostatic role*
- *Stress.*
- *Drugs and the ANS.*

Learning Outcomes

After studying Chapter 6 you should be able to:

- Name the divisions of the ANS.
- Compare and contrast anatomical features, neurotransmitters and functions of the divisions.
- Discuss the importance of the ANS in homeostatic mechanisms.
- Outline the effects of stress upon the ANS.
- Describe some strategies for coping with stress, and minimizing its effects.
- Outline the ways in which drugs influence the ANS.

Key Words

Acetylcholine – a neurotransmitter that functions in both divisions of the ANS.

Adrenaline – a catecholamine hormone released by the adrenal medulla which augments the effects of the sympathetic nervous system.

Anticholinergic – a drug that inhibits the action of acetylcholine.

Catecholamines – important physiological substances, e.g. adrenaline, noradrenaline and dopamine. They are formed from the amino acid tyrosine and act as neurotransmitters and hormones.

Craniosacral – the outflow of parasympathetic fibres from the central nervous system (CNS) via the cranial nerves and the sacral spinal cord.

Ganglion – a collection of nerve cell bodies in the peripheral nervous system (PNS).

Noradrenaline – the neurotransmitter functioning in part of the sympathetic division of the ANS. Also a hormone released

by the adrenal medulla.

Parasympathetic – the division of the ANS concerned mainly with resting functions of the body, e.g. digestion.

Parasympathomimetic (cholinergic) – a drug that stimulates parasympathetic action.

Preganglionic – refers to the autonomic neurone before the synapse in the autonomic ganglion. It runs from the CNS to the ganglion in the PNS.

Postganglionic – refers to the autonomic neurone after the synapse in the autonomic ganglion. It runs from the ganglion to the effector structure.

Sympathetic – the division of the ANS concerned mainly with the body functions adapted to stressful situations.

Sympathomimetic (adrenergic) – a drug that stimulates sympathetic activity.

Thoracolumbar – the outflow of sympathetic fibres from the CNS via the thoracic and lumbar spinal cord.

Introduction

The autonomic nervous system (ANS) is the part of the peripheral nervous system (PNS) that controls involuntary functions vital to homeostatic regulation of the internal environment, upon which everything we do depends, e.g. heart rate, blood pressure and digestive secretions. It provides the motor innervation to involuntary smooth muscle, cardiac muscle and glands.

The ANS has two divisions: the **sympathetic** (mainly involved with stressful situations) and **parasympathetic** (mainly involved with resting functions). These divisions are concerned with the many visceral reflexes which operate at subconscious levels in the central nervous system (CNS), e.g. in the medulla oblongata and spinal cord. Most of the time we are not aware of its workings; for example, without looking in a mirror you have no idea that your pupils have dilated or when fat is being broken down for energy. We are, however, aware of some of its effects, e.g. increased secretion of saliva in anticipation of a favourite meal. The two divisions are in general mutually antagonistic, i.e. one opposes the effects of the other. Normally, their combined activity produces a balanced situation, but as bodily needs change the balance swings one way or the other, as the appropriate division becomes dominant.

The activities of the ANS are influenced and regulated by information about internal and external conditions which it receives via sensory afferents from the viscera, spinal cord, higher centres, brainstem, reticular formation, hypothalamus and endocrine glands (see Chapter 8).

Early development of the ANS

The **postganglionic fibres** and ganglia (singular, **ganglion**) of the ANS are derived from special neural crest cells which detach themselves from the neural plate during early embryonic development (remember, the same cells give rise to the sensory nerves). Neural crest cells migrate, under the influence of nerve growth factor (NGF), to form the sympathetic chain, collateral ganglia and the middle part (medulla) of the adrenal gland. At this point you might find it helpful to have a quick look at the early development of nerve tissue in Chapter 3. The **craniosacral** parasympathetic ganglia are also derived from neural crest cells. **Preganglionic fibres** of the ANS develop from the neural tube in common with somatic motor nerves.

Structure and Function of the ANS

A basic unit of the ANS consists of two neurones, ganglia outside the CNS (within which the neurones synapse) and neuroglia. The synapses outside the CNS in the ANS are in complete contrast to the voluntary somatic motor system neurones which, you will remember, synapse in the spinal cord. The two divisions of the ANS also show differences in both structural and functional features (*Table 6.1*).

Some effector structures receive fibres from both divisions, e.g. the heart (which makes for complex interactions), others, such as the sweat glands, have mostly sympathetic fibres and the remaining structures are innervated mainly with parasympathetic fibres, e.g. gastrointestinal glands.

Table 6.1 Differences between the ANS divisions		
Features	**Sympathetic division**	**Parasympathetic division**
Outflow	Thoracolumbar	Craniosacral
General effects	Functions adapted for stressful situations Most are augmented by adrenal medulla	Functions adapted for resting situations
Neuro-transmitters	Noradrenaline Acetylcholine	Acetylcholine
Position of ganglia	Outside but close to the CNS	Inside or close to effector structure
Length of fibre	Short preganglionic Long postganglionic	Long preganglionic Short postganglionic

Table 6.1 Differences between the ANS divisions.

Sympathetic division

The sympathetic division is concerned with the functions which enable the body to respond rapidly to extreme or stressful situations – the so-called protective 'flight or fight' response. It is designed to provide you with the means to deal with unexpected circumstances which could endanger homeostatic balance.

Sympathetic fibres leave from the thoracic part of the spinal cord and the first part of the lumbar cord – the thoracolumbar outflow (see *Figure 6.1*). The preganglionic fibres, which have their cell bodies in the lateral horn of the spinal cord, exit as part of the spinal nerve (see Chapter 5). However, they very soon separate from the spinal nerve to form the white (myelinated) ramus communicans, which connects the preganglionic fibre with the chain of ganglia running either side of the vertebral column (the sympathetic chain or paravertebral ganglia). Here they may synapse with a second neurone, travel up or down the chain before synapsing or pass through the sympathetic chain to synapse in prevertebral or collateral ganglia which are situated in front of the vertebral column.

The postganglionic fibres leaving the sympathetic chain are unmyelinated and form the grey ramus communicans. They mostly rejoin the spinal nerves for their journey to the effector structures, which include the sweat glands and smooth muscle.

Sympathetic ganglia

Preganglionic fibres (first neurone) synapse with the postganglionic fibres (second neurone) within sympathetic ganglia (containing the nerve cell body of the second neurone). This occurs either in the sympathetic chain or in the prevertebral ganglia.

The sympathetic chain/paravertebral ganglia is a paired chain of ganglia joined by nerve fibres extending from the cervical to the lumbar region – an arrangement that enables sympathetic nerves (which only have thoracolumbar outflow) to supply a larger area of the body. The cervical ganglia (superior, middle and inferior) supply postganglionic fibres to the pupil of the eye, the salivary glands, blood vessels in the head, and the heart and lungs.

The lower (T5 and below) preganglionic fibres pass through the sympathetic chain to synapse in three prevertebral/collateral ganglia: the coeliac, superior and inferior mesenteric ganglia. The postganglionic fibres emerge to supply abdominal and pelvic structures such as the gastrointestinal tract, kidney, bladder and reproductive organs.

The sympathetic division and the adrenal medulla

At this point we should consider the relationship between the sympathetic division and the adrenal medulla (Chapter 8). Some fibres that pass through the coeliac ganglia without synapsing travel to the adrenal gland as very long preganglionic fibres (remember that preganglionic fibres are usually short). For simplicity we can regard the adrenal medulla as a sympathetic ganglion which has no postganglionic fibres. The adrenal medulla and sympathetic ganglia develop from the same embryonic tissue, which explains the close relationship (see page 122). The adrenal medulla augments (enhances) the functioning of the sympathetic division by releasing two **catecholamines – adrenaline** (hormone) and **noradrenaline** (neurotransmitter and hormone) – directly into the blood.

Parasympathetic division

The parasympathetic division is the part of the ANS concerned with body functions associated with normal 'at rest' situations. It is designed for low-energy processes that maintain the body, such as digestion. Using an everyday analogy, parasympathetic activity can be compared to planned food shopping whereas sympathetic activity equates with the panic discovery of having no milk and

---

Nursing Practice Application **Anxiety disorder – a mental health problem**

People with an anxiety disorder such as a phobia (e.g. agoraphobia – fear of open spaces/crowded places) or panic attacks will exhibit physical manifestations, many of which can be explained by excess autonomic (mainly sympathetic) activity and catecholamine secretion. Everyone feels anxious at times and this is a normal protective reaction to stressful situations – remember how you felt just before the interview for your nursing course. However, anxiety stops being normal when it interferes with everyday activities or is out of proportion to the situation. Imagine how disabling it would be if you were breathless, dizzy, sweaty and shaking when faced with the prospect of travelling on a crowded bus. Affected people also complain of headaches, palpitations (awareness of heart beat), diarrhoea and needing to void urine frequently. It is worth mentioning that people frequently think that these signs and symptoms are caused by physical disease – yet another reason for soaring anxiety levels.

rushing to the shop just before visitors are due. The cell bodies of its preganglionic fibres are situated in the brainstem and the lateral grey matter of the sacral part of the cord. Leaving the CNS with the cranial nerves and from the sacral region, the outflow is called craniosacral (*Figure 6.2*).

Generally, the parasympathetic division is structurally less complex than the sympathetic division; most of its long preganglionic fibres synapse in ganglia situated within the effector structure (cf. sympathetic division). There are, however, four special ganglia for the parasympathetic fibres of cranial nerves III, VII and IX: the ciliary, sphenopalatine, submandibular and otic ganglia. These fibres innervate structures in the head such as the salivary and lacrimal glands and the intrinsic eye muscles controlling lens shape and pupil size (see Chapter 4). The other part of the cranial outflow is the very important vagus nerve (X), which provides most of the parasympathetic fibres in the body. The vagus innervates the oesophagus, heart, bronchi and lungs in the chest and passes through the diaphragm to supply the stomach, intestine, liver, gallbladder, pancreas and kidney (see *Figure 5.5*). Some preganglionic fibres of the vagus synapse with postganglionic fibres in plexuses, e.g. those supplying the heart, to initiate widespread effects, and some synapse in ganglia within the walls of viscera, such as the gastrointestinal tract, where they initiate more local effects. In the latter example a very short postganglionic fibre supplies the organ concerned.

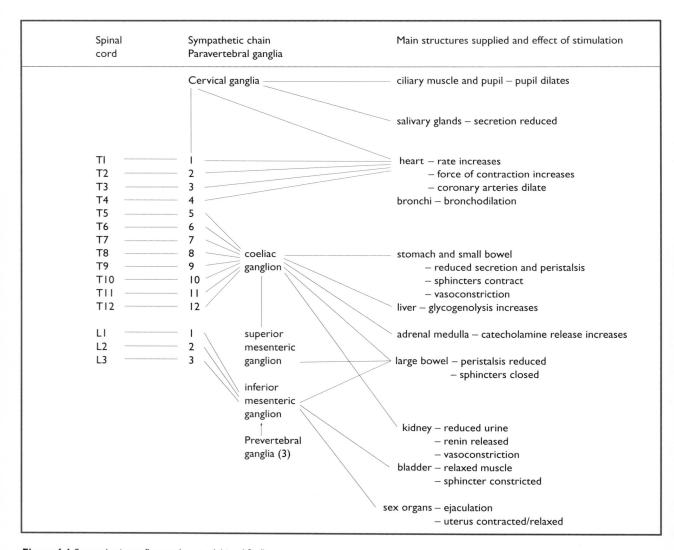

Figure 6.1 Sympathetic outflow and control (simplified).

The sacral parasympathetic outflow innervates the smooth muscle and glands of the large intestine, the bladder and the blood vessels of the genitalia. Preganglionic fibres (pelvic splanchnic nerves) synapse with postganglionic fibres in a plexus or ganglia situated in the walls of these structures. These fibres are important in the functioning of the anal and urinary sphincters and sexual functioning. The pelvic structures involved also have sympathetic and voluntary innervation. We are therefore able to exercise some voluntary control; for example, we can overcome bladder emptying during an exciting television programme until the adverts, but not indefinitely.

Neurotransmitters and the ANS

The two main neurotransmitters operating in the ANS are noradrenaline and **acetylcholine** (see flow charts and below). Other, mainly peptidic, substances, e.g. substance P, vasoactive intestinal peptide and enkephalins, may also have a role as neurotransmitters or in modulation (see Chapter 3). Neurotransmitters act by binding to specific receptors on the postsynaptic membrane of the postganglionic neurone or the effector structure. The ways in which neurotransmitters affect the ANS by receptor binding are complex, but a basic understanding will have numerous practice applications, e.g. responses to stress and drugs (see pages 127–130).

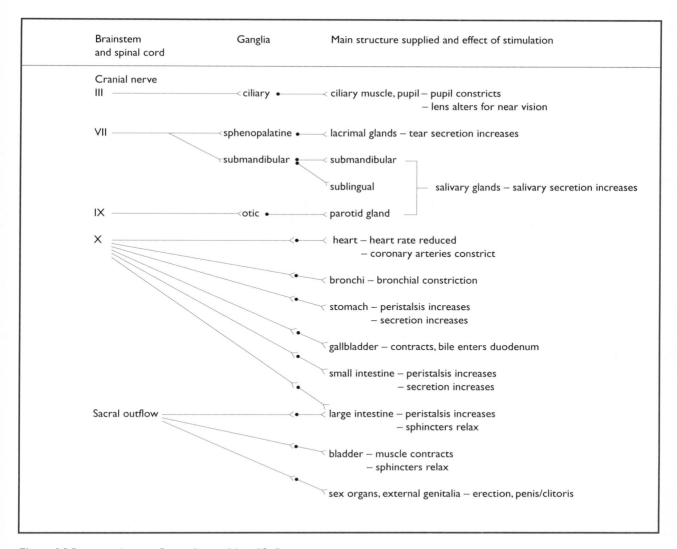

Figure 6.2 Parasympathetic outflow and control (simplified).

Sympathetic division — neurotransmitters

The sympathetic division synapses use both acetylcholine and noradrenaline. Acetylcholine is found at the preganglionic synapse (see below) and noradrenaline at the synapse between the postganglionic neurone and the effector structure.

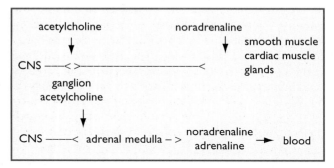

The postganglionic fibres using noradrenaline as their neurotransmitter are known as adrenergic nerves. There are two main types of adrenergic receptor found on effector structures – alpha (divided into α_1 and α_2) and beta (divided into β_1, β_2 and β_3), which react differently to the noradrenaline and adrenaline produced by the adrenal medulla and have different responses to various drugs. Alpha receptors are usually stimulated by noradrenaline or adrenaline and beta receptors are inhibited, but see below for an important exception to this generalization, e.g. the heart and β_1 receptors.

Location and main binding effects of noradrenaline and adrenaline on different adrenergic receptors (see Table 6.2 for effects).

α_1: Smooth muscle of blood vessels, bronchi, gastrointestinal and genitourinary tracts, etc. Liver and salivary glands. Mainly constriction and contraction. Promotes liver to release glucose from glycogen.

α_2: Blood vessels, platelets and adrenergic nerve terminals. Constricts blood vessels, causes platelet aggregation and decreases neurotransmitter release at nerve terminals.

β_1: Heart, non-sphincter gastrointestinal tract, adrenergic nerve terminals, salivary glands and kidney. Increases rate and force of heart beat. Stimulates renin release from kidney and neurotransmitter from nerve terminals.

β_2: Smooth muscle of blood vessels, bronchi and genitourinary tract. Skeletal muscle, mast cells, liver and pancreas. Mainly dilatation and relaxation, e.g. of bronchi and pregnant uterus. Prevents histamine release from mast cells. Promotes liver to release glucose from glycogen. Stimulates pancreas to secrete insulin.

β_3: Adipose tissue. Stimulates lipolysis (breakdown of fat) for energy.

It is important to note that some postganglionic sympathetic neurones use acetylcholine, e.g. the sweat glands (see below).

Parasympathetic division — neurotransmitters

Acetylcholine is the neurotransmitter used by all preganglionic and postganglionic neurones (synapse with the effector structure) in the parasympathetic division. It does, however, behave differently at each of the two sites. The sites can be classified as having nicotinic or muscarinic receptors, which simply tells which of the two chemicals – nicotine and muscarine – would bind to the receptor instead of acetylcholine, which they mimic. This is an important distinction when we consider the effects of drugs upon the ANS. Fibres that use acetylcholine are known as cholinergic nerves.

Remember that acetylcholine is also the neurotransmitter at the neuromuscular junction in skeletal muscle, sympathetic preganglionic neurones and a few sympathetic postganglionic neurones.

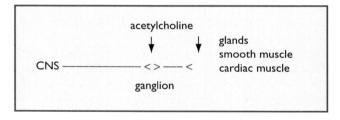

Location and main binding effects of acetylcholine on different cholinergic receptors (see Table 6.2 for effects)

Muscarinic receptors are found in all parasympathetic effector structures and a few sympathetic effector structures, e.g. the sweat glands and skeletal muscle blood vessels. Generally, they are excitatory in parasympathetic structures, but others, such as the heart, are inhibited. Muscarinic receptors cause sweat gland activity and dilate blood vessels in skeletal muscle by inhibition.

Nicotinic receptors are found in all autonomic postganglionic neurones (parasympathetic and sympathetic) and the neuromuscular junction of skeletal muscle cells. Always excitatory.

It is important to note that muscarinic and nicotinic receptors can be further subdivided into several subtypes, e.g. M1, M2 and M3. Readers can find details of these and their pharmacological variations in Rang *et al.* (1995).

ANS and homeostasis

It is worth restating the importance of the ANS to homeostatic regulation (see *Table 6.2*). The ANS, which is an entirely motor system, is influenced by sensory data from the muscle tissue and glands concerned, and the hypothalamus, cerebral cortex (higher centres), brainstem, reticular formation, spinal cord and endocrine glands. Just about every vital function you could mention, from blood pressure regulation to passing urine, requires the proper functioning of the ANS. The rest of the chapter outlines the effects of stress on the ANS, some of the disease processes occurring when homeostatic balance is lost, e.g. high blood pressure (hypertension), and an outline of how drugs influence autonomic function.

Although the functioning of the ANS is considered to be completely involuntary, there are learned techniques such as biofeedback (see Special Focus) and strategies used to promote relaxation which can influence some involuntary processes, e.g. heart rate and blood vessel dilatation.

Stress and the ANS

A variety of physiological, psychological and social stressors [a term used by Selye (1978) to describe factors which cause stress responses] affect the ANS and hence the homeostatic balance of the body. Selye (1978) described the local adaptation syndrome (LAS) in which part of the body responds to a stressor such as injury and the more generalized stress response or general adaptation syndrome (GAS). The GAS is a triphasic response to stressors:
(i) Alarm or initial response to the stressor.
(ii) Resistance/adaptation, where body systems stabilize as they adapt to the stressor, and if adaptation fails, the
(iii) Exhaustion phase, a situation where adaptation and resistance have failed, and which may result in chronic illness or death.

There is considerable interaction between LAS, ANS, endocrine glands and GAS – a severe LAS can cause GAS, and general stress can exacerbate LAS.

Basically, the functioning of the sympathetic division, adrenal gland (medulla and cortex) and, to a much lesser extent, the parasympathetic division produces effects which allow the body to adapt to a specific stressor, e.g. extreme cold, and maintain homeostasis. Initially, the adaptive heat-conserving mechanisms are stimulated by the sympathetic nerves; for example, vasoconstriction (constriction of blood vessels) in the skin slows heat loss. If these coping mechanisms fail to restore temperature homeostasis, the response to the stressor becomes non-adaptive, i.e. body temperature falls and metabolism slows (see hypothermia, Chapter 19). At this stage the individual is unlikely to survive without medical intervention.

The list of stressors is enormous and includes fear, pain, cold or heat, trauma, blood loss, infection, hunger, low blood sugar and a life crisis. The ability to cope with stressors varies between individuals and declines with age. Coping with physiological stress is also dependent on hormonal, nutritional and immunological factors (Clark, 1984).

A very intense stressor which places you in some danger, such as the fear you feel on being followed along a dark road, produces the 'fight or flight' response where predominantly sympathetic activity prepares you to cope by increasing the heart rate, dilating vessels in the skeletal muscle, dilating the bronchi and pupils, and releasing glucose into the blood (see *Table 6.2*). The response is usually short-lived, but if the stressor is severe or prolonged the person may progress to the resistance stage of GAS.

A less intense, but chronic, stressor causing anxiety over a period of time, such as a heavy workload, may result in maladaptive or 'unhealthy' physiological effects brought about by ANS and endocrine responses. The

Special Focus **Biofeedback**

The technique of biofeedback may, for some people, increase their conscious control over certain autonomic functions, such as the ability to lower blood pressure, reduce heart rate and influence blood vessel dilatation. The trick is to acquire a conscious awareness of when these functions are changing.

The technique involves the use of biofeedback information (displayed as an auditory or visual signal) gained from monitoring changes in an autonomic function, e.g. heart rate. The person learns to interpret these signals and becomes aware of alterations in that function. Once awareness has been

acquired the person attempts some conscious control over the function through achieving a calm and relaxed state. Biofeedback techniques may be helpful in reducing blood pressure, preventing migraine and managing stress, but it takes time, requires high levels of motivation and will not work for everyone.

Table 6.2 Autonomic effects - a summary

Effector structure	Sympathetic action	Parasympathetic action
Eye – pupil – ciliary muscle	Pupils dilate –	Pupils constrict Changes the shape of the lens (for close vision)
Lacrimal and nasal glands	Vasoconstriction No secretions	Secretion occurs; tears etc.
Salivary glands	Vasoconstriction No secretions	Saliva produced; watery with enzymes. Vasodilation
Oesophagus	Vasoconstriction	Secretion and increased motility/peristalsis
Stomach and small intestine	Vasoconstriction Reduced secretion and peristalsis Sphincters constricted	Secretion of digestive juices, peristalsis increased, sphincters relax
Liver	Glucose released into the blood (glycogenolysis)	–
Gallbladder	Relaxed	Contracts, causing bile to enter the duodenum
Pancreas (endocrine function)	Influences insulin secretion	
Large intestine/rectum/ anus	Reduced secretion and peristalsis Sphincters constricted	Secretion and peristalsis increased Sphincter relaxed – defecation
Bronchi/lungs	Bronchodilation	Bronchial constriction
Heart	Heart rate and force of contraction increases Coronary arteries dilate	Heart rate and force of contraction reduced Coronary arteries constrict
Kidney	Vasoconstriction, reduced urine output Renin production increased	–
Bladder	Relaxed muscle, sphincter constricted	Muscle contracts, sphincter relaxed – micturition

Genitalia
    – penis
    – clitoris
    – uterus
	
	Ejaculation
	–
	Muscular contraction/relaxation
		
		Vasodilation – erection
		Vasodilation – erection
		–

Adrenal medulla	Secretion – adrenaline and noradrenaline	–

Sweat glands
    – general
    – palms
	
	Sweating (cholinergic fibres)
	Sweating (alpha receptors)
		
		–
		–

Arrector pili muscles (hair follicles)	Muscles contract – hairs erect 'goose flesh'	–
Blood vessels	Most constrict so that heat is conserved, blood pressure increased and blood redirected to vital structures from skin and digestive organs. Vessels in skeletal muscle dilate during exercise (cholinergic fibres)	–
Adipose tissue	Lipolysis (fat breakdown for energy)	–

Table 6.2 Autonomic effects – a summary.

effects include: changes to blood chemistry with high levels of glucose and fatty acids, increased blood volume, increased blood pressure, rapid/irregular heart rate, indigestion caused by parasympathetic stimulation of gastric (stomach) secretion and headache as muscles tense. Prolonged maladaptive physiological responses to stress are implicated in the cause and maintenance of some very common (in developed economies) disease states, such as hypertension, coronary heart disease, diabetes mellitus and peptic ulceration (see Nursing Practice Application – Stress and anxiety in health-care situations, and Healthier Living – Coping with stress).

Nursing Practice Application **Stress and anxiety in health-care situations**

Apart from the events seen in extreme situations, e.g. shock caused by haemorrhage, the nurse will often observe the physiological effects of anxiety and stress. These effects include sweating, rapid pulse and restlessness, and may be seen in people anxious about admission to hospital or the results of investigations or treatment. A different, but especially intense and serious, response may be seen after people have been involved in a traumatic situation such as a natural disaster, violent crime, explosion or serious road accident. Individuals affected can develop post-traumatic stress disorder, which may present with headaches, poor memory and concentration, anxiety and sleep disorders such as nightmares.

Stress and anxiety, in all their forms, can affect anyone – children, adults, health-care workers and informal carers. It is vital that stress and anxiety are recognized and appropriate coping strategies implemented to prevent or minimize its effects (see the Healthier Living box) – Teasdale (1995) considers that nurses are well placed to assess the levels of anxiety associated with illness and help patients cope with this anxiety.

In health-care situations, stress-reducing measures such as counselling and giving information are useful – Boore (1978) found that stress indicators (urinary excretion of 17-hydroxycorticosteroid) in surgical patients could be reduced by giving information about care and treatment, and by teaching exercises preoperatively (see Chapter 8).

Informal carers, such as families caring for children with learning disabilities, may be especially at risk for stress. Courell (1996) describes the problems experienced by the family of a child who presents with challenging behaviour as being often caused by the inability to manage or cope with this behaviour. Similar situations are seen where families are caring for older adults or people with severe mental health problems at home. During observation and practice you will certainly come across many other examples of the stress that carers experience.

Stress and work pressures may affect standards of care, and all nurses have a responsibility to notice if the health or safety of colleagues is being adversely affected (UKCC Code of Professional Conduct, 1992). See Chapter 8 for further coverage of stress.

Healthier Living **Coping with stress**

We all need some degree of stress to function, but as already discussed (see pages 127, 129), prolonged or intense stress can have detrimental effects on health. There are numerous ways in which individuals can cope with the stressors in their lives – sometimes it is possible to completely eliminate the stressors, e.g. by reducing workloads through delegation or by learning to say no to people, but we may be stuck with the stressor. If the stressors cannot be altered we need to develop ways of minimizing the effects of stress. Coping strategies should help the person to regain his or her sense of control (Wallace, 1989).

Different people find different strategies effective. Some people use hobbies, exercise or sport to reduce stress effects, whereas others find that the opportunity to share their worries is very helpful – we should not underestimate the idea that 'a trouble shared is a trouble halved'.

A multitude of complementary therapies are used as coping strategies and many, such as yoga, meditation and massage, include relaxation techniques.

Other complementary therapies used in stress management include aromatherapy with essential oils, reflexology (foot massage), flower remedies, herbal medicine and acupuncture – readers requiring specific information are directed to Lynn (1996). People may use complementary therapies as coping strategies, but they can also be used as part of managing disease states, many of which are related to stress, e.g. migraine, hypertension, irritable bowel syndrome and asthma.

Drugs and the ANS

Many drugs have an influence on ANS function. *Table 6.3* gives a summary of the more commonly used substances plus some drugs that act centrally on neurotransmitters, but further examples will be seen during your own observation and practice.

Table 6.3 The effects of drugs on the ANS		
Drug group/example	**ANS division (S or P)/receptor**	**Effects/uses**
Sympathomimetic Adrenaline	S beta (mainly) agonist	Effect Sympathetic stimulation Uses Bronchodilation, allergy, anaphylaxis, cardiac arrest
Dopamine (noradrenaline precursor)	beta I agonist	Uses Cardiogenic shock to improve cardiac output
Selective adrenoceptor stimulant	S	Effect Selective sympathetic stimulation
Salbutamol	beta 2 agonist	Uses Bronchodilation, inhibition of premature labour
Sympathetic blocking agents/sympathetic inhibitors	S	Effect Sympathetic blockade (inhibition)
Alpha blocker – prazosin	alpha antagonist	Effect Vasodilation, reduces blood pressure Uses In hypertension
Beta blocker – atenolol	beta I antagonist	Effect Reduces heart rate and lowers blood pressure Uses Hypertension, angina and arrhythmias
Centrally acting drugs – methyldopa	Prevents the formation of noradrenaline	Effect Reduces blood pressure Uses Hypertension (rarely)
Antidepressants (acting centrally) Tricyclics – imipramine	Inhibits the re-uptake of noradrenaline and 5-HT and prolongs their action	Uses Depression
Monoamine oxidase inhibitors – phenelzine	Inhibits the enzymes which degrade monoamines, such as dopamine (CNS); leads to an increase in these neurotransmitters	Uses Depression
Selective 5-HT uptake inhibitors – fluoxetine	Selectively inhibits the uptake of 5-HT	Uses Depression
Parasympathomimetics (cholinergics) Neostigmine	P Inhibits the enzyme cholinesterase and prolongs the action of acetylcholine	Effect Enhance parasympathetic action Uses Mainly for its action on voluntary motor end plates in myasthenia gravis or to reverse certain muscle relaxants used in surgery
Carbachol	Acts like acetylcholine at muscarinic receptors. A muscarinic agonist which also acts at nicotinic receptors	Effect Contraction of bladder muscle Uses In unobstructed retention of urine
Anticholinergics Atropine	P Inhibits muscarinic receptors. A muscarinic antagonist	Effect Inhibits parasympathetic action Effects Relaxes smooth muscle and reduces salivary and bronchial secretions. Uses As part of premedication, can be used for colic but side effects may make it unacceptable, used in heart block, used in ophthalmology to dilate the pupil

NB Many centrally acting drugs have side effects that affect the ANS, e.g. tricyclics can cause dry mouth, constipation and blurring of vision.

Table 6.3 The effects of drugs on the ANS.

Summary/Check List

ANS Introduction – divisions, early development, structure, basic unit, differences between divisions.
Sympathetic division – function, outflow, structure, ganglia, relationship with adrenal medulla. Nursing Practice Application – anxiety disorder a mental health problem.
Parasympathetic division – function, outflow, structure, ganglia.
Neurotransmitters – Sympathetic – noradrenaline,
acetylcholine, adrenergic receptors. Parasympathetic – acetylcholine, cholinergic receptors.
ANS and homeostasis – influences on ANS. Special focus – biofeedback.
Stress and ANS – stressors, adaptive response, 'unhealthy' effects, disease. Nursing Practice Application – stress and anxiety in health care situations. Healthier Living – coping with stress.
Drugs and the ANS.

Self Test

1 Outline structure and functions of the sympathetic and parasympathetic divisions of the ANS.
2 Define the following: adrenergic, cholinergic, nicotinic, muscarinic.
3 Which of the following statements are true?
(a) Stressors are always physical.
(b) Most ANS response to stress is through the sympathetic division.
(c) The 'fight or flight' response results from an intense stressor.
(d) Prolonged exposure to stressors increases the risk for coronary heart disease.
4 How do beta-blocker drugs such as atenolol slow the heart rate?
5 What physical manifestations might alert you to the possibility of stress/anxiety in a patient awaiting a scan result?

Answers

1 See *Table 6.1*.
2 See page 126.
3 b, c, d.

4 They block β_1 receptors in the heart which normally respond to sympathetic nerves by increasing heart rate.
5 See page 129.

References

Boore JRP (1978) *Prescription for Recovery: the Effect of Pre-operative Preparation of Surgical Patients on Post-operative Stress, Recovery and Infection.* London: Royal College of Nursing.
Clark M (1984) Stress and coping: constructs for nursing. *J Adv Nurs*, **9**(1):3–13.
Courell D (1996) An approach to dealing with stress in carers. *Nurs Times*, **92**(8):44–46.
Selye H (1978) *The Stress of Life.* New York: McGraw-Hill.

Teasdale K (1995) The nurse's role in anxiety management. *Prof Nurs* **10**(8):509–512.
United Kingdom Central Council for Nursing, Midwifery and Health Visiting (1992) *Code of Professional Conduct for the Nurse, Midwife and Health Visitor*, 3rd edn. London: UKCC.
Wallace A (1989) An active role for patients in stress management. *Prof Nurs* **5**(2):65–72.

Further Reading

Bassett C (1995) Post-traumatic stress disorder: recognition and management. *Prof Nurs* **10**(11):709–710.
Lynn J (1996) The rising popularity of complementary therapies. *Prof Nurs* **11**(4):266–268.

Rang HP, Dale MM, Ritter JM (1995) *Pharmacology*, 3rd edn. Edinburgh: Churchill Livingstone.

The Special Senses

Chapter 7

Overview

- *The eye and vision.*
- *The ear and audition (hearing)/equilibrium (balance).*
- *Olfaction (smell).*
- *Gustation (taste).*

Learning Outcomes

After studying Chapter 7 you should be able to:

- Outline the early development of the eye.
- Describe how the eye is protected.
- Describe the structure and function of the parts of the eye.
- Define refraction and accommodation, and describe how light travels through the eye.
- Describe common problems with refraction and their correction.
- Describe how stereoscopic vision is produced.
- Explain how the retina adapts to dark and light.
- Outline how nerve impulses travel from the retina to the brain.
- Outline how visual acuity may be measured.
- Outline some of the changes in the eye associated with normal ageing.
- Outline the early development of the ear.
- Describe the structure and function of the parts of the ear.
- Describe the passage of sound waves through the ear.
- Outline how nerve impulses travel from the organ of Corti to the brain.
- Outline the ability of the ear to differentiate between sounds of different intensity and pitch, and to determine the direction of its source.
- Explain how the vestibular apparatus helps to maintain balance.
- Describe the changes in the ear associated with normal ageing.
- Describe the structure of the olfactory receptors and the mechanism of smell.
- Describe the structure of the taste buds and the mechanism of taste.
- Describe how smell and taste are affected by normal ageing.

Key Words

Accommodation – the ability of the eye to increase refraction by changing the shape of the lens as we focus on near objects.

Choroid – the middle coat of the eye. Contains pigment and blood vessels.

Cochlea – the spiral (snail-shaped) cavity of the inner ear. Contains the organ of Corti and endings of the vestibulocochlear nerve.

Olfactory epithelium – chemoreceptor cells in the nose which respond to inhaled chemicals to give the sense of olfaction (smell).

Key Words cont.

Organ of Corti – the organ of hearing within the cochlea.
Refraction – bending of light rays as they pass from one medium to another.
Retina – the inner coat of the eye. Contains rods and cones – the light-sensitive receptors.

Sclera – the fibrous outer coat of the eye.
Semicircular canals – three fluid-filled structures in the inner ear, concerned with equilibrium (balance).
Taste buds – the taste organs on the tongue containing chemoreceptor cells which respond to chemicals in food.

Introduction

The special senses are vision, hearing/balance, smell, taste, and touch or tactile sense (see Chapter 3, Sensory receptors, and Chapter 19, Skin). This chapter covers the structure and functioning of the eye, ear, **olfactory epithelium** and **taste buds**. These special sense organs are central to our ability to monitor and respond to environmental stimuli. Impulses from the sense organs are conveyed to the brain through the cranial nerves. These messages, along with those from other sensory receptors such as proprioceptors, allow the brain to form a comprehensive view of our immediate environment and to initiate appropriate responses.

As with other components of the nervous system, the special senses function as part of the whole system to facilitate the communication between the outside world and the central nervous system (CNS), which is essential for our protection, well-being and enjoyment. Try to imagine for a moment the complex neural processes involved when, on seeing a brightly coloured flower, you bend closer to enjoy its scent.

Vision – The Eye

A tremendous amount of information comes to us through the eyes. They contain photoreceptors, which respond to light from the environment. Light causes chemical changes in the photoreceptors, which in turn initiate electrical potentials in the axons of retinal ganglion cells. These impulses are transmitted through the optic nerves (II) and tracts to the brain for processing.

Early development of the eye

The eyes and optic nerves develop from optic vesicles [outgrowths from embryonic prosencephalon (forebrain)], starting around the fourth week of development. The optic vesicles invaginate to form double-layered optic cups into which the lens placode (plate) will eventually indent to form the lens – rather like pushing a ball into a partially inflated balloon. The double-layered optic cup will form the **retina**, and other parts of the eye will form from mesenchymal cells (embryonic connective tissue). The optic nerves develop from the proximal part of the optic vesicles known as the optic stalks. Later, the blood vessels supplying the eye will gain access through the optic stalk. Interestingly, the fetal eyelids are fused together during the middle part of the gestation period – weeks 10–26. During the first 4 months of pregnancy the developing eyes are vulnerable to damage from agents such as the rubella (German measles) virus, which may lead to cataract formation and blindness (see Healthier Living – Preventing congenital rubella syndrome).

Nursing Practice Application **Sensory problems and learning disabilities**

Some people with learning disabilities also have defects of vision, hearing and tactile sensations. These extra problems can increase the difficulties experienced by the person, their family and other carers. A child with a learning disability who also has poor sight or hearing will encounter difficulties in learning self-care skills required for some degree of independent living. Health professionals should take account of additional problems, and be imaginative and adaptable in their approach. It is vital that visual and/or hearing impairments be detected as early as possible, e.g. by health visitors in child development clinics, and where feasible the use of spectacles or hearing aid be started. Impaired vision and/or hearing obviously affects communication and may cause a level of frustration, which increases the challenging behaviour associated with some learning disabilities.

Healthier Living **Preventing congenital rubella syndrome**
....

During the first 4 months of pregnancy a maternal infection with rubella can damage the fetus in several ways – cataracts in the eyes (see page 139), ear damage resulting in sensorineural deafness (see page 148), heart defects (see Chapter 10) and brain damage. The earlier in pregnancy that the rubella infection occurs the higher the risk of congenital abnormalities. One way to prevent problems is to ensure that women of child-bearing age have immunity to rubella. However, the eradication of rubella infections from the whole pop-

ulation is the long-term goal. Eventually, this can be achieved by immunizing all babies (girls and boys) against rubella [together with measles and mumps (MMR); see Chapter 19] at 12–15 months and again at 3–5 years. As a 'back up' a single rubella immunization can be offered to girls aged 11–14 years who did not have MMR as infants. Also very important is a blood test to check rubella immunity as part of preconceptual planning – if no immunity exists women can be offered rubella vaccine and advised to avoid pregnancy for a fur-

ther 3 months. Women found to have no rubella immunity during pregnancy can be immunized soon after the birth of their baby. Health workers who have contact with pregnant women should also ensure that they have immunity to rubella to avoid being a source of infection. If rubella infection does occur early in pregnancy, the couple have the option of terminating the pregnancy if the risk of fetal abnormality is considered to exist. Alternatively, if termination is unacceptable, they can be offered an injection of immunoglobulin (see Chapter 19).

Accessory structures

The spherical eyeball is approximately 2 cm across. Most of the eyeball is protected within the bony orbit of the skull; only the very front portion is exposed. A pad of fat between the eyeball and the orbit also provides protection.

Other protective structures of the eyeball include the eyebrows, lashes, lids, conjunctiva and lacrimal apparatus (*Figure 7.1*).

Eyebrows

The eyebrows grow obliquely over the superior orbital ridges of the frontal bone (see Chapter 18). They protect the eye from sweat, foreign bodies and sunlight.

Eyelids and lashes

The upper and lower lids are thin, movable folds of tissue. They consist of an outer covering of skin, connective tissue, the tarsal plate, which supports two muscles – the levator palpebrae superioris and orbicularis oculi – that open and close the eye respectively (see Chapter 18), and a lining of conjunctiva. The lids converge at the medial and lateral margins of the eye to form the medial and lateral canthi (singular, canthus; literally, corner). At the medial canthus there is a small raised, fleshy structure called the caruncle. The medial canthus may be obscured by a skin fold (epicanthic fold), present in some Asian populations.

The eyelashes are curved hairs growing from the lid borders. Glands along the inner edge of the lid include the Meibomian glands; these are modified sebaceous glands (see Chapter 19) that secrete an oily fluid which helps to keep the eye lubricated. The eyelids close reflexly every few seconds; this moves secretions across the eye to prevent drying. This blink reflex is also initiated by situations which threaten the eye: bright lights (such as when you

put the main lights on after sitting with one small lamp) and if the lids or lashes are touched.

Conjunctiva

The conjunctiva is a vascular transparent membrane which lines the lids and is reflected over the front of the eyeball. Inferior and superior sacs are formed between the part of the conjunctiva lining the lid and that covering the eye. The conjunctival covering prevents drying and damage to the eyeball.

Lacrimal apparatus

The lacrimal gland is situated within the orbit above the lateral aspect of each eye (see *Figure 7.2*). The gland produces the watery fluid known as tears, which contains

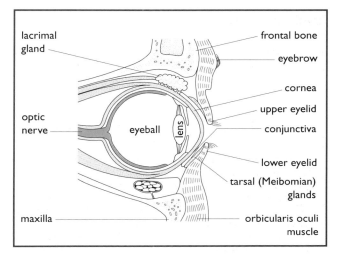

Figure 7.1 The eye and accessory structures.

Nursing Practice Application **Eye care**

Where the blink reflex or fluid secretion is impaired, such as in altered consciousness, measures to protect the eye and prevent corneal damage (see Healthier Living – Preventing occupational eye damage) may include taping the lids shut, eye covers and the instillation of prescribed medication into the inferior conjunctival sac – 'artificial tears', e.g. hypromellose drops – to keep the eye moist. From a small pilot study that compared two eye-care methods in ventilated patients (eye dressings with 'standard eye care') Laight (1996) concluded that although the outcomes were difficult to measure there was no sign of difference between the two methods. Although the study was small, the results supported the view that there was a need for eye care in these patients. Extra hygiene is also required when secretions are excessive or drainage obstructed, and when there is discharge from the eye.

---

water, mucus, salts and the antibacterial enzyme lysozyme (present in other body fluids). Tears leave the gland by a series of small ducts to be moved across the eyeball towards the medial canthus by blinking. Tears enter the two lacrimal canaliculi through openings called puncta (singular, punctum) which drain the tears into the lacrimal sac. This sac is continuous with the nasolacrimal duct, which drains into the nasal cavity (you need to blow your nose while crying).

The continual washing of tears across the eye keeps it moist and clean, and helps prevent bacterial infection. Excess tear production occurs when the eye is irritated by a foreign body or in response to some emotional situation. When the nasolacrimal ducts can no longer cope with the volume, tears overflow onto the face.

Tear production may diminish with age; affected individuals have dry eyes that are sore and susceptible to infection. Watery eye is caused by an obstruction in the drainage system. This may occur in newborn babies, during an upper respiratory tract infection, and in some older people.

Extrinsic (extraocular) muscles of the eye

Each eye is moved by six muscles (*Figure 7.3*). The muscles are attached to the orbit and the eyeball, and innervated (autonomically) by cranial nerves (see Chapter 5). This gives the precise control over eyeball movement and position that is essential for focusing on near or distant objects. Eyeball movement is also subject to voluntary control. The six muscles fall into two groups:

- Rectus muscles (four):
  The lateral rectus moves the eyeball outwards (VI nerve).
  The medial rectus moves the eyeball inwards (III nerve).
  The inferior rectus moves the eyeball downwards (III nerve).
  The superior rectus moves the eyeball upwards (III nerve).
- Oblique muscles (two):
  The superior oblique moves the eye out and downwards (IV nerve).
  The inferior oblique moves the eye out and upwards (III nerve).

The condition of strabismus (squint) occurs when the functioning of the six extrinsic (external) muscles and/or their nerve supply is impaired (see Chapter 5).

The Eyeball

Layers of the eyeball

The eyeball has three layers – outer, middle and inner (*Figure 7.4*).

Outer layer

An outer fibrous coat called the **sclera** forms the 'white of the eye'. The portion of outer coat over the very front of the eye is called the cornea. The cornea is a transparent avascular (without blood vessels) membrane which lets light into the eye. Its curved surface is the site of considerable light **refraction** (see pages 139–141). The avascularity of the cornea allows for corneal grafts without the need for tissue/blood type matches required for other transplants (see Chapter 19).

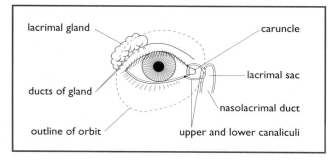

Figure 7.2 Lacrimal apparatus.

Healthier Living **Preventing occupational eye damage**

The cornea is very exposed and easily damaged (see also Nursing Practice Application, page 136) in the work situation. Every effort should be made to provide information regarding eye safety in the workplace. This should include the identification and safe handling of hazardous chemicals and materials, wearing eye protection where appropriate, being aware of first aid measures and having the appropriate equipment, e.g. eye irrigation solutions, easily accessible in the event of an accident. Nurses need to think about areas of their own practice which could be hazardous, e.g. the handling of disinfectants such as glutaraldehyde. It is imperative that all staff are familiar with local safety protocols and follow them at all times. Unfortunately, accidents do happen and all such occurrences should be reported to the appropriate authority. Information regarding specific risks are published by the Health and Safety Executive under the Control of Substances Hazardous to Health (COSHH) regulations 1994.

Middle layer

The middle layer (uvea) forms the **choroid**, ciliary body and iris. The choroid, found in the posterior five-sixths of the eye, is a highly vascular (many blood vessels) pigmented coat which absorbs light and prevents leakage or dissemination of light. At the front of the eye the uvea forms the ciliary body, which contains the ciliary muscles (intrinsic eye muscles) that control **accommodation**. Extending from the ciliary body is the suspensory ligament which supports the lens.

Blood vessels in the ciliary body processes produce a watery fluid, the aqueous humor, which fills the anterior and posterior chambers of the eye. Anterior to the ciliary body is the iris, which forms the coloured part of the eye (different amounts of brown pigment give blue, green, grey and brown eyes). The iris is a circular structure with muscle fibres (circular and radiating) which surround an opening, the pupil. The iris determines pupil size according to light intensity and emotional state – iris muscle fibres, you will remember, are reflexly controlled by fibres of the third (III) cranial nerve (see Chapters 5 and 6). Situated behind the cornea and in front of the lens, the iris forms the division between the anterior and posterior chambers.

Inner layer

The inner layer of the eyeball is the retina (see *Figures 7.5* and *7.6*), a two-layer complex of pigment cells and neurones (photoreceptors, ganglion cells and bipolar cells) which receives light rays and converts them chemically to nerve impulses.

If these two layers become torn and separated, a detached retina results, which leads to visual problems or blindness. Lasers or extremely low temperatures (cryosurgery) are used to 'weld' the two layers together, before vision is permanently impaired. The retina covers the posterior part of the eye, but only the part at the very back is photosensitive. There are two types of photoreceptor:

- Rods, which are more numerous and are responsible for peripheral and low light intensity vision (very sensitive to light), and contain the pigment rhodopsin (visual purple).
- Cones, which contain three other pigments and give high-definition colour vision in bright light (less sensitive to light than rods).

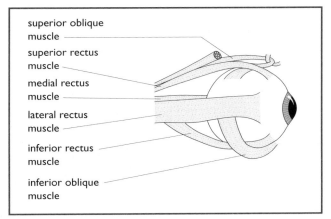

Figure 7.3 Extrinsic muscles.

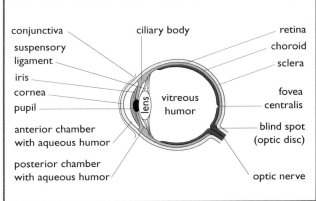

Figure 7.4 The eyeball.

There are distinct areas of the retina. The blind spot or optic disc (see *Figure 7.4*) is the point at which the optic nerve leaves the eye. As the name suggests, there is an absence of photoreceptors. This area contains many blood vessels and can be visualized using an ophthalmoscope (*Figure 7.6*). This can aid the diagnosis of conditions such as raised intracranial pressure (see Chapter 4), which causes the optic disc to bulge (papilloedema). At the lateral side of the optic disc is the macula lutea (yellow spot); this has a small depression, the fovea centralis, which contains only cones. The cones are concerned with colour vision and only function in bright light. The peripheral retina contains mainly rods, which explains the poor resolution images with indiscernible colour you receive 'out of the corner of your eye' or in reduced light, e.g. dusk. You can make sense of photoreceptor distribution if you think about what happens when you are out at night. You see something at the 'edge of sight' (using the rods in the peripheral retina), but when you turn to look directly at the object it disappears because the cones in the central retina cannot function in the dark.

The eye receives blood from a central artery and its venous blood drains through a central vein, both of which run in the middle of the optic nerve.

Inside the eye
The cavities/chambers
The anterior cavity of the eye is divided by the iris into the anterior and posterior chambers; both are filled with aqueous humor. Aqueous humor is produced by blood vessels in processes forming part of the ciliary body. The rate of production is determined by the intraocular (inside the eyeball) pressure. The correct volume is maintained by production being equal to the amount draining into the venous system via the canal of Schlemm in the angle between the iris and cornea (*Figure 7.7*). The process of aqueous humor production and drainage can be compared with that of cerebrospinal fluid (see Chapter 4). The aqueous humor maintains intraocular pressure at a constant level during health, transports nutrients and oxygen to structures such as the cornea and lens, and removes waste.

Posterior to the lens is the larger posterior cavity filled with the clear gel called vitreous humor. In contrast to the anterior cavity this is a closed system in which the vitre-

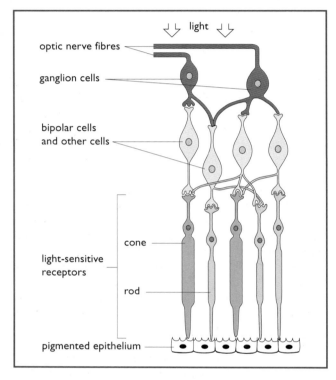

Figure 7.5 Cell layers of the retina (rods and cones).

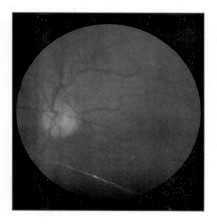

Figure 7.6 The retina viewed through an ophthalmoscope. (Bedford, M. (1990) *A Colour Atlas of Ophthalmological Diagnosis*, 2nd edn. Wolfe Medical Publications, Ltd. Reprinted with permission.)

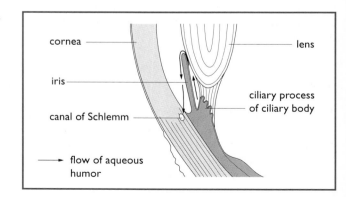

Figure 7.7 Production and drainage of aqueous humor (transverse section through part of the eye).

Nursing Practice Application Raised intraocular pressure and glaucoma

If fluid drainage is impaired or extra fluid is present, the intraocular pressure rises, resulting in glaucoma, which causes visual disturbances and blindness if untreated. Glaucoma, which may be primary or secondary to eye disease or trauma, is increasingly common in people aged 40 years or more. It is estimated to affect as many as 2% of this older population. Glaucoma can be detected by a simple eye examination and by measuring intraocular pressure. Most authorities, including the Royal National Institute for the Blind (RNIB) recommend regular screening in people over 40 years old (25 or over in Afro-Caribbean individuals) and where close relatives have glaucoma (RNIB., 1997), and nurses can encourage them to have these simple tests. Management of glaucoma depends upon its type and severity, but includes:

- Miotic eye drops which constrict the pupil and increase humor drainage, e.g. pilocarpine, a muscarinic agonist (parasympathomimetic) drug (see Chapter 6).
- Eye drops that reduce humor production, e.g. timolol, a beta adrenergic antagonist (beta blocker).
- Surgery or laser treatment to improve drainage.

ous humor, formed during embryonic development, is present for life. The vitreous humor contributes to intraocular pressure and helps to maintain eyeball shape and the position of the lens and retina.

The lens
The lens, which separates the anterior and posterior cavities, is an avascular, biconvex, transparent structure (it discolours with age as it becomes more dense) which alters shape to focus light onto the retina. The lens consists of epithelium on its anterior surface behind which successive layers of lens fibres containing special proteins called crystallins form the rest of the lens. It is supported by the suspensory ligaments and is enclosed in a capsule.

Cataract is an opacity or clouding of the lens; this is a common cause of impaired vision, but can be treated by removal/destruction of the lens. After removal of the affected lens, the ability to focus light is maintained by the implantation of a synthetic intraocular lens, or the use of contact lenses or glasses of the correct prescription. The proteins of the lens are normally isolated from the immune system because the lens is avascular. If the two should ever meet, e.g. after surgery or eye injury, the formation of autoantibodies (see Chapter 19) can damage the healthy eye.

Vision

The functioning of the eye can be compared with what happens when you take a photograph. Both the eye and the camera allow controlled amounts of light through a lens to be focused onto a photosensitive surface or film. The big difference comes when the image is processed; the image from the eye is interpreted and integrated by the (CNS), but the best you get from the camera is a photograph.

Light, refraction and the eye
At this stage it will be helpful to remind ourselves of a few basic but vital facts concerning light energy. You may also want to consult a basic physics book (see Further Reading).

Light travels in straight lines as waves of energy, arranged in 'parcels' known as photons, at the incredible rate of 300 000 km/s (186 000 miles/s). Our eyes can only respond to a range of wavelengths known as visible light, which forms a tiny part of the electromagnetic spectrum (*Figure 7.8*).

Visible light is split into the colours of the visible spectrum by passing it through a prism – the same effect is demonstrated when a rainbow is produced as sunlight passes through rain droplets (see *Figure 7.9*).

We see objects as coloured when that particular colour wavelength is being reflected; for example, grass reflects the green wavelength. Black objects appear so because they absorb all wavelengths; in contrast, white objects reflect all wavelengths.

Another property of light is refraction, or bending when it passes from one medium to another, e.g. air to water. This happens when light enters the eye (see *Figure 7.10*). Refraction can be demonstrated by placing a pen in a jar of water: the pen appears to bend as it enters the water. The eye uses refraction to bend the light so that it focuses correctly on the retina. Light is refracted by the cornea, aqueous humor, lens and vitreous humor. A biconvex lens causes convergence (as in the eye) of the light so that it is

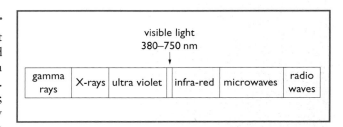

Figure 7.8 Electromagnetic spectrum.

focused onto a single point on the retina known as the focal point [see *Figure 7.10(a)*] whereas a biconcave lens causes divergence. The image produced on the retina is actually upside down and reversed, but is corrected by processing in the central nervous system. The distance between the lens and the focal point is called the focal length.

Just like the camera, we need to be able to focus light from both near and distant objects; more refraction occurs when focusing near objects.

Accommodation, distant and near vision

The ability of the lens to change shape (become more curved) and so increase refraction is known as accom-

modation. When we look at distant objects the ciliary muscle relaxes and the suspensory ligaments pull the lens flat; in this state there is little refraction at the lens (*Figure 7.11*). The distance (normally around 6 m) at which no accommodation is required for focusing on an object is called the far point. It is when we look at near objects that refraction is increased by contraction of the ciliary muscle, which reduces the pull on the suspensory ligaments and so allows the lens to bulge and become more curved. Ciliary muscle contraction occurs through parasympathetic stimulation via the oculomotor nerves.

The near point is the closest point at which we can focus clearly on objects. It is directly related to the ability of the lens to increase refraction by accommodation. As age increases (40–50) the lens loses elasticity and its ability to accommodate; this condition, known as presbyopia, moves the near point further from the eye, as demonstrated by an older person reading at arm's length. You can estimate your own near point by moving a page of print towards the eye until it starts to blur. The lens becomes less elastic and denser as fibres increase.

Looking at near objects also causes the pupil to constrict reflexly, which reduces light entry and directs light through the most curved part of the lens. Also required for focusing of near objects is the autonomic convergence of the eyeballs (ask a friend to look at the end of their nose – note how the eyes converge); this prevents the production of two images which would cause double vision (diplopia). Obviously the eye is working hardest for near vision, and prolonged close work can lead to 'tired eyes'.

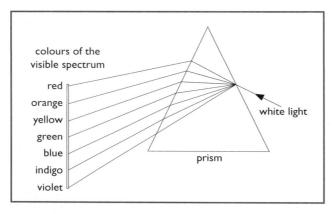

Figure 7.9 Visible spectrum.

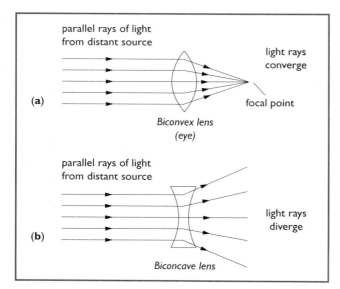

Figure 7.10 Refraction (**a**) Eye (biconvex); (**b**) for comparison, a biconcave lens.

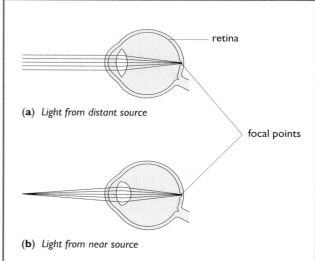

Figure 7.11 Distant and near vision.

Abnormal Function **Problems with refraction**

Myopia (short/near sight)
The eyeball is elongated or the lens over-refracts the light entering the eye (*Figure 7.12*). Near objects can be focused on the retina but distant objects are focused in front. Myopia is corrected by using a divergent biconcave lens.

Hypermetropia (long/far sight)
In this situation, the eyeball is shortened or the lens cannot refract the light sufficiently (*Figure 7.12*). Near objects are focused behind the retina and distant vision may require some lens accommodation. Correction is by the use of a convergent biconvex lens.

Astigmatism
Astigmatism is caused by defects in the curvature of the cornea. In this condition it is difficult to focus horizontal and vertical lines at the same time without blurring. Correction is with a cylindrical lens.

Retinal physiology

Sufficient amounts of visual pigments are required before the rods and cones can convert light energy to electrical impulses. The four visual pigments are formed from combinations of retinene (retinal) a light-sensitive molecule and a protein (opsin). Retinene is derived from vitamin A (retinol), lack of which can impair night vision (yes – carrots do help you see in the dark) and in severe cases cause blindness.

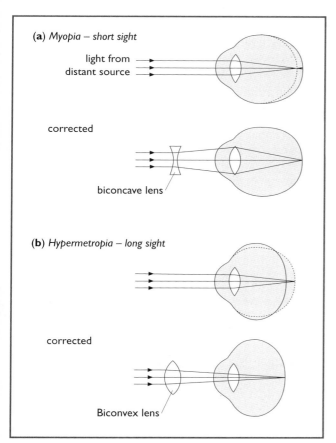

Figure 7.12 Problems with refraction and their correction.

Rods contain the pigment rhodopsin, which responds to dull light by changing shape and bleaching; this produces the receptor potential and triggers an impulse, which is transmitted to the optic nerve by bipolar and ganglion cells (see *Figure 7.5*). Cones have three visual pigments (chlorolabe, cyanolabe and erythrolabe), which contain retinene but have different proteins. These three cone types respond to bright light of the green, blue or red wavelengths. Impulses from the cones also find their way to the optic nerve fibres through bipolar and ganglion cells. Normal colour vision is inherited as a dominant gene (if present its characteristic is expressed) on the X chromosome.

Colour blindness caused by deficiency of one of these cone types often affects the red or green cones. Red–green colour blindness is inherited as a recessive gene (its characteristic is only expressed in the absence of a dominant gene on the homologus chromosome) on the X chromosome [one of the sex chromosomes – males have one X chromosome and one Y chromosome (XY); and females have two X chromosomes (XX)]. It follows that colour blindness is more common in males, who only have one X chromosome – they will be affected if they inherit the recessive gene. Females, however, because they have two X chromosomes, will only be colour blind if they inherit the recessive gene from both parents. Another example of this type of sex-linked inheritance is haemophilia (Chapter 9).

Adaptation

We live in an environment of variable light intensities and need mechanisms to cope with the changes. The visual pigments and pupil size are able to respond and adapt to different light intensities – when you enter a dark area from bright light and vice versa:

- Light ♦ Dark (at first we see nothing but blackness). The cones stop working, rhodopsin, which was bleached by the bright light, is formed and rod activity increases. Full adaptation may take several hours, but adequate vision is restored in minutes. In darkness the pupils are reflexly dilated to let more light enter the eye.

- Dark ◆ Light (we are initially 'blinded' or dazzled). Rhodopsin breakdown reduces retinal sensitivity, cone activity increases rapidly and within a few minutes we have high-quality colour vision. In bright light the pupils constrict to limit the light entering the eye.

Binocular vision

Having two eyes that transmit slightly different images to the brain from different, but overlapping, visual fields (*Figure 7.14*) gives us the advantage of three-dimensional or stereoscopic vision, which allows us to assess depth, speed and distance. You can test this by attempting to touch objects with one eye closed.

Visual acuity

Visual acuity is the ability to see the difference between two points of light. This gives visual clarity, 'sharpness' and the ability to perceive detail. Individual acuity differs and can be tested by use of a Snellen's type test chart (*Figure 7.13*), which has lines of different size letters. The letters are arranged in lines that can be read by a 'normal' (emmetropic) eye at 60, 36, 24, 18, 12, 9, 6 and 5 m. Visual acuity for each eye is tested separately by asking the person to read the letters from a distance of 6 m with one eye covered. The visual acuity for each eye is expressed as 6 over the small-

est line of letters that can be read; for example, visual acuity of a person able to read the 6 m line at 6 m distance is 6/6. Special E test-type charts (the letter E in different orientations) is available for children and others unable to read the English alphabet.

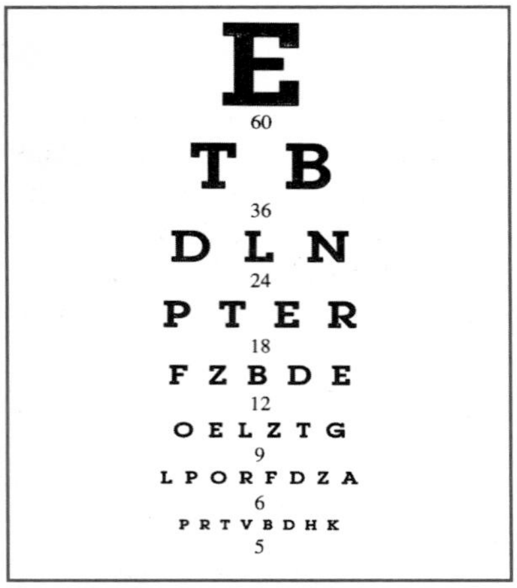

Visual acuity is underdeveloped at birth and infants have poor visual ability. It takes some years before full visual acuity is developed. At the other end of life our acuity decreases with the amount of light entering the eye; the lens loses its transparency and the pupils tend to constrict as iris function declines.

Visual pathway

Axons from retinal ganglion cells leave by the optic nerves, which merge and cross at the optic chiasma (*Figure 7.14*). Although some nerve fibres cross, it is important to note that only the fibres carrying impulses from the medial retina cross over; fibres from the lateral retina do not cross. This means that each side of the optic cortex receives impulses from both eyes. The visual fields overlap – light rays from the lateral (temporal) part of the visual field hit the medial retina on the same side and those from the central (nasal) part fall on the lateral retina of the opposite eye. This arrangement means that all the information from the right half of the visual field goes to the left optic cortex and vice versa. Overlap of the nasal parts of each field allows us binocular vision. Loss of different parts of the visual field, such as hemianopia or complete vision loss, depends on where the visual pathway is damaged.

Most impulses transmitted in the optic tracts synapse in the lateral geniculate body of the thalamus. Axons from the thalamus carry the impulses to the occipital lobes, which contain the visual cortex. It is here that the image is turned the right way up, reversed (right to left) and interpreted, all of which occurs almost instantly – no waiting for these prints. Other fibres travel from the retina to midbrain nuclei (pretectal and superior colliculi) to control visual reflexes such as the pupillary reflex and eye position.

Figure 7.13
Snellen's type test chart.

E
60
T B
36
D L N
24
P T E R
18
F Z B D E
12
O E L Z T G
9
L P O R F D Z A
6
P R T V B D H K
5

Abnormal Function **The causes of visual impairment (blindness)**

The causes of visual impairment worldwide include:
- Macular degeneration (loss of retinal pigment cells and damage to macula), which occurs with ageing and results in loss of colour vision and progression to blindness.
- Retinopathy (disease of the retina) associated with diabetes mellitus (see Chapter 8).
- Cataracts (see page 139), which may be congenital, due to rubella or part of ageing and disease, e.g. diabetes mellitus.
- Glaucoma (see page 139).
- Vitamin-A deficiency (see page 141).
- Trauma, e.g. chemical injury (see page 137).
- Tumours.
- Infections such as trachoma (caused by the organism *Chlamydia trachomatis*) and gonococcal ophthalmia (see Chapter 20). Both infections may occur during birth if the infant has contact with infected vaginal discharge.

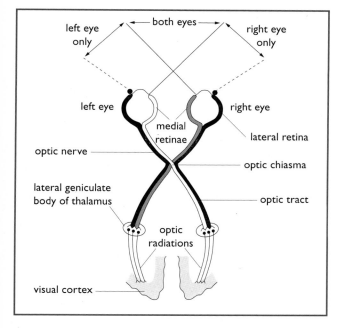

Figure 7.14 Visual pathways and fields.

Audition and Balance – The Ear

Our ears allow us to hear, respond to and enjoy a wide range of sounds, and help keep us upright. The ear has three main parts (*Figure 7.15*): the outer and middle ear, which are concerned with the transmission of sound waves to the inner ear, which contains mechanoreceptors that convert sound energy to electrical energy. The inner ear also contains the vestibular apparatus which maintains balance/equilibrium as mechanoreceptors respond to changes in head position and movement. Impulses travel through the vestibulocochlear nerves (VIII) to the brain for processing.

Early development of the ear

The inner ear develops from an otic placode (thickened surface ectoderm) on the hindbrain from around the fourth week of pregnancy. The otic placode invaginates to form a pit which eventually fuses to form an otic vesicle and the inner ear structures. Meanwhile, the middle ear structures develop from embryonic structures – the first

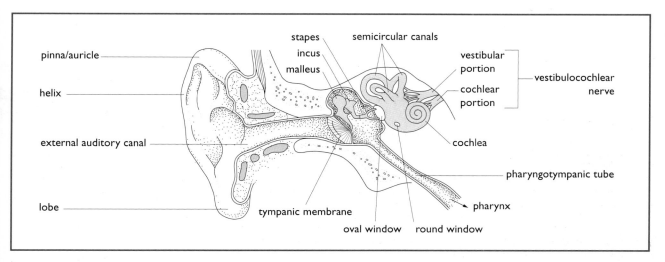

Figure 7.15 The ear.

and second pharyngeal pouches – and the outer ear develops from the first branchial groove (depression in the embryonic ectoderm). In common with the eye, the developing ear is vulnerable to damage during this early period from agents such as the rubella virus (see page 135).

Outer ear

The outer ear is formed from the pinna (auricle) and external auditory canal (meatus). The pinna consists of ridges of elastic cartilage covered with skin; the prominent outer ridge is called the helix and from this hangs the lobe, which has no cartilage. The pinna funnels sound waves into the ear and offers some protection to the auditory canal. In humans the pinna does not move, so we must move our head towards a sound; many animals, e.g. horses, move their pinnae towards the sound source.

The external auditory canal is about 2.5 cm in length and initially runs upwards and backwards to end at the tympanic membrane. The first part of the canal is cartilaginous and the inner two-thirds is within the temporal bone (see Chapter 18). The canal is lined with skin (see Chapter 19) containing sebaceous glands, hairs and modified sweat glands known as ceruminous glands, which produce cerumen (wax). The sticky yellow–brown wax traps dust and other foreign bodies which enter the ear. An excess of hardened wax can impede sound conduction and reduce hearing.

At the end of the canal the tympanic membrane (ear drum) forms a division between the outer and middle ear. This oval-shaped fibrous membrane is covered with skin on its outer surface and with mucous membrane on the internal surface, which is continuous with the middle ear lining. Sound waves cause the tympanic membrane to vibrate, which transmits sound energy to the middle ear structures.

Middle ear

The middle ear (tympanic cavity) is an air-filled cavity situated in the hard petrous ('stony') part of the temporal bone. The middle ear is lined with mucosa and bounded by the tympanic membrane, temporal bone and two openings: the oval window, which is occluded by the stapes (see below), and the round window, which is covered by fibrous tissue.

The middle ear communicates with the air cells (sinuses) of the mastoid process of the temporal bone and with the nasopharynx via a tube called the pharyngotympanic (auditory) tube (previously called the Eustachian tube). Air enters the middle ear through the pharyngotympanic tube to ensure that atmospheric pressure is maintained either side of the tympanic membrane; the equalization of pressure allows the tympanic membrane to vibrate correctly.

The pharyngotympanic tube is usually closed, but opens during swallowing, yawning, etc. to equalize the pressure. The lining of the pharyngotympanic tube is continuous with that of the nasopharynx. During air travel the 'ear popping' noises are caused by unequal pressures caused by an increase in altitude. To readjust the pressures it is necessary to swallow (hence suck a sweet). During childhood, microorganisms often gain access to the ear from the respiratory tract, through the shorter, more horizontal tube, to cause middle ear infections (otitis media).

Inside the middle ear are the three smallest bones of the body: the malleus (hammer), incus (anvil) and stapes (stirrup), known collectively as the middle ear ossicles (*Figure 7.16*).

The malleus is attached to the tympanic membrane and the stapes to the oval window; the incus, situated in the middle, articulates with both to complete the vibration system across the middle ear. When sound waves vibrate the tympanic membrane, the motion is transmitted through the ossicles to the oval window and hence to the fluid-filled inner ear. Sound conduction in the middle ear can be modified by two tiny muscles, the stapedius and tensor tympani,

Nursing Practice Application **Instilling ear medication**

When instilling ear medication, nurses should take account of the following points to ensure safety, efficacy of treatment and comfort:
- Check ear medication as in the usual procedure for drug administration.
- Give ear medications at room temperature to avoid dizziness and nausea caused by exposing inner ear structures

to temperature extremes.
- Avoid contact between the dropper and the ear (prevents contamination).
- Administer gently – the ear is very sensitive.
- Administration of fluid under pressure, into a blocked canal, may perforate the tympanic membrane.
- Remember that there are differences in

the external auditory canal between adults and children. Before giving ear medication it is first necessary to straighten the canal – in adults the pinna is pulled up and back, but in children the pinna is pulled down and back. Always report ear discharge before giving ear medication – the tympanic membrane may have perforated.

attached to the ossicles. Reflex contraction of these muscles (sound attenuation reflex) protects the ear from extremely loud noises by reducing conduction but, because of a time lag (a few milliseconds), damage may still occur.

Age changes in the middle ear include otosclerosis – the formation of new connective tissue causes the ossicles to adhere and the stapes to fuse to the oval window. The efficiency of sound conduction is reduced and hearing impaired.

Inner ear

The inner ear has two parts – the bony and membranous labyrinths (*Figure 7.17*). The bony labyrinth is formed by a complex arrangement of fluid-filled cavities within the temporal bone; it contains the auditory (hearing) and vestibular (balance) structures consisting of the **cochlea**, vestibule

and **semicircular canals**. Inside the bony labyrinth is a layer of fluid (perilymph) which separates the bony labyrinth from the membranous labyrinth which fits inside the bony labyrinth rather like an inner tube inside a tyre. The membranous labyrinth contains the fluid endolymph. The fluids of the inner ear (perilymph and endolymph) are discussed again on pages 146 and 147.

The cochlea (see *Figure 7.18*), which resembles a snail's shell, is a tube coiled around a central bony pillar (modiolus). It is divided into two chambers by the basilar membrane: the superior chamber, the scala vestibuli, which is in contact with the oval window, and the inferior chamber, the scala tympani, which is in contact with the round window. Both chambers are filled with perilymph. The basilar and Reissner's membranes enclose the scala media (cochlear duct), which contains endolymph and the auditory receptors ('hair cells') of the **organ of Corti** (see *Figure 7.18*). Fibres from the auditory receptors eventually form the cochlear branch of the vestibulocochlear nerves (VIII).

The central area of the bony labyrinth between the cochlea and semicircular canals is called the vestibule; its lateral wall contains the oval and round windows. The vestibule is filled with perilymph and contains two communicating membranous sacs: the saccule, which connects with the membranous part of the cochlea, and the utricle, which extends into the ampullae of the semicircular canals. The saccule and utricle contain the maculae (see *Figure 7.21*) – receptors concerned with equilibrium.

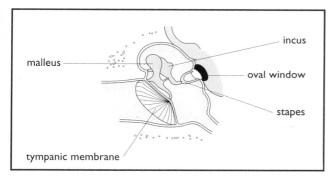

Figure 7.16 Middle ear ossicles.

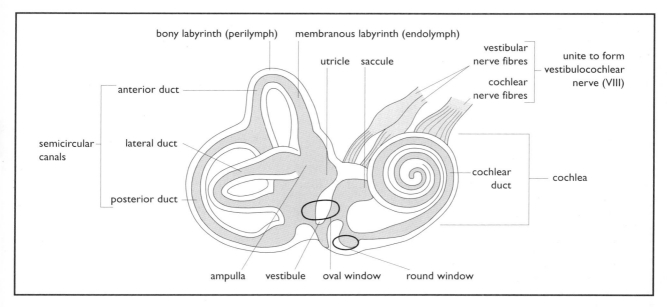

Figure 7.17 Inner ear.

Protruding from the vestibule are three semicircular canals, which are located in the three planes of space: anterior (superior), posterior and lateral. Like other parts of the inner ear, they have a bony portion filled with perilymph and membranous ducts filled with endolymph. The membranous ducts each have a distended area called the

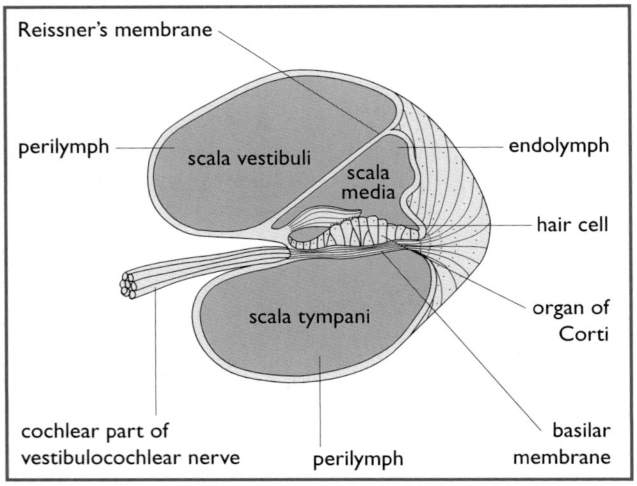

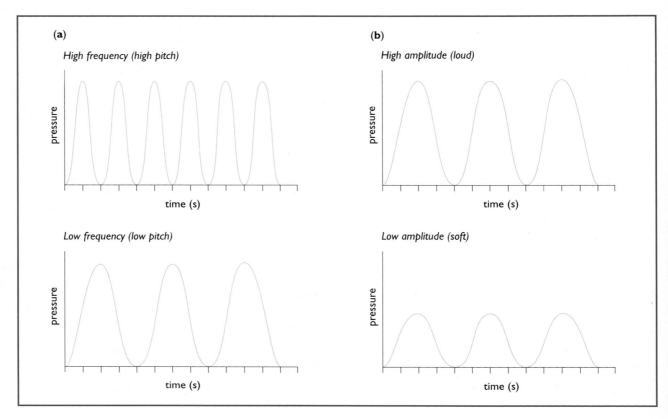

Figure 7.18 Cochlea and organ of Corti (section).

ampulla, which connects with the utricle and contains another type of equilibrium receptor – the crista ampullaris (see *Figure 7.21*). Nerve fibres from the ampullae, utricle and saccule eventually form the vestibular part of the vestibulocochlear nerves. To summarize, the inner ear has two parts – a bony labyrinth within which is fitted a membranous labyrinth. The space between the bony and membranous labyrinths is filled with perilymph, and endolymph fills the membranous labyrinth.

Audition (Hearing)

Hearing depends on vibrations caused by sound waves reaching the inner ear, where receptors convert the mechanical energy to electrical potentials which stimulate nerve impulses. Before looking at hearing, you may wish to consult a basic physics book (see Further Reading).

Sound and the ear

Sound is, in simple terms, the vibration of a medium, e.g. air, which causes a pressure change; the rate of vibration or frequency is measured in hertz (Hz) [*Figure 7.19(a)*]. At

Figure 7.19 Sound. (a) Frequency/pitch; (b) amplitude/intensity.

331 m/s, the passage of sound through air is slow (compare with light). This slowness accounts for the delay in hearing sounds; for example, the sound of the starting gun of a race may reach spectators after they see the runners have started. We hear different sound frequencies as differences in pitch; high pitched sounds have a high frequency and vice versa. Humans can hear sounds between 20 and 20 000 Hz, but the greatest sensitivity occurs in frequencies between 1000 and 4000 Hz. High-frequency hearing is lost with ageing, a condition known as presbycusis (see Chapter 21).

Sound also has amplitude – the degree of pressure change or vibration [*Figure 7.19 (b)*]. This accounts for the loudness (intensity) of the sound and is measured in decibels (dB). Normal hearing covers a range of about 120 dB; this allows us to hear sounds which are only just audible, such as whispering (10–20 dB), to a level which causes pain, e.g. a jet engine (130 dB). We can also detect small changes in sound intensity. Localization of sound depends upon nuclei in the brain stem which interpret impulses that reflect the response of the ear to sound intensity and timing.

Physiology of hearing

Sound waves directed by the pinna into the external auditory canal hit the tympanic membrane, which vibrates at that frequency. This movement is transferred by the ossicles to the oval window and hence to the inner ear. The fluids in the cochlea are displaced by the movement of the stapes on the oval window. Sounds within the audible range cause waves in the perilymph to be transmitted to the endolymph of the scala media, which causes the movement of the many cochlear 'hair cells' (mechanoreceptors) on the organ of Corti. The movement of the hairs causes action potentials, which in turn produce action potentials in the fibres of the cochlear branch of the VIII nerves.

> **Summary of events**
> Sound → Pinna → External canal → Tympanic membrane → Ossicles → Oval window → Perilymph → Endolymph → Organ of Corti → Nerve impulses.

Healthier Living **Noise levels – problems and solutions**

We are constantly exposed to noise – at work, in the home, and during leisure and recreation. Although the human ear can hear sounds at 130 dB, there is a risk of sustaining damage if exposed to sound levels between 85–90 dB. Loss of hearing will occur if the individual is exposed to noise over a prolonged period or at frequent intervals, e.g. machinery or loud music. Hearing loss will result because once the receptors of the organ of Corti have been destroyed they are never replaced. The ear will also be damaged by an isolated exposure of very high intensity, e.g. an explosion.

Other areas of behaviour affected by noise include:

- Loss of work efficiency; stress and irritability are linked to high noise levels.
- Stress at home; caused by noisy neighbours.
- Communication difficulties, e.g. using a public telephone on a busy road (heavy traffic can reach 85 dB).
- Sleep disruption, e.g. the noise levels in a hospital ward (see Chapter 4).

Where possible we should avoid high-intensity sounds or limit exposure by having frequent breaks. In the workplace it is vital to assess the risks to hearing from noise and employers have a duty to inform staff of the results (Payling, 1994).

Very important are measures to reduce noise levels (from all sources), which include: planning that removes heavy traffic from residential areas, developing quieter machinery, limiting time in noisy areas and working quietly on a ward at night.

At work proper ear protection should always be provided and worn for noisy jobs, with regular hearing tests for those involved, e.g. people working in heavy engineering or construction. Employers have a legal duty to protect their staff from the harmful effects of noise and an important part of this is through education and training.

Nursing Practice Application **Auditory hallucinations**

In Chapter 3 we mentioned that sometimes the perception of a sensation occurs without a stimulus, such as the hallucinations experienced by people with mental health problems, e.g. schizophrenia. Hallucinations can affect any sense, but often they involve 'voices' which may direct the person toward certain acts of self-destruction and violence to property or other people. Individuals may have some awareness that the voices are not real, but they can still be very frightening. Just having to cope with auditory hallucination may lead the individual to severe emotional problems and depression. Nurses who spend a great deal of time with people who have mental health problems are well placed to perform assessments to ascertain if auditory hallucinations are occurring and, if so, to what degree of severity.

Auditory pathway

Nerve impulses from the cochlea pass through the spiral ganglion and travel in the vestibulocochlear nerve to

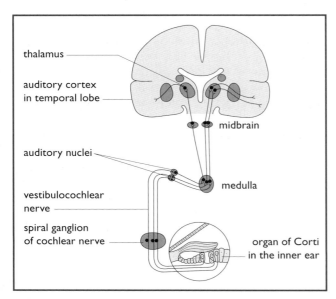

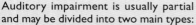

Figure 7.20 Auditory pathways (simplified).

synapse in the auditory (cochlear) nuclei of the medulla. Here some cross the midline, so that impulses from both ears travel to each auditory cortex. From the medulla they travel to the auditory cortex in the temporal lobe, having synapsed in the midbrain (inferior colliculi) and the thalamus *en route* (*Figure 7.20*). Impulses from the inferior colliculi connect with the superior colliculi (see page 142) to control combined auditory/visual reflexes. Certain fibres return to the middle ear muscles via cranial nerves (V and VII) to initiate the protective sound attenuation reflex (see pages 142–145). This rather complex arrangement provides the hearing abilities discussed earlier, such as the localization of sound.

Equilibrium (Balance)

The vestibular apparatus in the inner ear responds to changes in the position of the head and to rotational movement. Its reflex functioning, with sensory input from the eye and proprioceptors, helps to control balance and eye movements.

Abnormal Function **Auditory impairment (deafness)**

Auditory impairment is usually partial and may be divided into two main types:
• Conductive: conduction of sound is impaired, e.g. excess hardened wax (see page 144), otitis media (see page 144), otosclerosis (see page 145).
• Sensorineural (perceptive): caused by damage to hearing receptors, nerves or auditory cortex. It may be caused by maternal rubella during the first trimester (12 weeks) of pregnancy (see page 135), loss of receptors with increasing age, which leads to presbycusis (see

page 147), noise damage (see page 147), Meniere's disease (see page 149) and brain tumours.
• Mixed deafness: a combination of conductive and sensorineural deafness.
Tuning fork (512 Hz) tests (Rinne's and Weber's) may be helpful in differentiating between conductive and sensorineural hearing loss by testing air and bone sound conduction (see Further Reading, e.g. Bull, 1996).
Hearing ability can also be tested by pure tone audiometry, where the individual is

exposed to sounds of increasing frequency (Hz) and asked to indicate at what intensity (dB) the sound is heard. The test is performed in a soundproof area and each ear is tested separately. Sound conduction through air and bone can be tested during audiometry to determine the type of any hearing loss. With special equipment it is possible to test hearing in very small babies – early diagnosis of hearing impairment has obvious advantages for initiating strategies which minimize the effects on development and learning.

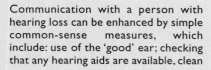

Nursing Practice Application **Auditory impairment**

Communication with a person with hearing loss can be enhanced by simple common-sense measures, which include: use of the 'good' ear; checking that any hearing aids are available, clean

and working; taking time and speaking clearly (not shouting); reducing the negative influence of background noise, e.g. turning down the television sound; ensuring that your mouth can be seen

for lip reading; any visual aids such as spectacles are used; sign language; and the use of other aids, such as printed information.

Physiology of equilibrium

The vestibular apparatus consists of the semicircular canals and the vestibule (maculae in utricle and saccule) [*Figure 7.21(a)*]. Changes in head position cause movement of the fluids within these structures, which affects the receptors. Activation of receptors stimulates action potentials in the vestibular branch of the vestibulocochlear nerves (VIII).

Static equilibrium

The maculae situated in the saccule and utricle contain hair cells. These receptors for static equilibrium respond to head position relative to gravity and to linear changes in speed and direction. The hair cells project into a gelatinous mass (cupula) containing chalky material called otoliths, which increase the weight of the cupula over the hair cells [*Figure 7.21(b)*]. When the head is upright, the maculae are vertical in the saccule and horizontal in the utricle; as the head tilts, the hair orientation changes. Movement of the hairs activates the receptor cells which stimulate the vestibular nerve fibres.

Dynamic equilibrium

Dynamic equilibrium is controlled by receptors called cristae, which are situated in the ampulla of the semicircular canals. These respond to rotational movements of the head, such as nodding, riding a bicycle or those experienced on a 'hair-raising' funfair ride. A crista ampullaris consists of hair cells which protrude into a cupula. As head position changes, the endolymph in one semicircular canal (one in each plane of space) moves over the cupula and reorientates the hairs. As before, hair movement activates the receptor cells which stimulate the vestibular nerve fibres [*Figure 7.21(c)*].

If you are rotated quickly and then stop you feel dizzy and nauseous, with loss of balance and nystagmus (lateral eyeball movements). This continues until your brain sorts out the incoming data from vestibular receptors, eyes and muscles.

A situation where the vestibular apparatus is at variance with the visual input may explain why some people suffer from the motion/travel sickness which makes any journey a nightmare. More seriously, excessive pressure in the endolymph leads to a condition called Meniere's disease, which is characterized by tinnitus (ringing in the ears), hearing loss, nausea, nystagmus and vertigo.

Vestibular pathway

Nerve impulses from the vestibular apparatus reach the

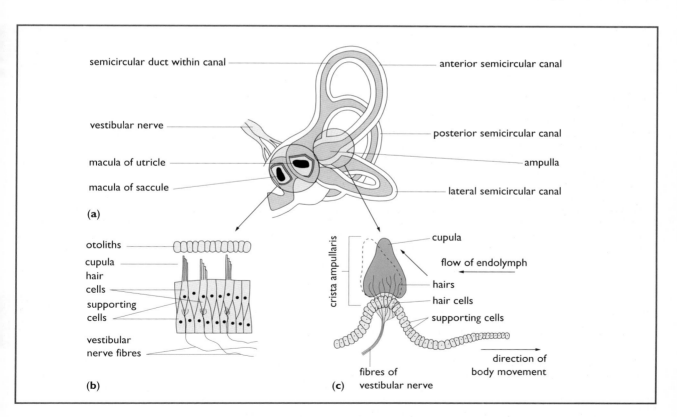

Figure 7.21 (**a**) Vestibular apparatus – vestibule and semicircular canals; (**b**) detail of receptors in saccule and utricle of the vestibule (static equilibrium); (**c**) detail of receptors in ampulla of the semicircular canals (dynamic equilibrium).

(CNS) through the vestibular ganglia, which connect with the hair cells (*Figure 7.22*). The fibres travel in the vestibular nerves to the vestibular nuclei in the medulla, from where some send axons to the cranial nerve nuclei (III, IV and VI) responsible for eye movement and the vestibulospinal tracts of the spinal cord. Some fibres travel to the cerebellum. Both the medulla and cerebellum receive information from the eyes and proprioceptors. All these impulses are integrated and the information is used to control eye movements, muscle tone and posture by reflexes. A few vestibular fibres terminate in the cerebral cortex – which permits us conscious awareness of changes in head position and speed.

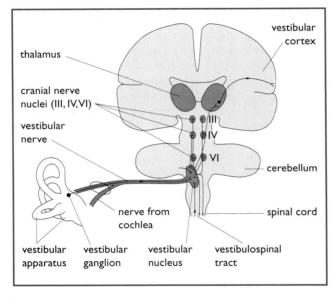

Figure 7.22 Vestibular pathway (simplified).

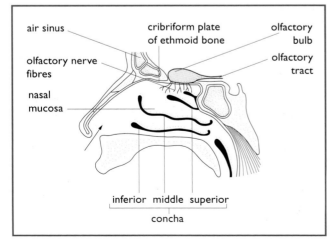

Figure 7.23 Olfactory structures.

Olfaction and Gustation – Chemical Senses

The chemical senses are olfaction (smell) and gustation (taste). Their receptors (chemoreceptors) respond to chemicals in the air and those in food or drink.

Olfaction

A sense of smell is important for protection – many harmful agents have a characteristic odour, e.g. rotten food or fire. Odours also provide experiences that enrich our lives, e.g. scented flowers in a city flat. In many species odours are vital for recognition between individuals and in reproductive behaviour. Our behaviour is also influenced by odours from chemicals called pheromones contained within sweat and other body secretions (see Chapter 19).

We have the ability to recognise thousands of odours and it is proposed that all odours are made up from seven primary odour classes – musky, floral, pepperminty, camphorous, pungent, ethereal and putrid, but larger numbers of 30–50 have been suggested. A strong link between olfaction, appetite and taste exists – appetite increases and food tastes better if it also smells good.

Physiology of olfaction

Specialized chemoreceptor cells are found within the olfactory epithelium, which forms part of the mucous membrane lining the roof of the nasal cavity (*Figure 7.23*). The receptors respond to minute amounts of chemical vapours which enter the nose during inspiration (breathing in); the concentration of chemical in contact with the receptor is greatly enhanced by sniffing.

Cilia (see Chapter 1) projecting from each olfactory receptor increase the surface area for contact with the odour molecule, which dissolves in mucus before contact.

Axons from the olfactory receptors form the fibres of the olfactory nerves (I) (*Figure 7.24*) which pass through the cribriform plate of the ethmoid bone (see Chapter 18) before synapsing in the olfactory bulbs. The olfactory bulbs contain cells that integrate and modify impulses. Olfactory tracts transmit impulses to the olfactory cortex in the temporal lobes of each hemisphere for interpretation and to areas of the limbic system (see Chapter 4) concerned with the emotional aspects of smell. A specific odour may stimulate memories; for example, the typical 'hospital smell' may remind you of a relative who died in hospital when you were a child.

Adaptation
Response to odours can be altered by processes in the brain. After a short exposure awareness of an odour will decrease

– a definite advantage when odours are unpleasant, and of practical benefit by making way for new odours.

Gustation

Being able to taste enhances appetite and the enjoyment of food (compare food which is bland with highly spiced dishes). Taste stimulates digestive processes, e.g. flow of saliva, and helps in homeostatic regulation by ensuring that we eat foods of different tastes which provide a balanced intake of minerals, vitamins and other nutrients. Rejection of harmful substances is assisted by their unpleasant taste (often bitter) and smell; we gag on 'bad food' or even vomit if swallowing does occur. Some individuals like bitter/salty foods such as olives, but they are definitely an 'acquired taste'.

Physiology of gustation

Taste buds are situated mainly on the tongue, although there are a few on the soft palate, cheeks, epiglottis and pharynx. They respond to chemicals dissolved in saliva and differentiate between four basic tastes: sweet, sour, salt and bitter. Taste buds are located in the tongue papillae, and the different areas of the tongue tend to detect different basic tastes (*Figure 7.25*), although there is some overlap: front (sweet and salt), sides (sour and salt), back (bitter).

Each taste bud (*Figure 7.26*) is a cluster of cells within the epithelium of the tongue; its 'hairs', or microvilli, which project through the pore, contain the chemoreceptors. A receptor response of sufficient strength stimulates an action potential in sensory fibres leaving the taste bud. Taste depends upon the concentration of the chemical in contact with the receptors and the temperature, texture and smell of the food. Adaptation to taste can occur within a few minutes.

Taste, and hence appetite, can be impaired if an upper respiratory tract infection affects the olfactory receptors in the nose. Taste is also affected when the mouth is dry or oral hygiene (see Chapter 13) declines, such as through dehydration (see Chapter 2). The nervous pathway (*Figure 7.27*) involves the facial (VII), the glossopharyngeal (IX) and to a limited extent the vagus (X) nerves. The nerve fibres synapse within the medulla and pass to the thalamus prior to travelling to the gustatory cortex of both parietal lobes for interpretation.

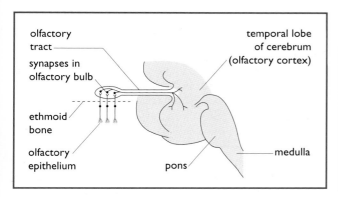

Figure 7.24 Olfactory pathway (simplified).

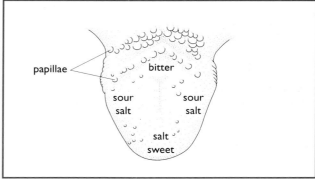

Figure 7.25 Taste regions of the tongue.

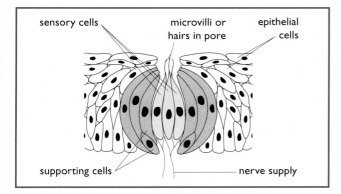

Figure 7.26 A taste bud.

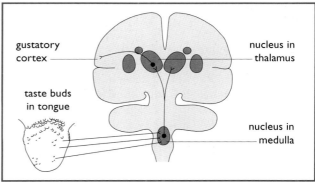

Figure 7.27 Gustatory pathways (simplified).

Nursing Practice Application **Changes in chemical senses**

The senses of taste and smell change with normal ageing; gradual loss of taste and olfactory receptors, starting in midlife accounts for the greatly diminished sense of taste and smell in older people. This may account for the common complaint voiced by older people that 'modern food' has no taste and contributes to a reduction in appetite. Nurses can encourage food intake by ascertaining preferences and making suggestions about stronger flavours and aromas, seasoning and interesting textures, and ensuring adequate oral hygiene and dental health. The loss of olfactory receptors impairs the ability to detect dangerous or unpleasant odours – the person may be unaware of food burning, body odours or environmental smells, e.g. from companion animals. Disturbances in smell or taste can occur as part of a disease state, including the aura experienced by some people with epilepsy (see Chapter 4) who perceive a strange smell or taste immediately before a seizure. Taste may also change in some malignant conditions and with drugs such as the muscle relaxants baclofen and methocarbamol (metallic taste).

Summary/Check List

Introduction – special senses. Nursing Practice Application – sensory problems and learning disabilities.

Vision – Eye (structure) – early development, Healthier Living – preventing congenital rubella syndrome, accessory structures, Nursing Practice Application – eye care. Extraocular muscles. Layers of the eyeball – sclera, Healthier Living – preventing occupational eye damage, uvea, retina (rods and cones). Inside the eye – cavities/chambers, Nursing Practice Application – raised intraocular pressure and glaucoma, lens. Vision (function). Light, refraction, accommodation. Problems with refraction. Retinal physiology – pigments, adaptation, binocular and stereoscopic vision, acuity, visual pathway. Visual impairment, Person-centred Study – Anwar.

Audition and balance – Ear (structure) – early development.

Outer ear, Nursing Practice Application – instilling ear medication. Middle ear. Inner ear. Audition (function). Sound, Healthier Living – noise levels – problems and solutions. Physiology of hearing. Nursing Practice Application – auditory hallucinations. Auditory pathway. Auditory impairment, Nursing Practice Application – auditory impairment. Equilibrium (balance) – vestibular apparatus. Physiology – static and dynamic equilibrium, vestibular pathway.

Olfaction (smell) – Nose, olfactory structures. Physiology of olfaction – olfactory pathway, adaptation.

Gustation (taste) – Taste buds. Physiology of gustation – gustatory pathway. Nursing Practice Application – changes in chemical senses.

Self Test

1 Put the following in their correct pairs:
   (a) tears;
   (b) posterior cavity;
   (c) aqueous humor;
   (d) lacrimal gland;
   (e) vitreous humor;
   (f) processes of ciliary body.
2 Which of the following statements are true?
   (a) The uvea consists of choroid, ciliary body and iris.
   (b) The vascular cornea covers the front of the eye.
   (c) Cones are colour vision receptors.
   (d) Pupil size is controlled by the oculomotor nerve.
3 Describe how light entering the eye is focused on the retina.
4 What changes are made to the image received by the visual cortex during interpretation?

5 Which of the following statements are true?
   (a) The pinna directs sound onto the tympanic membrane.
   (b) The middle ear communicates with the nasopharynx via the pharyngotympanic tube.
   (c) The stapes is attached to the round window.
   (d) The membranous labyrinth is surrounded by peri-lymph and contains endolymph.
6 What is the normal hearing range and what characteristics of sound can we determine?
7 Explain briefly how the vestibular apparatus helps to maintain balance.
8 Outline the benefits of having the chemical senses.
9 What changes in the chemical senses occur with normal ageing?

Answers

1   a–d, b–e and c–f.
2   a, c, d.
3   See pages 139–141.
4   See page 142.
5   a, b, d.

6   See page 147.
7   See pages 148–150.
8   See pages 150–152.
9   See page 152.

References

Laight SE (1996) The Efficacy of Eye Care for Ventilated Patients: Outline of an Experimental Comparative Research Pilot Study. *Intens Crit Care Nurs* **12**(1):16–26.

Payling KJ (1994) A hazard we can no longer ignore. Effects of excessive noise on wellbeing. *Prof Nurs* **9**(6):418–421.

Royal National Institute for the Blind (1997) *Half an hour could save your sight*, London: RNIB.

Further Reading

Breithaupt J (1995) *Understanding Physics for Advanced Level*, 3rd edn. Cheltenham: Stanley Thornes.

Bull PD (1996) *Lecture Notes on Diseases of the Ear, Nose and Throat*, 8th edn. Oxford: Blackwell Scientific Publications.

Freeland A (1989) *Deafness: the Facts*. Oxford: Oxford Medical Publications.

Johnson K (1991) *Physics for You* (GCSE level). Cheltenham: Stanley Thornes.

Martin FN (1986) *Introduction to Audiology*, 3rd edn. Englewood Cliffs, NJ: Prentice-Hall.

Sigler B, Schuring L (1994) *Ear, Nose and Throat Disorders*. London: Mosby.

Spalton D, Hitchings R, Hunter P (1994) *Atlas of Clinical Ophthalmology*, 2nd edn. London: Mosby.

Useful Addresses

Royal National Institute for the Blind
224 Great Portland Street
London W1N 6AA

Royal National Institute for the Deaf
105 Gower Street
London WC1E 6A

The Endocrine System: Hormonal Control and Regulation

Overview

- *Endocrine structures.*
- *Hormones.*
- *Detail: hypothalamus, pituitary, thyroid, parathyroids, adrenals, pancreas.*
- *Control and regulation of: growth, general metabolism, calcium homeostasis, water/electrolyte balance, stress response, blood glucose.*
- *Thymus and pineal body.*

Learning Outcomes

After studying Chapter 8 you should be able to:

- Describe endocrine system functions and its links with the nervous system.
- Describe the location of endocrine glands and other structures that produce hormones.
- Describe hormone structure and outline their actions on target cells.
- Explain the regulation of hormone secretion.
- Describe the relationship between the hypothalamus and the pituitary gland.
- List the hormones produced by the anterior pituitary and discuss their effects.
- Describe the function of the posterior pituitary.
- Describe how thyroid hormones control metabolism and help regulate calcium homeostasis.
- Discuss the role of parathyroid hormone in calcium homeostasis.
- Describe the physiological effects of the hormones secreted by the adrenal cortex and medulla.
- Discuss the role of the pancreatic hormones in the control of blood glucose.
- Outline the role of the thymus gland.
- Discuss the role of the pineal body.

Key Words

Cyclic adenosine monophosphate (cAMP) – the 'second messenger' substance formed from ATP. It initiates the effects of a hormone within its target cells in situations where the hormone does not enter the cell.

Endocrine gland/structure – a ductless glandular structure, its secretions (hormones) are discharged directly into the extracellular spaces to enter the blood or lymph.

Hormones – the chemical messengers produced by endocrine structures which regulate the functions of distant organs/structures. They are usually steroids or amino-acid-based, but other molecules also act as hormones.

Inhibiting hormone – a hypothalamic hormone that inhibits the secretion of a specific anterior pituitary hormone.

Metabolism – term used to describe all the biochemical processes occurring in the body. Anabolism (synthesis reactions) and catabolism (decomposition reactions).

Negative feedback – a mechanism by which hormone production is inhibited by high levels of that hormone in the blood. Regulates the release of most hormones.

Releasing factor/hormone – a hypothalamic hormone that stimulates the secretion of a specific anterior pituitary hormone.

Target cell – the specific cell type influenced by a particular hormone.

Introduction

The **endocrine structures** work closely with the nervous system to regulate body processes and maintain homeostasis. They function through the release of chemical hormones, which travel in the blood or lymph to **target cells** in distant organs (cf. Paracrine page 158). Onset of **hormone** action is usually slower than those initiated by the nervous system, but hormones often control longer-term functions, e.g. growth (cf. Reflex action, Chapter 3).

There are, however, exceptions; for example, blood glucose control is rapid. Although these two control systems are considered separately, there are several examples of their close links:

- The hypothalamus (see Chapter 4) is a dual purpose structure – both neural and endocrine (neuroendocrine).
- The posterior pituitary, which develops from the brain, stores and releases hypothalamic hormones.
- Anterior pituitary hormone production is regulated by hypothalamic **releasing/inhibiting hormones.**
- The adrenal medulla develops from the same embryonic tissue as the sympathetic ganglia. Its action augments the sympathetic division of the autonomic nervous system (ANS) and it can be considered to be a sympathetic ganglion without a postganglionic fibre (Chapter 6).
- Hormone levels affect behaviour and mood, e.g. the 'ups and downs' of puberty.
- Chemicals acting as hormones in one system may also function as a neurotransmitter, e.g. noradrenaline.

Endocrine structures secrete hormones directly into the extracellular spaces to enter the blood and lymph. They regulate the metabolic processes of most cells and influence growth, nutrition, energy utilization, fluid and electrolyte balance, stress responses and reproduction.

Endocrine Structures and Locations

The major 'classical' endocrine structures/glands and their locations are (*Figure 8.1*):

- Hypothalamus – brain.
- Pituitary gland – rests in fossa of sphenoid bone.
- Thyroid gland – neck.
- Parathyroid glands (four) – posterior aspect of thyroid gland.
- Adrenal glands (two) – one on top of each kidney.
- Islets of Langerhans in pancreas – abdominal cavity. The pancreas has both endocrine function (islets of Langerhans, page 170) and exocrine (secretions leave through a duct) function (Chapter 13).
- Gonads (two): ovaries (female) – pelvic cavity, testes (male) – scrotum (see Chapter 20).
- Pineal body – brain.
- Thymus – mediastinum (see Chapter 1).

Apart from the major endocrine structures, there are many other tissues which produce hormones in addition to their other functions (*Table 8.1*). These structures include the placenta, kidney, gastrointestinal tract and heart, all of which are discussed in the appropriate chapters.

Certain tumours may also produce hormones; for example, oat-cell lung cancers secrete substances which have similar effects to antidiuretic hormone (ADH) or adrenocorticotrophic hormone (ACTH).

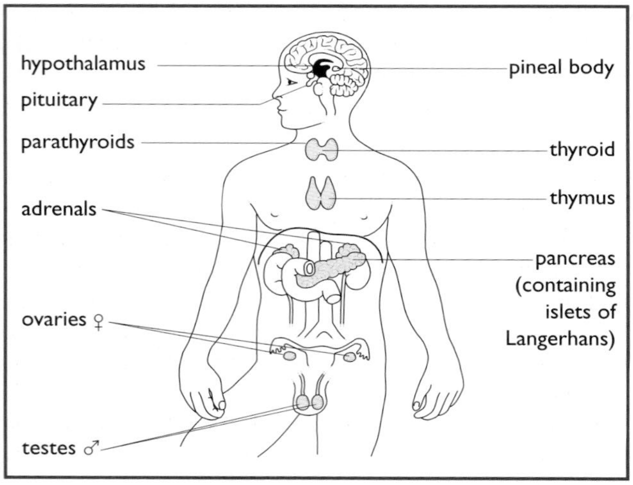

Figure 8.1 Location of major endocrine structures.

Table 8.1 Hormones produced by other structures

Structure	Hormone
Trophoblast –> Placenta	Human chorionic gonadotrophin (hCG), oestrogens, progesterones
Kidneys	A factor which activates erythropoietin, 1,25-dihydroxycholecalciferol
Gastrointestinal tract stomach small intestine	Gastrin, 5-hydroxytryptamine (5-HT) Secretin, cholecystokinin (CCK), enterogastrone and various other regulatory peptides
Heart	Atrial natriuretic peptides (ANP) (see Chapter 10)

Table 8.1 Hormones produced by other structures.

Early development of the endocrine structures – an overview

The endocrine structures are a very diverse group of tissues – so you will not be surprised to learn that all three embryonic germ layers are involved:

Ectoderm → neural ectoderm – the adrenal medulla, posterior pituitary; surface ectoderm – anterior pituitary

Mesoderm → the adrenal cortex and gonads

Endoderm → the thyroid, parathyroids, thymus, islets of Langerhans (pancreas)

A useful way to remember is that steroid-producing endocrine structures develop from mesoderm and those that produce amino-acid-based hormones or monoamines arise from endoderm or ectoderm. Further details are covered with the individual endocrine structures.

Hormones

Structure

Hormones can be divided into two major groups (see *Figure 8.2*): (i) amino-acid-based (amino-acid derivatives, peptides and proteins), e.g. thyroxine; and (ii) steroids derived from cholesterol, which include adrenocortical hormones and the sex hormones.

Action

A quick look at Chapter 1 (ATP, protein synthesis and cell membrane/internal receptors) would be helpful before continuing with hormone action.

Hormones change cellular activity by increasing or decreasing the **metabolism** of specific target cells which have receptor proteins (surface or internal) capable of binding the hormone. The binding of one hormone may also influence the availability of receptors for another hormone – the female sex hormones oestrogen and progesterone alter the number of each other's receptors and consequently affect responses. The ways in which target cell activity is changed by hormones include:

- Increased protein, e.g. enzymes, synthesis.
- Activation or deactivation of enzymes.
- Altering cell permeability by operating ion channels.
- Production of regulatory molecules.
- Secretion of molecules from cells.

- Influence on mitosis.
- Changing intracellular **cyclic adenosine monophosphate** (cAMP) levels (see below).

Some hormones act directly at gene level (DNA); for example, lipid-soluble steroid hormones and thyroxine enter the cell before binding to receptors, which then move into the nucleus to alter gene transcription and protein synthesis. The effects of hormones acting in this way tend to take some time to become apparent.

Other hormones act indirectly through regulatory intermediates called G proteins and 'second messengers' (see Chapter 1). Much like your telephone call for a 'take away' causes the activity which results in the delivery of your pizza. G proteins in the plasma membrane cause the formation of the second messenger which initiates the hormone effects in the target cell that the hormone itself is unable to enter (most of these hormones are amino acid-based.) One such second messenger is cAMP which, once formed, acts for the hormone (e.g. ACTH) by 'proxy'. Cyclic AMP induces intracellular processes whereby many chemical reactions are catalyzed simultaneously (enzyme cascade amplification) as several enzymes are activated which in turn stimulate still more. Enzyme cascades mean that some hormone effects can occur quickly in response to changing body needs; for example, glucagon increases blood glucose if levels fall too low (see page 170).

To summarize;

Hormone → intracellular receptor → nucleus → DNA transcription → mRNA formation → ribosomal protein synthesis

or

Hormone → membrane receptors → G proteins → second messenger – cAMP → chemical reactions (enzyme cascades) → change in cell activity

---

In addition to cAMP, there are other second messenger systems utilized by some hormones; for example, oxytocin uses the phosphoinositide system, which consists of two second messengers – diacylglycerol and inositol triphosphate. These second messengers work partly through enzymes or by releasing intracellular calcium ions (or 'third messenger'), which may combine with calmodulin (regulatory protein) or act directly on enzymes and calcium channels in the plasma membrane. The amount of intracellular calcium also influences the storage, secretion and action of many hormones.

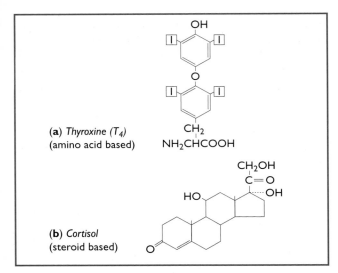

Figure 8.2 Hormone structure. (**a**) Amino acid based; (**b**) steroid based.

(**a**) *Thyroxine (T$_4$)* (amino acid based)

(**b**) *Cortisol* (steroid based)

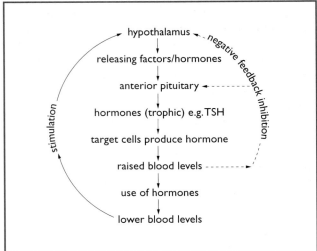

Figure 8.3 Negative feedback.

Direct and indirect modes of hormone action gives the flexibility (vital for homeostasis) which allows some hormone action to be rapid with immediate effects, e.g. adrenaline, or not be apparent for hours or in some cases days, e.g. cortisol.

Prostaglandins, prostacyclins, thromboxanes and leukotrienes

A large group of regulatory lipids also have hormone-like effects in the body. These include the prostaglandins, prostacyclins, thromboxanes and leukotrienes, which are all derived from fatty acids such as arachidonic acid (see Chapter 1). As a group, they influence processes as diverse as inflammation, blood clotting and reproduction. The ubiquitous, but vitally important, prostaglandins and related substances are produced in most tissues and initiate local effects, including gastric mucus secretion, inhibition of gastric acid production, inflammatory responses, pain, fever, vasoconstriction, platelet aggregation, menstruation and uterine muscle contraction. Prostaglandins, prostacyclins and thromboxanes are generally regarded as local hormones, or paracrines, because they act over a limited range in local target cells (cf. Hormones, page 156). Prostaglandins are very potent substances and tiny amounts initiate intense responses; however, their activity is extremely short-lived and they are broken down very effectively by lung enzymes.

Control of hormone secretion

Hormone secretion may be initiated by other hormones (hormonal), the concentration of substances in the extracellular fluid (humoral) or the nervous system (neural); it is, however, worth noting that some hormones use more than one control mechanism. Most hormone release is

regulated through **negative feedback**/inhibition (*Figure 8.3*). When the hormone level falls, release mechanisms are turned on; and when the hormone level rises, the mechanism is turned off (rather like cancelling the milk order when your refrigerator is full of milk). Positive feedback (uncommon) is demonstrated by the release of oxytocin during parturition (see Chapters 2 and 20). As you would expect, control mechanisms operate for hormones that respond to extracellular substances: high plasma levels of the substance inhibit hormone release. In these ways hormone levels, some of which are secreted in a rhythmic pattern, e.g. female sex hormones, are controlled within a preset range, usually with little variation in health.

Hormones have a specific half-life (the time taken for half the hormone to be removed from the plasma). When hormones are no longer needed they are degraded by enzymes in the liver, kidneys and lungs (see above), and excreted in bile or urine (see Chapters 14 and 15).

Hypothalamus and Pituitary Gland

The hypothalamus is central to the regulation of homeostasis. It controls pituitary function by producing the releasing/inhibiting hormones which regulate hormone secretion by the anterior pituitary, and synthesizing the two hormones stored and released by the posterior pituitary. The pituitary gland has been called the 'master gland', because it stimulates many other endocrine structures and metabolic processes.

Hypothalamic connections with other parts of the nervous system provide fine tuning for endocrine function. The tiny pituitary gland, or hypophysis, weighing about 0.5 g, is really two separate structures: the glandular anterior lobe (adenohypophysis), which develops from the surface ecto-derm of the embryonic mouth/pharynx (Rathke's pouch), and the posterior lobe (neurohypophysis), which grows down from the neural ectoderm of the embryonic dien-cephalon and consists of neural tissue. Some hormone pro-duction starts by week 9 of fetal development. The two lobes hang from the hypothalamus by a stalk (infundibulum) con-taining blood vessels (hypothalamohypophyseal portal system) and nerve fibres. The pituitary rests within the pitu-itary fossa of the sphenoid bone very close to the optic chi-asma (*Figure 8.4*). Tumours of the pituitary may cause visual problems if they press upon the optic nerves (Chapter 7).

Anterior lobe (adenohypophysis)

The anterior lobe of the pituitary gland produces several hormones, which are controlled by hypothalamic releas-ing and inhibiting hormones that travel in the portal system of blood vessels in the stalk (*Figure 8.5*). The six anterior lobe hormones are the four trophic hormones (stimulate other endocrine glands): adrenocorticotrophic hormone (ACTH), thyroid-stimulating hormone (TSH), and the gonadotrophins follicle-stimulating hormone (FSH) and luteinizing-hormone (LH); and two that act on other tissues: growth hormone (GH) and prolactin (PRL).

The anterior lobe also produces a large precursor mole-cule (prohormone) called pro-opiocortin, which forms sub-stances including ACTH and beta lipotrophin (LPH) –

considered to be the same as melanocyte-stimulating hor-mone (MSH), which acts with ACTH on the skin pigment cells (see Chapter 19). Skin pigmentation hormones are much more important in species that change colour, e.g. amphibians. LPH also forms beta endorphin, a natural opiate (see Chapters 3 and 4).

Problems with anterior pituitary hormones are diverse; there may be a complete failure (panhypopituitarism), oversecre-tion- or undersecretion of some hormones or a breakdown in hypothalamic control.

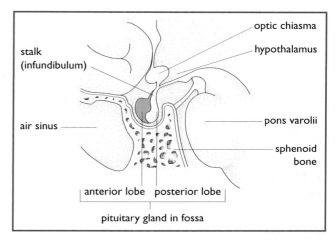

Figure 8.4 Hypothalamus and pituitary gland.

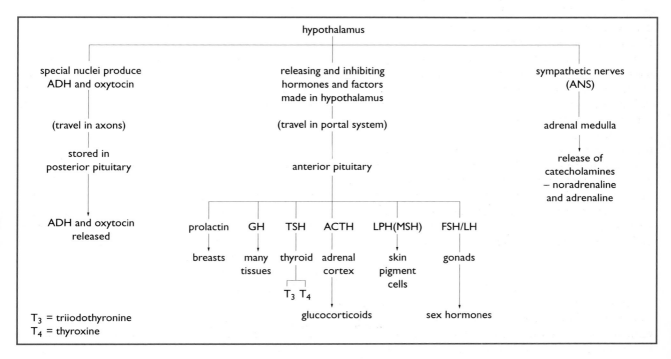

Figure 8.5 Flow diagram: the hypothalamus and pituitary gland – hormones and target organs.

Anterior lobe hormones – detail
Growth hormone (GH)

GH is a protein hormone with widespread effects on body tissues. Its secretion is regulated by two hypothalamic hormones: growth-hormone-releasing hormone (GHRH) and growth-hormone-inhibiting hormone (GHIH) or somatostatin, which is also produced to a limited extent by pancreatic and intestinal cells. GH stimulates the growth of bone, cartilage and muscle, and influences the metabolism of nutrients. It stimulates protein synthesis, causes fats to be broken down for use, which spares glucose, and promotes liver glycogen formation (see Chapters 1 and 13). Secretion of GH, which is greatest during childhood and adolescence, increases during sleep and after exercise, and is affected by emotions and nutrition. The effects of GH on certain target cells work through insulin-like growth factors or somatomedins (polypeptides), which are produced mainly by the liver and possibly also by other tissues.

Thyroid-stimulating hormone (TSH)

TSH is a glycoprotein which stimulates thyroid growth and secretion. Its secretion is stimulated by the hypothalamic hormone thyrotrophin-releasing hormone (TRH) and inhibited by high levels of thyroid hormones acting on the hypothalamus and pituitary.

Adrenocorticotrophic hormone (ACTH)

ACTH is a polypeptide which stimulates the secretion of glucocorticoid hormones from the adrenal cortex. Its release is stimulated by the hypothalamic factors – corticotrophin-releasing factor (CRF) and arginine vasopressin (AVP). Levels of ACTH tend to be highest in the early morning, but stressors (see Chapter 6), e.g cold, override the circadian (daily) rhythm. Release of CRF and ACTH is inhibited by high glucocorticoid levels.

Gonadotrophins (FSH and LH)

The gonadotrophins are glycoprotein hormones that affect the functioning of the gonads (ovaries or testes). FSH stimulates oocyte or spermatozoa` production. LH functions with FSH to stimulate ovulation and hormone release in the female and male hormone production. LH is also known as interstitial cell stimulating hormone–(ICSH) in the male. The hypothalamus starts to secrete gonadotrophin releasing hormone (GnRH) at puberty and the consequent gonadotrophin secretion stimulates maturation of the gonads.

The complex pattern of gonadotrophin production is stimulated by GnRH and inhibited by the gonadal steroid hormones and inhibin – a polypeptide produced by the gonads (see Chapter 20).

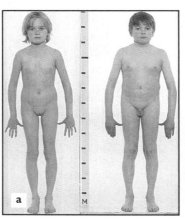
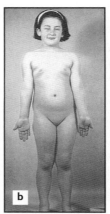
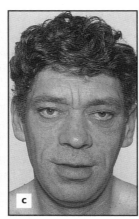

Figure 8.6 Growth problems. (a) Dwarfism in two siblings: a 15-year-old boy and a 13-year-old girl; (b) gigantism in a $4\frac{1}{2}$-year-old girl; (c) acromegaly. (Hall R, Evered DC (1990) *A Colour Atlas of Endocrinology*, 2nd edn. Wolfe Medical Publications Ltd. Reprinted with permission).

Abnormal Function Problems with GH secretion

Abnormal secretion of GH before bone growth is complete will influence eventual adult height (bone growth in length occurs from epiphyseal cartilage plates; see Chapter 16). Hyposecretion (undersecretion) limits growth and leads to dwarfism [*Figure 8.6 (a)*]; hypersecretion (oversecretion) causes gigantism [*Figure 8.6 (b)*]. Hypersecretion of GH after bone growth has ceased, i.e. when the epiphyseal plates have ossified (become bone), will cause acromegaly, which is characterized by enlargement of the bones of the feet, hands and face and internal structures, e.g. heart [*Figure 8.6 (c)*].

Prolactin

The protein hormone prolactin stimulates lactation (milk production). In males and non-lactating females its regulation is mainly inhibitory through the hypothalamic hormone prolactin inhibiting hormone, which has been identified as the neurotransmitter dopamine. Females show a small cyclical rise during the menstrual cycle – which may explain the breast changes familiar to many women just before menstruation. During pregnancy, prolactin levels are increased by a hypothalamic-releasing hormone (as yet unidentified) – prolactin-releasing hormone. The rise in prolactin leads to milk production, which is further stimulated by suckling (see Chapter 20).

High levels of prolactin (hyperprolactinaemia) due to a pituitary tumour can cause female infertility, and impotence or libido loss in males.

Please note that *Figure 8.3* illustrates the negative feedback control of anterior lobe hormones.

Posterior lobe (neurohypophysis)

The posterior lobe of the pituitary gland does not produce hormones – it stores and secretes oxytocin and ADH, also called vasopressin or arginine vasopressin (AVP). Both these hormones consist of nine amino acids; they differ by only two amino acids. The hormones are made in the paraventricular and supraoptic nuclei of the hypothalamus and travel in the nerve fibres of the stalk to the posterior lobe. Their release from the posterior pituitary is controlled by nerve impulses from the hypothalamus.

Hormones stored in the posterior lobe

Oxytocin

Oxytocin has a leading role in parturition (childbirth). During labour the rising blood levels of oxytocin stimulate the expulsive contractions of the uterine muscle which push the baby down on to the cervix. Oxytocin is also important for the 'let down' (ejection) of milk from lactating breasts. Reflex release of oxytocin occurs in response to suckling, which results in more milk being ejected – an example of positive feedback. During the early days of breast feeding some women experience cramp-like pains when the uterus contracts as oxytocin is released (see Chapter 20). Oxytocin and drugs with similar properties (oxytocics) are used to stimulate uterine contraction in the induction and active management of labour. In males and females who are neither pregnant nor lactating oxytocin appears to influence sexual responses.

Antidiuretic hormone

As its name suggests, ADH reduces diuresis (urine production) in the kidneys. Osmoreceptor cells in the hypothalamus monitor the osmolarity (see Chapter 2) of the blood. When blood osmolarity is high, because of, for example, insufficient fluids, or the blood pressure is low (monitored by baroreceptors), the posterior lobe releases ADH, which causes the kidney tubules to become more permeable to water (see Chapter 15). More water is reabsorbed by the kidney, urinary volume is reduced, and the volume and osmolarity of the blood returns to normal. High levels of ADH also increase blood pressure by its effect on the smooth muscle in blood vessels; this pressor (vasoconstriction) effect accounts for its other name, vasopressin, and is important in the long-term regulation of arterial blood pressure (see Chapter 10).

When blood osmolarity is low, e.g. after a large fluid intake, no ADH is released and excess water is excreted by the kidney. ADH secretion is also inhibited by atrial natriuretic peptides produced by the heart when atrial blood pressure increases. Fluid loss can be especially large following a copious intake of alcohol, which also inhibits ADH secretion – to produce the thirst and parched mouth associated with a 'hangover'. The ADH mechanism, with processes which include the action of the thirst centre (see Chapter 4), help to maintain fluid balance homeostasis.

Abnormal Function **Problems with ADH secretion**

Hyposecretion of ADH leads to a condition known as cranial diabetes insipidus, which may be genetic or may follow trauma, neurosurgery or meningitis. It results in the production of large volumes of dilute urine (up to 20 l/day). Homeostasis is still possible if fluid intake increases to match the loss, but life will be somewhat inconvenient for the unfortunate person who needs to drink copiously and spend considerable time in the toilet. Treatment with intranasal vasopressin analogues (similar substances with longer duration of action or lack of pressor effects) and other drugs is usually effective. Another form of diabetes insipidus occurs when the kidney tubules do not respond to ADH. Earlier we mentioned that some tumours, for example the lung, secrete high levels of ADH, which leads to water retention and electrolyte disturbances.

Thyroid Gland

The thyroid gland is situated in the anterior part of the neck. It has two lobes (joined by an isthmus of tissue) which lie one either side of the trachea and below the larynx [*Figure 8.7(a)*]. The thyroid is extremely well supplied with blood from branches of the external carotid and subclavian arteries (see *Figure 10.34*). The resultant vascularity increases the need for careful haemostasis during thyroid surgery. The venous blood returns to the heart by the jugular veins (see *Figure 10.36*).

Thyroid gland development starts around the fourth week of embryonic life. It forms from endodermal tissue of the pharynx and migrates to its final position in the neck by week 8. Its parafollicular cells (see below) are derived from neural ectoderm, and mesoderm containing many blood vessels which gradually permeate through the gland.

Structure

Each lobe of the thyroid has many follicles with walls of cuboidal epithelial cells, which produce thyroglobulin [*Figure 8.7(b)*]. Thyroglobulin is a colloidal (particles suspended in a liquid which do not settle out or pass through membranes) substance which forms two of the thyroid hormones (see below). It is stored in the follicles until required. A third hormone (calcitonin) is secreted by parafollicular cells found in the tissue between the follicles.

Thyroid hormones

The thyroid produces three hormones: thyroxine (T_4) (tetraiodothyronine) and triiodothyronine (T_3), which regulate metabolism; and calcitonin, which lowers serum calcium levels.

Thyroxine and triiodothyronine

Thyroxine (most abundant) and triiodothyronine are formed from the amino acid tyrosine with either four (T_4; thyroxine) or three (T_3; triiodothyronine) atoms of iodine. T_4 is formed from thyroglobulin by the addition of dietary iodine and is secreted from the follicles following enzyme action. Some T_4 is converted to T_3 (more active) in the follicles, although this usually occurs at the target cells. Thyroid hormones can be stored as colloid for several weeks. T_4 and T_3 travel in the blood to their target cells bound to a special protein, thyroxine-binding globulin (TBG). Thyroid hormones alter cell function by binding to receptors inside their target cells (see page 157). T_4 and T_3 are the major hormones controlling metabolism. Their effects include control and regulation of:

- Basal metabolic rate (BMR) – the rate at which cells consume oxygen.
- Maintenance of body temperature.
- Catabolism (breaking down) of glucose and use of fats to produce energy.
- Protein synthesis.
- Normal growth and development of skeletal and nervous systems.
- Functioning of adult nervous system.
- Reproductive function.

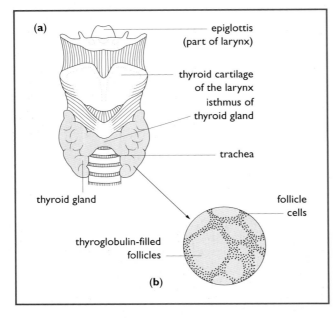

Figure 8.7 Thyroid gland. **(a)** Gross structure; **(b)** thyroglobulin-filled follicles.

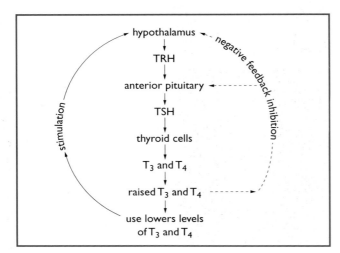

Figure 8.8 Negative feedback control of thyroid metabolic hormones.

Abnormal Function **Problems with thyroid function**

Underactivity of the thyroid, which reduces the metabolic rate, is known as hypothyroidism [Figure 8.9(a)]. In adults it is also called myxoedema. The congenital hypothyroidism occurring in infancy was previously called cretinism.

Hypothyroidism may be caused by:

- Severe iodine deficiency, with neck swelling (goitre). This occurs in isolated, mountainous regions of less-developed countries where the soil/plants are low in iodine and fish (contains iodine) is difficult to obtain. It was previously common in Derbyshire, UK – hence the term 'Derbyshire neck'.
- Lack of TSH or TRH.
- Autoimmune conditions where antibodies destroy the thyroid (see Chapter 19).
- Postoperatively if too much thyroid tissue is removed.

The effects of adult hypothyroidism include low body temperature, puffy eyes and face, bradycardia (slow pulse), weight gain, hair changes, dry, coarse skin and mental slowness. Hypothyroidism in children leads to stunted growth, brain damage and learning disabilities. Treatment involves the replacement of thyroid hormones or correction of iodine deficiency.

Overactivity has the opposite effects, with an increase in metabolic rate – known as hyperthyroidism (thyrotoxicosis) [*Figure 8.9 (b)*].

Hyperthyroid states may be caused by:

- Graves' disease or diffuse hyperplasia (see Chapter 1), caused by antibodies which act in place of TSH and abnormally stimulate thyroid hormone secretion.
- Hormone-secreting solitary nodule or multinodular goitre.
- Excess TSH secretion from a pituitary tumour.

Hyperthyroidism causes raised temperature and sweating, tachycardia (rapid pulse) and possibly cardiac failure, weight loss with good appetite, tremor, emotional lability and restlessness. Exophthalmos (eyeball protrusion), probably caused by changes in the tissue behind the eyeball and the extraocular muscles (see Chapter 7), may occur in Graves' disease. Eye damage can occur without eye protection and monitoring. Hyperthyroid states are treated with antithyroid drugs, surgery (subtotal thyroidectomy) or gland destruction with radioactive iodine (usually used for people aged over 40 years and never during pregnancy).

Swellings of the thyroid with or without excess hormone production may cause pressure effects: dysphagia (difficult swallowing), caused by pressure on the oesophagus, or dyspnoea (difficult breathing), caused by pressure on the trachea.

The synthesis and release of T_4 and T_3 is stimulated by TSH from the anterior pituitary, which in turn depends on the release of TRH from the hypothalamus. High levels of T_4/T_3 normally switch off TSH/TRH production (*Figure 8.8*) and reducing levels switches them on. Other factors influence thyroid hormone release, e.g. pregnancy, where extra energy is required, and it can be decreased by other hormones, e.g. glucocorticoids.

Calcitonin

Calcitonin is a polypeptide hormone secreted by the parafollicular cells (C cells) of the thyroid. As an antagonist (opposing) of the parathyroid hormone (see pages 164–165) it lowers serum calcium and phosphate levels by its action on bone and the kidneys. It inhibits calcium reabsorption from bone and favours its deposition, and increases urinary excretion of calcium and phosphates.

The release of calcitonin depends upon calcium levels in the blood: if calcium levels rise above normal (2.1–2.6 mmol/l), calcitonin is released. Calcitonin, with a half-life of 10 min, probably only has a fine-tuning role in calcium homeostasis (see Parathyroid glands, pages 164–165).

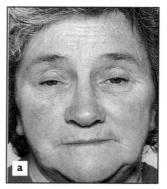

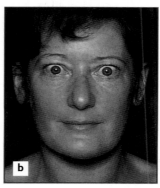

Figure 8.9 Problems with thyroid hormones. (**a**) Hypothyroidism; (**b**) hyperthyroidism. (Hall R, Evered DC (1990) *A Colour Atlas of Endocrinology*, 2nd edn. Wolfe Medical Publications, Ltd. Reprinted with permission).

Parathyroid Glands

These minute structures are only 6 mm in length. There are usually four situated on the posterior aspect of the thyroid (*Figure 8.10*). Some people, however, have more than four, and the extra glands may be located elsewhere in the neck, thorax or mediastinum.

During development the parathyroid glands form from the endoderm of the third and fourth pharyngeal pouches and mesoderm provides their blood vessels. The superior pair form on the posterior surface of the thyroid and the inferior pair migrate downwards, as the thymus gland moves down, to their position below the superior pair.

Structure

Each parathyroid gland is enclosed in a connective-tissue capsule and consists of cords of cells: chief cells, which secrete hormone, and oxyphil cells, the function of which is unknown. The cords are interspaced with vascular channels.

Parathyroid hormone

The parathyroid glands produce only one hormone, parathyroid hormone (PTH) (also called parathormone or parathyrin). This protein hormone is vital in maintaining serum calcium levels within the homeostatic range of 2.1–2.6 mmol/l. Calcium homeostasis (linked with phosphates) is maintained by cooperation between several different organs – the intestines, bone and the kidneys – along with PTH and vitamin D. The correct calcium level is essential for proper muscle contraction, nerve impulse transmission and blood clotting.

Figure 8.10 Parathyroid glands – gross structure and location (viewed from behind).

Figure 8.11 Parathyroid hormone – calcium and vitamin D metabolism.

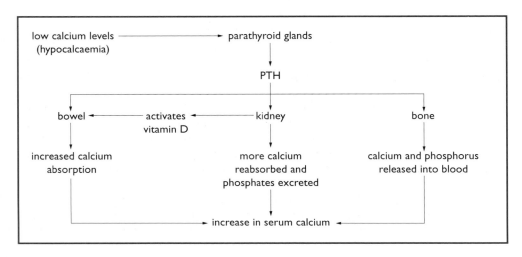

Nursing Practice Application **Tetany following thyroid surgery**

Postoperative care after thyroid surgery should include observations for tetany caused by hypocalcaemia. Initially the increase in nerve excitability will cause tingling around the mouth and in the hands and feet. There may also be painful carpopedal spasm (hands and feet) and more rarely laryngeal spasm and fits. Latent tetany may be detected by Trousseau's sign, where a sphygmomanometer cuff inflated around the upper arm induces forearm muscle spasm. Emergency medical management of tetany includes intravenous calcium gluconate and monitoring of serum calcium levels.

Nursing Practice Application **Hyperventilation and tetany**

The hyperventilation (overbreathing) that may occur with anxiety disorders can cause respiratory alkalosis and tetany. Nurses can help the individual to become calm and encourage compliance with the prescribed treatment. The initial treatment may include intravenous calcium gluconate and the inhalation of 5% carbon dioxide in oxygen or rebreathing expired air from a bag to increase carbon dioxide levels in the blood (acidic carbon dioxide makes the blood less alkaline, but remember that the blood is normally slightly alkaline at pH 7.4). Later, after physical causes of hyperventilation have been excluded, there should be interventions that identify the causes of the anxiety and help the person to find ways of controlling and coping with anxiety.

Abnormal Function **Problems with parathyroid function**

Parathyroid tumours cause hypersecretion of PTH (hyperparathyroidism). This results in hypercalcaemia, with muscle weakness, nerve conduction problems, weakened bones and kidney problems, e.g. stones and failure, as calcium is deposited in the kidneys.

Undersecretion of PTH may be caused by trauma or removal of parathyroid glands during thyroid surgery (see Nursing Practice Application), autoimmune disease and congenital defects. The resultant hypocalcaemia causes increased nerve excitability and muscle spasm, known as tetany. Other causes of hypocalcaemia include inadequate calcium intake which occurs in rickets, and when failing kidneys do not produce the active vitamin D required for calcium absorption.

Tetany can also result from changes in the blood pH – alkalosis (see Chapter 2). Although the serum calcium level is normal, the increased alkalinity reduces the amount of available ionized calcium. The alkalosis may be produced by hyperventilation (see Chapter 12 and Nursing Practice Application), persistent vomiting and excessive ingestion of alkalis (see Chapter 13). Management involves correcting the alkalosis as well as giving intravenous calcium gluconate.

PTH acts in a variety of ways to raise serum calcium levels and reduce phosphate levels (*Figure 8.11*):

- The kidney reabsorbs calcium and excretes phosphate. PTH also stimulates the kidney to convert vitamin D into its active form, 1,25-dihydroxycholecalciferol.
- 1,25-dihydroxycholecalciferol acts upon intestinal cells, causing increased absorption of calcium from food.
- PTH stimulates osteoclasts (see Chapter 16) in bone which reabsorb bone matrix, releasing calcium and phosphate into the blood.

PTH release is stimulated by low levels of calcium in the blood (hypocalcaemia) and inhibited by levels above normal (hypercalcaemia). For more on calcium metabolism, see Chapter 16.

Adrenal Glands

The two triangular adrenal glands are situated one on the upper pole of each kidney (see *Figure 8.12(a)*). Their position on top of the kidneys accounts for their alternative name, suprarenal glands. The adrenal glands derive arterial blood from a branch of the aorta and from the renal and phrenic arteries. Venous blood drains directly into the inferior vena cava from the right gland and into the renal vein from the left gland (see *Figures 10.42 and 10.44*)

The adrenal glands are divided into a middle part, the medulla, and the cortex around the outside [Figure 8.12(b)]. The medulla and cortex are really two separate endocrine structures which develop from different embryonic tissues. By the sixth week of embryonic

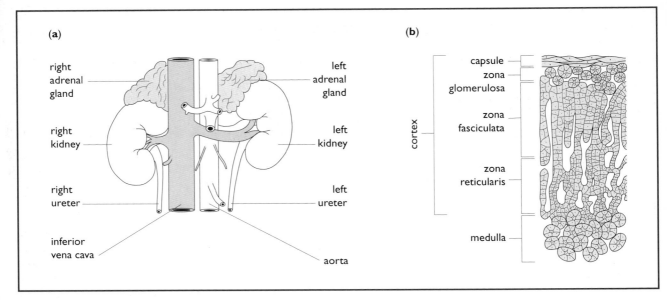

Figure 8.12 Adrenal glands. (**a**) Position; (**b**) layers through the adrenal gland.

development, the cortex is forming from mesoderm and the medulla from neural ectoderm which migrates from the sympathetic ganglia (the neuroendocrine link again). Gradually, the medulla is enveloped by two layers of developing cortex – fetal and adult. The fetal cortex persists during the first year of life.

Adrenal cortex

The adult cortex has an outer capsule and three distinct inner layers [*Figure 8.12(b)*] which produce the large group of steroid hormones derived from cholesterol known collectively as corticosteroids.

From the outside working in, the layers are:
- Zona glomerulosa, where clumps of cells secrete mineralocorticoids which regulate electrolyte/fluid balance.
- Zona fasciculata, the widest layer, in which cells arranged in parallel columns secrete glucocorticoids, which are important metabolic hormones.
- Zona reticularis, which consists of a network of cells producing small amounts of glucocorticoids and sex hormones.

The basic steroid structure (see Chapter 1) common to all corticosteroids means that different hormone groups will share some similarities of function, e.g. glucocorticoids have a slight mineralocorticoid effect.

Adrenal cortex hormones

The adrenal cortex secretes three hormone groups, glucocorticoids, mineralocorticoids and sex hormones.

Glucocorticoids

There are several glucocorticoids, but the most important is cortisol (hydrocortisone). Their role in many metabolic processes and stress responses make them essential for life. Glucocorticoid actions can be summarized as follows:
- Control and modification of carbohydrate metabolism by the stimulation of gluconeogenesis (production of glucose from non-carbohydrate sources, e.g. amino acids and glycerol) in the liver.
  Increasing the amount of glucose stored by the liver as glycogen (storage carbohydrate).
  Cortisol inhibits the uptake and use of glucose by voluntary muscle. These processes increase blood glucose levels which can be used by the brain.
- Increasing protein breakdown into amino acids for energy (by gluconeogenesis) and decreasing protein synthesis.
- Increasing the release of fatty acids and their oxidation for energy, again sparing glucose for the brain.
- Helping to convert noradrenaline to adrenaline in the adrenal medulla.
- High glucocorticoid levels cause some sodium and water reabsorption by kidney tubules.
- With adrenaline, initiating vasoconstriction, which increases blood pressure.
- Increasing calcium excretion by the kidney and inhibiting its absorption in the intestine.
- Suppressing inflammation, allergy and immune processes.
- Increasing secretion of gastric acid and enzymes.

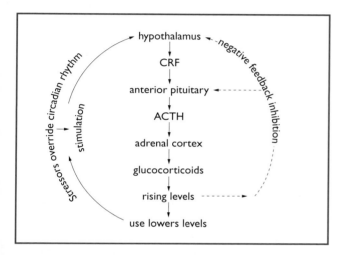

Figure 8.13 Control of adrenal cortex glucocorticoid secretion.

Glucocorticoid release is controlled by a negative feedback mechanism; CRF from the hypothalamus stimulates the anterior pituitary to secrete ACTH which in turn causes the release of glucocorticoids, e.g. cortisol, from the cortex. Rising levels of cortisol will inhibit both the hypothalamus and the pituitary (*Figure 8.13*). The release of glucocorticoids is not constant; a circadian rhythm exists, with an early morning peak and low levels in the evening. Low levels of cortisol overnight, with loss of anti-inflammatory effects, may partially explain the frequency of asthma attacks during the night and early morning. Other inflammatory diseases, such as rheumatoid arthritis, may also be affected by fluctuating levels of cortisol – with stiffness and immobility on waking.

Stressors such as pain and hypoglycaemia (low blood glucose) override the circadian rhythm, allowing the secretion of the extra glucocorticoids required for coping mechanisms (see pages 169-170 and Chapter 6). Glucocorticoids are mostly excreted in the urine after being changed chemically within the liver. Boore (1978) used the urinary excretion of 17-hydroxycorticosteroids as an indicator of physiological stress in her study of surgical patients (see also Chapter 6).

Mineralocorticoids

The mineralocorticoids form a group of hormones of which aldosterone is the most important. Aldosterone's main purpose is to regulate electrolyte (especially sodium) and fluid homeostasis by causing the distal kidney tubules to reabsorb sodium and water and eliminate potassium or hydrogen ions (see Chapter 15), and through this assist in long-term control of arterial blood pressure (see Chapter 10). The release of aldosterone has little to do with the hypothalamus or pituitary although ACTH has some effect in stress situations it depends on the concentration of ions in the blood, the osmolarity of the blood and the blood pressure. Aldosterone secretion increases when sodium and chloride levels are reduced or when potassium levels increase in the blood, and when the volume of extracellular fluid (see Chapter 2), and hence the blood pressure, is low.

Special cells in the kidney, the juxtaglomerular apparatus (JGA), respond to these changes by releasing the enzyme renin, which acts on the plasma protein angiotensinogen to form angiotensin I (see *Figure 8.14*). Angiotensin-converting enzyme (ACE) converts angiotensin I to angiotensin II and this stimulates the adrenal cortex to produce aldosterone, which acts upon the distal tubules (see Chapters 10 and 15). Angiotensin II also causes vasoconstriction, which raises the blood pressure. The renin–angiotensin–aldosterone response does not operate in isolation; it works closely with the osmoreceptors and ADH secretion (see page 161). Renin secretion is also stimulated by sympathetic nerves, and reduced sodium or increased potassium levels in the plasma stimulate the adrenal cortex directly. Atrial natriuretic peptides (ANPs) inhibit both renin and aldosterone to help reduce blood pressure.

Sex hormones

Compared with the gonads (ovaries and testes), the amounts of sex hormones secreted by the adrenal cortex are insignificant. They are mainly androgens (male hormones), with very small amounts of the female hormones oestrogens and progesterones. Their role is unclear, but levels are high during fetal life and again at puberty, when they probably stimulate the growth of pubic hair. Inappropriate secretion can lead to masculinization in females.

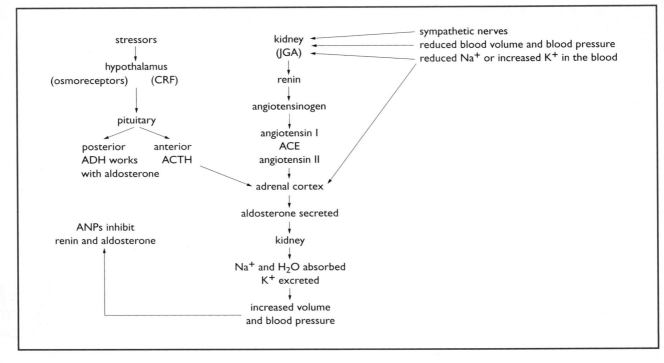

Figure 8.14 Renin–angiotensin–aldosterone response.

Abnormal Function **Problems with adrenal cortex secretion**

Hypersecretion of corticosteroids or Cushing's syndrome

The causes of Cushing's syndrome (*Figure 8.15*) include ACTH-producing pituitary tumour, adrenocortical hyperplasia or tumour, administration of ACTH and ectopic sources of ACTH, e.g. lung tumours. Similar effects are seen after high-dose corticosteroid drugs, e.g. prednisolone, are administered over a long period. The effects of hypersecretion, which may appear as exaggerations of physiological function, include:

- Hyperglycaemia (high blood glucose), caused by excessive gluconeogenesis, leading to diabetes mellitus (see page 171).
- Sodium and water retention, leading to hypertension (high blood pressure) and oedema. Muscle weakness caused by potassium loss.
- Changes in fat and protein metabolism, leading to typical 'moon' face, fat redistribution to the abdomen and back ('buffalo hump') and muscle wastage in the limbs.

- The suppression of the inflammatory response delays wound healing (see Chapter 19) and masks signs of infection. It can also cause the reactivation of tuberculosis.
- The skin becomes thin, fragile and easily damaged. Excessive bruising occurs and striae (stretch marks) appear on the abdomen and thighs. Special care is required postoperatively and in the prevention of skin breakdown (see Chapter 19).
- Hirsutism and acne.
- Menstrual cycle disturbance.
- Osteoporosis (see Chapters 16 and 21) and spontaneous fractures, especially vertebral collapse as calcium is lost.
- Peptic ulcer development linked to an increase in gastric acid secretion.
- Mood changes and serious psychotic illness – paranoia, euphoria and depression.

Adrenocortical insufficiency

This usually results in the hyposecretion of both glucocorticoids and mineralo-

corticoids. Primary hyposecretion is called Addison's disease and may be caused by autoimmune mechanisms or tuberculosis. Pituitary or hypothalamic defects are a secondary cause of hyposecretion. Loss of cortical hormones leads to the serious problems of dehydration, electrolyte imbalance, hypotension and hypoglycaemia. Those affected have weight loss and complain of gastrointestinal disturbances and weakness. Skin pigmentation is a feature where ACTH levels are high.

Aldosteronism

Excess secretion of aldosterone may result from an adrenal tumour (Conn's syndrome) or be secondary to conditions such as cardiac failure (see Chapter 10) or liver cirrhosis (see Chapter 14). Aldosteronism leads to retention of sodium and water, causing hypertension. Other problems include alkalosis, muscle weakness and cardiac arrhythmias, which are due to hypokalaemia caused by the loss of potassium in the urine.

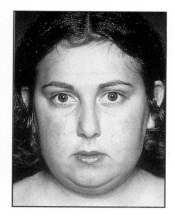

Figure 8.15 Cushing's syndrome. (Hall R, Evered DC (1990) *A Colour Atlas of Endocrinology*, 2nd edn. Wolfe Medical Publications Ltd. Reprinted with permission).

Adrenal medulla

The medulla forms the smaller part of the adrenal gland. It consists of chromaffin cells situated around blood vessels and sinusoids. The medullary cells produce two catecholamine hormones which augment the effects of the sympathetic nervous system in the 'fight or flight' response to stress (see Chapter 6).

Adrenal medulla hormones

The medullary hormones are adrenaline and noradrenaline, which, you will remember, is the postganglionic sympathetic neurotransmitter. Both are monoamines (having one amine group) derived from the amino acid tyrosine. More adrenaline than noradrenaline is produced (around 80% of production is adrenaline). Their metabolic effects are similar and include increase in heart rate, vasoconstriction, rise in

Abnormal Function **Problems with adrenal medulla secretion**

Hyposecretion is not a problem because the medulla is functionally part of the sympathetic nervous system. It is possible to live without the adrenal medulla – in fact, after removal of the adrenal glands it is only necessary to replace the cortical hormones.

Excess production of catecholamines produces a prolonged 'fight and flight' state with rapid heart rate and hypertension. This may result from prolonged exposure to a stressor or from a rare tumour of the medulla or sympathetic chain known as a phaeochromocytoma.

Tumours produce surges of catecholamines, with resultant swings in blood pressure, heart rate and sweating. Diagnosis of phaeochromocytoma may be confirmed by the presence of excess urinary metabolites.

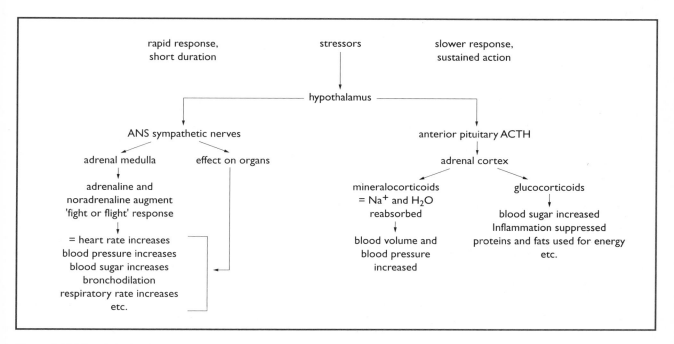

Figure 8.16 Adrenal gland and stress.

blood pressure, diversion of blood to the vital organs, increase in blood glucose, stimulation of respiration and bronchodilation. Adrenaline has most effect on the heart and noradrenaline on vasoconstriction and blood pressure. Release of medullary hormones is through sympathetic nerve stimulation in response to a stressor (see Chapter 6). The catecholamines have a short half-life; they are degraded by enzymes and their metabolites excreted in the urine.

Stress and adrenal response

The physiological responses to stressors have been covered with respect to the ANS functions (see Chapter 6). It is the sympathetic division (and, to a limited extent, the parasympathetic division) and both the adrenal medulla and cortex that allow the body to adapt to a specific stressor and maintain homeostasis. The ANS and medulla respond rapidly, usually for a short time to 'get you out of immediate trouble', whereas the cortex responds more slowly but its effects are more sustained (see *Figure 8.16*).

The Pancreas

Structure

The pancreas, a soft, tapering gland situated in the left upper abdomen, is around 23 cm in length and lies partly behind the stomach. It is a mixed gland, having both endocrine and exocrine functions (see Chapter 13). It receives arterial blood from the mesenteric and splenic arteries and its venous blood returns to the circulation by the hepatic portal vein and the liver [see *Figures 10.43(a)* and *10.45*].

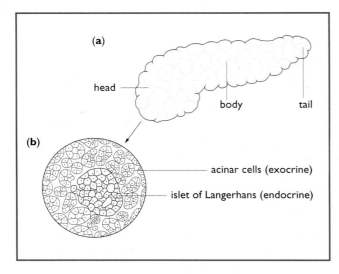

Figure 8.17 Pancreas. **(a)** Gross structure; **(b)** microscopic structure.

head

(a)

body   tail

(b)

acinar cells (exocrine)

islet of Langerhans (endocrine)

By the fifth week of embryonic development the pancreas is forming from two buds of endoderm from the primitive gut structures. The mesoderm provides the connective and supportive tissue of the gland.

The pancreas consists of (*Figure 8.17*):
- Exocrine acinar cells that produce digestive enzymes which leave the gland by ducts.
- Clusters of endocrine cells, known as the islets of Langerhans, scattered throughout the acinar cells like currants in a cake.

The pancreatic islets contain four types of hormone-producing cells: alpha (α) cells, which secrete glucagon; the more abundant beta (β) cells, which secrete insulin and amylin – a peptide which inhibits the secretion of insulin and opposes its effects (it is unclear whether amylin is of physiological significance); delta (δ) cells, which produce several substances, including somatostatin (GHIH; see page 160); and F cells, which secrete pancreatic polypeptide (regulates pancreatic exocrine secretion).

Pancreatic hormones

Glucagon and insulin are pivotal in carbohydrate metabolism and the control of blood glucose levels within the normal range: 3.6–5.8 mmol/litre after fasting to around 7–9 mmol/litre after food. The brain relies on a constant supply of glucose for energy and permanent damage can occur if it is deprived of glucose, such as may happen when blood glucose levels are low (hypoglycaemia).

Glucagon

Glucagon is a polypeptide hormone that acts on the liver to cause an elevation in blood glucose (hyperglycaemic hormone). Liver cells release glucose either by the conversion of stored glycogen to glucose (glycogenolysis) or the process of gluconeogenesis, which produces glucose from amino acids and glycerol. The most important stimulus to glucagon release is a reduction in blood glucose levels, such as during a period of fasting. It is also stimulated by certain amino acids and adrenaline. Glucagon release is inhibited by high blood glucose levels, fatty acids and somatostatin.

Insulin

The protein hormone insulin consists of two amino-acid chains joined by chemical bonds. It is formed as proinsulin and converted to insulin within the pancreatic cells. Broadly speaking, insulin is anabolic (favours synthesis/building up reactions) and anticatabolic (inhibits decomposition/breakdown reactions). Its major physiological effect is to reduce blood glucose levels (hypoglycaemic hormone), but it also affects fat and protein metabolism.

The reduction in blood glucose is achieved mainly by the effect of insulin on glucose transport across some cell membranes – it speeds up the entry of glucose into muscle and adipose but not liver, brain and kidney, which can 'pick up' glucose without its presence. Insulin also stimulates glucose metabolism within cells. There is increased use of glucose for energy and the conversion of the surplus to glycogen in liver and muscle cells. Insulin also enhances the entry of substances such as amino acids and potassium into the cell. Glycogenolysis and gluconeogenesis, both of which would increase blood glucose, are inhibited.

Insulin stimulates the storage of triglycerides (triacylglycerol-glycerol and three fatty acids; see Chapter 1) in adipose tissue and inhibits the breakdown of fatty acids. Protein synthesis from amino acids increases and the breakdown of proteins is inhibited. Insulin release is largely in

Abnormal Function **Problems with blood glucose**

The most common problem is that of diabetes mellitus – where an absolute or more often a relative lack of insulin causes hyperglycaemia and serious homeostatic imbalance as anabolism decreases and catabolism increases.

The aetiology of diabetes is complex and the following factors appear to be implicated: genetic predisposition, autoimmune mechanisms and environmental factors such as diet and exposure to certain viruses.

There are two main primary types of diabetes mellitus:

- Type I or insulin-dependent diabetes mellitus (IDDM), where there is usually an absolute lack of insulin. This type of diabetes usually occurs first in people aged under 40 years. Management currently centres around insulin injections and a diet modified to individual requirements. Recent developments have made it possible for whole pancreas or donor islet cells to be transplanted into some people with diabetes. The islet cells, once injected, take root in the liver, where they will hopefully start producing insulin. This type of management will not be suitable for all and still requires development and evaluation.
- Type II or non-insulin-dependent diabetes mellitus (NIDDM) is usually characterized by a relative lack of insulin caused by insulin resistance and is seen most commonly in overweight people aged over 50 years. This type of diabetes may be controlled by diet and sometimes drugs (oral hypoglycaemics) to reduce blood glucose, but sometimes insulin injections are required. Newer drugs such as acarbose (alpha glucosidase inhibitors) inhibit the intestinal breakdown of carbohydrates

into glucose. This slows absorption and helps to prevent hyperglycaemia after meals by smoothing out swings in blood glucose levels. In some individuals the diabetes will disappear with a return to their normal body weight. Hyperglycaemia can occur during pregnancy – so called 'gestational diabetes', where insulin levels are insufficient to meet the increased metabolic needs. Normally the pancreas increases insulin secretion to cope, but in women with a predisposition to diabetes this does not occur. It may disappear after delivery, but the majority of these women will subsequently develop IDDM or NIDDM.

Secondary diabetic states may follow pancreatitis (inflammation of the pancreas), corticosteroid therapy (see page 167) or administration of thiazide diuretics (see Chapter 15), and may be associated with other endocrine problems such as Cushing's syndrome (see page 168).

The pathophysiological effects of diabetes mellitus vary in severity between types and individuals, but include (see *Figure 8.19*):

- Hyperglycaemia. When glucose levels exceed the renal threshold (see Chapter 15) it is excreted in the urine (glycosuria). The glycosuria may result in pruritus (itching) caused by fungal infections, e.g. candidiasis (thrush).
- Polyuria (increased urinary volume). As glucose is excreted it takes water with it in an osmotic diuresis, resulting in serious water and sodium depletion.
- Polydipsia (intense thirst) and high fluid intake linked to the polyuria.
- Protein is broken down and converted into glucose by gluconeogenesis, which further increases blood glucose levels. It is important to note that,

although blood glucose is high, without insulin it is unavailable for cell use. Without available glucose the body will turn to other fuel molecules, e.g. fats. Loss of protein and fat utilization results in weight loss, tiredness and excess hunger (polyphagia).

- Fat breakdown releases fatty acids, which are metabolized to acetyl-CoA (see Chapter 13). Acidic ketones are formed from excess acetyl-CoA and in high quantities cause a fall in blood pH. This leads to ketoacidosis (acidosis caused by acidic ketones), which is more commonly seen in IDDM. Ketones are excreted by the lungs and in the urine to produce a characteristic odour of acetone. The 'anion gap' between measured cations and anions ($Na^+ + K^+$ is normally greater than $HCO_3^- + Cl^-$) increases as the acidic ketones pour into the blood. Remember that the person will also have serious fluid/electrolyte imbalance caused by the osmotic diuresis and changes in the composition of the ECF and ICF.

In NIDDM there is less risk of catabolic ketoacidosis, but individuals may present with hyperglycaemia and dehydration, known as non-ketotic hyperosmolar diabetic coma. It is important to note that lactic acidosis is another serious problem (over one-half may die) seen in some people treated with biguanide hypoglycaemic drugs – here there is severe acidosis but less dehydration.

- Altered consciousness and deep sighing respirations, or 'air hunger', as homeostatic mechanisms break down. Increased respiration is an attempt to remove more carbon dioxide and correct the metabolic acidosis (see Chapter 12).

response to a rise in blood glucose, but increasing amounts of fatty acids and amino acids, parasympathetic activity and gastrointestinal hormones also cause its release. Low blood glucose, sympathetic activity, adrenaline and somatostatin inhibit immediate insulin secretion.

Somatostatin

Somatostatin is the same substance as GHIH produced by the hypothalamus. Its secretion from the pancreas inhibits the release of glucagon, insulin and the pancreatic enzymes.

Blood glucose regulation – a summary

Having considered the major hormonal controls of blood glucose homeostasis, it is worth putting these together with other influences, including GH, glucocorticoids, adrenaline and thyroid hormones (*Figure 8.18*).

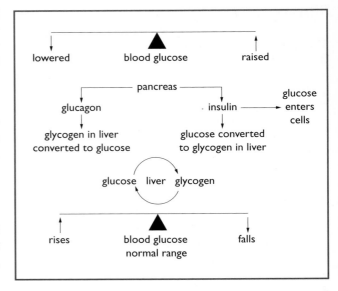

Figure 8.18 Regulation of blood glucose (other influences on blood glucose include diet, GH, somatostatin, gastrointestinal hormones, thyroid hormones, glucocorticoids, adrenaline and autonomic nervous system).

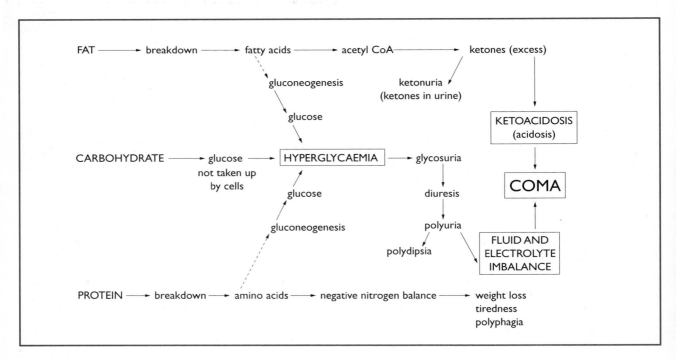

Figure 8.19 Pathophysiological changes associated with diabetes.

Thymus Gland

The thymus gland, which has two lobes, is situated in the mediastinum. Both lobes consist of many lobules, each with a medulla and cortex. The thymus, along with the inferior parathyroid glands, develops from endoderm of the third pharyngeal pouch and mesoderm which is pervaded by lymphoid stem cells by the tenth week of fetal development. It migrates to its final position in the mediastinum and continues to grow during infancy and childhood to reach a maximum during puberty, becoming smaller during adult life. It is gradually replaced by connective tissue in old age. Structurally the thymus is similar to the spleen and other lymphatic tissue (see Chapter 11). It contains many lymphocytes in the cortex and thymic corpuscles (Hassal's corpuscles), which are endodermal in origin, in the medulla.

The thymus produces peptide hormones, including thymosines and thymopoietins – these stimulate the proper development of T lymphocytes, which form part of the immune system (see Chapter 19).

Pineal Body

The pineal body is a small reddish structure in the brain, situated close to the third ventricle in the epithalamus (part of the diencephalon), which develops from the embryonic forebrain (see Chapter 4). It consists of nervous tissue and clusters of secretory cells. In humans its function is poorly understood, but it is known to produce melatonin and possibly the neurotransmitter 5-hydroxytryptamine (see Chapter 3). Other substances found in the pineal body include histamine and dopamine.

Melatonin secretion is linked to many cyclical biological functions such as sexual maturation/reproductive behaviour (see Chapters 20 and 21) and many that follow circadian (daily) cycles: sleep–wake patterns (see Chapter 4), appetite, mood and temperature (see Chapter 19).

Release of melatonin is on a circadian rhythm linked to the amount of light entering the eye; levels of melatonin are high at night and low during the day. High levels at night influence sleep–wake cycles by affecting the

Person-centred Study Andrew

Andrew is 19 and has just started an engineering course at university. He has felt tired and 'run down', which he thought was due to studying and late nights! More recently Andrew has lost weight, is always thirsty and seems to pass a lot of urine. When he visited the health centre the medical officer suspected a diagnosis of diabetes mellitus from the history plus the fact that Andrew had glucose in his urine – a random blood test showed that glucose levels were raised (15 mmol/l).

Once the diagnosis has been confirmed the obvious priority for Andrew is the stabilization of his diabetes, but this will require the identification and careful consideration of his lifestyle and individual needs. Initially Andrew may be admitted to hospital; however, stabilization is more easily achieved in the community with him undertaking normal activities. Andrew and his family will be involved with a multidisciplinary team whose aim will be to help them understand and cope with the diabetes. The team includes a specialist diabetic nurse, medical staff, dietitians and the staff at the university health centre. Callaghan and Williams (1994) stress the importance of having access to a specialist diabetic nurse even though patients have accepted responsi-

bility for managing their own diabetes.

Andrew and his family need information and education covering the following aspects:

- Physiology of blood glucose control and changes in diabetes.
- Monitoring blood glucose and regular contact with the 'team'.
- Insulin injections: technique, care of equipment and storage of insulin.
- Diet modification: a high-fibre/unrefined carbohydrate, reduced fat diet which provides adequate energy and the correct nutrients (healthy diet for everyone). High-fibre diets are useful in the control of diabetes because fibre ensures a slow and even absorption of nutrients from food, thereby avoiding sudden swings in blood glucose.
- Sport and exercise: effects on energy requirements.
- Recognition and management of hypoglycaemia.
- Recognition of ketoacidosis and hyperglycaemia, which may be precipitated by stressors such as infections.
- Support from groups such as the British Diabetic Association.
- Future developments, e.g. insulin implants which deliver insulin into the blood when needed and transdermal (through the skin) delivery systems

which use electricity or ultrasound to administer insulin without needles and eventually a modified insulin (protected from digestive enzymes) taken orally.

Nurses should ensure that the education programme is designed to enable Andrew to resume a normal healthy lifestyle despite his chronic condition. The long-term vascular complications, increased infection risk and neuropathy should be discussed with particular reference to healthy eating, hygiene, foot and skin care.

Vascular disease, e.g. atherosclerosis, occurs more frequently in diabetics and increases the incidence of peripheral vascular disease and gangrene, myocardial infarction (see Chapter 10) and strokes (see Chapter 4). Small vessel disease (microangiopathy) results in retinopathy (see Chapter 7), leading to blindness and nephropathy with renal failure (see Chapter 15).

Sensory problems caused by peripheral neuropathy may lead to the diabetic being unaware of fairly minor foot damage which, because of a poor blood supply and infection, could lead to gangrene.

The importance of good blood glucose control should be stressed as the major way to reduce the risks.

hypothalamic suprachiasmatic nucleus or 'biological clock'; it enhances sleep and synchronizes circadian rhythms (Haimov *et al.*,1994).

Melatonin appears to inhibit the release of gonadotrophin-releasing hormone, which influences the production of gonadotrophins and the timing of puberty and reproductive function. Certainly the amount of light (day length) is known to influence mating and reproduction in other animal species, especially those who breed in the spring. The link between melatonin and the timing of puberty in humans is supported by the fact that melatonin levels are high during childhood and that some secreting tumours of the pineal gland delay the onset of puberty while disease processes that destroy the pineal may lead to abnormally early puberty.

Apart from the influences on sleep, reproduction and mood, we mentioned earlier that the secretion of melatonin may have links with other circadian rhythms – appetite and temperature. Changes to these rhythms and hormone levels would account for some of the physiological upsets associated with travel through time zones ('jet lag') and shift work – which is a particular problem for health professionals, who need to function at a consistently high level.

It only remains to stress the following points about endocrine function:

• The importance of endocrine activity for maintaining homeostasis.
• The inseparable neuroendocrine links.
• Hormone levels are central to many circadian rhythms.

Healthier Living **Seasonal affective disorder (SAD)**

Aspects of behaviour, such as mood, may be linked to the secretion of melatonin. Some types of depression, e.g. SAD, become more frequent as the days shorten and winter approaches. Individuals feel lethargic and sleepy, and may crave carbohydrate foods. Some people affected in this way can be helped by phototherapy with special white light, which presumably inhibits melatonin secretion. SAD may be a particular problem for individuals working or living in areas with no natural light, such as those in residential care. Where possible, it is important to plan adequate time outside to benefit from natural daylight.

Summary/Check List

Introduction, links with nervous system.
Major endocrine glands – location, other hormone-producing structures.
Hormones – structure, action, control of secretion.
Hypothalamus and pituitary – releasing/inhibiting hormones. Anterior lobe – hormones, growth problems. Posterior lobe – hormones, problems with ADH.
Thyroid – structure, hormones, Nursing Practice Application – checking for congenital hypothyroidism, problems with secretion.
Parathyroids – structure, hormone, calcium homeostasis, problems with secretion, Nursing Practice Application – tetany following thyroid surgery. Nursing Practice Application

– hyperventilation and tetany.
Adrenals – cortex, hormones – glucocorticoids, mineralocorticoids, sex hormones, Nursing Practice Application – glucocorticoid therapy. Problems with cortical secretion. Medulla, hormones (catecholamines). Problems with medullary secretion. Stress and adrenal responses.
Pancreas – structure, hormones – glucagon, insulin, somatostatin. Blood glucose regulation. Problems with blood glucose – diabetes mellitus, Person-centred Study – Andrew.
Thymus – immune response.
Pineal – melatonin, sleep, puberty, mood, Healthier Living – seasonal affective disorder.

Self Test

1   Outline the ways in which the hypothalamus controls pituitary function.
2   Which of the following statements are true?
    (a) ADH and oxytocin are made in the neurohypophysis.
    (b) Prostaglandins are derived from arachidonic acid.
    (c) ACTH is controlled by positive feedback.
    (d) GHIH is also known as somatostatin.
3   Which of the following would result from thyroid hypersecretion?
    (a) sweating;
    (b) weight loss;
    (c) mental slowness;
    (d) bradycardia;
    (e) tetany;
    (f) restlessness.
4   Outline how PTH raises the serum calcium.

5   (a) Which adrenal hormones regulate carbohydrate metabolism?
    (b) Which 'fight or flight' hormone has most effect upon the heart?
    (c) Which adrenal hormone release is controlled by ion concentration and blood pressure?
6   Explain how diabetes mellitus causes dehydration and ketoacidosis.
7   Which of the following do not affect blood glucose levels?
    (a) prolactin;
    (b) glucagon;
    (c) cortisol;
    (d) calcitonin;
    (e) insulin.
8   Trevor, who is housebound, asks you why he feels depressed and tired as the days shorten during November. How would you explain?

Answers

1   See pages 158–159.
2   b, d.
3   a, b, f.
4   See page 165.

5   (a) Glucocorticoids; (b) adrenaline; (c) aldosterone.
6   See page 171.
7   a, d.
8   See page 174.

References

Boore JR (1978) *Prescription for Recovery: the Effect of Preoperative Preparation of Surgical Patients on Post-operative Stress, Recovery and Infection.* RCN Research Report. London: Royal College of Nursing.

Callaghan D, Williams A (1994) Living with diabetes: issues for nursing practice. *J Adv Nurs* **20**(1):132–9.

Edwards CRW, Bouchier IAD, Haslett C et al. Eds (1995) *Davidson's Principles and Practice of Medicine,* 17th edn. Edinburgh: Churchill Livingstone.

Haimov I, Laudon M, Zisapel N et al. (1994) Sleep disorders and melatonin rhythms in elderly people. *BMJ* **309**:167.

Further Reading

Besser G, Thorner M (1994) *Clinical Endocrinology,* 2nd edn. London: Mosby.

Guthrie D, Guthrie R (1991) *Nursing Management of Diabetes Mellitus,* 3rd edn. New York: Springer.

Haire-Joshu D (1992) *Management of Diabetes Mellitus: Perspectives Across the Lifespan.* London: Mosby.

Lowes L, Davis R (1997) Minimizing hospitalization: children with newly diagnosed diabetes. *Br J Nurs* **6**(1), 28–33.

Young M (1997) Problems affecting Asian women with diabetes. *Prof Nurs* **12**(8):565–567.

Useful Addresses

British Diabetic Association
10 Queen Anne Street
London W1M 0BD

Blood

Overview

- *Composition and functions of blood.*
- *Plasma.*
- *Blood cells – erythrocytes, leucocytes, platelets.*
- *Haemostasis.*
- *Blood groups and transfusion.*

Learning Outcomes

After studying Chapter 9 you should be able to:

- Describe the major components and physical properties of blood.
- List the functions of blood.
- Discuss the importance of precautions required for the safe handling of blood and body fluids.
- Describe the composition and functions of plasma.
- Outline the formation of blood cells.
- Describe the structure and functions of erythrocytes.
- Discuss the requirements for healthy erythrocyte production.
- Describe the structure, functions and breakdown of haemoglobin.
- Outline the types of anaemia and discuss its effects.
- Describe sickle-cell disease and thalassaemia (haemoglobinopathies).
- Describe the various types of leucocyte, their production and functions.
- Discuss altered leucocyte production and the problems resulting from abnormal leucocyte counts.
- Describe the production and functions of platelets.
- Outline the processes involved in haemostasis.
- Describe abnormal haemostasis: thrombosis, bleeding disorders, etc.
- Describe ABO and rhesus blood groups.
- Discuss rhesus incompatibility and haemolytic disease of the newborn and their prophylaxis.
- Outline the indications for transfusion of blood and blood products.
- Describe measures taken to ensure safe transfusion.
- Describe major complications of blood transfusion.

Key Words

Agglutination – abnormal 'clumping' or 'sticking together' of cells, which may occur with a mismatched blood transfusion.

Anticoagulant – substance that prevents or delays coagulation (clotting).

Clotting factors – substances that control the process of blood clotting/coagulation.

Coagulation – blood clotting; the last stage of haemostasis.

Erythrocyte (red cell) – blood cells containing haemoglobin; they carry gases and buffer pH change.

Key Words cont.

Erythropoiesis – formation of erythrocytes in the bone marrow.
Haematology – the science of the blood.
Haemoglobin – complex molecule of iron-containing pigment and protein. Found in erythrocytes.
Haemopoiesis – formation of blood cells.
Haemostasis – the processes which prevent inappropriate bleeding from small vessels.
Leucocyte (white cell) – the generic name given to the different blood cells concerned with immunity and protection against infection.
Leucopoiesis – formation of leucocytes.

Phagocytosis – process of enveloping and destroying bacteria and other particles by certain leucocytes, e.g. polymorphonuclear cells.
Plasma – the fluid part of the blood in which the cells are suspended.
Platelet (thrombocyte) – non-nucleated (without a nucleus), disc-shaped cellular fragment derived from large multinucleate (more than one nucleus) cells. Platelets are concerned with haemostasis.
Serum – clear fluid produced after blood has coagulated; plasma – clotting factors = serum.
Thrombosis – inappropriate intravascular clotting; formation of a thrombus (clot) in the heart or blood vessels.

Introduction

The blood (flowing within a network of vessels) and the heart (maintaining circulation by pumping a steady flow of blood) form the main transport system of the body. Blood is carried around the body by a branching system of vessels comprising arteries (from the heart), veins (to the heart) and thin-walled capillaries which facilitate the exchange of substances between blood, interstitial fluid and cells. The various substances and oxygen carried by the blood cross the capillary wall and enter the interstitial fluid (fluid surrounding the cells); conversely, waste and other molecules leave the interstitial fluid and enter the capillary. This molecular exchange is vital to homeostatic regulation.

Excess interstitial fluid is collected by vessels of the lymphatic system – the remaining part of body transport (see Chapter 11) – and returns it to the circulation (see Chapter 10) to maintain a constant blood volume. The fluid within the lymphatic vessels, known as lymph, is also concerned with the transport of substances around the body. The other vital roles of the lymphatic system – body defence and immunity – are discussed in Chapter 19.

Composition and Functions of Blood

Composition

Blood, a fluid connective tissue (see Chapter 1), is a sticky red liquid which appears uniform, but really consists of many cellular components suspended in fluid. Blood is slightly alkaline, with a normal pH range of 7.35–7.45 (see Chapter 2).

The blood cells – **erythrocytes** (red cells – the most abundant cell), **leucocytes** (white cells) and **platelets** (thrombocytes) – form about 45% of the blood volume, with the fluid **plasma** forming the remaining 55%. The proportion of erythrocytes to plasma is termed the packed cell volume (PCV), or haematocrit. A sample of blood in a test tube normally forms a clot surrounded by **serum**. A sample of blood spun in a centrifuge or exposed to **anticoagulants**, however, separates into three layers: the erythrocytes form the thick bottom layer; there is then a thin layer of leucocytes and platelets, called the buffy coat; and finally the plasma (*Figure 9.1*).

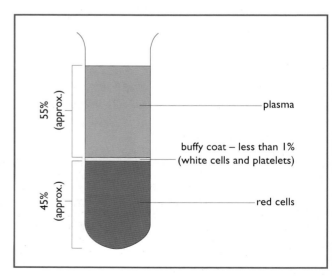

Figure 9.1 Blood components.

In adults blood forms approximately 7–8% of the body weight; females have 4–5 l and males 5–6 l. Blood as a percentage of body weight is higher in children and lower in overweight individuals (adipose tissue contains less blood).

Functions

Blood is vital in maintaining the internal environment and homeostasis. It performs the following functions:

- Carries oxygen and nutrients to cells.
- Removes waste carbon dioxide to the lungs and nitrogenous waste to the kidneys.
- Maintains body temperature by heat distribution.
- Transports enzymes and hormones to their areas of action.
- Maintains pH, fluid and electrolyte balance.
- Protects against infection with leucocytes and antibodies.
- Prevents severe haemorrhage by clot production (coagulation).

Unfortunately, blood may also provide the means by which harmful agents, e.g. parasites, micro-organisms and to a lesser extent malignant cells, travel around the body.

Plasma

Plasma is the pale yellow (straw-coloured), slightly alkaline fluid that forms approximately 55% of the blood volume. It consists of water, plasma proteins, inorganic ions and all the substances normally transported by the blood. Plasma is:

- 90–91% water.
- 7–8% plasma proteins, e.g. albumin, globulin, fibrinogen and many more (see below).
- 1–2% inorganic ions, hormones, enzymes, nutrients and waste, e.g. urea.

Plasma proteins

There are between 60 and 80 g of plasma proteins in every litre of blood. They are concerned with exerting the osmotic pressure that maintains fluid compartment volumes, contributing to blood viscosity and blood pressure, carriage of substances (e.g. hormones), buffering pH changes, inflammatory and immune responses, blood coagulation and providing a protein reserve.

Nursing Practice Application **Blood supply – healing and infection**

Overweight (body mass index greater than 25 – see Chapter 13) individuals are at increased risk for delayed healing and wound infections after surgery because adipose tissue, with its poor blood supply, may not receive the nutrients needed for healing and infection-fighting leucocytes may not reach the wound in sufficient quantities. Nursing interventions should take account of the increased risk.

Nursing Practice Application **Safe handling of blood**

Micro-organisms such as human immunodeficiency virus (HIV), which causes acquired immune deficiency syndrome (AIDS), and hepatitis B virus (HBV) are present in the blood and body fluids of affected individuals. According to Oakley (1994) it is safest to assume that a person carries an infective agent in their blood. A vaccine for HBV which provides a high level of protection is currently available for high-risk groups, which includes health care workers. However, it is essential that current Department of Health guidelines for universal precautions and local protocols are followed where exposure to blood or body fluids is a possibility. Health-care workers need to exercise care when handling blood, other body fluids and potentially contaminated items, such as used needles, syringes, intravenous equipment and linen. This care should include:

- The appropriate use of gloves, plastic aprons, masks and in special circumstances gowns and eye protection.
- Correct disposal of used items – especially 'sharps'.
- Dealing safely with spillages.
- Following proper procedures when accidents occur which involve 'needle stick' injuries and contamination of mucous membranes/conjunctiva by blood or body fluids.

Albumin (35–50 g/l)

Albumin is made in the liver. It has a molecular weight (see Chapter 2) of 69 000, which means it is too large to pass through the capillaries of a healthy kidney; its presence in the urine indicates that renal physiology is disordered, as may occur in kidney inflammation (see Chapter 15). Albumin is important in maintaining the osmotic pressure of plasma, which ensures that water mostly stays in the blood (small amounts of water and protein do leak into the interstitial fluid and are returned to the blood via the lymphatics). Reduced albumin levels, which may be caused by liver malfunction, result in oedema (see Chapters 2 and 10) as excess water leaks out of the blood vessels and 'waterlogs' the interstitial spaces. Remember that ions such as sodium also contribute to osmotic pressure (see Chapter 2).

Albumin makes plasma viscous, or sticky. Blood is definitely 'thicker than water' by a factor of four and therefore contributes to blood pressure (see Chapter 10). Protein molecules such as albumin act as buffers to limit pH changes (see Chapter 2). Albumin also carries the substances bilirubin, bile acids, calcium and drugs, e.g. aspirin. These substances are bound chemically to albumin before transportation.

Globulins (23–35 g/litre)

The globulins can be divided into three fractions; alpha (α), beta (β) and gamma (γ). Alpha and beta globulins are made in the liver, but gamma globulin is produced by cells of the immune system. Alpha globulins transport many hormones, including cortisol and thyroxine (see Chapter 8). The beta globulins are important in the transport of lipids, e.g. cholesterol, fat-soluble vitamins (A, D and K), insulin and iron. Our ability to fight infection depends on the gamma globulins (immunoglobulins) (see Chapter 19).

Fibrinogen (1.5–4.0 g/litre)

Fibrinogen, made in the liver, is one of the **clotting factors.** During coagulation soluble fibrinogen is converted to insoluble fibrin to form a clot (see page 191). Fibrin also 'seals off' areas of inflammation and prevents the spread of bacterial infection.

Other plasma proteins

These include:
- Other clotting factors, e.g. prothrombin.
- Complement, a complex of several proteins involved in the immune and inflammatory responses (see Chapter 19).
- Kinins, e.g. bradykinin (cause pain by stimulating nerve endings), which are inflammatory proteins.

Inorganic ions/electrolytes

The main plasma ions are sodium, chloride, potassium, calcium, hydrogen carbonate, phosphate and magnesium (see Chapter 2). The ions assist in maintaining blood pH and osmotic pressure.

Gases

Oxygen is carried mainly by the erythrocytes, although a small amount is dissolved in the plasma. Carbon dioxide is much more soluble than oxygen and most is carried as hydrogen carbonate (bicarbonate) ions in the plasma, although erythrocytes carry small amounts.

Hormones and enzymes

Hormones and enzymes form a variable component of the plasma, depending on what substances are actually in transit. Hormones are secreted into the blood by endocrine glands (see Chapter 8) and transported to their target tissues.

Some enzymes are part of the functioning of the blood, e.g. clotting; whereas others, which are produced by cell breakdown, e.g. aspartate aminotransferase from damaged cardiac muscle after a myocardial infarction (see Chapter 10), are merely being transported.

Nutrients

Glucose, amino acids, vitamins and some lipids are absorbed from the gastrointestinal tract and distributed around the body.

Metabolic waste

The plasma carries nitrogenous waste – urea, uric acid and creatinine – to the kidneys for excretion. Other waste products include bilirubin (bound to albumin) and the metabolites of drugs and hormones.

Blood Cells

Earlier we mentioned that cells form approximately 45% of the blood volume. The majority are erythrocytes, followed by platelets, with the least numerous being the leucocytes.

Blood cell formation – haemopoiesis

All blood cells develop from a pluripotent stem cell (formed during embryonic life) found in the bone marrow. This stem cell, or haemocytoblast, gives rise to multipotent cells and then to committed cells (proerythroblast, megakaryoblast, myeloid stem cells – myeloblast and monoblast, lymphoid stem cell – lymphoblast) that eventually become erythrocytes, platelets and several varieties of leucocytes (*Figure 9.2* and page 187). Various growth factors – erythropoietin, colony-stimulating factors and interleukins, control the development of each cell type. Some leucocytes are further processed by lymphoid tissues and thymus (see Chapter 19 and *Figure 19.6*).

Early development of haemopoietic tissue and formation of blood cells

Primitive blood cell (and vessel) development starts in mesenchymal cells from the mesoderm layer of the yolk sac and chorion (see Chapters 20 and 21) during the third week of embryonic development. Islands of haemopoietic (blood-producing) tissue develop in the liver followed by the spleen, and by 12 weeks they have found their way to the bone marrow. At the time of birth all blood production has shifted to the red marrow present in the medullary cavities of the bones (see Chapter 16).

Red marrow is gradually replaced by fatty yellow marrow during childhood, until in adults the only haemopoietic sites are the skull, ribs, sternum, vertebrae, pelvis and ends of the long bones. At times of extra demand, such as severe anaemia, the body compensates by extending haemopoietic marrow and reviving hepatic (liver) haemopoiesis. Detailed discussion of haemopoiesis is included with individual cell types.

Erythrocytes (Red Cells)

Normal mature erythrocytes are non-nucleated biconcave discs, measuring 7–8 μm in diameter, which contain haemoglobin (see *Figure 9.3*). Differentiation (see Chapter 1) occurring during development ensures that the mature erythrocyte is well adapted to its primary function of gas carriage – mainly of oxygen with some carbon dioxide. The haemoglobin also buffers pH changes. Erythrocytes have very few organelles – just a plasma membrane enclosing the haemoglobin. The glycoproteins that determine blood group (see page 196) are situated on the membrane surface. The shape and large surface area of erythrocytes means that all areas are near the surface and can engage in gaseous exchange. Erythrocytes can distort to travel along narrow capillaries. This ability to distort is due to the surface area:size ratio and the presence of special proteins, e.g. spectrin, in the membrane. Spectrin and other proteins are able to control and stabilize erythrocyte shape.

The normal range for erythrocyte numbers is 3.8–5.8 $\times$ 10^{12}/l in females and 4.5–6.5 $\times$ 10^{12}/l in males. Gender differences in erythrocyte numbers and haemoglobin concentration may be explained by menstrual blood loss and stimulation of erythrocyte production by androgens (male hormones).

Erythrocyte formation – erythropoiesis

Erythrocytes are produced in the red marrow from proerythroblasts. These are committed cells (i.e. they can only become erythrocytes), which develop from stem cells

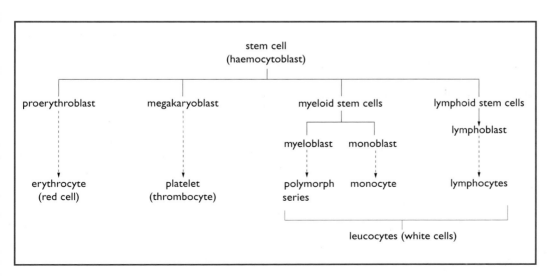

Figure 9.2 Formation of blood cells.

(haemocytoblasts). The developing erythrocytes pass through several stages during which immature blast cells lose organelles and nucleus, fill with haemoglobin and become smaller. The 'young' erythrocyte, or reticulocyte, is produced in about 3–4 days. Reticulocytes mature after they have been released into the blood (*Figure 9.4*). In adults, reticulocytes normally form less than 2% of the circulating erythrocytes, but this rises when demand for erythrocytes increases, e.g. after severe bleeding, as extra immature cells are released.

Erythrocyte numbers remain fairly constant; cells at the end of their lifespan (remember, erythrocytes cannot divide) are replaced by new cells. Replacement involves the production of many millions of cells every minute. The red marrow forms erythrocytes as a result of direct stimulation by the growth factor erythropoietin, a glycoprotein hormone produced mainly by the kidney, in response to hypoxia (lack of oxygen). Renal erythropoietic factor (REF), produced by the hypoxic kidney, acts upon a plasma protein to form active erythropoietin within the kidney prior to its release (*Figure 9.5*). Some erythropoietin is also produced by the liver. Other hormones known to stimulate erythropoiesis include androgens (see page 181), corticosteroids, thyroid hormones and growth hormone.

Erythropoietin production and hence erythropoiesis is increased at high altitudes, where the partial pressure of atmospheric oxygen is low. Shortage of oxygen with chronic respiratory diseases also increases erythropoiesis as the body compensates. These situations lead to the production of extra erythrocytes, or secondary polycythaemia.

Dietary requirements for healthy erythrocytes

To keep pace with erythrocyte production the body needs a constant supply of dietary raw materials, including:

- Iron for the haem part of haemoglobin.
- Protein for the globin part of haemoglobin and other erythrocyte proteins.
- Vitamin B_{12} (cobalt-containing cobalamins) and folic acid (folate) for DNA synthesis (see Chapter 1) and erythrocyte growth.
- Vitamin C for the absorption and utilization of iron and folate.
- Trace elements, e.g. copper.

Iron metabolism

The importance of iron in erythropoiesis merits further consideration. An adult body contains about 4 g of iron. Most is in haemoglobin and some is stored in the liver and spleen. Iron is toxic and for this reason is combined with proteins to form storage complexes called ferritin and haemosiderin. While in transit around the body, iron is bound to the protein transferrin.

Iron absorption from food is enhanced by:

- Intake of foods rich in available iron, e.g. meat, eggs and green vegetables.
- Adequate vitamin C (often destroyed in cooking).
- Ethanol (in alcoholic drinks).
- Gastric acid (converts ferric iron into the absorbable ferrous state).

An adult male needs to absorb just over 1 mg of iron daily to replace the losses in urine, faeces and sweat. Females require at least 2 mg daily to replace that lost during menstruation and the extra demands of pregnancy. Although these amounts appear small, you should note that only about 15% of dietary iron is absorbed. This means that actual intakes must be higher; for example, for males aged

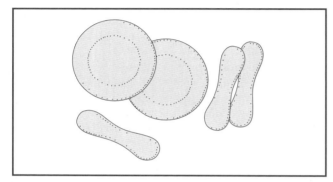

Figure 9.3 Erythrocytes.

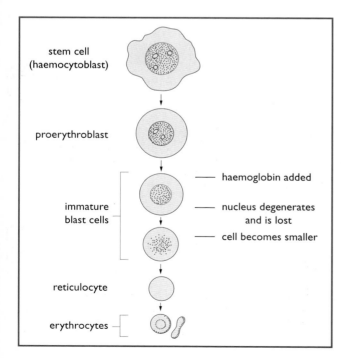

stem cell (haemocytoblast)

proerythroblast

immature blast cells

— haemoglobin added

— nucleus degenerates and is lost

— cell becomes smaller

reticulocyte

erythrocytes

Figure 9.4 Formation of erythrocytes.

19–50 years, 8.7 mg/day is sufficient for 97% of people in the group. During childhood the requirement for iron is comparatively high – a child aged 1–3 years needs an intake of 6.9 mg/day.

Absorption of iron can be inhibited by phytic acid and phosphates in cereals and tannin in tea. Vegetarians and those with a high fibre or tea intake should ensure that they have adequate iron.

Iron deficiency caused by inadequate intake, malabsorption or excess loss causes anaemia. This and the effects of B vitamin deficiency are considered later.

Conversely, excess iron may cause problems. Normal function is disrupted as iron is deposited in the liver, heart and other organs. Excess iron storage, known as siderosis, may be caused by repeated blood transfusion, high iron intake and abnormal absorption.

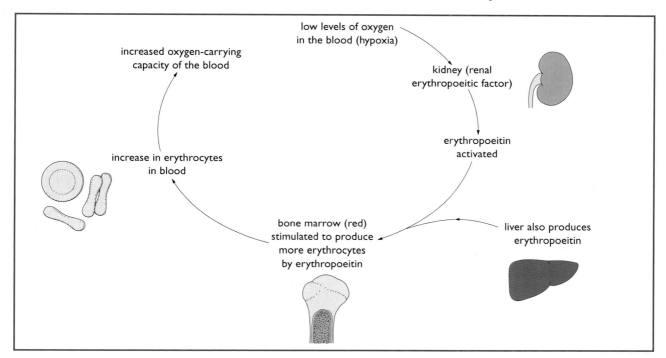

Figure 9.5 Erythropoietin and erythropoiesis.

Nursing Practice Application **Erythropoietin and anaemia**

Erythropoietin production can be decreased by kidney (renal) disease, which explains why people with chronic renal failure are usually anaemic. The use of dialysis further exacerbates the anaemia through blood loss. It is possible, however, to alleviate some effects of anaemia – extreme tiredness and breathlessness – by injections of recombinant ('genetically engineered') human erythropoietin or epoietin. Possible future uses for epoietin include anaemias associated with chronic inflammatory diseases such as arthritis.

Nursing Practice Application **Iron deficiency during childhood**

Poor iron intakes coupled with high demand during growth can result in low haemoglobin levels and anaemia during childhood. The iron deficiency is commonly seen in communities where babies are weaned late and given diets deficient in available iron. Nurses should be alert to vulnerable groups and be able to give culturally sensitive nutritional information. Various studies, such as that carried out by Ehrhardt (1986), have found that children of Asian parents have a higher incidence of anaemia than white children.

Haemoglobin (Hb)

Haemoglobin is the red iron-containing pigment–protein complex contained in erythrocytes. A molecule of haemoglobin (molecular weight 68 000) consists of four haem groups, each with an atom of ferrous iron (Fe^{2+}), and four globin chains (*Figure 9.6*). Several forms of haemoglobin exist, differing in their globin chain composition. Fetal haemoglobin (HbF) has two alpha (α) chains and two gamma (γ) chains. There are two forms of adult haemoglobin (HbA and HbA_2). The major form, HbA, has two alpha (α) chains and two beta (β) chains, and the minor form, HbA_2, has two alpha (α) chains and two delta (δ) chains.

Each molecule of haemoglobin combines reversibly with four molecules of oxygen to form oxyhaemoglobin, which is bright red (see Chapter 12). The affinity of haemoglobin for oxygen changes as the four molecules of oxygen combine sequentially, giving rise to the sigmoid shape of haemoglobin's oxygen dissociation curve (see *Figure 12.19*). Dark red reduced haemoglobin, having given up its oxygen in the tissues, carries some carbon dioxide bound to the globin as carbaminohaemoglobin (see Chapter 12). Haemoglobin is an important component of the buffer systems which limit pH changes in the blood (see Chapters 2 and 12).

In the fetus, the special haemoglobin (HbF) has a high oxygen affinity which overcomes the low partial pressure of oxygen in the placenta (the fetus is receiving 'second-hand' oxygen from the maternal circulation). By early childhood HbF has been mostly replaced by the adult haemoglobins (HbA and HbA_2). Normally adults have 11.5–18 g of haemoglobin in every 100 ml of blood (11.5–18 g/dl). Males have a higher concentration for reasons already discussed. For haematological indices see *Table 9.1*.

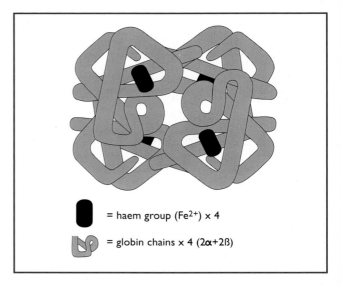

= haem group (Fe^{2+}) x 4

= globin chains x 4 ($2\alpha + 2\beta$)

Figure 9.6 Structure of haemoglobin.

Table 9.1 Haematological values.

Table 9.1 Haematological values.		
Measurement	**Male**	**Female**
Red cell count	$4.5–6.5 \times 10^{12}$/l	$3.8–5.8 \times 10^{12}$/l
Packed cell volume (PCV)	40–54%	35–47%
Haemoglobin (Hb)	13–18 g/dl (130–180g/litre)	11.5–16.5 g/dl (115–165g/litre)
Mean cell volume (MCV)	←———— 78–95 fl ————→	
Mean cell haemoglobin concentration (MCHC)	←———— 30–35 g/dl ————→	
Mean cell haemoglobin (MCH)	←———— 27–32 pg ————→	
Erythrocyte sedimentation rate (ESR) - results depend on age, gender and method	normal uncertain abnormal	0–7 mm/h 8–20 mm/h >20 mm/h

Abnormal Function **Disordered erythrocyte function**

Anaemia

Anaemia means a reduction in erythrocyte numbers, a reduction in haemoglobin, or both, which leads to diminished oxygen-carrying capacity. It is important to remember that anaemia is a 'symptom' of underlying disease. Causes of anaemia may be:

• *Haemorrhagic.* Acute blood loss, e.g. after a road accident, or more insidious loss caused by chronic bleeding, e.g. peptic ulcer or heavy menstrual loss. Management involves treating the cause, and possibly blood transfusion.

• *Deficiency:* of iron may result from inadequate intake, poor absorption or chronic blood loss. Iron deficiency results in small erythrocytes (microcytes) with reduced haemoglobin. Iron supplements are given, and transfusion if the anaemia is severe.

Lack of vitamin B_{12} and folate give rise to a macrocytic or megaloblastic anaemia (see *Figure 9.7*), so called because megaloblasts (abnormal erythrocyte precursors) are produced by the marrow. With vitamin B_{12} and folate deficiency, the erythrocytes are large (macrocytes).

Vitamin B_{12} may be lacking in the diet of strict vegans, but deficiency is usually caused by problems with absorption, which requires the intrinsic factor (gastric glycoprotein essential for absorption of vitamin B_{12}). This is missing in pernicious anaemia, where the stomach lining atrophies, or after gastrectomy (removal of part or all of the stomach). There may be problems with absorption in the small bowel.

Folate may be lacking in the diet when intake does not meet demand, such as during pregnancy, and some drugs prevent the use of folate, e.g. methotrexate (cytotoxic antimetabolite) and antiepileptic drugs. See Chapter 4 for details regarding folate and nervous system development.

Where vitamin B_{12} is deficient there may also be nerve changes, e.g. demyelination (see Chapter 3). The effects of deficiency may take time to develop as the liver stores reserves of folate (sufficient for some months) and vitamin B_{12} (enough for 3–5 years). Treatment is based on supplements of vitamin B_{12}

(injection if the intrinsic factor is absent) and oral folate.

• *Haemolytic.* Some anaemias are caused by the excessive breakdown (haemolysis) of erythrocytes. Causes include drugs, abnormal erythrocytes, overactive spleen, severe infections, haemoglobinopathies (see below) and mismatched blood transfusion (see pages 196 and 199–200).

• *Aplastic.* The bone marrow is destroyed and ceases to produce erythrocytes, leucocytes and platelets. This increases the risk for infection and the tendency to bleed, in addition to anaemia. Causes of marrow aplasia include cytotoxic drugs, e.g. busulphan, radiation and bone cancers.

Each type of anaemia is characterized by specific pathophysiological effects, but all cause changes due to reduced oxygen-carrying capacity (see Person-centred Study – Kate page 186).

Polycythaemia

In addition to secondary polycythaemia (page 182), there is a condition known as primary polycythaemia vera whereby erythrocytes increase without any physiological stimulus. It is a serious condition in which increased PCV and blood viscosity lead to abnormal clotting. Primary polycythaemia is one of a group of myeloproliferative disorders and can progress to leukaemia. Management includes venesection, radiotherapy and cytotoxic drugs.

Haemoglobinopathies

Of the many abnormal haemoglobins, sickle-cell disease and thalassaemia are the most common. These are genetic conditions where the amino acid sequence in the globin chains (see page 184) is abnormal or globin production is reduced. The haemoglobin structure is abnormal, which in turn alters the shape of the red cell and its functioning.

Sickle-cell disease affects people from areas where falciparum malaria is common (equatorial Africa, parts of India and part of the Eastern Mediterranean) and their descendants in the USA, West Indies and Europe. People who are heterozygous (see below) for the sickle-cell

gene have an increased ability to withstand the malaria parasite.

People with sickle-cell disease produce a different type of haemoglobin (HbS, for sickle-cell) from normal adult haemoglobin. All people in at-risk groups should be screened for HbS before procedures that may cause hypoxia, e.g. anaesthesia. The condition occurs in individuals who are homozygous for the sickle gene, i.e. inherited from both parents (see *Figure 9.8*). Their erythrocytes become 'sickle-shaped', leading to reduced oxygen-carrying capacity, blockage of blood vessels with pain and tissue death (infarction), and rapid erythrocyte destruction by the spleen, causing haemolytic anaemia (see earlier text). During sickle-cell crisis the immediate need is for hydration and pain control.

Sickle-cell trait occurs in heterozygous individuals who have inherited one abnormal gene (cf. homozygous, above). People with sickle-cell trait can pass the abnormal gene to their children and may themselves show signs when hypoxic.

Thalassaemia affects populations around the Mediterranean, in the Middle East, on the Indian subcontinent and in the Far East. Abnormal globin production results in fragile erythrocytes with reduced oxygen carriage. Excessive erythrocyte breakdown in the spleen results in haemolytic anaemia and iron overload. Homozygous individuals have the severe thalassaemia major whereas heterozygotes have the much milder thalassaemia minor.

The management and prevention of haemoglobinopathies depend on the type and severity but may include:

• Avoidance of stressors, e.g. cold and hypoxia.
• Folate supplements.
• Red cell/whole-blood transfusion.
• Chelating agents for iron overload.
• Splenectomy (removal of the spleen).
• Symptom control.
• Antimicrobial drugs.
• Bone marrow transplant.
• Identification of carrier status.
• Genetic counselling.
• Antenatal diagnosis with termination of pregnancy offered if the fetus is affected.

Person-Centred Study **Kate**

Kate is retired and has lived alone since her friend died 6 months ago. They were always busy with the house and garden, but now Kate cannot be bothered. She feels tired and gets breathless after the slightest exertion. Cooking is a real chore and she tends to make do with toast. Kate decided to visit her GP when she became dizzy and had palpitations. Kate's doctor noted her pallor and felt that her history suggested anaemia. The signs and symptoms experienced by Kate can be explained by the diminished oxygen-carrying capacity of her blood and the reduced supply of oxygen reaching the tissues:

Tiredness: reduced oxygen for muscles causes fatigue.
Breathlessness: the respiratory rate increases on slight exertion in an attempt to supply more oxygen to hypoxic tissues.
Dizziness: some degree of cerebral hypoxia as the brain receives less oxygen.
Palpitations: heart rate increases and the person becomes aware of their heart beating as the body tries to circulate more oxygenated blood to the tissues.
Pallor: the skin is paler than normal. This is because haemoglobin, which normally contributes to the 'pinkish' skin colour (in Caucasians), may be reduced.

A blood test (see *Table 9.1*) confirmed that Kate had iron deficiency anaemia: her Hb level was down to 9.0 g/dl; MCV, MCHC and MCH were all reduced; in the blood film her erythrocytes were microcytic and hypochromic (pale); and her serum iron was reduced. Two factors have contributed to Kate's anaemia: inadequate iron intake and bereavement-linked depression, which has caused Kate to neglect her needs. Kate is prescribed oral iron and the practice nurse arranges an appointment to discuss nutrition. Recently the practice has employed a counsellor and Kate is referred for help regarding her bereavement.

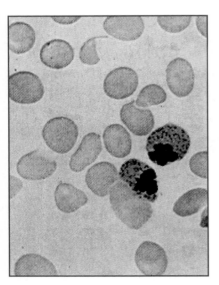

Figure 9.7 Abnormal erythrocytes – macrocytic anaemia with megaloblasts. (Hayhoe FGJ, Flemans RJ (1991) *A Colour Atlas of Haematological Cytology*, 3rd edn. Wolfe Medical Publications Ltd. Reprinted with permission).

Summary – erythrocyte functions

- Carriage of oxygen.
- Buffering pH changes.
- Carriage of some carbon dioxide.

Destruction of erythrocytes/haemoglobin

Erythrocytes have a lifespan of 100–120 days in the blood – without a nucleus they are unable to synthesize proteins or divide. Old or damaged erythrocytes are destroyed by macrophages – the phagocytic cells found in the spleen and liver. This liberates iron and protein, which are recycled, and haem. The degradation of haem produces the pigments bilirubin and biliverdin. These are bound (conjugated) to glucuronic acid in the liver and then pass into the intestine via the bile (see Chapter 14).

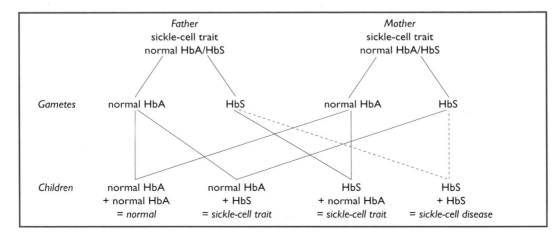

Figure 9.8 Inheritance of sickle-cell disease (HbA, adult haemoglobin; HbS, sickle-cell haemoglobin).

Leucocytes (White Cells)

All leucocytes are concerned in some way with body defences. Leucocytes are the least numerous of the blood cells; normally there are 4–11 × 10^9/l (see *Table 9.2*). Unlike erythrocytes they contain nuclei and other organelles, and are mobile. Some have the ability to pass through capillary walls into the tissues – a process called diapedesis. This means that they can locate and move to areas of inflammation. Their ability to move through the tissues in response to chemicals released at the site of inflammation is known as positive chemotaxis. Bacterial or viral infections cause the levels of certain leucocytes to increase rapidly in the blood. This rise above normal is called leucocytosis. Inflammation caused by tissue damage has a similar effect.

The main types of leucocytes are (*Figure 9.9*):

• Polymorphonuclear cells (polymorphs), or granulocytes, which have a many-lobed nucleus and granules in their cytoplasm, e.g. neutrophils, basophils and eosinophils.
• Agranulocytes, which have no granules, e.g. monocytes and lymphocytes.

The nomenclature is somewhat complex, especially where the same cell gets renamed on moving into the tissues. The functioning of different leucocytes is interrelated.

Polymorphonuclear leucocytes (granulocytes)

Development in the marrow takes a few days. The mature polymorph is approximately 12 μm in diameter.

Following release they have a lifespan of a few hours to several days.

Neutrophils

Neutrophils are the most abundant of the leucocytes and, as their name suggests, they take up neutral dye in the laboratory to stain violet. Some of their granules store lytic enzymes such as peroxidases and other antimicrobial substances, e.g. lysozyme. Neutrophils are phagocytic (*Figure 9.10*) and their main function is to engulf and destroy foreign particles, e.g. bacteria. They are attracted to inflamed areas by chemicals and, after engulfing the bacteria, destroy them with enzymes. The effectiveness of **phagocytosis** is enhanced by the presence of complement proteins and immunoglobulins (antibodies), which coat the 'invader' in a process called opsonization (see Chapters 1 and 19). Pus resulting from bacterial infection is a mixture of dead neutrophils, cellular debris, fluid and bacteria.

Basophils

Basophils take up basic dye in the laboratory to stain blue/black, and are the least abundant of the leucocytes. Their granules contain histamine and heparin. Histamine causes smooth muscle contraction, vasodilation and increased vessel permeability, all of which attract leucocytes to the area. Heparin is an anticoagulant, but its role in inflammation is unclear. Basophils which migrate to the tissues are known as mast cells. They are found around small blood vessels, where they bind to antibodies [immunoglobulin E (IgE)] before releasing chemicals involved in anaphylactic reactions and inflammation (see Chapter 19).

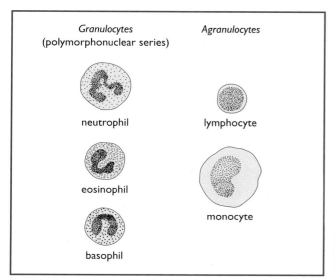

Figure 9.9 Types of leucocytes.

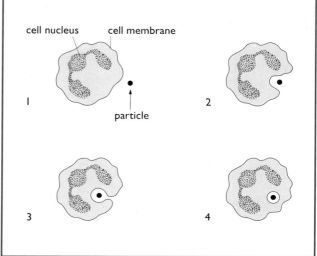

Figure 9.10 Phagocytosis.

Table 9.2 Leucocyte count and differential	
Measurement	Value
Total leucocyte (white blood cell) count	$4-11 \times 10^9/l$
Polymorphonuclear cells (granulocytes): neutrophils basophils eosinophils	 $2.5-7.5 \times 10^9/l$ (40-75%) $0.01-0.1 \times 10^9/l$ (0-1%) $0.04-0.4 \times 10^9/l$ (1-6%)
Agranulocytes: monocytes lymphocytes	 $0.2-0.8 \times 10^9/l$ (2-10%) $1.0-3.5 \times 10^9/l$ (20-45%)

Table 9.2 Leucocyte count and differential.

Eosinophils

Eosinophils are mobile, phagocytic cells which take up acid dye in the laboratory to stain red. They are present in the blood, respiratory and intestinal mucosa, and skin. Eosinophils are important in immune processes involving IgE and allergic reactions. They remove antigen–antibody complexes and foreign proteins by phagocytosis and have a role in reducing the effects of some inflammatory chemicals. Blood levels increase in parasitic conditions, e.g. worms, and allergies such as asthma. Glucocorticoid hormones which suppress inflammatory and allergic responses reduce eosinophil numbers (see Chapter 8).

Agranulocytes
Monocytes

Monocytes are large phagocytic cells up to 18 μm in diameter. They develop in the marrow over 2–3 days and, when released into the blood, have a large kidney-shaped nucleus. Monocytes move into the tissues, where they differentiate into macrophages (also called histiocytes) that may remain active for months. Macrophages ('big eaters') live up to their name as the phagocytic cells of the liver, spleen, lymph nodes and marrow, which form the mononuclear phagocytic system (previously called reticuloendothelial) concerned with body defences (see Chapters 1 and 19). Macrophages have an important defensive role, are responsible for phagocytosis of bacteria and debris, and, in the immune response, are required for T lymphocyte function.

Lymphocytes

Lymphocytes have a large spherical nucleus. There are two basic types, large (10–14 μm) and small (5–10 μm). Their development in the marrow takes only 1 or 2 days. Immature lymphocytes released into the blood migrate to the lymphoid tissue and the thymus for further development

(see Chapter 19). This produces two distinct functional groups of lymphocytes: T lymphocytes, which are involved in cell-mediated immune responses, e.g. destruction of virus-infected cells and rejection of transplants; and B lymphocytes, which are part of humoral immunity, developing into plasma cells which produce antibodies (immunoglobulins). During their lifespan, which may be days or years, lymphocytes spend most of their time in the lymphoid tissues, moving from there to the blood via lymphatic vessels (see Chapters 11 and 19).

Summary – leucocyte functions

- Phagocytosis – polymorphonuclear cells especially neutrophils, and monocytes.
- Production of antibacterial enzymes – neutrophils.
- Release of inflammatory chemicals – basophils.
- Involvement in anaphylaxis and inflammation – basophils.
- Reduce effects of some inflammatory chemicals – eosinophils.
- Process antigens for T lymphocyte action – monocytes.
- Humoral immunity through antibodies – B lymphocytes.
- Cell-mediated immunity – T lymphocytes (see also Chapter 19).

Leucocyte formation – leucopoiesis

In common with erythrocytes and platelets, the leucocytes develop in the marrow from the uncommitted pluripotent haemocytoblasts. Myeloid stem cells give rise to the polymorph series (through myeloblast, promyelocyte and myelocytes) and monocytes (through monoblast and promonocyte), and lymphoid stem cells develop (through lymphoblast and prolymphocyte) into lymphocytes (*Figure 9.11*). Knowledge of growth factors that stimulate leucopoiesis is increasing – several hormonal colony-stimulating factors (CSFs), such as granulocyte–macrophage-CSF (GM-CSF), and interleukins have now been identified. They are produced by a variety of cells including many leucocytes, possibly as part of the immune response. Not only do the CSFs stimulate leucocyte precursor maturation, but they also appear to make existing leucocytes more 'powerful' in their defence roles. As with erythropoietin (page 183), there are recombinant forms of CSFs in use clinically which:

- Counter decreases in neutrophil and platelet counts after cancer chemotherapy with cytotoxic drugs and the neutropenia following some anti-AIDS drugs.
- Stimulate the production of immature blood cells which can be collected and given instead of, or in conjunction with, bone marrow transplants.

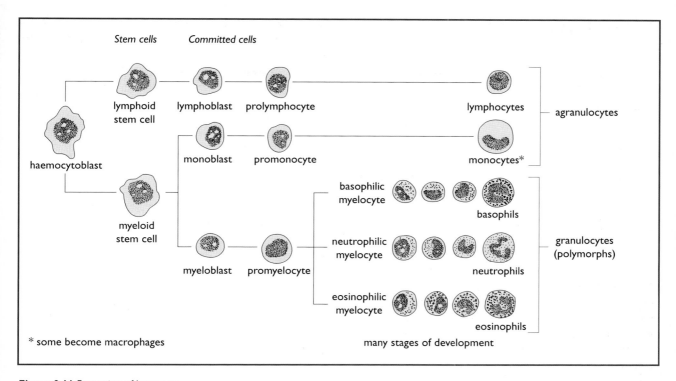

Figure 9.11 Formation of leucocytes.

Abnormal Function **Problems with leucocytes**

Leucocytosis

Leucocytosis is a normal physiological increase in leucocytes in response to infection. It can, however, be accompanied by abnormal leucocytes; for example, in infectious mononucleosis (glandular fever) or leukaemia, where atypical and immature cells are produced. The increase can affect any of the cell types.

Leukaemia

A malignant condition of leucopoietic tissue, leukaemia is characterized by proliferation of immature and abnormal leucocytes. The aetiological factors associated with leukaemia include: exposure to ionizing radiation, viruses, previous treatment with some cytotoxic drugs, some industrial chemicals, immunodeficiency and a genetic link. Interestingly, people with Down syndrome and those who have the abnormal Philadelphia (Ph) chromosome in their leucocytes show an increased incidence of leukaemia. Leukaemia can affect myeloid cells or lymphoblasts/lymphocytes and may be acute, usually affecting children, or chronic,

where older adults are affected. Different types are named for the leucocyte or precursor involved, e.g. acute lymphoblastic leukaemia (ALL), where lymphoblasts proliferate, and chronic myeloid leukaemia, where granulocyte precursors predominant. Overproduction of leucocytes disrupts other haemopoiesis, resulting in anaemia and a tendency to bleed. The huge numbers of abnormal leucocytes 'crowd out' the erythrocytes and platelets. Although leucocyte numbers are often very high ($200 \times 10^9/l$), the affected person is vulnerable to infection as immature leucocytes do not function correctly.

Leukaemia is diagnosed by examination of the blood and marrow (if the product is faulty it makes sense to check the factory). This is obtained from a suitable site, e.g. ilium or sternum, by bone marrow puncture.

Leukaemia management depends on type and stage, but includes chemotherapy with cytotoxic drugs, radiotherapy, bone marrow transplant (BMT), alpha interferon, protection from infection,

antibiotics, blood and platelet transfusion, and drugs to reduce uric acid levels (which rise as cells are destroyed by cytotoxic drugs). Recent research trials have indicated that pluripotent fetal stem cells, collected from the umbilical cord, may be a viable alternative to bone marrow transplant in some types of adult leukaemia.

It is now possible to produce a remission of several years in some types of leukaemia, but for others treatment is palliative (alleviates the symptoms but does not cure). The prognosis in children with certain types of leukaemia is often very good, reflecting the successful development of effective chemotherapy and BMT.

Leucopenia

Leucopenia is a reduction in leucocyte numbers and is associated with increased susceptibility to infection. Causes include radiation, cytotoxic and other drugs, chemicals or general marrow suppression (pancytopenia) (see aplastic anaemia, page 185).

Nursing Practice Application **Leukaemia**

Nursing interventions should be planned to minimize the effects of disordered haemopoiesis (infection risk, anaemia and bleeding), e.g. protective isolation and rigorous attention to hygiene, meticulous observation for infection, planning which prevents fatigue, and oral or intravenous medication (often via a central line) to avoid intramuscular injections.

The aggressive treatment of leukaemia can cause distressing side-effects, e.g. vomiting and alopecia (hair loss); nurses should ensure that this is fully explained and, where possible, satisfactory solutions found for the problems. The person, and his or her family and friends will need support and information at all stages.

Platelets (Thrombocytes)

Platelets are cellular fragments vital in **haemostasis**. They are formed in the bone marrow from the large multinucleate cells known as megakaryocytes which develop from the megakaryoblast (see *Figure 9.2*). Non-nucleated disc-shaped platelets break from the cytoplasm of the megakaryocytes and are released into the blood (*Figure 9.12*).

Platelets measure 2–4 μm in diameter. Their lifespan is about 10 days, after which they are destroyed by macrophages in the spleen and liver. The platelet count in adults is normally $150–400 \times 10^9/l$. This range alters very little in health, suggesting that a homeostatic mechanism controls thrombopoiesis (production of thrombocytes). Production is controlled by platelet numbers and the hormone thrombopoietin.

Platelets contain a contractile protein in microtubules and microfilaments which cause clot retraction. The platelet membrane and cytoplasmic granules contain substances, e.g. enzymes, inflammatory chemicals, phospholipid clotting factors, 5-hydroxytryptamine (5-HT), adenosine diphosphate (ADP), platelet-derived growth factor (PDGF) and prostaglandin derivatives (see Chapter 8) involved in platelet aggregation and clotting.

The process of haemostasis depends on platelet aggregation, plug formation and release of chemicals required during clotting.

Haemostasis

Haemostasis is the physiological process by which bleeding from small blood vessels is controlled. If the endothelial lining of a blood vessel is damaged, a complex series of events is initiated by substances found in the blood and others that are released by tissue damage and platelets. Haemostasis involves four overlapping processes: vasoconstriction, platelet plug formation, clotting (coagulation) and fibrinolysis.

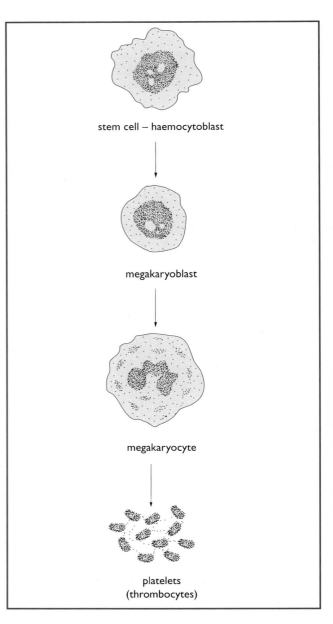

stem cell – haemocytoblast

megakaryoblast

megakaryocyte

platelets
(thrombocytes)

Figure 9.12 Megakaryocytes and the formation of platelets.

Vasoconstriction (vasospasm)

A few seconds after an injury, blood vessel constriction occurs through reflexes and in response to chemicals released by the endothelial cells and platelets, e.g. 5-HT and the prostaglandin derivative thromboxane A_2. Vasoconstriction, which can last for 20–30 min, limits blood flow and loss while a platelet plug forms and clotting occurs, i.e. it 'buys the time' needed before other processes can stop the bleeding.

Platelet plug formation

Platelets do not normally adhere to undamaged blood vessels. Substances such as collagen, exposed when damage occurs, cause platelets to become sticky and adhere at the damage site. When platelets adhere to the vessel wall they cause the release of ADP from the vessel wall itself, from platelet granules and from other blood cells. Platelet aggregation is increased by this release of ADP. The presence of thromboxane A_2 and 5-HT, which are released by platelet degranulation (break-up of granules with the release of chemicals), further increases aggregation and vasoconstriction. Platelets attracted to the area form a plug which closes the vessel defect on a temporary basis (*Figure 9.13*).

The events of platelet aggregation and plug formation illustrates positive feedback control of homeostasis (see Chapter 2).

Degranulation also produces factors that initiate thrombin formation (thrombin also encourages platelet aggregation) and clotting.

Another prostaglandin derivative, prostacyclin (PGI_2), produced by cells in the vessel, inhibits platelet aggregation and causes vasodilation. Opposing thromboxane A_2, it is probably important in preventing intravascular clotting (clotting inside a blood vessel).

Aspirin and other substances that inhibit the synthesis of prostaglandins are prescribed to reduce platelet adhesion and thrombus (clot) formation after myocardial infarction. There is, however, a risk of bleeding, especially from the gastrointestinal tract. Drugs, such as dipyridamole, which augment the action of prostacyclin and inhibit thromboxane synthesis can also be used to minimize the risk of thrombus formation in a variety of situations, e.g. following the insertion of prosthetic heart valves.

Clotting/coagulation (fibrin clot formation)

The coagulation of blood is an extremely complex process. It relies on enzyme cascade amplification (the product of one reaction triggers the next reaction) to produce a fibrin clot. Information regarding the 12 clotting/coagulation factors is provided in *Table 9.3*. In addition to these factors, clotting depends upon phospholipids such as PF_3 released when platelets aggregate.

There are two coagulation pathways (see flow chart, page 193): (i) intrinsic, which is initiated by the exposure of factor XII and platelets to collagen and platelet breakdown; and (ii) extrinsic, which depends on tissue damage and thromboplastin release. Both pathways are required for normal clotting and in the body are usually both activated by the event that initiates clotting. The extrinsic pathway has fewer stages and is quicker, but both mechanisms converge to follow a final common pathway (see *Figure 9.14*).

Detailed discussion of these separate mechanisms is not included and readers requiring more information are directed to Further Reading, e.g. Cotton (1992).

The stages of both pathways culminate in the activation of factor X. Prothrombin activator is formed when factor X complexes with platelet phospholipids or thromboplastin, calcium and factor V. In the next step, prothrombin activator converts inactive prothrombin into the active enzyme thrombin. This proteolytic enzyme (breaks down protein) changes fibrinogen, the soluble plasma protein, into a network of fibrin strands. Platelets and other blood cells become trapped in the mesh to form a fibrin clot which is stabilized by factor XIII. The stages of clotting normally take 3–8 min to complete.

In health, blood clots only when a blood vessel is damaged and anticoagulant substances normally present in the blood – antithrombin III, heparin, PGI_2 – and protein C from the liver, which is activated by thrombin, help to limit the action of clotting factors to areas where coagulation is needed.

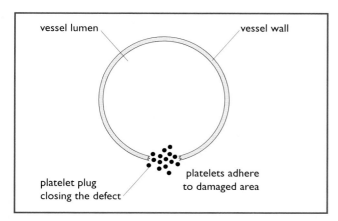

Figure 9.13 Platelet plug.

	Table 9.3 Coagulation factors		
Number	**Name**	**Origin**	**Action**
I	Fibrinogen	Plasma protein made by liver	Converted to fibrin
II	Prothrombin*	Plasma protein made by liver	Converted to thrombin
III	Thromboplastin	Released by damaged tissues	Joins with other factors to activate X
IV	Calcium ions	Obtained from diet or from bone	Required for most stages of clotting
V	Labile factor (proaccelerin)	Plasma protein made by liver	Required by intrinsic and extrinsic pathways to form prothrombin activator
VI	No longer in use		
VII	Stable factor* (proconvertin)	Plasma protein made by liver	Extrinsic pathway
VIII	Antihaemophilic globulin (AHG), Antihaemophilic factor A	Globulin made by liver	Intrinsic pathway Lack causes haemophilia A
IX	Christmas factor* (Antihaemophilic factor B), Plasma thromboplastin component	Plasma protein made by liver	Intrinsic pathway Lack causes haemophilia B (Christmas disease)
X	Stuart-Prower* factor	Plasma protein made by liver	Vital for both pathways
XI	Plasma thromboplastin antecedent (PTA)	Plasma protein made by liver	Intrinsic pathway
XII	Hageman factor	Plasma protein	Intrinsic pathway. Activation of other enzyme systems in the plasma
XIII	Fibrin stabilizing factor (FSF)	Protein found in plasma and platelets	Forms insoluble fibrin

NB *Although numbered the factors do not react in this sequence.*
* needs Vitamin K.

Table 9.3 Coagulation factors.

Fibrinolysis

Discussion of haemostasis would be incomplete without details of how the body deals with clots after healing. A new clot is rather soft and sticky, but within an hour it has become smaller and firmer. This is clot retraction, a process involving the contractile protein thrombosthenin (or actomyosin) in platelets. The edges of the damaged area are held more closely together, promoting healing. The healing process is further assisted by PDGF, which encourages the cell division needed to repair the hole in the vessel wall.

When healing is complete, the proteolytic enzyme plasmin breaks down the fibrin clot and phagocytic cells remove the debris. Plasmin is derived from the activation of plasminogen, a plasma protein made by the liver. Sources of plasminogen activators include clotting factors, blood cells at the clot site, and tissues, e.g. endothelium,

which produce tissue plasminogen activator (t-PA), lung and kidney. In this way the homeostatic balance between clotting and vessel patency (vessel remains open) is maintained. The activation of protein C which we mentioned earlier can also initiate fibrinolysis. During menstruation the uterine lining produces anticoagulants which prevent the coagulation of blood within the uterus (see Chapter 20).

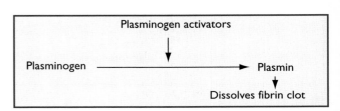

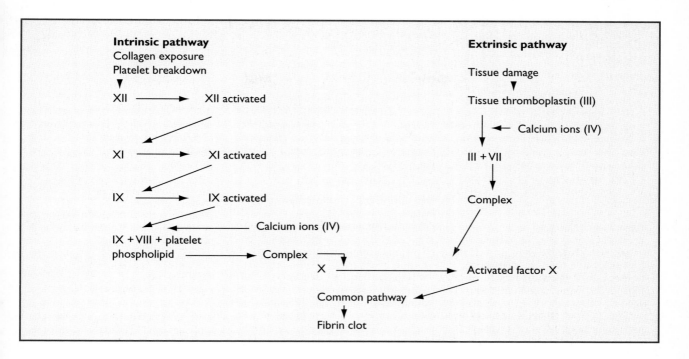

Intrinsic pathway
Collagen exposure
Platelet breakdown

XII ──────▶ XII activated

XI ──────▶ XI activated

IX ──────▶ IX activated

Calcium ions (IV)

IX + VIII + platelet
phospholipid ──────▶ Complex

X ──────▶ Activated factor X

Common pathway

Fibrin clot

Extrinsic pathway

Tissue damage

Tissue thromboplastin (III)

◀── Calcium ions (IV)

III + VII

Complex

Figure 9.14 Final common pathway of coagulation (X → fibrin clot).

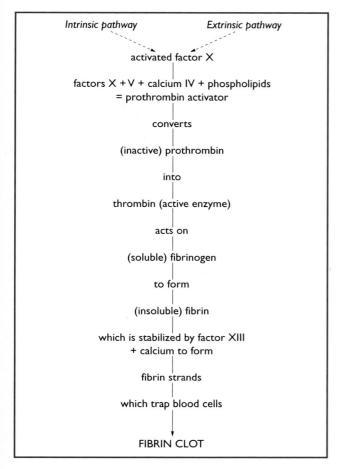

Intrinsic pathway   *Extrinsic pathway*

activated factor X

factors X + V + calcium IV + phospholipids
= prothrombin activator

converts

(inactive) prothrombin

into

thrombin (active enzyme)

acts on

(soluble) fibrinogen

to form

(insoluble) fibrin

which is stabilized by factor XIII
+ calcium to form

fibrin strands

which trap blood cells

FIBRIN CLOT

Abnormal Function **Problems with haemostasis**

Thrombocytopenia

Thrombocytopenia is a reduced number of platelets in the blood. Causes include marrow depression (due to drugs, chemicals, radiation, cancer or infection), leukaemia and hypersplenism. Many cases, however, are idiopathic (cause unknown). Affected people bleed easily; they bruise and develop small purple/red spots on the skin (petechiae). Platelet transfusions may be required.

Reduced clotting factors

Production of clotting factors depends largely upon healthy liver function and the absorption of fat-soluble vitamin K from the small intestine. Severe liver malfunction or malabsorption of vitamin K will both cause clotting factor deficiency. The presence of bile in the intestine is needed for the absorption of vitamin K.

Haemophilias

The two bleeding disorders, haemophilia A (lack of factor VIII) and Christmas disease (lack of factor IX), are inherited as sex-linked (X-chromosome) recessive genes (*Figure 9.15*). The inheritance of this type of sex-linked recessive condition is also discussed in Chapter 7 in relation to red–green colour blindness.

Asymptomatic females carry the gene which they transmit to some of their offspring; theoretically 50% of males will have haemophilia and 50% of females will be carriers. All the daughters of an affected male will be carriers, but his sons will be unaffected. Genetic counselling and antenatal diagnosis are available for affected families.

It is important to note that it is possible for a female to have haemophilia – if a female carrier and a male haemophiliac have a female child she could inherit the defective gene from both parents. For further details of haemophilia inheritance, readers are directed to the genetics text in Further Reading (Mueller and Young, 1995).

The haemophilias cause bleeding of variable severity and are managed with intravenous injections of the missing coagulation factor, blood transfusion and lifestyle modification, e.g. avoiding hazardous activities. In the UK preparations of factors VIII and IX are now heat-treated to destroy harmful agents, e.g. human immunodeficiency virus (HIV). Unfortunately, in

the early 1980s many people were supplied with infected blood products, became HIV-positive and have since developed acquired immune deficiency syndrome (AIDS) (see Chapter 19). People with haemophilia were also infected with the hepatitis C virus (HCV) before the regular screening of blood donors for this virus (see Chapter 14).

Disseminated intravascular coagulation

Disseminated intravascular coagulation (DIC) is a life-threatening complication of various other conditions, e.g. intrauterine death and severe trauma. Widespread clotting occurs in small vessels with consequent depletion of fibrinogen and platelets. This leads to bleeding, which is controlled by transfusion of fibrinogen, platelets and fresh blood in conjunction with heparin to inhibit further clotting.

Thromboembolic conditions – caused by intravascular clotting

The body normally controls clotting by limiting it to areas of vessel damage and by fibrinolysis. Inappropriate coagulation leads to thrombus (plural, thrombi) formation. If the thrombus detaches from the vessel to travel in the circulation it is known as an embolus (plural, emboli).

Problems arise when a thrombus or embolus is large enough to occlude (block) a blood vessel. Tissue deprived of blood and hence oxygen cannot function and eventually dies. The area of devitalized tissue is called an infarction. The majority of adult deaths in developed countries are caused by thromboembolic events affecting the brain (cerebral thrombosis/embolism – stroke), heart (coronary **thrombosis**) or lungs (pulmonary embolism).

The conditions that predispose to inappropriate coagulation include:

- Blood stasis, e.g. associated with immobility or heart failure. It may cause deep vein thrombosis (DVT) with clots in leg and pelvic veins. Prevention is achieved through early ambulation, leg exercises and deep breathing, prophylactic heparin and elastic compression stockings, which must be selected and fitted with care. In a study of 15 types of below-the-knee compression hosiery only five were found to be effective, i.e.

had significant linear trend graduated compression (Cornwall *et al.* 1987). Nurses can improve compliance by educating people about the purpose of compression hosiery (Dale and Gibson, 1992). The danger with DVT is a clot breaking off, which then travels in the circulation through the heart (right side), to the lungs. Here it causes pulmonary infarction, or death if a major vessel is blocked.

- Vessel wall disease and/or damage, e.g. atheroma (see Chapter 10), trauma and infection.
- Changes in the blood that increase coagulation, e.g. polycythaemia vera (see page 185) and excess platelets.

Drugs used in the prophylaxis and treatment of thromboembolic conditions include anticoagulant drugs (*Table 9.4*) and plasminogen activators (fibrinolytic drugs). Plasminogen activators, such as alteplase (recombinant t-PA), urokinase (produced by kidney) and the bacterial streptokinase, increase fibrinolysis and restore vessel patency. The plasminogen activators are effective if commenced within an hour of a pulmonary embolism or preferably within 6 hours of myocardial infarction. Improved results are obtained by using fibrinolytics in a regimen which includes aspirin and possibly anticoagulants (trial results have differed about the advantage or not of giving anticoagulants).

There are problems associated with the use of fibrinolytics, which include:

- Some are antigenic; for example, streptokinase can cause antibody production with hypersensitivity and allergic reactions.
- They may cause a fall in blood pressure, which would be 'bad news' for someone who was already hypotensive after a myocardial infarction.
- They can cause bleeding, which can be managed by antifibrinolytic agents, such as tranexamic acid, that inhibit plasminogen activators and transfusion of blood/coagulation factors.

It is important to note that tranexamic acid can be used to stop bleeding in other situations, e.g. peptic ulceration (see Chapter 13), and to minimize the risk of severe bleeding in haemophiliacs needing surgery.

Fibrinolytic agents and arterial disease are discussed further in Chapter 10.

Nursing Practice Application **Oral anticoagulant therapy**

It is important that people taking anti-coagulants are monitored carefully for bleeding and have regular prothrombin time blood tests. Many drugs, including aspirin, should not be taken unless specifically prescribed. Discharge planning should include education about the drug and its effects — especially bleeding, the need to carry an anticoagulant card and to tell all health professionals about taking anticoagulants, and, where possible, the need to avoid hazards at work or during leisure activities.

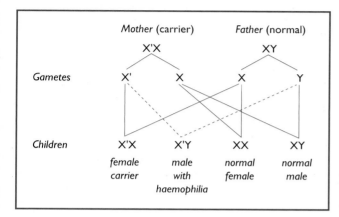

Figure 9.15 Inheritance of haemophilia.

Table 9.4 Anticoagulants		
Drug	**Action**	**Antidote**
Heparin	Inhibits thrombin, active at once	Protamine sulphate
Warfarin (coumarins)	Vitamin K inhibition effective after 36-48 hours	Vitamin K
Ancrod (derived from pit viper venom)	Reduces fibrin formation	Antivenom

Table 9.4 Anticoagulants.

Blood Groups

The surface membrane of erythrocytes and other blood cells contain glycoprotein antigens (a molecule or part molecule which is recognized by the body defences and stimulates an immune response) which determine blood groups. Individuals inherit many different antigens, including ABO, rhesus, Lewis, MNSs, Kell, Duffy, Lutheran and Kidd; however, for most purposes only ABO and rhesus (Rh) groups are clinically significant (except where repeat transfusions are needed).

Table 9.5 Antigens and antibodies.		
Group	**Erythrocyte (antigen)**	**Plasma (antibody)**
A	A	Anti-B
B	B	Anti-A
O	None	Anti-A and anti-B
AB	A and B	None

Table 9.5 Antigens and antibodies.

ABO groups

The presence of two antigens (A and B), the basis of ABO groups, was discovered by Landsteiner in 1900. Blood group depends on whether these antigens are present or not. The presence of A antigen denotes group A, whereas group B has B antigen, group O has neither antigen and group AB has both antigens (*Table 9.5*).

Before Landsteiner's work, blood transfusion carried a high risk of fatal incompatibility. Safety improved to some extent, but transfusion reactions still occurred until rhesus groups were identified some 40 years later.

We inherit one blood group gene from each parent (*Table 9.6*). The genes for antigens A and B are co-dominant over the gene for O. The inheritance of two A genes results in group A and two B genes in group B. If the A or B gene is inherited with an O gene, the blood group will still be A or B. This occurs because A and B, being co-dominant, will determine the blood group in both homozygous (A + A, B + B) and heterozygous (A + O, B + O) states. If a person inherits an A and B gene they will be group AB. The commonest group, O, will only result if an individual inherits two O genes – they must be homozygous for the O gene (O + O).

ABO antigens, which are present on the erythrocyte at birth, are also known as agglutinogens because they cause erythrocyte **agglutination** (clumping together) if exposed to the specific antibody (a protein which binds to and inactivates a specific antigen). The antibody or agglutinin is not present at birth, but is produced during the first months of life (*Table 9.5*). An antibody that acts against the antigen not present on the individual's erythrocyte (it would be crazy to have an antibody against your own erythrocyte) forms in the plasma. This production of preformed antibodies (iso-antibodies) is unusual in that it occurs without exposure to the appropriate antigen. After considerable debate it now seems likely that antibody production is stimulated by proteins taken orally (which are absorbed in the first few days of life) and by micro-organisms in the gut. The level of antibody peaks around 10 years of age and gradually decreases throughout adult life.

Before a transfusion of blood it is vital to know that the donor blood is compatible with that of the recipient. In the vast majority of cases (except in an extreme emergency) a blood sample is taken from the recipient for group and cross-match. This involves ascertaining the recipient's group (ABO/rhesus) and ensuring compatibility by mixing donor erythrocytes with recipient serum to check for agglutination (direct cross-match). Obviously only blood that shows no agglutination is transfused (*Figure 9.16*)

Generally, group O, having no antigens, can be given to any group, and group AB, with no antibodies, can receive blood from any group, providing that other groups, e.g. rhesus, are compatible. Individuals from groups A and B can receive their own group and O. The terms 'universal donor and recipient', which only apply to ABO groups, have little relevance and should be discarded.

In most transfusions it is not necessary to consider reactions between recipient erythrocyte antigens and donor antibodies because they are sufficiently diluted by the recipient's blood.

If ABO-incompatible blood is transfused, antibody in the recipient's plasma will agglutinate the donated erythrocytes with disastrous results. Erythrocytes clump together and block small blood vessels. Later the clumps undergo haemolysis and haemoglobin is released. Organs such as the kidney are damaged by the 'free' haemoglobin, resulting in renal failure (see Special Focus – transfusion of blood and blood products, page 199).

Rhesus group

The other important antigen on erythrocytes is the rhesus factor (Rh), identified in 1940 by Landsteiner and Weiner. There are several genes for Rh antigens, including those designated CDE/cde. CDE are dominant over cde. Only D (d has not been identified), however, is really important for clinical purposes. The presence of D antigen (genes DD or Dd) makes the individual Rh-positive (85% in UK are positive) and those without the D antigen (genes dd) are Rh-negative. The inheritance of Rh factor is shown in *Figure 9.17*.

In contrast to the ABO system, there are no preformed antibodies (agglutinins) to D antigen. Formation of anti-D requires the exposure of a Rh-negative person to Rh-positive blood. This will occur if Rh-positive blood is transfused to a Rh-negative person or a Rh-negative woman is pregnant with a Rh-positive fetus. Antibodies are formed after the first exposure and these cause reactions at second or subsequent exposures (see rhesus incompatibility and *Figure 9.18*).

Table 9.6 Inheritance of ABO groups and distribution in Caucasian population in United Kingdom.			
Genes inherited	Genotype	Group (phenotype)	%
O+O	OO	O	46
A+A or A+O	AA, AO	A	42
B+B or B+O	BB, BO	B	9
A+B	AB	AB	3

Table 9.6 Inheritance of ABO groups and distribution in Caucasian population in the UK.

Figure 9.16 ABO compatibility for transfusion.

		recipient			
	group	A	B	O	AB
donor	A	✓	✗	✗	✓
	B	✗	✓	✗	✓
	AB	✗	✗	✗	✓
	O	✓	✓	✓	✓

✓ = compatible

✗ = not compatible

Problems occur when fetal Rh-positive erythrocytes enter the maternal (Rh-negative) circulation through the placenta. This occurs with a full-term pregnancy, during childbirth or when a pregnancy ends in spontaneous miscarriage or termination. The woman makes anti-D in response to the Rh-positive cells. Next time she is pregnant with a Rh-positive fetus anti-D (rarely anti-C) crosses the placenta to cause haemolysis of fetal blood. The fetus will be anaemic, hypoxic and jaundiced (bilirubin released from erythrocytes). If severe, this will lead to brain damage or death (the baby is stillborn or dies soon after birth). This is haemolytic disease of the newborn (HDN) or erythroblastosis fetalis. Intrauterine transfusion and exchange transfusions after birth (with Rh-negative blood – remember that anti-D is already 'searching' for Rh-positive cells) are used for affected babies.

It is important to note that haemolytic disease of the newborn caused by ABO incompatibility between mother and fetus is a much milder condition and again it is usually second or subsequent pregnancies which are affected.

Nursing Practice Application **HDN prophylaxis with anti-D immunoglobulin**

Anti-D immunoglobulin (an intramuscular injection) given to Rh-negative women within 72 hours of delivery, miscarriage (including threatened miscarriage with bleeding) or termination destroys any fetal erythrocytes in the circulation before the woman's immune system is stimulated to produce her own anti-D. In some situations the Rh group of the infant is determined and anti-D is only given to the woman if the infant is Rh-positive.

At-risk Rh-negative women of childbearing age require education regarding Rh-incompatibility and the need for anti-D immunoglobulin after each pregnancy where a risk exists. Nurses should be aware of at-risk women in their care and ensure that they receive the correct information and treatment (see Chapter 19).

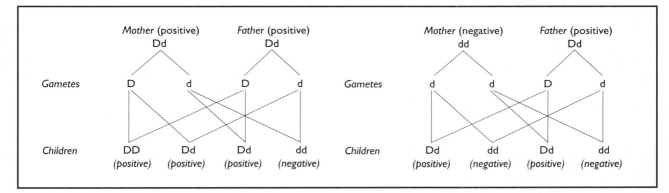

Figure 9.17 Inheritance of rhesus factor. Dd, positive (heterozygous); DD, positive (homozygous); dd, negative.

At a basic level we now have eight groups, as each ABO group may be rhesus-positive or negative (A Rh-positive, A Rh-negative, B Rh-positive, B Rh-negative, O Rh-positive, O Rh-negative, AB Rh-positive and AB Rh-negative).

Tests for Rh-compatibility before transfusion are similar to those for ABO groups. Rh-positive individuals may receive Rh-positive or Rh-negative (remember no preformed antibodies) blood, but Rh-negative people must only receive Rh-negative blood.

Blood transfusion

The transfusion of blood and blood products is a commonly used therapeutic measure in situations such as anaemia, trauma, surgery, leukaemia, burns, leucopenia and thrombocytopenia.

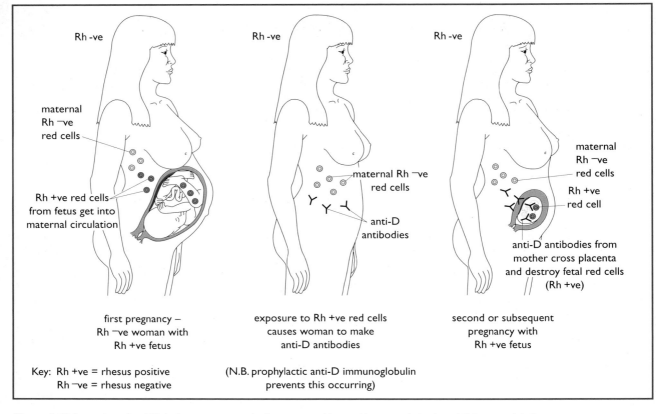

Figure 9.18 Formation of anti-D during pregnancy and subsequent problems without prophylactic anti-D immunoglobulin.

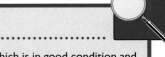

Special Focus **Transfusion of blood and blood products**

Although blood transfusion is an everyday procedure, there are potential hazards which must be anticipated and prevented where possible. Transfusion of blood or blood products may be indicated in situations which include:

Haemorrhage: whole blood replacing volume and cells.

Anaemia: plasma-reduced blood (packed cells) replacing cells rather than volume.

Thrombocytopenia: platelets to treat bleeding.

Leucopenia: granulocytes to combat infection in marrow suppression.

Plasma: used to replace that lost from major burns. Plasma substitutes, e.g. gelatin and dextran, are used in the short term to expand the blood volume. They also reduce the risk of plasma transmitted disease.

Plasma components: e.g. factors used in haemophilia (Factor VIII), fibrinogen and albumin.

Blood Transfusion Safety
(see page 179 for risks to health-care workers) - Precautions

- Donors screened for disease, e.g. haemoglobin levels, HIV – those in high-risk groups are asked not to donate.
- According to Drugs and Therapeutics Bulletin (1993), all donated blood is screened for HBV, HCV, HIV 1 and 2, and syphilis, some is tested for cytomegalovirus (CMV) and in some areas an additional check for malaria is made.
- Sterile, single-use equipment is used.
- Blood is anticoagulated and stored at 4°C for a maximum of 35 days (whole blood).
- Group and cross-match tests.
- The intravenous infusion is started with 0.9% saline before blood is transfused.
- Vigorous checking procedures to ensure the person receives the correct

blood, which is in good condition and in date.
- Blood should be removed from refrigeration 30 minutes before use and allowed to reach room temperature. When large volumes are to be transfused quickly it can be warmed in a special blood warmer. A transfusion of cold blood could reduce body temperature and cause cardiac problems.
- Careful monitoring of recipient's vital signs, etc. – see Nursing Practice Application.
- Complete records kept of blood used, and blood bags retained in case of reaction.
- Administration sets changed at regular intervals to minimize infection risk – at least every 24 hours and on completion of transfusion.
- Filters used where appropriate to prevent micro-aggregates being transfused.

Abnormal Function **Selected transfusion complications/problems**

Haemolytic reactions due to erythrocyte incompatibility – immediate
Erythrocyte incompatibility, such as ABO mismatch, causes an extremely serious reaction produced by the agglutination and haemolysis of the mismatched donor erythrocytes (see page 196). Soon after incompatible blood is transfused the following may occur: anaphylaxis, pyrexia (fever) and rigors, rashes, breathing difficulties, hypotension, rapid pulse, discomfort at the infusion site, loin pain, haemoglobin in the urine, reduced urine output and, possibly, renal failure. Other manifestations may include flushing, vomiting and diarrhoea.

Haemolytic reaction – delayed
Delayed haemolytic reaction resulting in anaemia and jaundice can occur around 1 week after transfusion, which may be missed if the person has been discharged home. This type of reaction is caused by immune antibodies and affects people needing multiple transfusions. With the increased exposure to blood components they produce antibodies to erythrocyte antigens other than ABO, leucocytes, platelets and plasma proteins. The person having multiple transfusions who produces antibodies such as anti-Duffy has an extra problem as compatible blood becomes more difficult to find (Dodsworth, 1995).

Febrile – allergic/pyrogenic reaction
Allergic reactions occurring in response to donated blood may cause effects ranging from minor urticarial rashes and pyrexia to laryngeal swelling with airway obstruction (see Chapter 12). Pyrogens (which can increase temperature) present in the blood or equipment may cause a rise in temperature.

Circulatory overload
Circulatory overload may occur if whole blood is used to treat anaemia, especially in older adults or those with cardiac problems. It causes pulmonary oedema (fluid in the lung) with rapid respiration, frothy sputum, chest pain and rapid pulse.

Infected blood and transmission of specific diseases (see Special Focus, Transfusion of blood and blood products)
Bacteria may contaminate the blood or equipment. This results in septicaemia with pyrexia, rigors and shock (hypotension), which may be fatal. Specific viral infections such as CMV, HIV, HBV and HCV have been transmitted via infected blood/blood products.

Thrombophlebitis
Thrombophlebitis is inflammation of vein with thrombus formation. Phlebitis is the most common complication of intravenous infusion/blood transfusion (Francombe, 1988).

Cold blood
Cold blood may cause cardiac arrhythmias (abnormal heart rhythm) and may lower core temperature.

Storage problems
Platelets and clotting factors do not store well – people having large transfusions may have problems with haemostasis.

Leucocytes deteriorate quickly (granulocytes die within hours) after transfusion of stored blood and a fresh transfusion is needed if leucocytes are required to treat leucopenia.

Some people develop jaundice following transfusion as many donor erythrocytes at the end of their lifespan are broken down and release bilirubin.

During storage, potassium leaks from the erythrocytes. This may cause hyperkalaemia (raised levels of potassium in the blood) and a risk of cardiac arrhythmias for which cardiac monitoring may be required.

Large transfusions may produce hypocalcaemia and tetany (see Chapter 8). Available calcium levels are reduced after the transfusion of large amounts of citrated (anticoagulant) stored blood.

Iron overload
This can be a problem for people requiring regular transfusions, e.g. those with haemoglobinopathies (see pages 185 and 186).

Nursing Practice Application **Observations and blood transfusion**

Pre-transfusion baseline vital signs should be available for comparison during transfusion – temperature, pulse, blood pressure and respiration, plus colour and general condition. At the start of transfusion the blood is generally administered slowly and the nurse stays with the person to monitor vital signs and general condition. Observations are done every 5 minutes (with local variations) because reactions are more likely to occur in the early stages. If the observations are satisfactory for at least 15 minutes the frequency can be reduced according to local procedures, e.g. hourly throughout the transfusion, and the transfusion rate adjusted as ordered. In addition, it is important to record fluid balance, test urine for blood and observe for rashes, rigors, pain (chest, loin or transfusion site), inflammation at the site, jaundice, signs of bleeding and any other abnormalities. Early detection of both immediate and late-onset complications with prompt reporting to medical staff and treatment saves lives (see *Figure 9.19*).

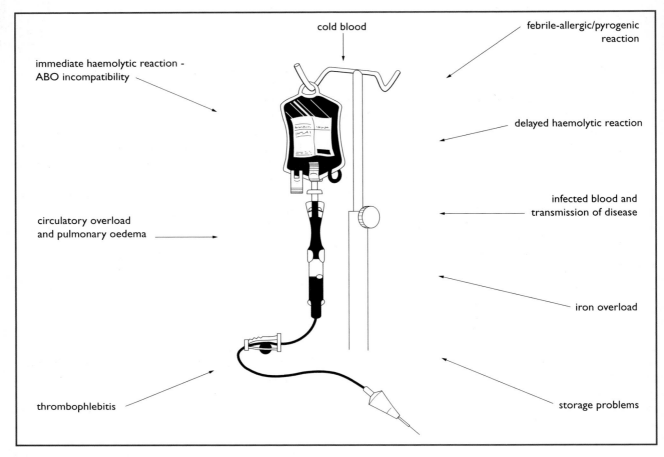

immediate haemolytic reaction - ABO incompatibility

cold blood

febrile-allergic/pyrogenic reaction

delayed haemolytic reaction

circulatory overload and pulmonary oedema

infected blood and transmission of disease

iron overload

thrombophlebitis

storage problems

Figure 9.19 Complications and problems of blood transfusion.

Summary/Check List

Introduction.
Composition and functions of blood – composition, Nursing Practice Application – blood supply – healing and infection, functions, Nursing Practice Application – safe handling of blood.
Plasma contents – proteins, ions, gases, hormones, enzymes, nutrients, waste.
Blood cells – haemopoiesis.
Erythrocytes – structure, erythropoiesis, Nursing Practice Application – erythropoietin and anaemia, dietary requirements, iron metabolism, Nursing Practice Application – iron deficiency during childhood, Healthier Living – accidental acute iron poisoning, haemoglobin, destruction of erythrocytes, disordered erythrocyte function – anaemia, Person-Centred Study – Kate, polycythaemia, haemoglobinopathies – sickle-cell disease and thalassaemia.
Leucocytes. Polymorphonuclear cells (granulocytes) –

neutrophils, basophils, eosinophils. Agranulocytes – monocytes, lymphocytes. Leucopoiesis. Problems with leucocytes – leucocytosis, leukaemia, Nursing Practice Application – leukaemia, leucopenia.
Platelets – thrombopoiesis, structure, function.
Haemostasis – vasoconstriction, platelet plug formation, clotting, fibrinolysis. Problems with haemostasis – thrombocytopenia, reduced clotting factors, haemophilias, DIC, thromboembolic conditions, Nursing Practice Application – anticoagulants.
Blood groups – ABO, inheritance and distribution, cross-match/compatibility. Rhesus group – inheritance, rhesus incompatibility, Nursing Practice Application – HDN prophylaxis with anti-D immunoglobulin, Special Focus – transfusion of blood and blood products. Complications of transfusion, Nursing Practice Application – observations and blood transfusion.

Self Test

1 Which of the following describes plasma?
  (a) Red alkaline fluid forming 55% of blood volume.
  (b) Straw-coloured neutral fluid forming 45% of blood volume.
  (c) Red neutral fluid forming 45% of blood volume.
  (d) Straw-coloured alkaline fluid forming 55% of blood volume.

2 Describe how erythrocyte structure is adapted to oxygen carriage.

3 Which of the following statements are true?
  (a) Leucocyte is the general name for all white cells.
  (b) Neutrophils are phagocytic.
  (c) Leucocytes are not produced in the marrow.
  (d) The normal white count is $4–11 \times 10^9$/litre.

4 Outline the role of platelets in haemostasis.

5 Put the following in the correct order:
  (a) Clotting;
  (b) Vasoconstriction;
  (c) Fibrinolysis;
  (d) Platelet plug.

6 Explain how a man (A Rh-positive) and a woman (B Rh-positive) can have children who are group O Rh-positive.

7 What would cause an Rh-negative woman to produce anti-D?

8 Which of the following transfusions are compatible?
  Donor   *Recipient*
  (a) A Rh-negative   AB Rh-positive
  (b) O Rh-positive   O Rh-negative
  (c) B Rh-positive   A Rh-positive
  (d) O Rh-positive   B Rh-positive.

Answers

1 d.
2 See page 181.
3 a, b, d.
4 See pages 190–193.
5 b, d, a, c.
6 See pages 195–197.
7 Transfusion of Rh-positive blood, pregnant with a Rh-positive fetus.
8 a, d.

References

Cornwall JV, Dore CJ, Lewis D (1987) Graduated compression and its relation to venous filling times. *BMJ* **295**:1087–90.

Dale JJ, Gibson B (1992) Information will enhance compliance: informing clients about compression hosiery. *Prof Nurs* **7**(11):755–760.

Dodsworth H (1995) Making sense of the use of blood and blood products. *Nurs Times* **91**(1): 25–7.

Drugs and Therapeutics Bulletin (1993) The risks and uses of donated blood. *Drugs and Therapeutics Bulletin* **31**(28):89–92.

Ehrhardt P (1986) Iron deficiency in young Bradford children from different ethnic groups. *BMJ* 292:90–3.

Francombe P (1988) Intravenous filters and phlebitis. *Nurs Times* **84**(26):34–5.

Oakley K (1994) Making sense of universal precautions. *Nurs Times* **90**(27):35–6.

Further Reading

Belcher A (1993) *Blood Disorders*. London: Mosby.

Cotton RE, Ed (1992) *Lecture Notes on Pathology*, 4th edn. Oxford: Blackwell Scientific.

Department of Health (1993) *Protecting Health-care Workers and Patients from Hepatitis B: Recommendations of the Advisory Group on Hepatitis*. London: HMSO.

Love C (1990) Deep vein thrombosis – threat to recovery. *Nurs Times* **86**(5):40–3.

Love C (1990) Deep vein thrombosis – methods of prevention. *Nurs Times* **86**(6):52–5.

Mueller RF, Young I (1995) *Emery's Elements of Medical Genetics*, 9th edn. Edinburgh: Churchill Livingstone.

Royal College of Nursing Oncology Nursing Society (1989) *Safe Practice with Cytotoxics*. Harrow: Scutari Press.

Royal College of Nursing (1994) *Universal Precautions Against Hepatitis B and AIDS*. London: RCN.

Useful Addresses

Haemophilia Society
123 Westminister Bridge Road
London SE1 7HR

Leukaemia Care Society
14 Kingfisher Court
Venny Bridge
Pinhoe
Exeter EX4 8JN

Cardiovascular System: Heart, Vessels and Circulation

Overview

- *Cardiac structure.*
- *Cardiac physiology.*
- *Blood vessel structure.*
- *Circulatory physiology.*
- *Circulatory pathways.*

Learning Outcomes

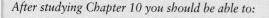

After studying Chapter 10 you should be able to:

- Describe the location, size and shape of the heart.
- Describe the heart wall, relating structure to function.
- Outline the properties of cardiac muscle.
- Describe the chambers and valves of the heart.
- Describe the coronary circulation.
- Discuss the multifactorial causation of coronary heart disease.
- Describe strategies for reducing heart disease risk.
- Describe blood flow through the heart.
- Describe the cardiac conduction system.
- Explain the normal electrocardiogram and describe some common abnormalities.
- Describe the cardiac cycle.
- Outline the regulation of cardiac output, heart rate and stroke volume.
- Describe the structure of arteries, veins and capillaries, and how each is adapted to function.
- Explain blood flow, peripheral resistance and blood pressure.
- Outline how blood vessel size and flow are controlled.
- Describe the factors which influence and control blood pressure.
- Outline the pathophysiological changes occurring in shock and describe its causes.
- Explain the role of the capillary bed in exchange.
- Describe pulmonary circulation and gaseous exchange.
- Describe the major vessels of the systemic circulation.
- Describe the hepatic portal circulation and explain its role.

Key Words

Artery – vessel carrying blood away from the heart.

Atria – two thin-walled upper receiving chambers of the heart.

Blood pressure – force exerted by the blood on the vessel walls.

Capillaries – network of tiny vessels linking arteries with veins. Their structure allows the exchange of molecules between blood and cells.

Cardiac output – amount of blood pumped out by each ventricle per minute.

Key Words cont.

Cardiovascular system (CVS) – the heart and blood vessels.
Diastole – relaxation phase of the cardiac cycle when the heart fills with blood.
Mediastinum – the space in the chest, between the lungs, containing the heart and blood vessels.
Peripheral resistance – friction or resistance between the blood and the arteriolar (small arteries) walls.

Stroke volume – amount of blood pumped out by each ventricular contraction.
Systole – contraction phase of the cardiac cycle when the heart pumps blood into the arteries.
Vein – vessel carrying blood to the heart.
Ventricles – two thick-walled lower chambers of the heart which pump blood into the circulation.

Introduction

The heart and the circulation of blood within the network of blood vessels is vital in homeostatic control. Cells constantly need oxygen and nutrients for metabolism and the waste produced must be removed. Homeostasis is maintained by the ability of the **cardiovascular system** (CVS) to adapt to changes in physiological conditions and needs. This feature of the CVS is easy to take for granted, but without this response an individual would faint on getting out of bed, would have no chance running for a bus and would have difficulty digesting a large meal.

Heart

Popular opinion perceives the heart to be the location of emotion, as illustrated by expressions such as 'sweetheart'

and 'heartbreak'. Not so – the bounding heart before your driving test is caused by hormones and the autonomic nervous system. It is simply a double pump which circulates fluid around a system of pipes (*Figure 10.1*).

The heart is two super-efficient mechanical pumps acting in unison: one circulates blood around the body in the systemic circulation and the other pumps blood through the lungs. Most of the time we are unaware of its efforts or the scale of these labours; during a lifetime of 70 years the heart beats some 3000 million times at an average rate of 80/min.

Early development of the heart

During embryonic life the heart develops from two endothelial tubes derived from mesoderm, which initially form a single chamber. As early as the fourth week this primitive structure is pumping blood.

Figure 10.1 The heart, great vessels and lungs.

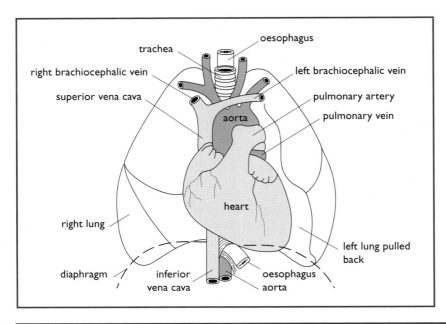

During the next 3–4 weeks the single-chamber heart rotates and undergoes the structural changes which produce the double-pump heart with four chambers. There are, however, several structural modifications to the fetal heart and circulation (see page 206 and Chapter 21).

Cardiac development during the vital early weeks may be adversely affected by maternal rubella, alcohol misuse or drugs. Damage during development may result in structural problems, such as septal defects ('hole in the heart'; see page 206) or valve or vessel narrowing, e.g. coarctation of the aorta. Some heart defects are associated with chromosomal anomalies such as Down syndrome (see above).

Location, shape and size of the heart

The heart is a hollow organ, situated in the **mediastinum** and behind the sternum. It is roughly cone shaped, with its base uppermost and the apex inclined to the left. Protection for the heart is provided by the thoracic cage (ribs and sternum).

The heart is of roughly the same proportions as the person's fist; it measures around 10–12 cm from base to apex and weighs approximately 300 g. The base is level with the second costal cartilage and the apex can normally be located just medial to the midclavicular line in the fifth intercostal space (*Figure 10.2*).

Functions of the heart

- Circulates oxygenated blood to the tissues through the high pressure (systemic) general circulation.
- Pumps deoxygenated blood to the lungs through the low pressure pulmonary circulation, where gaseous exchange occurs (see Chapters 9 and 12).

Forget St Valentine's Day – the heart has nothing to do with 'love'.

Structure of the heart wall

Endocardium

The endocardium (see *Figure 10.5*) is endothelial tissue which lines the chambers of the heart and extends to cover the valves. It also forms the lining of the vessels joining and leaving the heart. In health this smooth tissue allows blood flow without turbulence which would damage the vessel walls (an eroded river bank is further damaged by the turbulent flow of water).

Myocardium

The middle layer of the heart wall consists of highly specialized muscular tissue known as the myocardium. Cardiac muscle has features in common with both skeletal and smooth muscle (see Chapter 17). It has striations, is involuntary and has an internal control system or pacemaker.

The fibres are short, with one or two nuclei and many mitochondria, which reflect the high metabolic activity. Boundaries between individual cells are not well defined, and darkly staining intercalated discs (containing gap junctions and desmosomes – see Chapter 1) join the cells together (see *Figure 10.3*). This means that ions can exchange freely across the muscle cell plasma membrane, allowing the action potential (see Chapters 3 and 17) and hence the wave of contraction to pass easily across the myocardium, which behaves like a single unit or syncitium. A strategically located fibrous tissue network within the myocardium helps to strengthen the muscle, prevents overstretching and directs the action potentials to well-defined routes through excitable cells.

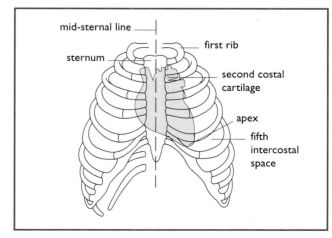

Figure 10.2 Position of the heart.

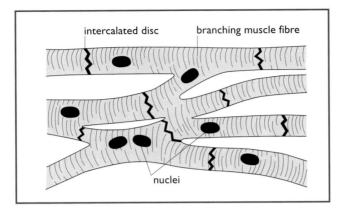

Figure 10.3 Cardiac muscle.

The myocardium depends on aerobic (oxygen-requiring) respiration for its energy requirements and its performance is rapidly impaired by oxygen deficiency. Skeletal muscle can build up an 'oxygen debt' and switch to anaerobic respiration (see Chapters 12 and 13), e.g. when you decide to sprint for the train. Not so the heart, which needs a constant supply of oxygen to use fuel molecules (e.g. glucose, lactic acid, fatty acids) to produce ATP. It is protected from fatigue (you cannot really have a 'tired' heart) and tetanic contraction (see Chapter 17), where pumping would cease, by a refractory period (see Chapter 3). This may be absolute, when contraction is not possible, or relative, when a sufficiently large stimulus will cause contraction.

The myocardium reaches maximal thickness over the apex (**ventricles**), which has to exert sufficient power to pump blood to all areas of the body. The force of the myocardial contraction is proportional to the degree of stretching of the ventricular muscle fibres (within physiological limits). As the heart fills with blood during **diastole** (relaxation phase) the fibres are stretched and the next contraction is more powerful. This relationship between length and tension, known as Starling's law of the heart, helps to ensure that output from both ventricles is equal. We shall discuss Starling's law later in this chapter in relation to preload and **stroke volume**.

Pericardium

The heart is surrounded by a double-layer sac called the pericardium. The outer sac enclosing the heart is known as the fibrous pericardium. It is lined with an inner serous layer – the parietal pericardium. The visceral pericardium (epicardium) is a second serous layer found as part of the cardiac wall. A potential space between the two serous layers contains serous fluid, which lubricates and prevents friction as the heart contracts (see Chapter 1). The heart is protected from damage and over-distension with blood by the outer fibrous layer, which also attaches it to the diaphragm, vessels and chest wall.

Chambers of the heart

The heart consists of four chambers: two upper receiving chambers called **atria** (singular atrium) and two lower chambers, which pump blood into the circulation, called ventricles. Between the atria and ventricles are valves, and the right and left sides of the heart are divided by a septum (*Figure 10.5*). Before birth an opening between the atria, the foramen ovale, allows blood to bypass the fetal lungs (see Chapter 21). There is normally no communication between right and left sides after birth. Defects in the atrial septum (ASD) or ventricular septum (VSD) present after birth can be successfully repaired by surgery.

The atria receive deoxygenated blood returning from the tissues (right atrium) and oxygenated blood from the lungs (left atrium). Each atrium has a small appendage known as the auricular appendage or auricle, which marginally increases atrial volume. The ventricles are much larger chambers with thick muscle which contracts to pump blood out into the general (left ventricle) and pulmonary circulation (right ventricle).

Heart valves

Blood flow through the heart is controlled by valves derived from endothelium. They allow flow in one direction only, by preventing backflow. Atrioventricular (AV) valves between atria and ventricles stop backflow of blood into the atria when the ventricles contract. The valve between the right atrium and right ventricle is the tricuspid, which has three cusps or flaps. On the left side the mitral (shaped like a bishop's mitre), or bicuspid valve, has two cusps. Both valves are stabilized by cords (chordae tendineae) which fix the cusps to papillary muscle in the ventricular wall [*Figure 10.4(a)*]. This arrangement prevents the valve being blown inside out – like securing a tent against strong winds. Rising pressure in the ventricles during **systole** (contraction phase) causes the AV valve to close.

Two semilunar (half-moon shape) valves guard the entrance to the great vessels from the ventricles [*Figure 10.4(b)*]: the aortic valve, between left ventricle and aorta, and the pulmonary valve, between right ventricle and pulmonary **artery**. They open during ventricular contraction, to allow blood into the circulation, and close as the pressure in the aorta and pulmonary artery rises.

The heart sounds, heard when a stethoscope is placed against the chest wall, are the sounds of the valves closing (similarly, the sound is heard when you slam a door, not when it is opened). The first sound ('Lub') is the AV valves

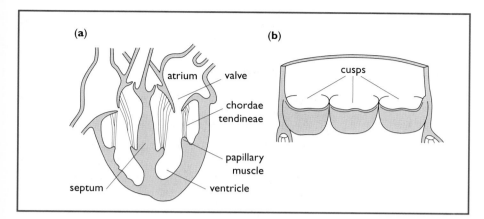

Figure 10.4 Heart valves. (**a**) AV valve; (**b**) semilunar valve.

(a)

atrium valve

chordae tendineae

papillary muscle

septum ventricle

(b)

cusps

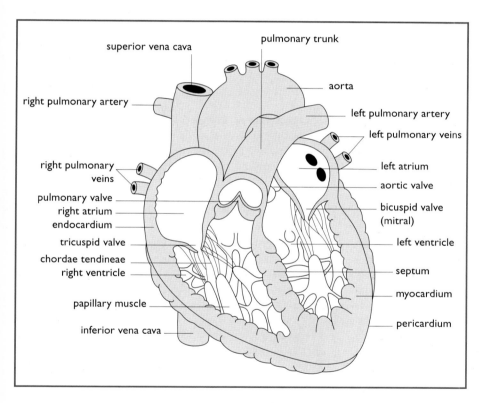

Figure 10.5 Interior of the heart to show layers, chambers and valves.

superior vena cava

pulmonary trunk

right pulmonary artery

aorta

left pulmonary artery

left pulmonary veins

right pulmonary veins

left atrium

aortic valve

pulmonary valve

right atrium

endocardium

bicuspid valve (mitral)

tricuspid valve

left ventricle

chordae tendineae

right ventricle

septum

papillary muscle

myocardium

inferior vena cava

pericardium

closing and the second sound ('Dup') is heard as the semilunar valves close.

The action of heart valves is important for the efficiency of the heart. Damage to the valves resulting from diseases such as rheumatic fever or endocarditis (endocardial inflammation) may cause incompetence, where the valve is 'leaky', or stenosis, where the valve is narrow and stiff. This valvular damage may produce abnormal heart sounds or murmurs caused by turbulence, as blood leaks back into the heart or is forced through the narrowed valve. Both incompetent and stenosed valves lead to increased cardiac work, loss of efficiency and eventual

heart failure. The mitral and aortic valves are most often affected, but can be treated surgically.

Coronary circulation

The myocardium receives its blood supply from the right and left coronary arteries, which are the first branches from the aorta. These two arteries divide into smaller branches which run in grooves on the surface of the heart. The left coronary artery forms the circumflex and anterior interventricular arteries and the right coronary artery the marginal and posterior interventricular arteries (see *Figure 10.6*).

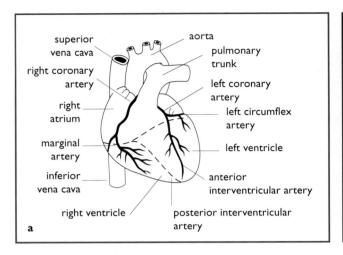

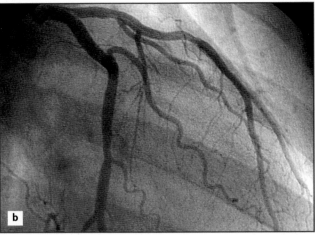

Figure 10.6 (a) Coronary circulation; **(b)** left coronary arteriogram – injection of left coronary artery. (Weir J, Abrahams PH (1997) *Imaging Atlas of Human Anatomy, 2nd edition*. Published by Mosby-Wolfe, an imprint of Times Mirror International Publishers Ltd. Reprinted with permission.)

This arrangement of arteries, which encloses the heart like a crown (hence coronary), ensures that myocardial cells are supplied with adequate oxygen and nutrients for their continuous functioning. With the body at rest, the myocardium receives about 250 ml of blood per minute, which is a lot for an organ weighing less than 0.5 kg. Myocardial cells extract more oxygen from the blood than other body structures. Most of the blood reaches the myocardium during diastole as the coronary vessels are compressed during systole. When the myocardium needs more oxygen, such as during exercise, the coronary vessels dilate and the blood flow increases. Various factors influence blood flow changes, including lack of oxygen, high levels of carbon dioxide, the ANS (see Chapter 6) and the pressure in the aorta, which depends on myocardial contraction.

Deoxygenated blood leaves the myocardium through cardiac veins. Some of these form the coronary sinus, which returns most of the blood to the right atrium. The remainder drains directly into the right atrium through cardiac veins.

Blood flow through the heart

Venous blood (low in oxygen and rich in carbon dioxide) returns to the heart through the superior and inferior venae cavae and the coronary sinus (see *Figure 10.8*). Blood enters the right atrium and passes through the tricuspid valve into the right ventricle. It is pumped from the ventricle, through the semilunar valve, into the pulmonary artery, which transports blood to the lungs. In the pulmonary circulation the close proximity between the **capillaries** and the alveoli (air sacs in the lungs) allows gaseous exchange between blood and alveolar air; carbon dioxide from the blood moves into the alveoli and oxygen moves into the blood (see Chapter 12).

Blood rich in oxygen and low in carbon dioxide returns to the left atrium via four pulmonary veins (two from each lung) and passes through the bicuspid valve into the left ventricle. Contraction of the ventricle moves blood through the semilunar valve into the aorta and then to all parts of the body through the systemic circulation.

Nursing Practice Application
Low birth weight and later coronary artery disease (CHD) risk

In a recent study Fall *et al.* (1995) found evidence that CHD is linked to growth early in life. An earlier study showed that most deaths from CHD occurred in the group of men with the lowest birth weight and weight at 1 year. These findings provide yet another good reason for planning strategies that reduce low birth weights, e.g. encouraging women to stop smoking during pregnancy. It is also important that babies receive the essential nutrients in the correct quantities and that their growth is monitored during the all important first year. Midwives and health visitors have an important role in preventing problems through education and in monitoring growth and development during pregnancy and the early years.

Cardiac conduction system

Heart muscle has the ability to contract without nervous stimulation. The coordinated contraction of the heart depends upon a conduction system formed from specialized non-contractile muscle cells and is facilitated by the specialized structure of the myocardium (see pages 205–206). This allows an impulse to spread from atria to ventricles in an orderly manner. The intrinsic conduction system consists

---

Special Focus **Coronary heart/artery disease (CHD/CAD)**

Cardiac muscle is totally dependent on adequate supplies of oxygen for its proper function (relies on aerobic respiration). When blood flow and oxygen levels are inadequate the myocardial fibres become ischaemic (lacking blood). This, if severe, will cause cell death (infarction).

Myocardial blood flow is reduced if the coronary arteries are narrowed by the atheromatous plaques of atherosclerosis (see Chapter 9 and page 221) or arterial spasm. The results of this narrowing may be angina pectoris, characterized by chest pain on exertion, myocardial infarction or sudden death if a major coronary vessel is occluded by a thrombosis.

Coronary heart disease (CHD) is the 'plague' of developed economies, where it most commonly affects people in the least affluent social groups. The UK has the unenviable distinction of having one of the highest death rates due to CHD, with over 160 000 deaths in 1985 (Ball and Mann, 1988). In 1991 26% of deaths in England were due to CHD (DoH, 1993).

The risk factors linked to the development of atherosclerosis, which include smoking, hypertension and elevated blood lipid levels, are discussed on page 221 within the context of arterial disease. Associated health promotion issues are addressed in Healthier Living – Reducing the risk of CHD (page 211).

Angina pectoris

Angina pectoris is caused by a gradual build-up of atheroma within the coronary arteries. It gives rise to pain in the chest, neck and left arm (see Chapter 4, referred pain). The pain is experienced in stressful situations, such as exertion or emotion, when myocardial demand for extra oxygen is not met, but usually disappears after rest. A person with angina is usually treated with drugs:

- Nitrates, e.g. glyceryl trinitrate, which reduce preload and cardiac output (see pages 215–216), reduce myocardial oxygen demand and divert coronary blood flow to ischaemic areas via collateral vessels, can be used when pain occurs or is anticipated.
- Beta blockers, e.g atenolol (see Chapter 6), which reduce cardiac work and hence myocardial oxygen demands.
- Calcium-channel blockers, e.g. nifedipine, prevent the influx of calcium through ion channels which relaxes smooth muscle and dilates coronary and peripheral vessels.
- Aspirin, which prevents platelet aggregation by altering the balance between thromboxane A_2 and prostacyclin (see Chapter 9), is used in unstable angina to reduce the risk of myocardial infarction. Nurses should ensure that the person has sufficient information regarding his or her condition and drug regimen, and understands the importance of compliance, safe storage and common side-effects. Simple measures, such as avoiding sudden exertion, especially after a meal, and keeping warm, will help to reduce pain attacks.

Severe angina may be treated surgically by coronary artery bypass graft. Recently techniques involving inflated balloon angioplasty or laser to open up the narrowed vessel have been developed. These techniques do not stop the vessel 'furring up' again, but stent insertion may keep it open longer.

Individuals with angina need help and encouragement to change certain aspects of their lifestyles: they should stop/reduce smoking, take regular gentle exercise, reduce intake of saturated fat, increase fibre intake, maintain normal weight, reduce alcohol intake and take active measures to manage stress, e.g. relaxation (see Chapter 6).

Myocardial infarction (*Figure 10.7*)

Myocardial infarction is the 'heart attack' or 'coronary' of lay terminology. It usually occurs when a coronary artery is occluded by extensive atheroma, a thrombosis which forms on the damaged vessel wall or an embolus. Men are more commonly affected than women until after the menopause, when this gender difference disappears. Recent studies, however, indicate that the replacement of oestrogen (see Chapter 21) in healthy postmenopausal women may prevent or reduce CAD (King and Ross Kerr, 1996).

The area of myocardium normally supplied by the occluded vessel becomes ischaemic, cells die and form an infarction. The wedge-shaped infarcted region eventually becomes fibrous scar tissue because cardiac muscle fibres do not regenerate.

The prognosis following myocardial infarction depends on the size and location of the area affected. Many people recover completely as collateral vessels develop to carry blood to the muscle fibres, but some will have permanent loss of function which may lead to heart failure (see page 218). Where a large area of myocardium is affected the person may die at once or within a few hours because of alterations in heart rhythm.

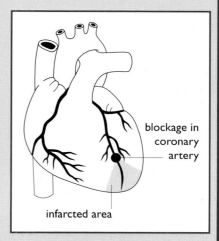

Figure 10.7 Myocardial infarction.

blockage in coronary artery

infarcted area

---

of a sinoatrial (SA) node, an atrioventricular (AV) node, an atrioventricular bundle (bundle of His), the bundle branches and Purkinje fibres (*Figure 10.9*).

The impulse is developed by the SA node situated in the right atrium, close to the opening of the superior vena cava. The cells of the SA node are autorhythmic, i.e. changes in membrane ion permeability, as sodium and calcium channels open and close, cause depolarization and production of an action potential without innervation (see Chapter 3). Cells of the SA node depolarize more frequently than those in other areas. This sets the heart rate (usually of 60–80 beats/min) and for this reason is known as the 'pacemaker'; however, without external neural or hormonal influences the SA node depolarizes about 100 times/min. The impulse from the SA node spreads through both atria, causing depolarization and contraction.

Person-Centred Study **Derek**

Derek is 51 and has a pig farm, which he manages with his wife and son. He has had angina pectoris for about 3 years – usually controlled by nitrates and beta blockers. Today, while doing the accounts, he experienced severe pain in his chest and left arm. When Derek gained no relief from the usual regimen of sublingual glyceryl trinitrate spray and a rest on the bed his wife called their GP, who provisionally diagnosed (by portable ECG) a myocardial infarction, gave Derek oral aspirin and intramuscular morphine for the pain, and arranged for his admission to hospital. When he arrived in the Accident and Emergency department the staff noted the following clinical features:

- Crushing chest pain resulting from the ischaemic changes in the myocardium.
- Pallor caused by poor skin perfusion.
- Sweating caused by sympathetic activity in response to pain and anxiety (see Chapter 6).
- Nausea and vomiting, occurring as blood is diverted from the digestive tract to the vital structures.
- Tachycardia (rapid heart rate), caused in part by pain and anxiety, but also in an attempt to maintain an adequate circulation.
- Hypotension (low blood pressure), which occurs because the infarcted left ventricle is unable to maintain an adequate cardiac output (see page 215).
- Breathlessness, caused by lack of oxygen, which may be exacerbated by some degree of left ventricular failure causing a build-up of blood in the lungs and pulmonary oedema (see page 218).

An electrocardiogram (ECG) showed early changes that indicated an infarction – ST elevation, smaller R wave and later T wave inversion (see page 212) and

blood was taken to estimate cardiac enzyme levels. Damaged cardiac muscle (and other tissues) releases enzymes into the blood which can be measured and used with clinical features and ECG changes to confirm the diagnosis. The enzymes usually measured are: creatine kinase (CK) and its specific myocardial isoenzyme (CK-MB), aspartate aminotransferase (AST) and lactate dehydrogenase (LD). All these rise and peak at different intervals following an infarction or some other muscle damage. This can complicate interpretation, so measurements are usually taken over consecutive days. In addition, Derek's leucocytes and erythrocyte sedimentation rate will increase in response to the inflammation associated with the infarcted area.

Before transfer to the coronary care unit Derek is given further pain relief and an antiemetic for the vomiting. An intravenous infusion is sited and fibrinolytic/thrombolytic treatment is commenced with alteplase, a plasminogen activator, to increase fibrinolysis/thrombus degradation (see Chapter 9). The importance of early fibrinolytic treatment cannot be stressed too strongly – it saves lives.

The initial nursing responsibilities include:

- Pain relief.
- Information and explanation for Derek and his family to reduce anxiety. A study by Thompson (1989) suggests that counselling after the first infarction reduces anxiety and depression in the individual and anxiety in the individual's partner.
- Planning care that minimizes cardiac work and ensures rest.
- Monitoring blood pressure, pulse, colour, respirations, temperature, urinary output and heart rhythm to detect potentially life-threatening arrhythmias (see *Figure 10.12*).

- Administration of prescribed drugs and oxygen.

Later the nurse, with Derek and other members of the care team, will have a vital role in planning a rehabilitation programme and preparing Derek and his family for discharge. Increased activity, driving, travel, return to work and resumption of sexual activity all depend upon the individual concerned and the severity of the infarct. The programme will also include provision of relevant health education information (see healthier living) and support for the family in making lifestyle changes (Deans and Hoskins, 1987). Longer term medical management and treatment may include:

- Lifestyle adaptations (see reducing the risk).
- Continued treatment with beta blockers.
- Possibly drugs to lower serum cholesterol where hyperlipidaemia (high levels of blood lipids) exists.
- Antiplatelet drugs, such as aspirin, which reduce the risk of further myocardial infarctions.
- Coronary artery bypass graft using a leg vein (or the internal mammary artery).
- Omega-3 fatty acids (certain fish oils), which may have a beneficial effect in individuals who have suffered a myocardial infarction (Siess et al. 1980; Hay et al. 1982). The results of a trial by Burr et al. (1989) also suggested that a modest intake of fatty fish (2–3 portions/week) reduces the mortality in men who have had a myocardial infarction. Further work, by Daviglus et al. (1997) showed that men who had consumed 35 g (or more) of fish each day were nearly 50% less likely to die from a heart attack than those who had not eaten fish daily.

The next area to receive the impulse is the AV node at the bottom of the right atrium. Conduction through the AV node is delayed by 0.1 s, allowing time for the completion of atrial systole. The impulse passes from the AV node down the AV bundle and right and left bundles to the apex of each ventricle. It travels rapidly through the Purkinje fibres to the ventricular muscle cells, which contract simultaneously to produce a coordinated ventricular systole.

We have looked at the intrinsic control of cardiac contraction; however, the autonomic nerves and hormones also influence heart rate (see Chapters 6 and 8). The parasympathetic vagus nerve acts as a 'brake' on heart rate and the sympathetic nerves, adrenaline and thyroxine all accelerate heart rate. The regulation of heart rate is further considered on pages 217–218.

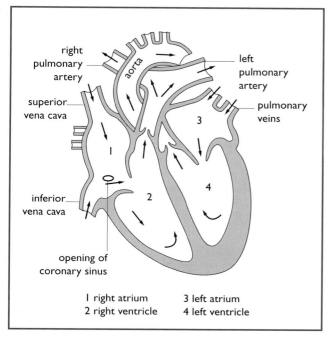

Figure 10.8 Blood flow direction.

1 right atrium   3 left atrium
2 right ventricle 4 left ventricle

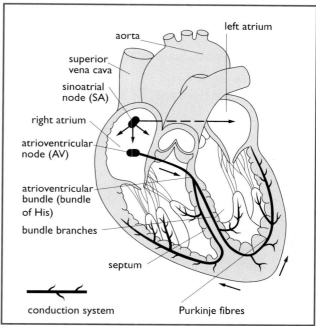

Figure 10.9 Conduction through the heart.

Healthier Living **Reducing the risk of CHD/CAD**

The aetiology of arterial disease, including that affecting the coronary arteries, is multifactorial. Some risk factors such as smoking have been proved, but for others the link is more tenuous (see page 221). A study of people following myocardial infarction revealed that the main causes of heart attack were thought, by the subjects, to be overwork and worry rather than physical causes (Murray, 1989). Sensible measures and changes in lifestyle which reduce the risks are:

- Stop or reduce smoking.
- Regular exercise.
- Avoid obesity.
- Reduce the intake of saturated fats; these tend to increase blood cholesterol levels and alter the ratio between high- and low-density lipids (see page 221).
- Increase unrefined carbohydrate intake (fibre), especially the gel-forming type.
- Ensure adequate intake of antioxidant vitamins and minerals (see Chapter 1).

- Reduce alcohol to recommended levels (see Chapter 14). Recent studies indicate that a moderate intake of alcohol may have a protective role against CHD.
- Most authorities recommend that salt intake be restricted – particularly in older people with hypertension.
- Regular blood pressure checks – early detection of hypertension and initiation of treatment.
- Development of stress management strategies.

Abnormal Function **Problems with conduction**

Problems with the conducting system lead to cardiac arrhythmias (without proper rhythm – irregular or abnormal heart rhythm; see *Figure 10.12*), which include:

*   Ectopic beats – where a heartbeat is initiated in the wrong place. Note that any part of the conducting system can produce a heartbeat if exposed to an irritable focus such as ischaemia.
*   Fibrillation (see page 214).

*   Various degrees of heart block where the rate is slow, e.g. 40/min in complete heart block. Some types of heart block are treated with drugs such as atropine (see Chapters 3 and 6), but others need the insertion of an electronic pacemaker. This may be temporary, with wires attached to an external pulse generator being introduced into the right ventricle through the veins. It is also possible

to 'pace' the heart indirectly with wires placed in the oesophagus or directly through the chest wall into the myocardium. These methods are unsuitable for long-term use because of the external pulse generator. When a permanent pacemaker is required the pacemaking device is sited under the skin of the chest wall.

Electrocardiography

It is possible to record the electrical events that occur in the myocardium during conduction and contraction using skin electrodes. The electrical impulses are picked up using an electrocardiograph, which produces the electrocardiogram (ECG), displayed graphically on an oscilloscope or as a paper tracing. The impulses, which spread to all parts of the body, can be 'picked up' by electrodes placed on the limbs and chest wall. This allows different 'views' of the heart as voltage differences between two points, or zero and a single point, can be measured. Being able to do this provides a much more comprehensive picture of how each part of the heart is performing – much like witnesses of a traffic accident give slightly different accounts depending on their position, which collectively build a complete picture. The 12-lead ECG which provides an all-inclusive 12 views of the heart consists of:

*   Six limb leads (frontal plane views), comprising three standard bipolar leads (I, II and III) which form a triangle [see *Figure 10.10(a)*] to measure voltage difference between the arms, and the left leg and the arms, and three unipolar leads (aVR, aVL and aVF) to measure voltage differences between zero and the limbs.
*   Six precordial or chest leads (horizontal plane views). These are unipolar leads (V_{1-6}) to measure voltage, against zero, at different points of the heart, e.g. V_1 records activity in the right ventricle [see *Figure 10.10(b)*].

The normal heart produces a typical waveform (different for each lead), or sinus rhythm, which consists of five deflection waves, known universally as P, Q, R, S and T (see *Figure 10.11*). The PQRST complex, which lasts about 0.8 s, represents a complete cardiac cycle.

The small P wave represents the atrial depolarization (see Chapter 3) caused by conduction of the impulse from the SA node across the atria. After a short pause

(0.1 s) the atria contract. The next three waves, which come close together, are the large QRS complex. This represents ventricular depolarization, which immediately precedes contraction. The T wave represents ventricular repolarization. Atrial repolarization is not usually represented in waveform as it is hidden by the much larger QRS complex. The PR interval (really PQ, but the Q wave is often very small) is the time taken for impulse conduction from the SA node, through the atria, to the AV node and on to the ventricles. The period from the start of ventricular depolarization through contraction to repolarization is termed the Q–T interval. The short ST segment represents a period of inactivity and ventricular depolarization after the QRS complex.

Normal changes in the sinus rate may occur with respiration – decreasing on expiration and increasing on inspiration. This is known as sinus arrhythmia.

Alterations in the waveform pattern or time intervals may indicate problems with the conduction system or myocardial function (see *Figure 10.12*). The 12-lead ECG is a very useful diagnostic aid following myocardial infarction, heart failure, drug toxicity and many other situations.

Cardiac cycle

The cardiac cycle (see *Figure 10.13*) describes the events occurring during one heart beat. It lasts around 0.8 s when the heart rate is 75/min. It is divided into diastole and systole, and usually refers to ventricular activity. Although we will describe events in stages, you should remember that it is a continuous process.

Late diastole

The heart is completely relaxed and pressures are low. Blood enters from the circulation, and flows through the atria and into the ventricles. At this stage the AV valves are open and the semilunar valves are closed. Near the end of diastole the SA node 'fires', atrial systole occurs and the ventricles receive the remaining 30% of blood.

Systole

The atria are relaxed and the pressure rises in the ventricles until the AV valves close. For a brief time the ventricles are closed chambers, a period called isovolumetric contraction. Soon the ventricular pressure is greater than that in the aorta and pulmonary artery, and the semilunar valves open to allow blood to leave the ventricles – the ventricular ejection phase. This is the period of maximum pressure in the left ventricle and aorta (see systolic **blood pressure**, pages 225–228).

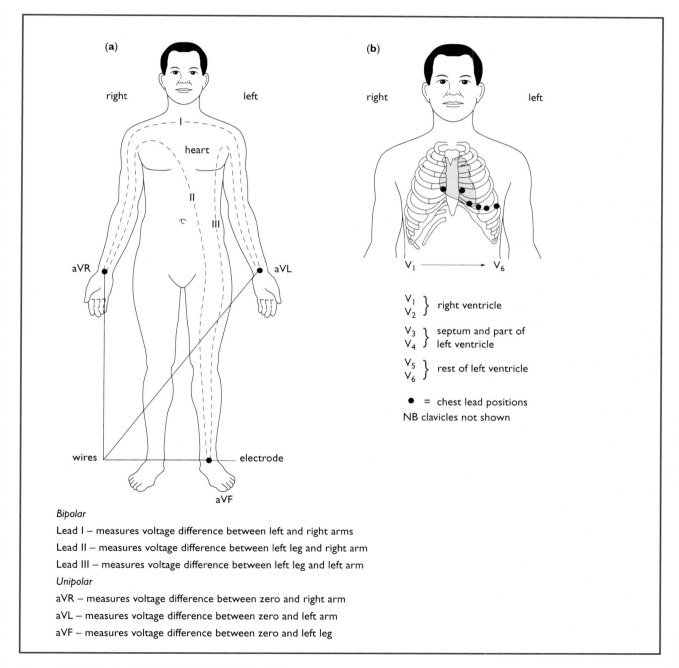

Bipolar

Lead I – measures voltage difference between left and right arms

Lead II – measures voltage difference between left leg and right arm

Lead III – measures voltage difference between left leg and left arm

Unipolar

aVR – measures voltage difference between zero and right arm

aVL – measures voltage difference between zero and left arm

aVF – measures voltage difference between zero and left leg

Figure 10.10 Twelve-lead ECG. (**a**) Limb leads; (**b**) chest leads.

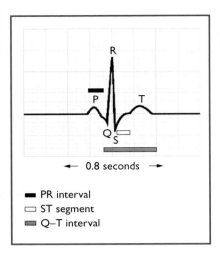

Figure 10.11 Normal electrocardiogram tracing (PQRST complex).

Early diastole

The ventricles relax, ventricular pressure falls and back-pressure in the great vessels causes the semilunar valves to close. The ventricles are again closed chambers – the isovolumetric relaxation phase. Meanwhile, the atria have been filling with blood (atrial diastole). The rising pressure eventually forces open the AV valves and blood flows into the ventricles, which is where we started. The cycle is complete.

Earlier we mentioned that the cardiac cycle lasts for 0.8 s when the heart rate is around 75/min. Diastole lasts 0.5 s and ventricular systole 0.3 s. When the heart rate increases, diastole becomes shorter, which may become a problem when the rate is very fast and the ventricles have no time to

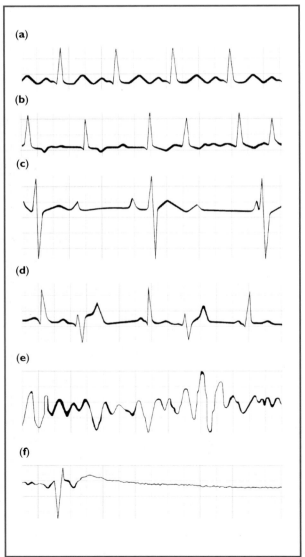

Figure 10.12 Normal and abnormal heart rhythms
(a) Sinus rhythm.
(b) Atrial fibrillation: atrial rate is rapid and irregular, with no proper P wave. Ventricular rate is irregular and produces an irregular pulse.
(c) Complete heart block (third-degree AV block): no impulses from the AV node reach the ventricles. Atrial contraction is regular, but the slower ventricular contraction is initiated by fibres in the AV bundle or ventricle.
(d) Ventricular ectopic beats: these are wide QRS complexes without a P wave. They can occur in healthy people, being associated with an excess of tea, coffee or alcohol. They may also be a feature of disease such as myocardial infarction.
(e) Ventricular fibrillation: a completely disordered pattern of irregular QRS complexes which produce no cardiac output. This is the usual reason for cardiac arrest and is the commonest cause of sudden death. It requires the commencement of immediate resuscitation.
(f) Asystole: in this case no QRS complexes are seen. Again, this is a cardiac arrest situation which requires immediate resuscitation.

fill with blood between systoles. All the events of the cardiac cycle – pressures, valves open/shut, heart sounds and ECG – are shown in *Figure 10.13*.

Cardiac output

The blood volume pumped by each ventricle in 1 minute is termed the cardiac output (CO). It depends upon heart rate (HR) and stroke volume (SV, the amount of blood pumped out with each ventricular contraction).

The cardiac output is altered by changes in rate and stroke volume. During exercise an average person can raise his or her output to, for example, 25 l/min by increasing the stroke volume to 200 ml and the heart rate to 125 beats/min. The heart's facility to do this is called the cardiac reserve. In very fit people cardiac output may increase to as much as 35 l/min. Cardiac output is an important factor in the regulation of arterial blood pressure and is discussed when we look at blood pressure (page 225), but now we should consider the regulation of stroke volume and heart rate.

Stroke volume

Stroke volume is the difference between ventricular end diastolic volume (EDV) and end systolic volume (ESV):

$$CO = HR \times SV$$
e.g. at rest:
$70/min \times 70\ ml = 4900\ ml \therefore CO = 4900\ ml/min$

$$SV = EDV - ESV$$
e.g.
$130\ ml - 60\ ml = 70\ ml \therefore SV = 70\ ml$

Nursing Practice Application **Cardiac arrest and resuscitation in the hospital situation**

Cardiac arrest is the cessation of an effective heart beat and cardiac output caused by ventricular fibrillation, asystole or electromechanical dissociation (EMD – where QRS complexes are present without cardiac output). Causes include myocardial ischaemia, electrocution and alterations in serum potassium. If an effective circulation is not restored within 2–3 min, the brain will be irreversibly damaged (see Chapter 3). Cardiac arrest is characterized by death-like appearance, unconsciousness, absent major pulse such as the carotid, gasping or absent respiration, dilated pupils and cyanosis or pallor.

Immediate resuscitation must be initiated by the person discovering the arrest. Nurses need to be competent in cardiopulmonary resuscitation (CPR) and be fully conversant with local emergency procedures as they will be required to start treatment before the arrival of the specialist cardiac arrest team ('crash team'). The importance of every nurse receiving the same training and using the same manoeuvres in CPR is stressed in an article by Eastwick-Field (1996).

Resuscitation

Airway: must be opened and cleared of any obstruction, e.g. vomit, displaced dentures.
Breathing: expired air mouth-to-mouth or mouth-to-nose ventilation. Where available a Brook's airway or airway with a bag and face mask is used. Later, when the team arrive, ventilation is maintained by endotracheal intubation.
Circulation: maintained by external cardiac massage, where the heart is compressed between the sternum and spine to produce an output of blood. Where the arrest was witnessed a precordial blow to the lower end of the sternum may be sufficient to restart the heart.

Advanced life support measures – when the team arrives

Drugs and defibrillation: an intravenous line is sited for the administration of drugs and the correction of the metabolic acidosis (see Chapters 2 and 12) with sodium hydrogen carbonate solution. The specific management depends on the cause of the arrest; for example, in ventricular fibrillation the heart is defibrillated by passing direct current electricity through the ventricles by paddles applied to the chest wall. Drugs used depend on the ECG (see below) and include adrenaline and atropine
Electrocardiogram: needed to determine the cause – ventricular fibrillation, asystole or EMD.

Readers requiring general information regarding resuscitation are directed to the References and Further Reading, e.g. Eastwick-Field (1996), Edwards et al. (1995) and European Resuscitation Council (1996).

NB It is vitally important that resuscitation techniques are modified for infants and small children – to avoid damage, less expired air is used for lung inflation and cardiac massage requires much less sternal depression than for an adult. Articles detailing paediatric resuscitation techniques are included in Further Reading, e.g. Simpson (1994a, b).

Earlier we discussed the relationship between myocardial fibre stretch and the force of contraction – Starling's law of the heart (see page 206) – much like needing a well-stretched elastic band to propel a paper pellet across a room. When venous return to the heart increases, such as with slow heart rate, the myocardial fibres stretch and the next contraction is more powerful, resulting in an increased output. The degree of stretch present in the myocardial fibres, which depends on the EDV, is known as the preload. However, if the venous return is reduced, e.g. in shock, there is a reduction in stretch or preload and consequently in stroke volume and output. Two other factors that influence stroke volume are muscle fibre contractility (its force of contraction) and afterload, which is the backpressure of blood in the aorta

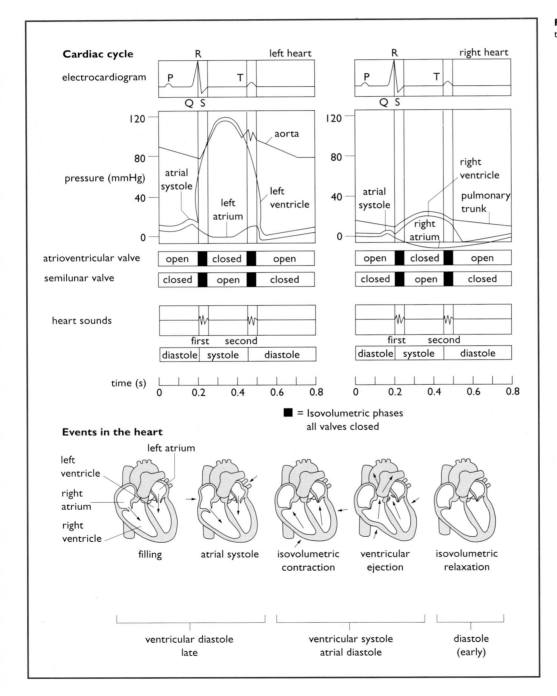

Figure 10.13 Events of the cardiac cycle.

and pulmonary artery creating a resistance which ventricular contraction must overcome to pump blood into the circulation. The higher the afterload the harder the heart muscle has to work – this is particularly so where the arterial blood pressure is abnormally high (hypertension – see page 228). In health the balance between right and left is ensured: if the output of one side of the heart increases, the other side will receive more blood causing its output to increase.

Stroke volume is also influenced by external factors such as sympathetic nerves and the adrenal hormones – adrenaline and noradrenaline (see Chapters 6 and 8) – and thyroxine. These all increase myocardial contractility, enhancing the force of ventricular contraction. Stroke volume increases as the ventricles empty more efficiently. Inotropic drugs, used to treat heart disease, affect myocardial contractility; digoxin, which increases contractility, is said to be positively inotropic whereas contractility is decreased by beta blockers such as atenolol, which is negatively inotropic (see page 219). Ion levels and pH of the blood also affect contractility; calcium ions increase contractility and increasing potassium levels and acidosis are both negatively inotropic.

Heart rate

The adult heart rate is normally 60–80 beats/min, but this can be altered by several factors in response to changing body needs (*Figure 10.14*). Clearly you need different effort from the heart while sleeping and during a game of squash. The heart rate, which is much faster at birth (120–140/min), slows during childhood to reach the adult level and then slows in older adults. Women tend to have faster heart rates than men. A resting rate greater than 100/min is termed tachycardia and a rate less than 60/min is known as bradycardia.

The cardiovascular centre (CVC), situated in the medulla, consists of the cardiac centre which controls rate and force of contraction and the vasomotor centre which controls blood vessel size and blood pressure, but there is some overlap of function. The CVC controls heart rate via the ANS; the parasympathetic vagus nerves act as a brake on the SA node to slow heart rate whereas stimulation of sympathetic nerves (beta receptors), with release of adrenaline and noradrenaline, increases heart rate. A cardiac mechanism called the Bainbridge reflex, which involves stretch receptors in the right atrium, can increase heart rate by 15%

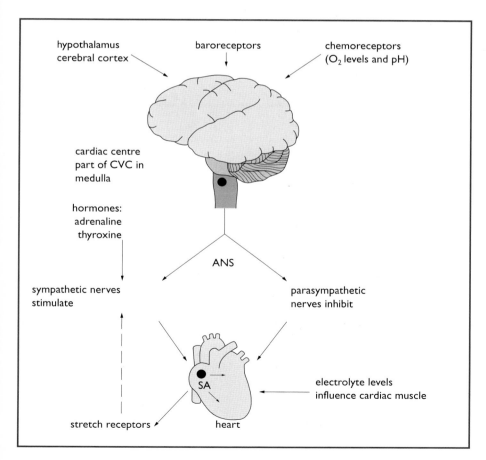

Figure 10.14 Regulation of heart rate (SA, sinoatrial node; ANS, autonomic nervous system; CVC, cardiovascular centre).

Abnormal Function **Problems with cardiac output**

The breakdown of homeostatic controls on cardiac output has profound effects on cells and their functioning. The results of poor tissue oxygenation eventually affect the efficiency of every body system:

• **Acute circulatory failure:** cardiac output is insufficient to maintain blood pressure and tissue perfusion. It is seen in various types of shock (see page 229).

• **Heart failure:** a chronic inability of either the left or right side of the heart to pump effectively and produce a cardiac output sufficient for the person's needs. One side may fail initially, but both sides may eventually be affected to produce congestive cardiac failure. If the output of the heart is reduced while blood is still returning, obviously there will be congestion and a backlog of blood in the vessels trying to empty blood into the heart.

A useful analogy is what happens when a motorway accident causes traffic congestion which eventually spreads to smaller roads leading to the motorway, and to the towns and villages nearby.

At first the heart tries to compensate, by hypertrophy and enlargement (see Chapter 1), in an attempt to increase output. If cardiac function continues to deteriorate, a point is reached when the

failure is decompensated. This is a serious state where overstretching and dilation cause further output reduction, multi-organ failure and death.

Left heart failure leads to high pressure in the pulmonary veins, pulmonary congestion and pulmonary oedema, in which fluid from the pulmonary capillaries leaks out into the alveoli. As you can imagine, these are not the ideal conditions for gaseous exchange and result in orthopnoea (breathlessness relieved by an upright position) and cyanosis (blue coloration). Another feature is paroxysmal nocturnal dyspnoea, whereby the person suffers sudden breathless attacks in the night. The causes of left-sided failure include hypertension, infarction affecting the left ventricle, cardiomyopathy (disease of myocardium), and mitral or aortic valve malfunction.

If the right side fails there is widespread venous congestion, which will eventually affect most tissues. Its effects include oedema (see page 230 and Chapter 11) in dependent areas such as the ankles or sacral area, anorexia, nausea, constipation and reduced urinary volume. Right-side failure may be caused by problems in the heart such as pulmonary or tricuspid valve

malfunction, but more commonly it follows left-sided failure. Here the right ventricle is exhausted trying to pump blood into the congested lungs. Chronic lung diseases may also increase the work required by the right ventricle to the point where it no longer achieves an adequate output; this type of heart failure is called cor pulmonale.

The management of heart failure includes drugs to improve contractility and cardiac output, e.g. digoxin; diuretics to reduce congestion; and angiotensin-converting enzyme (ACE) inhibitors (prevents the conversion of angiotensin I to angiotensin II; see Chapters 8 and 15), such as catopril, to decrease afterload. For some individuals with severe heart failure, heart transplantation may be an option. Other treatments for heart failure include short-term circulatory support with intra-aortic balloon counterpulsation to help push blood along the aorta, and trials continue on various mechanical left ventricular assist devices which can be used while a donor heart is sought. Possible long-term developments are the production of tiny assist devices which can be used instead of transplants, and surgical reduction of left ventricular hypertrophy.

---

through sympathetic stimulation. At rest both parts of the ANS influence the heart, but inhibition by parasympathetic nerves is the more important – they reduce the inherent firing rate of the SA node by around 25% to produce a heart rate of about 75 beats/min.

The many factors influencing the CVC include peripheral chemoreceptors (monitoring oxygen levels), baroreceptors (monitoring blood pressure), and data from the cerebral cortex and hypothalamus. This well-coordinated control mechanism allows us to respond to changes in oxygen demand by increasing heart rate and cardiac output.

When needed, heart rate can be altered as we respond to posture, exercise and stressors, such as cold, pain, anxiety, fever and anger or fear (adrenal hormones – the 'fight or flight' response). Abnormal blood electrolyte levels can have serious effects on cardiac contraction, especially calcium and potassium levels, which may lead to life-threatening arrhythmias.

It is important to remember that cardiac output, stroke

volume and heart rate are interrelated components which should be viewed as a whole unit. The associated topics of blood pressure and peripheral resistance are covered later in this chapter.

Blood Vessels

Having discussed the heart in detail, we now need to look at the 'plumbing' (the blood vessels) and the many mechanisms that control their size, blood flow and pressure (circulation – see pages 224–225).

Blood vessels form a closed network. Within this network blood circulates around the body. There are three basic types of vessel: arteries, which carry blood away from the heart; veins, which carry blood back to the heart; and capillaries, where substance exchange between blood and cells occurs – which is the purpose of the circulation. Capillaries form the link between the arterioles (small arteries) and venules (small veins).

Nursing Practice Application **Cardiac glycosides – digoxin**

Many people with cardiac conditions, e.g. heart failure with atrial fibrillation and other atrial arrhythmias, are treated with digoxin (derived from the foxglove). Digoxin slows heart rate by increasing vagal activity and by partially blocking AV conduction, it inhibits the Na^+/K^+ pump, causing Ca^{2+} to accumulate in the myocardial fibres, which increases contractility and improves cardiac output. Digoxin is a very useful therapeutic agent,

but has serious side-effects which must be anticipated.

An important nursing role, apart from teaching people about their drugs and the need for compliance, is careful observation for side effects. Digoxin may cause bradycardia and apex beat/radial pulse should be determined before administration (see Nursing Practice Application – Pulse and apex beat). Should the apical rate fall below 60/min

the dose is withheld and medical advice is sought. Digoxin may cause other serious arrhythmias such as ventricular tachycardia, which can progress to life-threatening ventricular fibrillation. Other toxic effects include confusion and disorientation, which are easy to attribute to another cause in older adults, and gastrointestinal problems such as anorexia, nausea and abdominal pain.

Early development of blood vessels

Primitive blood vessel (along with blood cells) development starts in mesenchymal cells from the mesoderm layer of the yolk sac and chorion (see Chapters 20 and 21) during the third week of embryonic development. Initially, the vessels consist of just an endothelial tube, but later the mesenchymal cells form the muscle and connective-tissue layers of arteries and veins. As these vessels grow they will eventually fuse to form a comprehensive network with each other and the heart to supply blood to most parts of the body – remember, some areas such as the lens of the eye are avascular. The special vascular structures, used only during fetal life, are also formed, e.g. umbilical vessels and ductus venosus (see Chapter 21).

Blood vessel structure

Capillaries have the least complicated structure. They comprise one layer of endothelial cells, which is ideally suited to their role in molecular exchange (see *Figure 10.15*).

Arteries and veins are more complex, but both have the same basic three-layer structure. The outside layer, or tunica adventitia, made of fibrous tissue and collagen fibres, covers and protects the vessel. A network of tiny blood vessels, the vasa vasorum, supplies blood to the outer layer of larger veins and arteries. The variable middle layer, or tunica media, consists of elastic fibres and involuntary muscle innervated by sympathetic nerve fibres. This layer, thickest in the arteries, is responsible for alterations in vessel lumen size. When the muscle is relaxed the vessel opens (vasodilation) and when it contracts the vessel narrows (vasoconstriction). The inner layer, the tunica intima, comprises a very smooth endothelium and a basement membrane, which reduces friction. The endothelium is continuous with that lining the heart.

The variations in structure between vessels of different size or type reflect their specific functions; for example, large arteries such as the aorta are well supplied with elastic tissue, which allows for expansion as the left ventricle contracts.

Arteries

The arteries, which carry blood away from the heart, include the large elastic arteries (conducting), medium-sized muscular arteries (distributing) and tiny arterioles which feed into the capillary network.

Many structures receive blood from more than one artery; these may anastomose (communicate) to form a network of vessels, e.g. the circle of Willis that supplies the brain. This has an obvious advantage as, when one vessel is occluded, the rest of the structure still receives blood through a collateral circulation.

Some arteries are end arteries, e.g the central artery of the retina. If these are occluded there are no alternative vessels and the structure normally supplied with blood is irreversibly damaged.

Large elastic arteries, such as the aorta and its main branches, have elastic fibres within the tunica media. The aorta has a diameter of 2.5 cm, which importantly offers a low resistance to flow. It distends readily as the elastic fibres stretch when blood is ejected during ventricular systole. It maintains blood flow during diastole by the recoil of the elastic fibres. These properties help to produce a steady arterial flow, rather than sudden gushes of blood (which would not help you maintain homeostasis – try watering the garden with someone turning the water on and off).

During normal ageing these vessels lose their elasticity, resulting in increased resistance and blood pressure. Large

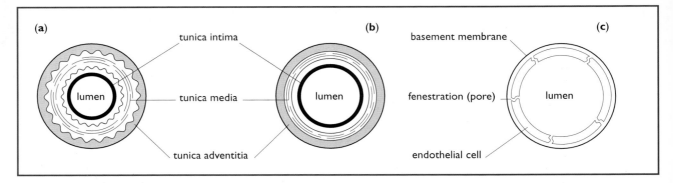

Figure 10.15 Blood vessel structure. (**a**) Artery; (**b**) vein; (**c**) capillary.

arteries have considerable smooth muscle, but are not subject to much nervous vasoconstriction.

The medium arteries have more muscle and less elastic tissue in their tunica media. These arteries, which generally supply specific organs, are subject to more vasoconstriction.

The smallest arteries, the arterioles, have a thick layer of smooth muscle – their structure is well related to function. Resistance to flow in these vessels is high and the arterioles are important in determining overall peripheral resistance (see page 225). Vasoconstriction and vasodilation change vessel diameter in response to nervous and local chemical stimuli. This ability to constrict or dilate, and the presence of smooth muscle precapillary sphincters between the terminal arterioles and capillaries, control blood flow through the capillary network.

Arterial pulse
The pulse is the wave of expansion felt in the arteries as the left ventricle contracts. It is most conveniently felt where an artery passes over a bone, e.g. the radial artery felt at the wrist (*Figure 10.16*).

Capillaries
The exchange of substances occurring in the capillaries is the whole point of having the circulation – it is about getting substances to the cells and removing waste through the capillaries.

Capillaries are minute vessels forming the dense network found in most tissues, but some connective tissues, such as tendons, have very few capillaries, and the cornea and lens of the eye have none at all. Capillaries, which on average measure 750 μm in length and 8 μm in diameter, provide a delivery and waste collection service for individual cells. They consist of a single layer of endothelial cells, the tunica intima, and a basement membrane, which allows oxygen

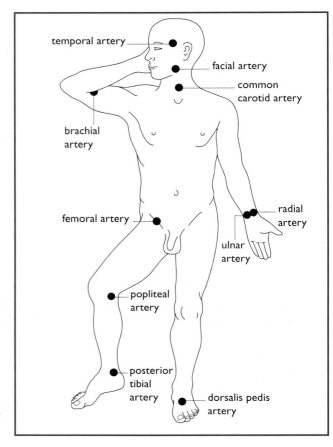

Figure 10.16 Arterial pulses and pressure points for the arrest of haemorrhage.

and small-molecular-weight nutrients to pass from blood to cell and waste such as carbon dioxide to move in the opposite direction. Molecular movement across the capillary membrane occurs by direct diffusion or through fenestrations, via clefts or by endocytosis and exocytosis.

Special Focus Arterial diseases

Atherosclerosis

Atherosclerosis (see thromboembolic conditions Chapter 9, Special Focus, page 209, and Person-Centred Study, page 210) is a degenerative process which results in structural changes in arteries. Most adults aged over 40 years have some degree of arterial change and, as already mentioned, atherosclerotic disease is a major cause of death in developed countries.

Stages in development are:
- The appearance of fatty streaks on the tunica intima.
- Formation of a fatty plaque of atheroma containing cholesterol and low-density lipoproteins (LDL) with thickening of the tunica intima.
- The atheromatous plaque enlarges with fibrosis and calcification, the media is disrupted and ulceration of the endothelium may occur.

This severe later stage results in vessel narrowing and ischaemia. The roughened lining gives rise to turbulent flow, abnormal haemostasis and thrombus/embolus formation. Damage to the vessel wall may eventually lead to the development of an aneurysm or dilatation of the wall (see *Figure 10.17*).

There is considerable information available regarding factors that may predispose to arterial change, but some of the evidence fails to prove direct causal relationships. Unfortunately, media coverage of isolated and unsubstantiated work leads to confusion and conflict about how we should promote healthy cardiovascular function.

It is generally accepted that atherosclerosis does not have a single cause but results from the damaging effects of several factors operating together (multifactorial aetiology). Atherosclerosis causes CHD (see page 209), strokes (see Chapter 4) and peripheral vascular disease necessitating limb amputation.

Factors linked to the development of atherosclerosis:
- Increasing age.
- Gender – it is more common in males than females until after the menopause (see page 209 and Chapter 21).
- Family history of arterial disease (both genetic and environmental factors).
- Inherited hypercholesterolaemia, e.g. familial hyperlipidaemias.
- Ethnic origin – in the UK people of Asian origin have an increased incidence of atherosclerosis compared with Caucasians (possible link with their predisposition to diabetes mellitus).
- Hypertension damaging the arterial lining.
- High blood levels of LDLs and cholesterol are linked to the development of atherosclerosis. For reduced risk it is important to have a high ratio of high-density lipoproteins (HDL) to LDL. The HDLs, such as omega-3 fatty acids (see page 210), are thought to have a protective role in reducing thrombus formation. Intake of polyunsaturated fats tends to lower blood cholesterol/LDL levels, whereas a high intake of saturated fats tends to increase cholesterol/LDLs. Information about the structure, absorption and metabolism of lipids can be found in Chapters 1 and 13. However, the relationship between dietary intake of fats (saturated and polyunsaturated), blood lipid levels and risk is extremely complex. Before you become agitated about your cholesterol intake remember that you need it as a precursor for the steroid hormones and that the body is able to make it as well as ingest it.
- Smoking – some chemicals in tobacco (carbon monoxide and nicotine) can damage endothelium, increase platelet adhesion and cause vasoconstriction.
- Sedentary lifestyle, lack of exercise, excess alcohol and obesity all lead to an unfavourable HDL:LDL ratio and hypertension.
- A stressful lifestyle or job may be linked with atherosclerosis.
- Personality type may have some influence – type A personalities, characterized by aggressive, restless behaviour,
- Diabetes mellitus.
- Inadequate intake of antioxidants – vitamins A, C and E, and selenium, which cells use to counter the damaging effects of free radicals (see Chapter 1).

Aneurysm

Aneurysm is a permanent dilatation of an artery with disruption of the inner and middle coats. Those occurring in the aorta are often caused by atherosclerosis and are associated with hypertension. Where the defect has been diagnosed, elective surgical treatment can be very effective. Sometimes, however, the aneurysm 'dissects' and bleeding occurs between the vessel layers; this may require surgery. If an aortic aneurysm ruptures, the result, as you can imagine, will be disastrous unless immediate advanced life support and specialist surgery is available

The 'berry' aneurysms which affect vessels of the circle of Willis result from a congenital vessel defect. Rupture, which leads to subarachnoid or intracerebral haemorrhage (see Chapter 4), is also associated with hypertension.

Most capillaries are of the continuous type, with tight junctions between adjacent cells; limited small molecule exchange occurs through minute clefts. The tight junctions in the brain capillaries really are 'tight', which renders them virtually impermeable (see Blood–brain barrier, Chapter 4). Some capillaries (fenestrated) have pores or fenestrations in their wall which increase permeability. This structural feature is useful in the gut, for nutrient absorption, and in the kidneys, where waste is removed from the blood. Another type of capillary (sinusoid) is a large-diameter channel. Lined or associated with phagocytic macrophages, they connect arterioles and venules in organs such as the liver (macrophages called Kupffer cells), spleen and some endocrine structures. Blood flow through sinusoids is slower, allowing time for phagocytosis of microorganisms and metabolism of nutrients. Sinusoids are often fenestrated and, having fewer tight junctions, are

Nursing Practice Application **Pulse and apex beat**

Counting the pulse is used to determine the heart rate, with which the pulse should correspond. Heart rate changes through the lifespan – 120–140 beats/min in newborns, gradually decreasing during childhood to reach the adult resting rate of 60–80 beats/min. Rate obviously depends on activity and health status. An abnormally rapid pulse (tachycardia) may be caused by anxiety, pain (see Chapter 4), hyperthyroidism (see Chapter 8), infections, heart disease or severe haemorrhage. Abnormal slowing of the rate (bradycardia) may be caused by heart block, drug side effects, hypothyroidism (see Chapter 8) or raised intracranial pressure (see Chapter 4).

Characteristics other than rate should be noted when monitoring pulse rate.

These include the rhythm (normally regular), the volume (which may be bounding or thready) and the elasticity of the artery.

Although accessibility of the radial pulse makes it the first choice for routine use in adults, it may be necessary to use other arteries or record the apex beat. Other arteries used include the temporal (small babies), carotid, facial, brachial (children), ulnar, femoral, popliteal, posterior tibial and dorsalis pedis (see *Figure 10.16*). These alternative sites might be required, for instance, if both wrists were injured or to check vessel patency after surgery to clear an occlusion, e.g. dorsalis pedis used after femoral artery surgery. Knowledge of these arteries is also important as they form the pressure points used to arrest

haemorrhage; for example, the posterior tibial or dorsalis pedis are compressed to stop bleeding from the foot.

Generally heart rate is determined by counting the radial pulse, but in some situations, e.g. atrial fibrillation, the radial pulse may be inaccurate, as some beats are too weak to reach the wrist. It is then necessary to listen to the apex beat. This is best heard in the mid-clavicular line at the level of the fifth intercostal space. Apex beat is also used during treatment with certain drugs, e.g. digoxin. Two nurses perform simultaneous recordings of apex and radial pulse prior to drug administration. The simultaneous recordings remove any difficulties in interpretation caused by changes in heart rate between separate recordings.

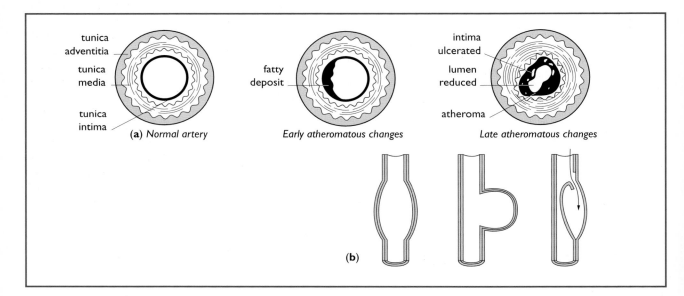

Figure 10.17 Arterial disease. (**a**) Atherosclerosis; (**b**) aneurysm.

'leaky' to larger molecules such as hormones and other proteins, and sometimes to blood cells.

As already mentioned, blood flow into the capillaries is controlled by the radius of the arterioles and by precapillary sphincters in the arterioles feeding into the capillary network or bed (*Figure 10.18*). Not all the capillaries are open and functional at the same time. When they are shut blood passes through arteriovenous shunts or anastomoses and takes no part in molecular exchange. These shunts provide a direct link between

the arterioles and venules, thereby bypassing the capillary network. These mechanisms are important in diverting blood from one area to another as physiological needs change. For example, after a meal the capillaries of the gastrointestinal tract are full of blood, but between meals they close; capillaries in skeletal muscle open during exercise; and those in the skin open when heat loss is required.

The capillaries/sinusoids eventually join up with the tiny venules which form the first part of the venous system.

Abnormal Function **Problems with varicose veins**
....

These dilated and meandering veins occur when the valves are damaged by the high pressure which builds-up if venous return from the legs is impeded [*Figure 10.19(b)*]. Standing for long periods at work, pregnancy, abdominal tumours and obesity can all cause this high pressure. Usually it is the superficial leg veins which are affected. Varicose veins are unsightly, and cause swelling and discomfort. They bleed if traumatized and in severe cases lead to ulcers which are notoriously resistant to treatment.

Veins

Blood leaves the capillary network through venules, which unite to form veins. These eventually merge to become the venae cavae. Veins have the same basic three coats as arteries, but with less elastic tissue, a thinner muscle layer and a thicker tunica adventitia. They are easily distended and, because they have a large diameter, offer very little resistance to blood flow. Veins are capacitance (able to hold a lot of blood) vessels and generally contain 60–65% of the blood volume. This capacity is variable because vessel size can be changed by the venomotor tone, which is produced as the muscle layer contracts or relaxes in response to sympathetic activity. When veins are partially empty they flatten and become elliptical in shape.

Blood flow in the veins depends on small pressure gradients, but these require help, in addition to the venomotor tone, to provide a venous return sufficient for the heart to produce an adequate cardiac output. In the veins of the limbs the endothelial lining is modified to form valves which allow flow in one direction only (*Figure 10.19(a)*). Valves allow us to overcome the effects of gravity while standing upright, by helping to prevent pooling of blood in the leg veins. Contraction of skeletal muscles in the leg squeezes blood from valve to valve. When standing for any length of time it is prudent to operate this 'skeletal muscle pump' by wiggling your toes to aid venous return and prevent pooling of blood in the leg veins and fainting. Numerous anastomoses between veins provide alternative routes for blood; skeletal muscle contracts to push blood from the superficial veins through these communicating channels into the deep veins of the legs and on to the heart. Pressure changes in the thorax and abdomen during breathing, known as the 'respiratory pump', also aid venous return. On inspiration, rising abdominal pressure

Figure 10.18 Capillary network and arteriovenous shunt.

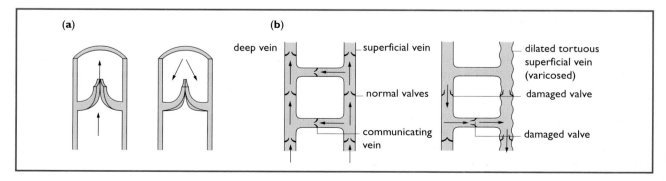

Figure 10.19 (a) Valves in veins; (b) varicosities.

squeezes the veins, and the concomitant fall in thoracic and right atrial pressure 'sucks' blood back to the heart.

Specialized venous structures called venous sinuses are present in the heart and brain. In the heart they drain venous blood from the myocardium. Those in the brain drain venous blood and are involved in the absorption of cerebrospinal fluid (see Chapter 4). They are thin-walled channels supported by external connective tissue.

Circulatory Physiology

The circulation of blood is a continuous and dynamic process influenced by many factors that enable the CVS to respond appropriately to changing needs. Circulation of blood around the closed CVS depends upon flow, pressure and resistance.

Before considering the individual factors, we should

first emphasize the relationship between blood flow, pressure and resistance:

Flow is directly proportional to differences in pres-

$$\text{Flow} = \frac{\text{Difference in blood pressure along a vessel}}{\text{Peripheral resistance}}$$

sure – when pressure increases so does flow and *vice versa*. Peripheral resistance, however, is the factor with most influence. Flow is inversely proportional to peripheral resistance – when peripheral resistance decreases, as vessels dilate, then flow increases, even if pressure falls.

Blood flow

The blood flow is the amount of blood moving within the

circulation (which equals cardiac output) or through an individual structure. The flow rate of any fluid (not just blood) depends on resistance to flow and pressure differences along the tube/pipe (vessel) – see above.

Flow in blood vessels is usually smooth or laminar, but fast flow, large vessels and heart valves, reduced blood viscosity or damage to the endothelium, e.g. atheromatous plaques, can all produce turbulence.

Obviously flow rates alter as body activities and needs change; for example, at rest the skeletal muscles receive about 20% of the resting cardiac output, but during strenuous exercise most of the increased cardiac output is diverted to the muscles. Many structures regulate their own blood flow by controlling arterioles, sphincters and flow through capillary networks, e.g. heart, kidney, skeletal muscle. This autoregulation is based on local chemical conditions, such as pH and potassium, carbon dioxide and oxygen levels, and the release of substances from cells, e.g. lactic acid. This causes vasodilation and increased flow, which is known as active hyperaemia. In this way, metabolically active tissues can receive more blood and therefore more oxygen and nutrients, and waste can be removed.

Pressure

All fluids exert pressure on the walls of their container (hydrostatic pressure). The force exerted by blood on the vessel walls is called blood pressure. Blood only flows around the circulation if pressure gradients exist within the CVS. The heart initiates the pressure which powers the circulation, but pressure needs to fall between the left ventricle and the tissues and again between the tissues and the right atrium (*Figure 10.20*).

Pressure also falls between the right ventricle, the pulmonary vessels and the left atrium. The pressure within different vessels varies, but when we talk about blood pressure we generally mean the pressure within large arteries close to the heart (see page 225).

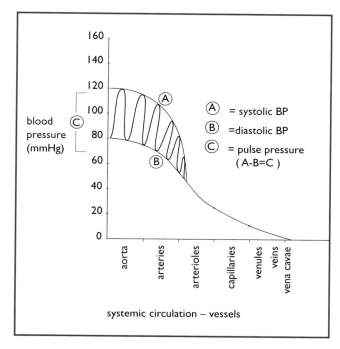

Figure 10.20 Blood pressure in the major types of vessels in the systemic circulation.

Resistance

Resistance is the degree of friction experienced by the blood as it flows through the vessels. Most of this resistance occurs in the small peripheral arterioles and is known as the peripheral resistance (PR).

The factors which produce resistance are:
- Vessel length.
- Vessel diameter.
- Blood viscosity (determined by PCV see Chapter 9).

Resistance to flow increases with the length of the vessel, as vessels narrow (small diameter vessels produce more resistance – think what happens if you kink a hosepipe even with the tap full on) and when blood becomes more viscous/sticky (sticky fluids create more resistance to flow). Vessel length and blood viscosity are relatively stable in health and alterations in PR are mainly caused by changes in vessel diameter. We can use the following to illustrate these relationships in a simple system where flow is laminar:

$$R = \frac{Ln}{r^4}$$

R = resistance to flow, L = vessel length, n = blood viscosity, r = vessel radius

Earlier we said that PR was the most important factor influencing flow – this is because a small increase in vessel radius causes a big decrease in PR, which allows a large increase in flow. Chemical stimuli, hormones, inflammatory chemicals and sympathetic nerves cause the smooth muscle of arterioles to contract (vasoconstrict), increasing PR, or to relax (vasodilate), decreasing PR.

The nervous control is through the vasomotor centre (VMC), which is part of the cardiovascular centre in the brain (see page 217). It transmits impulses through sympathetic nerves which constrict the blood vessels (see *Figure 10.21*). The level of activity in the VMC depends on the amount of inhibition by the baroreceptors. These are sensory receptors responding to pressure changes in the carotid sinus and aortic arch (see *Figures 10.32* and *10.34*). When pressure is normal the baroreceptors partially inhibit the VMC, which sends sufficient impulses to maintain normal vasomotor tone (partial constriction). Low pressure reduces baroreceptor inhibition of the VMC, which sends more impulses to the vessels, which constrict. High pressure results in complete inhibition of the VMC and vasodilation. Baroreceptor/VMC mechanisms are vital in the regulation of arterial blood pressure. They also affect heart rate and contractility through functional overlap with the cardiac centre.

Arterial blood pressure

Pressure is exerted by the blood on the arterial walls as the left ventricle pumps blood into the aorta. The pressure is produced when flow meets resistance, which can be summarized as:

Blood pressure (BP) =
Peripheral resistance (PR) × Cardiac output (CO)

Blood pressure is generally measured in millimetres of mercury (mmHg), although the SI unit for pressure is the pascal (Pa) or kilopascal (kPa). It has two readings: systolic, representing the highest pressure reached in the arteries after ventricular systole; and diastolic, which is the lowest pressure during ventricular filling. A 'typical' blood pressure for a young adult would be 120/70 mmHg (16/9.3 kPa). Blood pressure in babies and children is lower than in adults and has more to do with their body size than age. You might be wondering why the diastolic pressure does not fall to zero – this is because the arteries are never completely empty and the

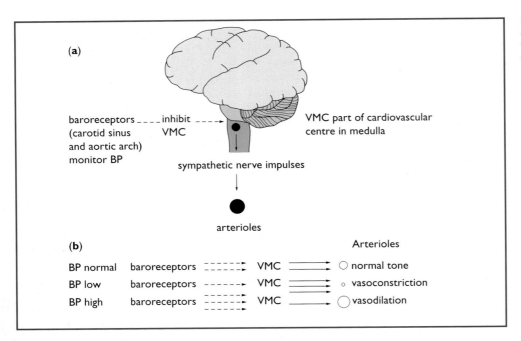

next systole occurs before the pressure can fall further. The difference between systolic and diastolic pressures is termed the pulse pressure. Variations in blood pressure occur in healthy individuals as their situation changes, e.g. posture, exercise, stress causing the release of adrenal hormones and general level of activity.

Blood pressure also varies between racial groups, and in Western countries it usually rises with ageing. In general, men have higher blood pressure than women.

Factors contributing to blood pressure:
- Peripheral resistance (page 225).
- Cardiac output (page 215).
- Blood volume – a low volume reduces blood pressure, e.g. after haemorrhage, and *vice versa*.
- Venous return (pages 223–224).
- Blood viscosity, which affects peripheral resistance (Chapter 9 and page 225).
- Elasticity of large arteries; arterial disease will cause blood pressure to rise as blood is forced into non-distending vessels (pages 219–220 and Special Focus).

Controlling blood pressure

Being able to change blood pressure in response to an altered situation is vital to homeostasis. Various mechanisms originating in the CVS, brain and very importantly the kidneys control blood pressure by modifying peripheral resistance, blood volume and cardiac output, both in the short-term and long-term.

Short-term mechanisms

Neural and chemical mechanisms that control blood pressure in the short-term include:
- Baroreceptors reflex through the VMC (see page 225).
- Chemoreceptors (see Chapter 12) responding to pH, oxygen (O_2) and carbon dioxide (CO_2) levels in the blood influence the VMC and cardiac centre; for example, reduced O_2 or increased CO_2 and acidosis cause vasoconstriction, increased heart rate and stroke volume with a rise in blood pressure.
- A fall in blood pressure and the 'fight or flight' response through the medulla oblongata, with some higher centre influences, initiates sympathetic activity and the release of the hormones noradrenaline and adrenaline. This in turn raises blood pressure by increasing heart rate, stroke volume and vasoconstriction.
- Angiotensin II (see Chapters 8 and 15), which is part of the renin–angiotensin–aldosterone response important in long-term blood pressure control, can raise blood pressure in the short term through its powerful vasoconstrictor properties.
- Antidiuretic hormone (ADH; see Chapters 8 and 15) prevents renal water loss and raises blood pressure in the long term, but high levels raise blood pressure through its pressor (vasoconstriction) effect on vessel smooth muscle.
- Atrial natriuretic peptides (ANPs; see Chapter 8) are hormones produced by the atria when the blood pressure rises. They inhibit ADH and aldosterone, resulting in increased water and sodium loss by the kidneys.

This, with some general vasodilation, reduces the blood pressure.

- Many vasoactive chemicals influence blood pressure: inflammatory chemicals such as histamine lower blood pressure through vasodilation, as in severe allergic reactions; and peptides produced by the endothelium, e.g. endothelin, are very powerful vasoconstrictors through their action on smooth muscle and nitric oxide (see Chapter 1 – free radicals and Chapter 3 – neurotransmitters/modulators), which causes vasodilation and may have a role in blood pressure control.

Long-term mechanisms

This is where the kidney really 'comes into its own', with two major mechanisms for long-term blood pressure control (see Chapters 2, 8 and 15):

- The renin–angiotensin–aldosterone response occurs when the volume of extracellular fluid, and hence the blood pressure, is low. Special kidney cells, known as the juxtaglomerular apparatus (JGA), respond by releasing the enzyme renin, which initiates a series of reactions to convert angiotensinogen to angiotensin II. We have already looked at the vasoconstriction and increased blood pressure caused by angiotensin II, but it also stimulates the adrenal cortex to produce aldosterone, which increases sodium reabsorption by the kidney. Remember that water always follows sodium – which increases blood volume and with it the blood pressure.

- When blood pressure is low (monitored by baroreceptors) or blood osmolarity is high (monitored by hypothalamic osmoreceptor cells), the neurohypophysis releases ADH, which causes the kidney tubules to become more permeable to water. More water is reabsorbed and the blood volume and blood pressure returns to normal.

Nursing Practice Application **Recording blood pressure**

Measuring blood pressure is a skill and nurses should be aware of and take account of the factors which affect accuracy and consistency. The person should be at rest and children under 5 years should lie down. Their arm is supported at heart level without tight clothing constricting the upper part (*Figure 10.22*). It seems rather obvious that the equipment should be working, but a study in a general hospital found that only a third of the sphygmomanometers (sample 110) were working properly (Bell and Siklos, 1984). Where a portable boxed sphygmomanometer is used, it should be on a flat surface and the observer's eye should be level with the column of mercury. The cuff should be of the correct size and applied correctly over the brachial artery. Accurate recording of blood pressure in children is difficult and having a selection of smaller cuffs is of particular importance. More consistent results are obtained if one nurse records blood pressure for an individual patient over the whole duty shift; this is important if frequent observations are required for assessment, e.g. head injury (see Chapter 4). The environment should be quiet if possible.

It is essential to implement a nursing policy regarding which phase of Korotkoff sounds (sounds heard whilst recording blood pressure) will represent diastolic pressure in different groups – this is generally phase 4 in children and phase 5 in teenagers and adults (see *Figure 10.23*). Adequate knowledge and training in recording blood pressure is fundamental – in a two-centre study Kemp et al. (1994) found that only 23% of respondents could correctly describe Korotkoff sounds and only 18% knew that diastolic in adults was Korotkoff phase 5.

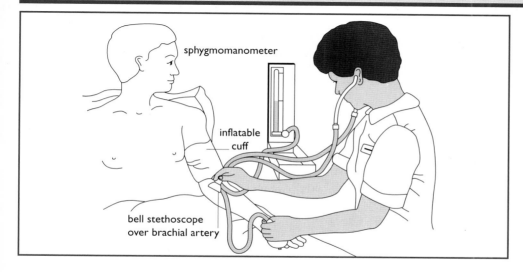

Figure 10.22 Measuring blood pressure.

sphygmomanometer

inflatable cuff

bell stethoscope over brachial artery

Abnormal Function **Problems with blood pressure**

Hypertension

Blood pressure sustained above the 'normal' level for age and gender is known as hypertension. The general concensus is that a BP of 160/95 mmHg at 50 years is abnormally high. Drug therapy, which may include diuretics, beta blockers, antihypertensives, calcium channel blockers, ACE inhibitors and possibly prophylactic aspirin, can be effective in reducing BP and associated cardiovascular disease such as stroke. Affected individuals should also be encouraged to adopt a healthier lifestyle, especially reducing salt (sodium) intake (see page 211).

Around 20–30% of adults in developed countries have an elevated blood pressure – in the UK hypertension is six times more common in Afro-Caribbeans than in Caucasians, and it is frequently seen in the Japanese and in African Americans. Many people will be asymptomatic and the high BP will be discovered by screening before problems arise. In around 90–95% of people the hypertension is essential (primary), and of unknown cause; only rarely is it secondary to conditions such as renal disease, coarctation of the aorta or the rare adrenal medulla tumour (phaeochromocytoma; Chapter 8). High blood pressure can result in arterial disease, leading to stroke and myocardial infarction, cardiac failure, renal failure and retinopathy.

Hypotension

Many people function perfectly well on a blood pressure lower than the average values. Systolic pressure below 100 mmHg is usually accepted as hypotension. A chronically low BP may be caused by adrenal failure (Addison's disease; see Chapter 8) or nutritional inadequacies. Sudden falls in BP cause fainting if cerebral blood flow is inadequate. This may be a transitory event associated with rising quickly (especially in older adults where the CVS takes longer to adjust), standing in the heat, lack of food or intense excitement. Much more serious are the events causing shock (see page 229), where the blood pressure is too low to maintain circulation and organ perfusion, e.g. after major haemorrhage.

phase	blood pressure (mmHg)	
	120	systolic
1	sharp thud	
	110	
2	blowing or swishing	
	100	
3	soft thud	
	90	first diastolic
4	soft blowing that muffles	
	80	second diastolic
5	no sound	

Figure 10.23 Korotkoff sounds.

Capillary bed and exchange of molecules

It is within the capillary network that oxygen and nutrients move from the blood through the interstitial fluid to the cells. Waste products of cell metabolism make the reverse journey. All this depends on the delicate balance between hydrostatic and osmotic pressure (see *Figure 10.26*).

The hydrostatic pressure (see page 224) at the arterial end of the capillary is sufficiently high to overcome the osmotic pressure (see Chapter 2) of the blood exerted by the non-diffusible plasma proteins (mainly albumin) and some inorganic ions (see Chapter 9). As there is very little interstitial fluid present, its hydrostatic pressure can be taken as zero. Fluid and nutrients consequently move through the selectively permeable capillary wall into the interstitial spaces. Net effective hydrostatic pressure falls across the capillary network and at the venous end the hydrostatic pressure is lower than the osmotic pressure (which is unchanged across the capillary network). This results in fluid and waste being drawn back into the capillary. The minimal amount of fluid and some proteins remaining within the interstitial compartment drain into lymphatic vessels and are returned to the circulation by the vital functioning of the lymphatic system (see Chapter 11).

Molecules cross the plasma membrane, to enter and leave cells (see *Figure 10.27*), by various processes, including osmosis, diffusion, and active and bulk transport (see Chapters 1 and 2). Slow blood flow through the capillary network gives time for these processes to occur. Autoregulatory mechanisms (see page 224) ensure that capillary flow is appropriate for local cellular needs.

Abnormal Function **Shock**

Shock (see *Figure 10.24*) is a syndrome (collection of signs and symptoms) in which there is a reduction in the effective circulating blood volume with impaired tissue perfusion. It is characterized by clinical features that include:

- Hypotension: caused by reduced cardiac output and circulating blood volume, a late sign in some types of shock.
- Tachycardia/weak pulse: heart rate increases in an attempt to increase output.
- Increased respiration: as lactic acid, produced by cells short of oxygen, causes a fall in blood pH.
- Pallor: sympathetic peripheral vasoconstriction diverts blood flow to vital organs, e.g. heart and brain.
- Cyanosis (blue colour seen first in the nail beds and lips): poor oxygenation of the blood and peripheral vasoconstriction.
- Skin cold and clammy: peripheral vasoconstriction and sweating caused by sympathetic activity.
- Oliguria: renin–angiotensin–aldosterone response initiated by reduced renal perfusion and the release of ADH reduce fluid loss in urine (see before).
- Thirst: as the hypothalamic thirst centre responds to reduced blood volume.
- Altered consciousness/restlessness/confusion: inadequate oxygenated blood reaches the brain, which is also depressed by pH changes.

The body attempts to minimize the effects of shock through baroreceptor, chemoreceptor and sympathetic activity, which increase:

- Vasoconstriction.
- Peripheral resistance.
- Blood volume (fluid drawn from cells).
- Venous return.
- Heart rate.
- Cardiac output.

Adrenaline and noradrenaline enhance sympathetic effects and the release of corticosteroids ensures a supply of energy. Fluid-conserving mechanisms involving ADH and angiotensin are initiated – remember that they are also powerful vasoconstrictors. Autoregulatory processes help to ensure that 'vital' organs are perfused.

If the state of shock is not reversed the cells become hypoxic (deficient in oxygen), dilation of the capillary network occurs and the vessels become permeable, allowing fluid to leak from the blood. This loss of fluid increases the degree of shock by further reducing the circulating blood volume and blood pressure. Irreversible cell damage and eventual death from multi-organ failure will occur if this 'vicious circle' of events remains unbroken. The events occurring in shock can be described by using the stages of the triphasic stress response (see Chapter 6).

Types and causes of shock

There are several ways of classifying types of shock, but for our purposes a straightforward approach has been adopted.

Hypovolaemic (decreased blood volume) The causes of hypovolaemia include:

- Haemorrhage.
- Loss of other body fluids, e.g. plasma lost from burns, vomiting or diarrhoea.
- Diabetic ketoacidosis.

Cardiogenic (pump failure) Causes of cardiogenic shock include extensive myocardial infarction, pericardial tamponade (pericardial collection of blood obstructing heart movements) and pulmonary embolus.

Vascular (normal volume) Septic shock (septicaemia with bacteria/toxins within the blood) or anaphylaxis (shock caused by an intense antigen–antibody reaction – see Chapter 19) causes vasodilation and eventual movement of fluid from the vascular compartment as vessel permeability increases. Vasodilation increases the capacity of the circulation and movement of fluid from the blood results in poor circulation and tissue perfusion. BP falls early in vascular shock, especially where bacterial toxins reduce vasomotor tone and peripheral resistance.

Neural mechanisms may operate in other situations to reduce vasomotor tone and cause shock. It may follow some anaesthetics and events such as witnessing a major road accident or receiving very bad news, where its effects may be transitory.

Nursing Practice Application **Monitoring condition in shock**

The vital signs normally used to monitor an individual's condition may be inadequate in shock – blood pressure may only be affected in the late stages and can be inaccurate (see above). Kidney function is monitored through measuring urinary output. Skin temperature can give an indication of peripheral blood flow, and blood oxygen saturation levels are useful.

Central venous pressure (CVP), which measures pressure in the right atrium, is a useful guide to condition and fluid requirements. A catheter passed into the right atrium through the subclavian or jugular vein is attached to an intravenous (IV) administration set with a manometer and

a three-way tap (see *Figure 10.25*). This arrangement with a three-way tap allows direct communication between catheter and manometer. The level of fluid in the manometer in cmH_2O pressure represents the CVP. When measurements are not being taken the tap position is changed and the IV fluid infusion resumed.

Where an individual has serious cardiopulmonary malfunction, e.g. after extensive myocardial infarction or massive pulmonary embolus, the CVP is not always a dependable indicator of left heart function. Where it is helpful to have accurate information about left heart function a Swan–Gantz catheter passed through the

veins into the right atrium is allowed to float through the ventricle to wedge in a small pulmonary artery. Inflation of a small balloon at its tip wedges the catheter and blocks off the pulmonary artery behind the balloon. Now the pressure in the pulmonary capillaries, and hence the left atrium and ventricle, is measured. The catheter, which is attached to a pressure transducer, records pulmonary capillary wedge pressure (PCWP), giving information regarding left ventricular pressure at the end of diastole. PCWP is recorded at intervals and between measurements, when the balloon is deflated, it records pulmonary artery pressure.

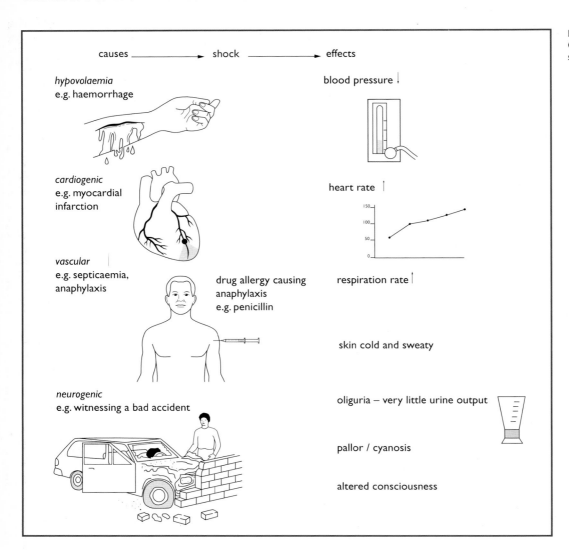

Figure 10.24
Causes and effects of shock.

causes ⟶ shock ⟶ effects

hypovolaemia
e.g. haemorrhage

blood pressure ↓

cardiogenic
e.g. myocardial
infarction

heart rate ↑

vascular
e.g. septicaemia,
anaphylaxis

drug allergy causing
anaphylaxis
e.g. penicillin

respiration rate ↑

skin cold and sweaty

neurogenic
e.g. witnessing a bad accident

oliguria – very little urine output

pallor / cyanosis

altered consciousness

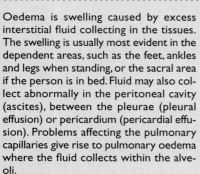

Abnormal Function **Homeostatic imbalance – oedema**

Oedema is swelling caused by excess interstitial fluid collecting in the tissues. The swelling is usually most evident in the dependent areas, such as the feet, ankles and legs when standing, or the sacral area if the person is in bed. Fluid may also collect abnormally in the peritoneal cavity (ascites), between the pleurae (pleural effusion) or pericardium (pericardial effusion). Problems affecting the pulmonary capillaries give rise to pulmonary oedema where the fluid collects within the alveoli.

Oedema will result from a failure of any part of the homeostatic mechanisms involved in maintaining the fluid compartments. Oedematous tissue becomes hypoxic and metabolites accumulate, which renders the tissues more susceptible to injury. This has serious implications for nursing practice as this waterlogged, poorly oxygenated tissue is more likely to break down and develop pressure sores (see Chapter 19).

Main causes of oedema
Figure 10.28 illustrates the possible causes of oedema:
- Reduced osmotic pressure in the blood caused by a decrease in plasma protein levels (hypoproteinaemia). This may be caused by liver disease, starvation or protein loss from the kidneys.
- Increased venous hydrostatic pressure such as in congestive cardiac failure (see page 218), increased blood volume of pregnancy, fluid or sodium retention and varicose veins.
- Increased capillary permeability such as that caused by inflammatory chemicals.
- Obstruction in the lymphatic vessels; for example, malignant cells from the breast may block the arm lymphatics, causing oedema. This happens because excess fluid in the interstitial space is unable to drain away.

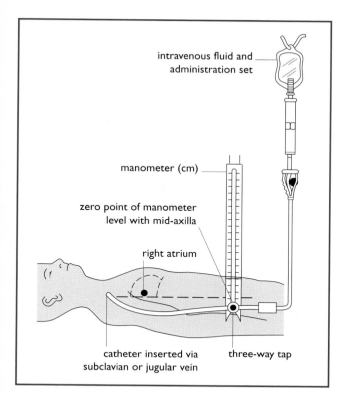

Figure 10.25 Central venous pressure.

intravenous fluid and administration set

manometer (cm)

zero point of manometer level with mid-axilla

right atrium

catheter inserted via subclavian or jugular vein

three-way tap

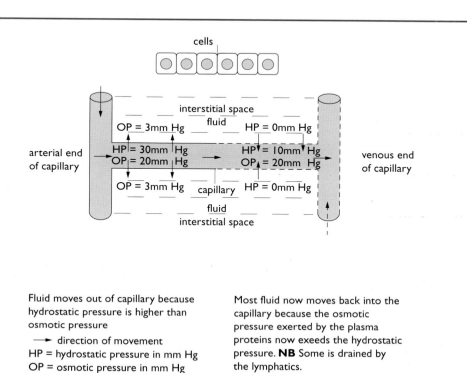

Figure 10.26 Formation of interstitial fluid (tissue fluid) – hydrostatic and osmotic pressure.

cells

interstitial space
fluid

OP = 3mm Hg   HP = 0mm Hg

arterial end of capillary   HP = 30mm Hg   HP = 10mm Hg   venous end of capillary
OP = 20mm Hg   OP = 20mm Hg

OP = 3mm Hg   capillary   HP = 0mm Hg
fluid
interstitial space

Fluid moves out of capillary because hydrostatic pressure is higher than osmotic pressure

→ direction of movement
HP = hydrostatic pressure in mm Hg
OP = osmotic pressure in mm Hg

Most fluid now moves back into the capillary because the osmotic pressure exerted by the plasma proteins now exeeds the hydrostatic pressure. **NB** Some is drained by the lymphatics.

NB There is a small amount of protein in the interstitial fluid which produces a small OP

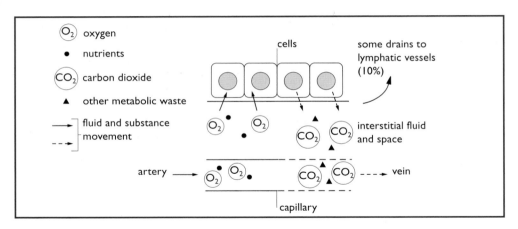

Figure 10.27 Exchange of molecules between blood and cells.

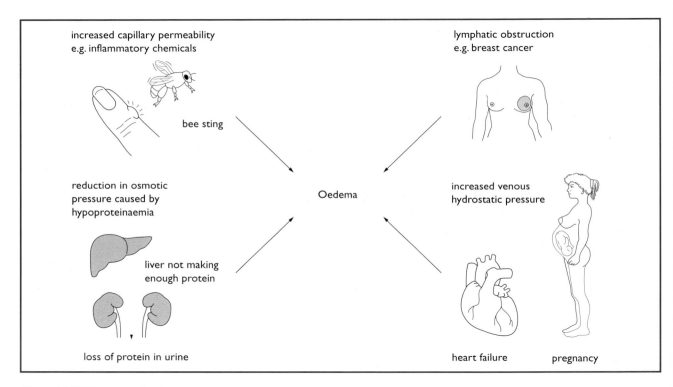

Figure 10.28 The causes of oedema.

Circulation

Circulation consists of two main systems – the low-pressure pulmonary circulation through the lungs and the high-pressure systemic circulation, which supplies blood to most cells. You do not need to memorize details of every vessel, and with this in mind, a brief coverage of major vessels is included. This should be sufficient for your nursing practice, but where more information is needed readers are directed to Further Reading, e.g. Williams *et al.*, (1995).

Pulmonary circulation

The pulmonary circulation transports blood low in oxygen and high in carbon dioxide to the lungs, where it gains oxygen and loses carbon dioxide. Dark red venous blood returning to the right side of the heart is pumped into the pulmonary trunk. This large artery divides into the right and left pulmonary arteries, one going to each lung. These further divide and eventually feed into a capillary network. Here the intimate contact between capillaries and alveoli allows the exchange of gases. Gases diffuse down pressure gradients, which means that oxygen passes from alveolar air into the blood and carbon dioxide moves in the opposite direction – a process known as external respiration (see Chapter 12).

The high oxygen/low carbon dioxide blood is transported by venules to veins which eventually form four pulmonary veins (two from each lung). The pulmonary veins return the bright red oxygenated blood to the left atrium, completing the pulmonary circuit (*Figure 10.29*).

It is important to note that the pulmonary circulation does not supply lung tissue with arterial blood (see page 238).

Systemic or general circulation

The systemic circulation circulates blood rich in oxygen through the main artery (aorta) and its branches (see *Figure 10.30*). These branches eventually form the arterioles, which supply individual capillary networks in organs and tissues. Internal respiration or gaseous exchange between blood and cells ensures that there is oxygen for cellular respiration (energy production) and that carbon dioxide is removed from the tissues. Venules collecting the blood low in oxygen become veins that form the venae cavae, which drain into the right atrium to complete the circuit (see *Figure 10.31*).

The general circulation is rather more complex than this and more detail is needed – first a consideration of the arterial supply to a particular area and, where appropriate, the corresponding venous return.

Aorta

The aorta ascends from the left ventricle, arches over and descends behind the heart to pass through the thorax and abdomen. Branches of paired or single arteries exit from the aorta, of which many are named for the organ supplied. The first branches from the ascending aorta supply the myocardium – the coronary arteries (see *Figure 10.6*). Venous blood from the myocardium returns to the right atrium through the coronary sinus and cardiac veins (see page 208). Baroreceptors concerned with blood pressure regulation are situated in the aortic arch, as are the peripheral chemoreceptors which regulate respiratory rate (see pages 225–226, *Figure 10.21* and Chapter 12).

Aortic arch

Three arteries branch from the aortic arch (see *Figure 10.32*):
- Left common carotid.
- Left subclavian.
- Brachiocephalic (innominate) which becomes the right subclavian and right common carotid.

They supply the neck, head and upper extremities.

Superior vena cava and venous return

Venous return is through the superior vena cava, formed from the right and left brachiocephalic veins which are derived from the subclavian and internal jugular veins (see *Figure 10.33*).

Blood vessels of the head and neck
Arteries

The main arteries supplying the head and neck are the two common carotids which run one up each side of the neck. Baroreceptors are found where the arteries divide into

Figure 10.29 Pulmonary circulation.

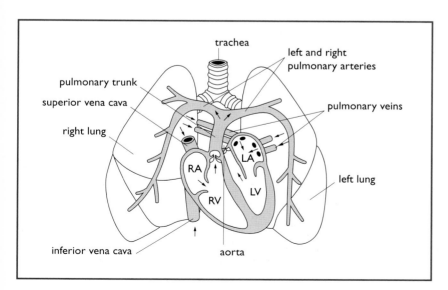

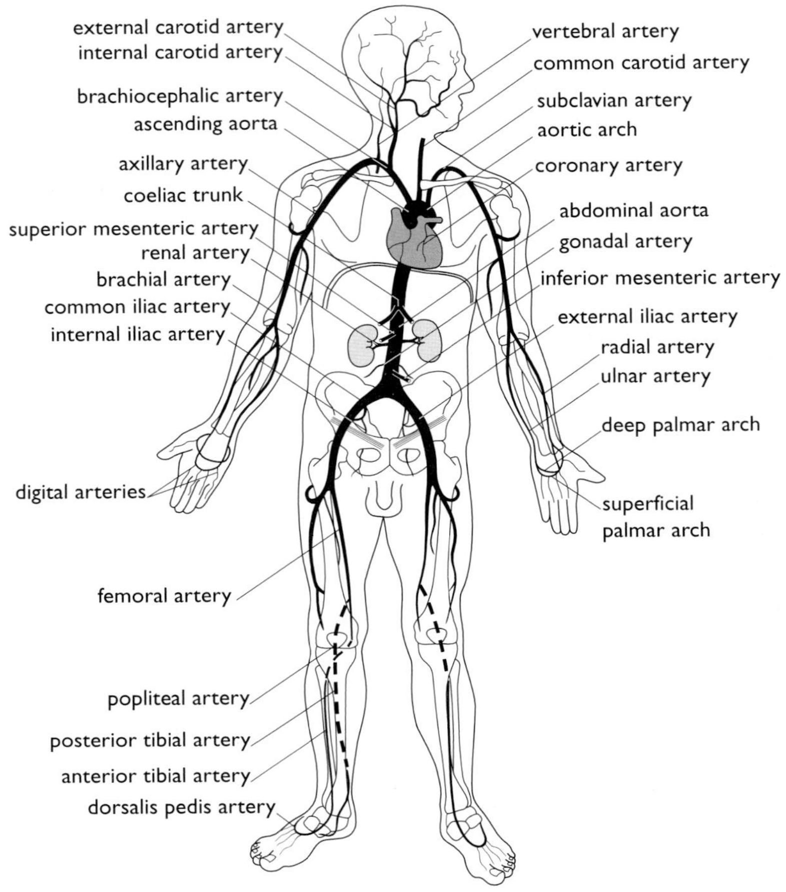

Figure 10.30 Main arteries.

internal and external carotid arteries – the carotid sinus and the nearby carotid bodies, which contain chemoreceptors.

The external carotid forms arteries to the face (the facial artery), tongue (lingual), scalp (temporal/occipital), muscles of mastication (maxillary), bones of the skull and dura (middle meningeal), and neck and associated structures, e.g. thyroid (see *Figure 10.34*).

The internal carotid arteries enter the skull through the temporal bones. They contribute to the circle of Willis (see *Figure 10.35*) and form the ophthalmic artery (supplies the eye). The circle of Willis (an arterial anastomosis – see Chapter 4) supplying the brain is formed from the anterior cerebral arteries (internal carotids), communicating arteries and posterior cerebral arteries formed from the basilar artery. The basilar artery is formed from a unification of two vertebral arteries (from the subclavian arteries) which enter the skull through the foramen magnum. The brainstem is also supplied by the basilar artery.

Venous return

Most blood from superficial areas drains through veins (the names of which correspond with the arteries branching from the external carotid) which form the external jugular veins in the neck. The external jugular veins pass over the sternocleidomastoid muscles, behind the clavicles to empty into the subclavian veins (see *Figure 10.36*).

Venous blood from the brain empties into venous sinuses (see Figure 10.37) enclosed in fibrous dura mater. The main venous sinuses include the superior and inferior sagittal sinuses, straight sinus, two transverse sinuses, sigmoid sinus and cavernous sinuses – which drain into two internal jugular veins. Arachnoid granulations projecting into the superior sagittal sinus return cerebrospinal fluid to the circulation (see Chapter 4).

The internal jugular veins also receive blood from the deep structures of the face and neck as they pass behind the sternocleidomastoid muscles before entering the subclavian veins to form the two brachiocephalic veins.

Figure 10.31 Main veins.

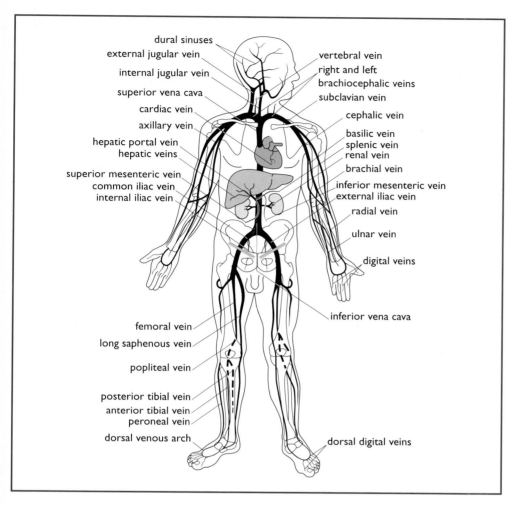

- dural sinuses
- external jugular vein
- internal jugular vein
- superior vena cava
- cardiac vein
- axillary vein
- hepatic portal vein
- hepatic veins
- superior mesenteric vein
- common iliac vein
- internal iliac vein

- vertebral vein
- right and left brachiocephalic veins
- subclavian vein
- cephalic vein
- basilic vein
- splenic vein
- renal vein
- brachial vein
- inferior mesenteric vein
- external iliac vein
- radial vein
- ulnar vein
- digital veins
- inferior vena cava

- femoral vein
- long saphenous vein
- popliteal vein
- posterior tibial vein
- anterior tibial vein
- peroneal vein
- dorsal venous arch
- dorsal digital veins

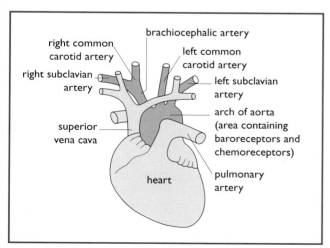

- right common carotid artery
- right subclavian artery
- superior vena cava
- brachiocephalic artery
- left common carotid artery
- left subclavian artery
- arch of aorta (area containing baroreceptors and chemoreceptors)
- heart
- pulmonary artery

Figure 10.32 Aortic arch.

- right brachiocephalic vein
- right internal jugular vein
- right subclavian vein
- superior vena cava
- left brachiocephalic vein
- left internal jugular vein
- left subclavian vein
- aorta
- heart
- pulmonary artery

Figure 10.33 Superior vena cava.

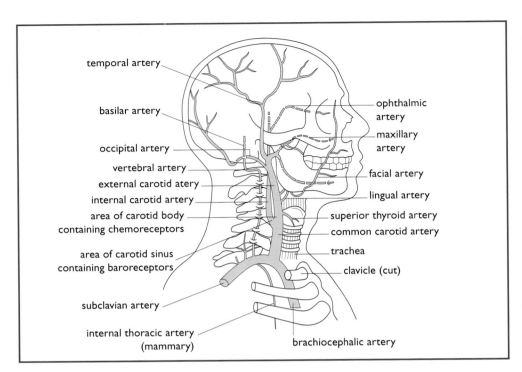

Figure 10.34 Arteries – head and neck.

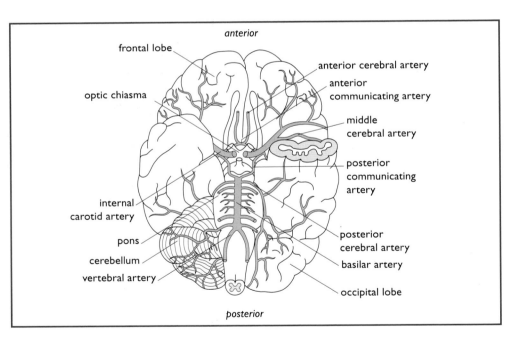

Figure 10.35 Circle of Willis.

Blood vessels of the upper extremity
Arteries

The subclavian artery branches to the neck, thoracic cavity and breast (internal mammary artery) before passing between the clavicles and first rib to enter the axilla. Now called the axillary artery, it provides branches to the shoulder, axilla and chest muscles. On entering the arm it becomes the brachial artery, supplying the upper arm. As it passes over the inner aspect of the elbow joint it provides a convenient point for measuring blood pressure (see *Figure 10.22*). Below the elbow it divides into the radial and ulnar arteries, which supply the lateral

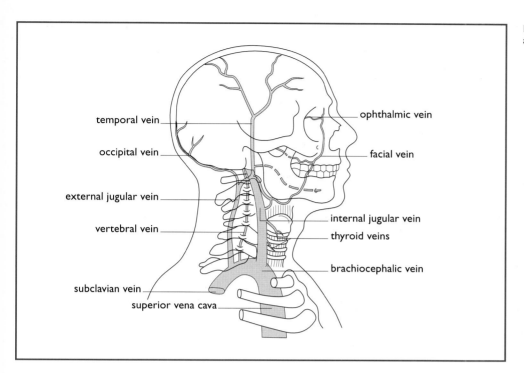

Figure 10.36 Veins — head and neck.

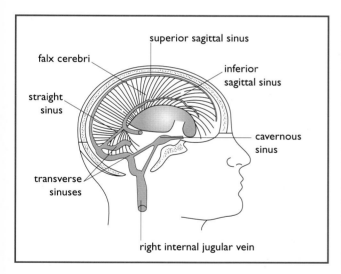

Figure 10.37 Venous sinuses of the brain.

and medial aspects of the forearm. Where the radial artery surfaces at the wrist it can be used to count pulse rate (see page 222). The radial and ulnar arteries anastomose to form the arteries supplying the hand: the superficial and deep palmar arches and the digital arteries (*Figure 10.38*).

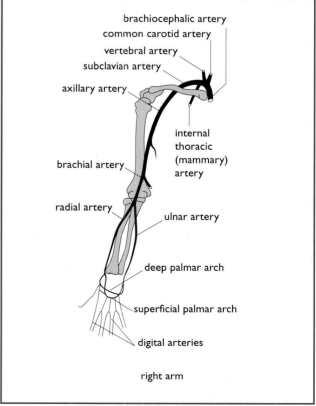

Figure 10.38 Arteries of the upper extremity.

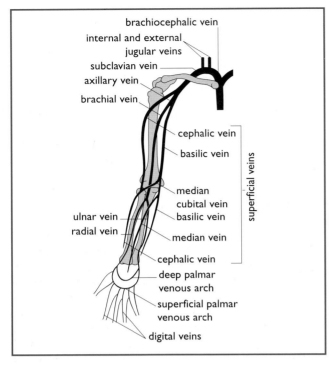

Figure 10.39 Veins of the upper extremity.

Venous return

There are two groups of veins within the arm (*Figure 10.39*):

- Deep veins, which take the name of the arteries and follow the same route: deep and superficial palmar arches, ulnar, radial, brachial and axillary veins, which empty in the subclavian veins.
- Superficial veins: median, cephalic, basilic and median cubital veins. Running close to the surface, they are used to gain vascular access for blood samples, infusions or injection.

Thoracic blood vessels and descending aorta

The aorta passes behind the heart and travels through the thoracic cavity, with branches spreading to the chest wall (the posterior intercostal arteries). Many branches leave the thoracic aorta and include those supplying the oesophagus (oesophageal arteries), lungs/bronchi and pleura (bronchial arteries) and pericardium (the pericardial artery) (*Figure 10.40*).

Venous return from the thorax

Major veins, which include intercostal, oesophageal and bronchial veins (not shown on *Figure 10.41*), empty into the azygos system of veins which run up the sides of the vertebral column. The hemiazygos vein joins the azygos vein,

Figure 10.40 Thoracic aorta.

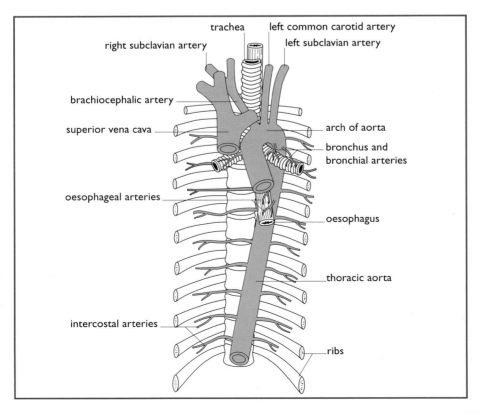

which empties into the superior vena cava. An accessory hemiazygos vein also drains the thorax. In addition, the azygos system of veins receives blood from the abdominal cavity through the ascending lumbar veins (*Figure 10.41*).

It is important to note that the lower oesophageal veins drain into the hepatic portal system.

Abdominal aorta and branches

The thoracic aorta passes through the diaphragm to become the abdominal aorta. Travelling down the posterior abdominal wall to the level of the fourth lumbar vertebra, it divides into two common iliac arteries. Branches from the abdominal aorta include (see *Figure 10.42*):

- Unpaired coeliac, superior and inferior mesenteric arteries.
- Paired arteries supplying the diaphragm (inferior phrenic arteries) and the posterior abdominal wall (four lumbar arteries).
- Paired visceral arteries supplying the adrenals (the suprarenal arteries), kidneys (renal arteries) and the gonads (ovarian or testicular arteries).

Arterial supply to the gastrointestinal tract and liver

The coeliac artery (trunk) divides into three branches [see *Figure 10.43(a)*]:

- The left gastric artery, supplying the stomach and lower oesophagus.
- A common hepatic artery, which branches to the stomach, duodenum and pancreas before dividing into the right and left hepatic arteries, supplying the liver and gallbladder (see Chapter 14).
- The splenic artery, which branches to the stomach, pancreas and spleen.

The superior mesenteric artery and its branches supply the pancreas, the entire small bowel and the proximal part of the large bowel. The inferior mesenteric artery and its branches supply the distal large bowel and most of the rectum [see *Figure 10.43(b)*].

Venous return from the abdominal cavity

Most of the venous blood from the structures supplied by paired arteries drains into veins of the same name emptying into the inferior vena cava (IVC) (see *Figure 10.44*). The IVC, formed by the two common iliac veins, carries blood from the lower part of the body and passes through the diaphragm to the right atrium. The renal, lumbar, right suprarenal and right gonadal veins all drain directly into the IVC, but the left suprarenal and gonadal veins drain into the left renal vein. The hepatic veins drain venous blood from the liver directly into the IVC.

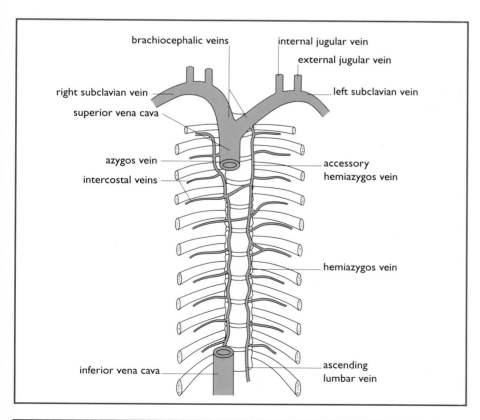

Figure 10.41 Venous return from the thorax.

brachiocephalic veins

internal jugular vein

external jugular vein

right subclavian vein

left subclavian vein

superior vena cava

azygos vein

accessory hemiazygos vein

intercostal veins

hemiazygos vein

inferior vena cava

ascending lumbar vein

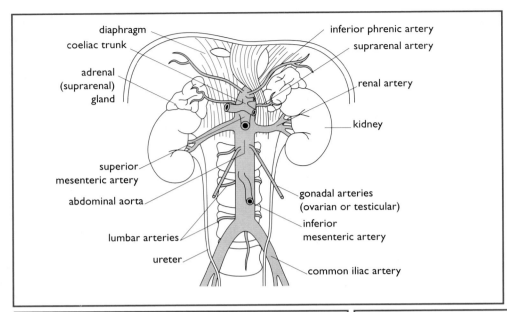

Figure 10.42 Abdominal aorta.

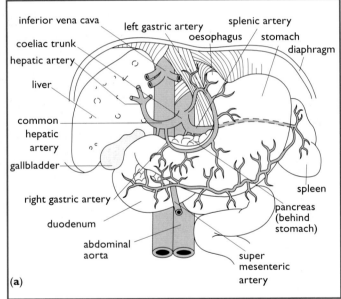

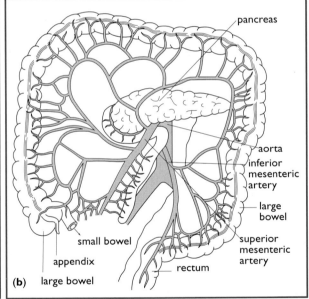

Figure 10.43 Arteries of the gastrointestinal organs. (**a**) Coeliac artery; (**b**) mesenteric arteries.

It is important to note that venous blood from structures supplied by the coeliac and mesenteric arteries passes through the liver before entering the IVC (see hepatic portal circulation).

Hepatic portal circulation
The veins carrying blood from the lower oesophagus, stomach, spleen, pancreas, small bowel and large bowel/rectum drain into a common vessel called the hepatic portal vein (*Figure 10.45*). The major vessels which form the hepatic portal vein include:

- Oesophageal veins – lower oesophagus (draining into gastric veins).
- Gastric veins – stomach.
- Splenic vein – spleen and part of stomach and pancreas.
- Superior mesenteric vein – small bowel and proximal large bowel.
- Inferior mesenteric vein – distal large bowel and rectum.

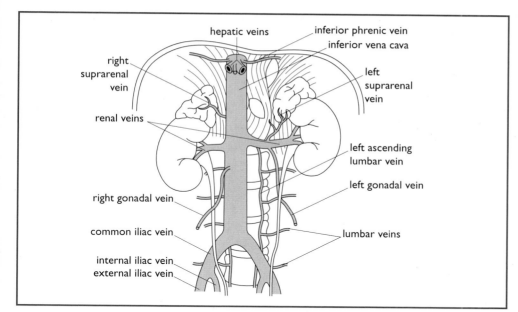

Figure 10.44 Venous return from the abdominal cavity.

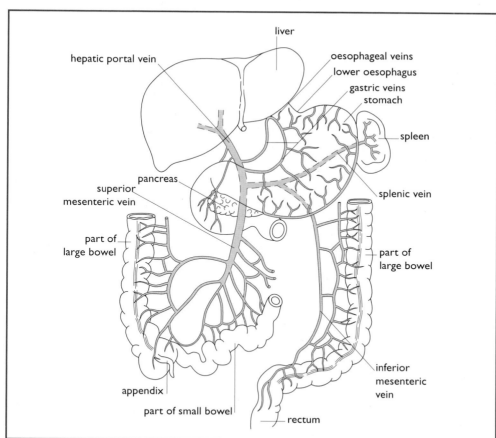

Figure 10.45 Venous drainage from the gastrointestinal tract and the hepatic portal vein.

This portal system ensures that venous blood passes through a second capillary bed (liver sinusoids) before returning to the general circulation. This complex arrangement makes considerable sense, as nutrients absorbed from the gastrointestinal tract and hormones from the pancreas are conveyed directly to the liver for processing.

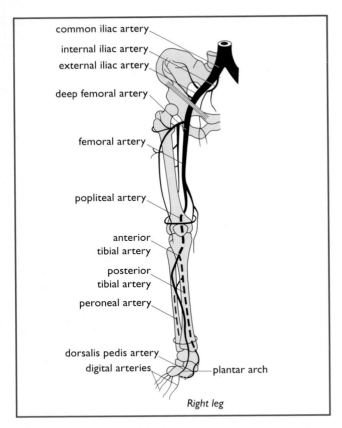

common iliac artery
internal iliac artery
external iliac artery
deep femoral artery
femoral artery
popliteal artery
anterior tibial artery
posterior tibial artery
peroneal artery
dorsalis pedis artery
digital arteries
plantar arch

Right leg

Figure 10.46 Arteries of the pelvis and lower extremities.

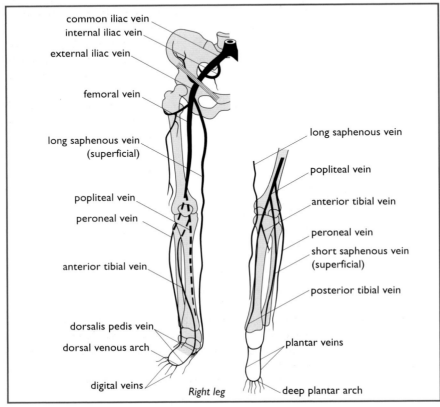

common iliac vein
internal iliac vein
external iliac vein
femoral vein
long saphenous vein (superficial)
popliteal vein
peroneal vein
anterior tibial vein
dorsalis pedis vein
dorsal venous arch
digital veins

long saphenous vein
popliteal vein
anterior tibial vein
peroneal vein
short saphenous vein (superficial)
posterior tibial vein
plantar veins
deep plantar arch

Right leg

Figure 10.47 Veins of the lower extremities and pelvis.

Abnormal Function **Hepatic portal dysfunction**

Problems occur when blood pressure rises in the hepatic portal vein (portal hypertension). This may be caused by liver cirrhosis (see Chapter 14) and leads to back pressure being transmitted to areas where the hepatic portal and systemic circulations anastomose.

Varicosities develop at these points, which include the gastro-oesophageal junction (oesophageal varices) and the rectum. Massive haemorrhage from oesophageal varices is the main complication of portal hypertension.

Blood vessels of the pelvis and lower extremities

Arteries

The aorta divides to form the right and left common iliac arteries, which supply blood to the lower abdomen, pelvic structures and legs. At the level of the sacroiliac joints the common iliac arteries split into the internal and external iliac arteries (*Figure 10.46*).

Branches of the paired internal iliac arteries supply the pelvis, lower rectum, bladder, uterus, vagina, prostate and external genitalia. The right and left external iliac arteries supply the legs. In each leg, the external iliac arteries pass behind the inguinal ligament in the groin to become the femoral artery supplying the groin and thigh. The femoral artery passes down the anterior thigh until, near the knee, it moves posteriorly to enter the popliteal fossa. Now known as the popliteal artery, it divides into the posterior and anterior tibial arteries. The posterior tibial artery supplies the back of the leg and branches to form the peroneal artery, which supplies the lateral aspects. It becomes the plantar and digital arteries, supplying the sole and toes. The anterior tibial artery supplies the front of the leg and at the ankle forms the dorsalis pedis artery (see Pulses, page 222). This supplies the dorsal aspect of the foot. With the plantar arteries it forms the plantar arch.

Venous return

The veins of the leg are deep or superficial. The deep veins of the leg generally accompany and have the same names as the arteries (*Figure 10.47*). Digital and plantar veins drain the foot. They form the posterior tibial vein, which travels deep within the calf muscles. An anterior tibial vein runs up the front of the leg to the knee, where it joins the posterior tibial vein to become the popliteal vein and eventually the femoral vein. This travels up the thigh and passes behind the inguinal ligament to form the external iliac vein. Internal iliac veins drain the pelvic structures. The external and internal iliac veins join to become common iliac veins which unite to form the IVC. These deep veins of the leg and pelvis are a frequent site for the formation of deep vein thrombosis (see Chapter 9).

The two superficial vessels – the long (great) and short (small) saphenous veins – run from the dorsal venous arch up the leg, draining the superficial structures. Many communicating vessels allow blood to pass between the superficial and deep systems. The long saphenous, which is the longest vein in the body, joins the femoral vein just before the inguinal ligament. The many valves present in the saphenous veins are easily damaged by high pressure, resulting in varicosities (see page 223). The long saphenous vein is used as a graft when diseased coronary arteries are bypassed (see pages 209 and 210). The short saphenous vein drains into the deep system at the popliteal vein.

Summary/Check List

Introduction – CVS.
Heart – development. Nursing Practice Application – congenital heart defects and Down syndrome. Location. Shape. Size. Functions. Structure – wall, chambers, valves. Coronary circulation, Special Focus – coronary heart/artery disease, Nursing Practice Application – low birth weight and later CHD risk, Person-Centred Study – Derek. Healthier Living – reducing the risk of CHD/CAD. Blood flow direction. Conduction system – problems, pacemakers. ECG – normal and abnormal, Nursing Practice Application – cardiac arrest and resuscitation. Cardiac cycle. Cardiac output, stroke volume, heart rate. Problems with cardiac output, Nursing

Practice Application – cardiac glycosides.
Vessels – general structure. Arteries – pulse, Nursing Practice Application – pulse and apex beat. Special Focus – arterial disease. Capillaries. Veins, valves, Nursing Practice Application – venous return, varicose veins.
Circulatory physiology – blood flow, pressure, resistance. Arterial blood pressure, Nursing Practice Application – recording blood pressure, problems with blood pressure. Shock, Nursing Practice Application – monitoring condition in shock. Capillary bed and exchange. Oedema.
Circulation – Pulmonary. Systemic. Hepatic portal.

Self Test

1 How does the myocardium receive its blood supply?
2 Draw a diagram to show the direction of blood flow through the heart.
3 Put the components of the conduction system in the correct sequence for receiving the impulse:
   (a) Bundle of His;
   (b) SA node;
   (c) Purkinje fibres;
   (d) AV node;
   (e) Bundle branches.
4 Explain the isovolumetric contraction and relaxation phases of the cardiac cycle.
5 Complete the following:
   (a) CO = ? x SV
   (b) EDV – ESV = ?
6 Relate the structure of arteries, capillaries and veins to function.
7 Mikhail asks about preventing CHD. What would you suggest?
8 Which factors contribute to arterial blood pressure?
9 Explain how a low serum albumin level causes oedema.
10 Which of the following statements are true?
   (a) Arteries always carry oxygen-rich blood.
   (b) Venous blood from the brain drains via venous sinuses.
   (c) The pulmonary artery supplies blood to the lungs.
   (d) The hepatic veins carry venous blood from the liver.

Answers

1 Via coronary arteries.
2 Figure 10.8.
3 b, d, a, e, c.
4 Pages 213–214.
5 (a) HR;
   (b) SV.
6 Pages 219–223.
7 Pages 211.
8 Page 226.
9 Pages 228, 230–231.
10 b, d.

References

Ball M, Mann J (1988) *Lipids and heart disease: a practical approach.* Oxford: Oxford University Press.

Bell M, Siklos P (1984) Recording blood pressure: accuracy of staff and equipment. *Nurs Times* **80**(26):32–4.

Burr M, Gilbert J, Holliday R *et al.* (1989) Effects of changes in fat, fish and fibre intakes on death and myocardial reinfarction: Diet and reinfarction trial (DART). *Lancet,* **ii**:757–61.

Deans W, Hoskins, R (1987) Preventing coronary heart disease. *Prof Nurs* **2**(10):328–9.

Department of Health (DoH) (1993) *The health of the nation. Key area handbook. Coronary heart disease and stroke.* London: HMSO.

Daviglus ML, Stamler J, Orenica AJ *et al.* (1997) Fish consumption and the 30-year risk of fatal myocardial infarction. *New Eng J Med* **336**(15):1046–53.

Eastwick-Field P (1996) Resuscitation: basic life support. *Nurs Stand* **10**(34):49–53. Continuing education article.

Fall C, Vijayakumar M , Barker D *et al.* (1995) Weight in infancy and the prevalence of coronary heart disease in adult life. *BMJ* **310**:17–19.

Hay C, Durber A, Saynor R (1982) Effect of fish oil on platelet kinetics in patients with ischaemic heart disease. *Lancet,* **i**:1269–72.

Kemp F, Foster C, McKinlay S (1994) How effective is training for blood pressure measurement? *Prof Nurs* **9**(8):521–4.

King K, Ross Kerr J (1996) The women's health agenda: evolution of hormone replacement therapy as treatment and prophylaxis for coronary artery disease. *J Adv Nurs* **23**(5):984–91.

Murray P (1989) Rehabilitation information and health beliefs in post-coronary patients: do we meet their information needs? *J Adv Nurs* **14**(8):686–93.

Siess W, Roth P, Scherer B *et al.* (1980) Platelet-membrane fatty, acids, platelet aggregation and thromboxane formation during a mackerel diet. *Lancet* **i**:441–4.

Thompson D (1989) A randomized controlled trial of in-hospital nursing support for first time myocardial infarction patients and their partners: effects on anxiety and depression. *J Adv Nurs* **14**(4):291–7.

Further Reading

Darbyshire P (1988) Making sense of central venous pressure monitoring. *Nurs Times* **84**(6):36–8.

DoH (1991) *Dietary reference values for food energy and nutrients for the United Kingdom. Report on Health and Social Subjects*, no. 41. London: HMSO.

DoH (1994) *Nutritional aspects of cardiovascular disease. Report on health and social subjects*, no. 46. London: HMSO.

Edwards CRW, Bouchier IAD, Haslett C et al., Eds (1995) *Davidson's Principles and Practice of Medicine*, 17th edn. Edinburgh: Churchill Livingstone.

European Resuscitation Council (1996) *Guidelines for resuscitation.* Antwerp: ERC.

National Heart Forum (1997) *Preventing coronary heart disease: The role of antioxidants, vegatables and fruit.* London: Stationery Office.

Simpson S (1994a) Paediatric basic life support – an update. *Nurs Times* **90**(21):40–2.

Simpson S (1994b) Paediatric advanced life support – an update. *Nurs Times* **90**(27):37–9.

Williams PL, Warwick R, Dyson M et al., (1995) *Gray's Anatomy*, 38th edn. Edinburgh: Churchill Livingstone.

Useful Address

British Heart Foundation
14 Fitzhardinge Street
London W1H 4DH

Lymphatic System: Vessels, Nodes and Tissues

Overview

- *Lymphatic vessels, lymph formation and transport.*
- *Lymph nodes.*
- *Lymphoid tissues/organs – spleen.*

Learning Outcomes

After studying Chapter 11 you should be able to:

- Describe the structure of lymphatic vessels.
- Name the major lymphatic vessels.
- Outline the formation and transport of lymph.
- Describe lymph node structure and location.
- Outline the functions of the lymph nodes.
- Give examples of lymphoid tissues and their location.
- Outline lymphoid tissue functions.
- Describe the structure and functions of the spleen.

Key Words

Lymph – fluid, derived from interstitial fluid, found within the lymph vessels.
Lymphatic system – the lymph vessels, lymph nodes and lymphoid tissues/organs.
Lymphatics – a general term which describes the network of

lymph vessels conveying lymph.
Lymph capillaries – tiny vessels that convey fluid (lymph) from the interstitial spaces to larger lymphatic vessels and ducts.
Lymph nodes – small masses of lymphoid tissue found along lymph vessels with collections at strategic points, e.g. axilla.

Introduction

Our look at body transport systems is completed by consideration of the **lymphatic system**. Often overlooked, the lymphatic system is vital for cardiovascular functioning, absorption and transport of fats, and the immune system. It returns interstitial fluid (at a rate of 3 l/day) and proteins to the cardiovascular system, and forms an important component of the defence strategies initiated by the immune system (see Chapter 19). Without the lymphatic system the cardiovascular system would 'grind to a halt' and the body would be vulnerable to attack from malignant cells and micro-organisms.

Development of the lymphatic system

Development starts by week 5–6 of embryonic life from lymph sacs (jugular and iliac) which form from primitive veins. The lymphatic vessels, which grow out from the sacs to form the network of vessels, and the **lymph nodes** arise from the sac mesoderm. The lymphoid tissues/organs are mostly mesodermal in origin formed as mesenchymal cells migrate to designated areas; the exception is the thymus (see Chapter 8), which is endodermal. Only the spleen, which develops during weeks 6–7 from the fusion of mesodermal masses, is well formed at birth – other lymphoid tissues and lymph nodes continue to develop during infancy and childhood. Lymphocytes infiltrate the lymph nodes and other lymphoid tissues soon after birth, the thymus grows throughout childhood to reach a maximum during puberty and the tonsils reach full size around 5–6 years, after which they become smaller.

The Lymphatic Vessels

Tiny blind-ended **lymph capillaries** drain fluid (called **lymph** after it enters the **lymphatics**) from the interstitial spaces (interstitium) (*Figure 11.2*). Lymph capillaries are found in most parts of the body except the central nervous system and some connective tissues, e.g. bone. Their endothelial walls are highly permeable – the endothelial cells overlay each other in a way that can be pulled apart to produce gaps which allow the movement of water, waste, certain nutrients, hormones, proteins, malignant cells, micro-organisms and assorted debris into the lymph capillaries. The overlap between cells will cover the gaps to stop fluid escaping the other way when the lymph capillary is full. Lymph capillaries in the small bowel mucosa, called lacteals (see Chapter 13), are modified to absorb digested fats and carry the creamy lymph, known as chyle,

to the blood. The network of lymph capillaries unites to form the larger lymph vessels, which are similar in structure to veins, but with many more valves to prevent backflow (see Chapter 10).

The lymphatic vessels convey the lymph to two main ducts which return lymph to the circulation through connections originating from embryonic development. Lymph vessels from the right arm, right side of the head and chest drain into the right lymphatic duct [*Figure 11.1(b)*], which empties into the great veins in the neck, right subclavian and internal jugular veins [*Figure 11.1(a)*]. The rest of the body drains lymph through the thoracic duct [*Figure 11.1(b)*], commencing at the level of the L2–T12 vertebrae with a dilation called the cisterna chyli, which receives lymph from the legs and digestive tract. The thoracic duct passes through the diaphragm accepting lymph from the left thorax, arm and head before to emptying into the junction between the left subclavian and internal jugular veins [*Figure 11.1(a)*].

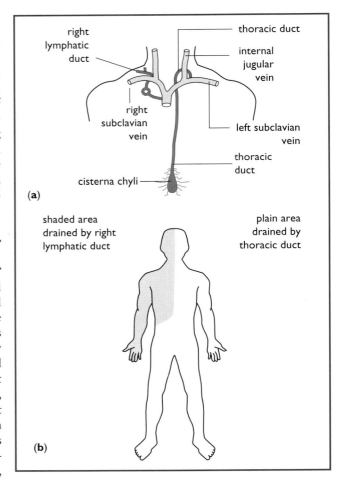

Figure 11.1 (a) Right lymphatic and thoracic ducts; **(b)** areas drained by each duct.

Lymph: formation and transportation

In Chapter 10 we considered the formation of interstitial fluid from plasma in the capillary network. Most fluid is drawn back at the venous end of the capillary by the osmotic pressure of the blood, but the 3 l remaining daily in the interstitium forms the lymph (*Figure 11.2*).

Lymph, which consists of water, proteins and cellular waste, may on occasions contain fats, hormones and cell debris. If malignant cells have developed or microorganisms are present in the body they, too, may appear in the lymph.

Lymph flows in one direction only – away from the periphery, towards the heart. This flow is achieved without a pump such as the heart – muscular contraction squeezes the vessels and the 'thoracic pump', which aids venous return, also operates for lymph. Pulsation in adjacent arteries helps to move lymph, as does contraction of the smooth muscle coat of the larger lymph vessels. It follows that sufficient exercise and movement is required for lymph transportation and its return to the circulation.

Lymph Nodes

Structure and location

Lymph nodes are divided by connective-tissue trabeculae (fibrous bands) into segments containing a supporting stroma (network) of reticular fibres (see Chapter 1), blood vessels, lymphocytes (which move between blood and lymph nodes) and phagocytic macrophages (see *Figure 11.3* and Chapter 9). Enclosed within a fibrous capsule, the lymph nodes are kidney-shaped, with a cortex and medulla. They vary from a few millimetres to 2.5 cm in diameter.

Several afferent lymphatic vessels lead into each node, but lymph leaves the node in a single efferent vessel – which ensures that lymph stays in the node long enough for the macrophages and lymphocytes to work on foreign particles in the lymph.

Many hundreds of lymph nodes are located throughout the system and lymph passes through several nodes (see *Figure 11.4*). There are collections of nodes at certain strategic points, which include the deep nodes, found in the abdomen, thorax and neck, and the superficial inguinal, axillary, occipital and cervical nodes. These strategically placed lymph nodes provide points where extraneous particles, such as bacteria, can be intercepted before reaching the blood. When you have a sore throat and 'cold' the cervical nodes enlarge in response to the infection, which is why they can be felt in the neck. People often say that their 'glands are up', but please note lymph nodes are not glands (do not secrete or excrete). If the lymphatic vessel becomes inflamed (lymphangitis) it may be visible, in superficial vessels, as a red streak tracking to the next set of lymph nodes, e.g. from an infected finger to the nodes in the axilla.

Lymph node functions

As part of the surveillance system of the body, lymph nodes 'filter' lymph and remove extraneous particles such as bacteria, viruses and malignant cells. Hopefully, these particles will be destroyed by the macrophages, but if the node is inundated, bacteria can infect the node, which becomes swollen and painful. Malignant cells are likewise destroyed in small numbers, but the lymph nodes can themselves become the site of metastatic cancer (see Chapter 1) – in which case the lymph node is swollen but usually painless. The lymph vessels can also provide a route by which malignancy spreads from the primary site to other organs; for example, breast cancer (see Chapter 20) frequently shows lymphatic spread (see Nursing Practice Application – Lymphoedema).

Lymph nodes provide a site for the proliferation of T and B lymphocytes and the production of antibodies (see Chapter 19).

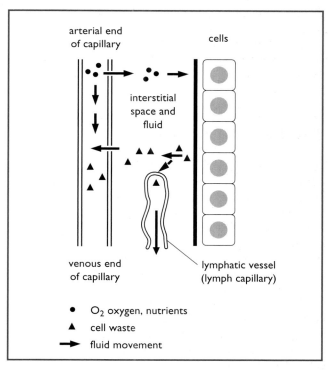

Figure 11.2 Formation of lymph.

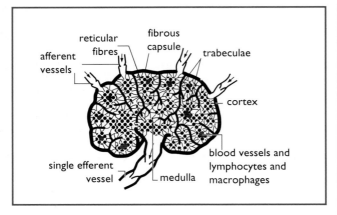

Figure 11.3 A lymph node.

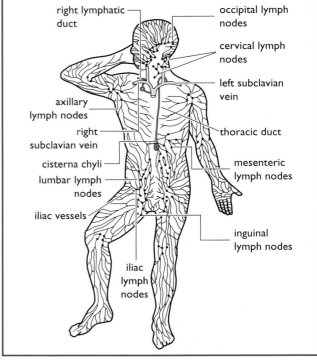

Figure 11.4 Lymphatic system: location of vessels and nodes.

Abnormal Function **Problems: lymph vessels and nodes**

Infectious mononucleosis

Infectious mononucleosis (glandular fever) is caused by the Epstein–Barr virus, which affects the B lymphocytes and causes an increase in atypical lymphocytes in the blood. It occurs mainly in teenagers and young adults (you probably know someone who had it at school or on your nursing course), and is spread through oral (saliva) contact – 'kissing disease'. The affected person may have:

- Lymphadenopathy (enlarged lymph nodes).
- Splenomegaly (enlarged spleen).
- Sore throat.
- Headache.
- Rash.
- Pyrexia (fever).
- Chronic tiredness and lethargy.

There is no specific treatment and only symptomatic measures are available. Most people recover in around 6 weeks, but some individuals can take months to return to normal – particularly difficult during examinations, a new course or job.

Lymphomas

Lymphomas are a group of primary malignant diseases affecting the lymph nodes. One of the most common is Hodgkin's disease, which is characterized by - painless lymph node enlargement, hepatosplenomegaly (enlargement of liver and spleen), pyrexia, weight loss, weakness and anaemia. The prognosis has been greatly improved by developments in diagnosis, by determining the extent of disease (staging) and by selecting the treatment modalities most effective for the stage identified. Treatment is based on radiotherapy, chemotherapy with combinations of cytotoxic drugs, and supportive measures, such as blood transfusion. For a person with very early-stage disease (stage IA) the 5-year survival, with radiotherapy, is over 90% (Edwards *et al.* 1995). Bone-marrow transplants are used in the management of some types/stages of lymphoma, but with varying degrees of success.

The Epstein–Barr virus mentioned earlier, as the cause of infectious mononucleosis, appears to be implicated in the aetiology of Burkitt's lymphoma. This is a form of non-Hodgkin's lymphoma which affects young children in tropical Africa and other areas. Interestingly, many of those affected show a chromosome translocation abnormality (see Chapter 21).

Vessel obstruction

If lymph vessels/nodes become blocked, the interstitial fluid is unable to drain away as lymph. The increased protein content and osmotic pressure of the interstital fluid causes more fluid to collect in the extracellular spaces as lymphoedema (see Chapter 10). Causes of lymphatic obstruction include metastatic malignant cells, damage from surgery or radiotherapy, and parasitic diseases, such as filariasis (infestation with tiny parasitic thread-like worms).

Nursing Practice Application **Lymphoedema**

Lymphoedema is an important health problem, especially for women treated for breast cancer – Logan (1995) puts its prevalence as high as 25–28% in this group. Problems of lymphoedema include: heavy/painful arm; skin tightness; swelling, causing difficulties with clothes and mobility; and further alteration in body image (in addition to breast surgery) with loss of self esteem. According to Kirshbaum (1996), the management of lymphoedema consists of: skin care, compression, massage, advice on activities, exercise and psychological support. It is difficult to assess the effectiveness of treatment and Badger (1996) suggests that limb volume measurements, using fluid displacement, is the only objective assessment.

Other Lymphoid Tissues/Organs

Other collections of lymphoid tissue, similar in structure to the lymph nodes, are found in sites other than the lymphatics. These include the spleen, tonsils, thymus (which has no reticular tissue), bone marrow, liver, small bowel (Peyer's patches) and appendix (*Figure 11.5*).

In common with lymph nodes, these lymphoid accumulations form part of the body defences – they provide sites for lymphocyte proliferation and contain macrophages which remove unwanted material from the blood, but they do not filter lymph. In addition, some structures have other, more specialized roles; for example, the spleen degrades old blood cells. More detailed accounts of some structures can be found in the relevant chapters (thymus, Chapter 8; tonsils, Chapter 12; bowel, Chapter 13; liver, Chapter 14; and Chapter 19 deals with body defences). The spleen will, however, be covered within this chapter.

The spleen

The spleen, situated below the diaphragm in the left upper abdomen, is the most extensive lymphoid organ (see *Figure 11.6*). Some people have more than one – during embryonic development small accessory spleens can form in the peritoneum. However, the normal spleen is a vascular structure weighing around 200 g. It receives blood from the splenic artery and its venous blood drains through the splenic vein into the hepatic portal vein (see Chapter 10). These vessels, plus autonomic nerves and lymphatic vessels, enter or leave the spleen at the hilum. A fibrous capsule encloses the splenic tissue which contains lymphocytes, macrophages, erythrocytes and reticular fibres divided into compartments by trabeculae. Splenic tissue is of two types:

- Red pulp, containing reticular tissue, erythrocytes, macrophages and venous sinuses, which is concerned with phagocytosis and erythrocyte breakdown.
- Areas concerned with immune functions – the white

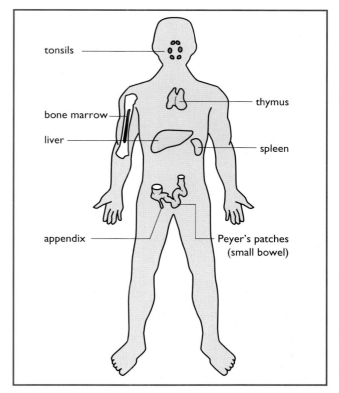

Figure 11.5 Lymphoid tissues: location.

pulp, consisting of reticular fibres which support numerous lymphocytes grouped around branches of the splenic artery.

Sinusoids (see Chapter 10) within the spleen allow the intimate contact between blood and pulp needed to fulfil its roles.

Functions of the spleen

- Filters blood and destroys, by phagocytosis, any micro-organisms, toxins and debris.
- Site of lymphocyte proliferation and antibody production.

- Site of fetal haemopoiesis (peaks between weeks 12–20 of development) and can produce erythrocytes in times of increased need after birth.
- Destruction, by macrophages, of old or defective erythrocytes and platelets (see Chapter 9).
- Storage of erythrocyte breakdown products, e.g. iron, for recycling in new haemoglobin.
- Platelet storage.

- Reservoir for blood – important in some mammals, but is of limited significance in humans.

All this sounds rather impressive, but it is entirely possible to function without a spleen. This is reassuring, as its removal may be required to treat conditions such as haemolytic anaemia or after trauma (see Nursing Practice Application – Splenectomy).

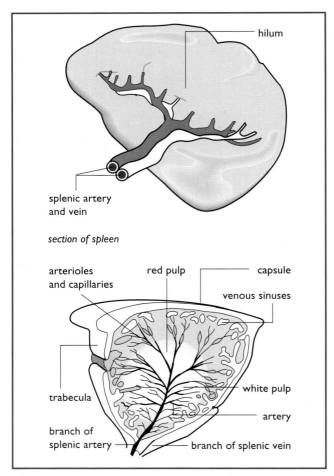

section of spleen

Figure 11.6 Spleen.

Nursing Practice Application **Splenectomy**

The spleen is often damaged during road accidents, with severe internal haemorrhage and shock. After diagnosis, the person's condition is stabilized, e.g. with blood transfusion, before surgical removal of the spleen (splenectomy). Once bleeding has been controlled, the person soon recovers. A common anxiety for the person concerned is 'how can I live without my spleen'? Nurses can anticipate and prevent this anxiety by explaining how macrophages in other areas (marrow and liver) take over and that there is plenty of other lymphoid tissue to cope with its immune role.

Summary/Check List

Introduction.
Lymphatic vessels – lymph capillaries, vessels and main ducts. Lymph – formation and transportation.
Lymph nodes – structure, location, functions.

Lymphatic problems – mononucleosis, lymphomas and obstruction. Nursing Practice Application – lymphoedema.
Lymphoid tissues/organs – structure and location. Spleen. Nursing Practice Application – splenectomy.

Self Test

1 Which of the following statements are true?
  (a) Cardiovascular system function depends upon the lymphatics.
  (b) Lacteals are lymph capillaries of the large bowel.
  (c) Lymphatic vessels from the legs and digestive tract empty into cisterna chyli.
  (d) The thoracic duct empties into the veins in the left side of the neck.

2 Describe the mechanisms involved in lymph transport.
3 Outline the role of lymph nodes.
4 Relate the structure of the spleen to its functions.
5 What would you say to Keith, a health-care assistant, who asks how it is possible to live without a spleen?

Answers

1 a, c, d.
2 See page 249.
3 See page 249.
4 See pages 251–252.
5 Lymphoid tissue in the liver, marrow and other sites take on its role.

References

Badger C (1996) Treating lymphoedema. *Nurs Times* **92**(11): 84–8.
Edwards CRW, Bouchier IAD, Haslett C *et al.* eds (1995) *Davidson's Principles and Practice of Medicine,* 17th edn. Edinburgh: Churchill Livingstone.
Kirshbaum M (1996) Using massage in the relief of lymphoedema. *Prof Nurs* **11**(4):230–2.
Logan V (1995) Incidence and prevalence of lymphoedema: a literature review. *J Clin Nurs* **4**(4):213–19.

Further Reading

Kirshbaum M (1996) *Clinical practice guidelines:The management of lymphoedema after treatment for breast cancer.* London: HMSO.
Staines NA, Brostoff J, James K (1993) *Introducing Immunology,* 2nd edn. London: Mosby.
Williams A (1997) Lymphoedema. *Prof Nurs* **12**(9):645–8

Respiration

Overview

- *Respiratory tract structure and function.*
- *Breathing/ventilation.*
- *Gaseous exchange.*
- *Gas transport.*
- *Control of ventilation.*
- *Respiration and pH regulation.*

Learning Outcomes

After studying Chapter 12 you should be able to:

- Describe the respiratory tract, relating structure to function.
- Explain the mechanism of breathing.
- Describe intrathoracic pressure changes during breathing.
- Use your physiological knowledge in the assessment of breathing.
- Outline factors which influence airflow and pulmonary ventilation.
- Describe lung volumes and pulmonary function tests.
- Define alveolar ventilation.
- Outline the behaviour of gases.
- State the composition of atmospheric, alveolar and expired air.
- Explain how gaseous exchange occurs.
- Explain differences in the oxygen and carbon dioxide content of arterial and venous blood.
- Outline the importance of the ventilation–perfusion relationship.
- Describe oxygen transport.
- Explain the oxygen dissociation curve.
- Describe carbon dioxide transport.
- Explain how ventilation is controlled.
- Outline the effects of altitude and exercise upon ventilation.
- Describe respiratory regulation of blood pH.

Key Words

Expiration – breathing out.

External respiration – gaseous exchange between alveolar air and blood.

Gaseous exchange – the interchange/movement of gases in the body occurring by diffusion through the tissues and by bulk flow.

Inspiration – breathing in.

Internal respiration – gaseous exchange between blood and cells through the interstitial fluid.

Oxygenation – combine or saturate with oxygen.

PCO_2 – the partial pressure (P), measured in kilopascals (kPa), of carbon dioxide (CO_2). $PaCO_2$ = partial pressure of carbon dioxide in arterial blood.

PO_2 – the partial pressure (P), measured in kilopascals (kPa), of oxygen (O_2). PaO_2 = partial pressure of oxygen in arterial blood.

Key Words *cont.*

Pulmonary – relating to the lungs.
Respiration – the processes that supply oxygen to cells for cellular respiration, involving the oxidation of fuel molecules, and removes carbon dioxide.

Ventilation – mechanical process of breathing.

Introduction

The functions of the respiratory tract are to provide oxygen for cellular metabolism of fuel molecules and to remove waste carbon dioxide. This is achieved by **ventilation, external respiration**, gas transport and **internal respiration.** These processes, vital to life, involve close links with the cardiovascular system and the blood (see Chapters 9 and 10). Reduced functional efficiency leads to insufficient oxygen reaching the tissues, a build-up of carbon dioxide in the body and possibly pH disturbance. We survive for only a few minutes if no oxygen reaches the brain.

Respiratory Structures

The respiratory structures include the nasal cavity (nose), pharynx, larynx, trachea, bronchi and smaller bronchioles which warm, moisten and filter air *en route* to the lungs (*Figure 12.1*). **Gaseous exchange** occurs in the system of tiny ducts and alveoli (singular, alveolus) within the two lungs.

Early development

Formation of the respiratory tract commences during the fifth week of embryonic development as a groove in the wall of the pharynx, which soon forms an enclosed tube. This tube divides to form two tubes, one of which becomes the larynx and trachea while the other forms the oesophagus. This close developmental relationship means that failures in oesophageal development can result in an abnormal opening (fistula) between the trachea and the oesophagus (tracheo-oesophageal fistula).

Tiny lung buds, or outgrowths, which form on the lower end of the trachea will eventually develop into the lungs, bronchi and alveoli. The primitive endoderm layer forms the epithelium of the respiratory tract and the pleurae are derived from mesoderm. Before birth the fluid-filled fetal lungs (respiratory movements suck in amniotic fluid) play no part in gaseous exchange. Before lung inflation, which commences with the infant's first breath (takes

some days to complete), all gaseous exchange occurs through the placenta (see Chapter 20). Although the respiratory structures may be formed, a lack of surfactant, (fluid produced by weeks 24–28 that reduces surface tension in the alveoli), in the lungs of preterm babies causes problems with lung inflation and respiratory distress syndrome (pages 263 and 271). The newborn has only 12–16% of adult alveoli numbers and development continues well into childhood.

Nose

Much more than a convenient place to balance your 'specs', the nose is a respiratory structure that also helps to produce speech and contains the olfactory receptors (see Chapter 7). It is the only part of the respiratory tract that you can see externally.

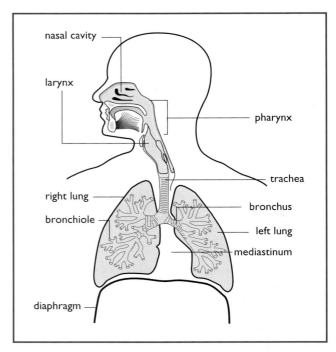

Figure 12.1 Respiratory structures.

The nasal cavity is formed from the bones of the face and skull, the nasal bone and hyaline cartilage [see *Figure 18.10 (b, c)*]. It is irregular in shape and is divided in the midline by a septum formed by the vomer and ethmoid bones (posteriorly) and nasal cartilage (anteriorly). The roof of the cavity consists of the cribriform plate (part of ethmoid bone) and the sphenoid, frontal and nasal bones; its lateral walls are the ethmoid, maxilla and conchae, and inferiorly it is separated from the oral cavity by the hard and soft palates (see Chapter 13).

Air enters through two anterior nares (the nostrils), which open into the nasal vestibule. This part of the nose is lined with skin and contains hairs which trap large foreign particles entering the nose. The internal part of the cavity is lined with highly vascular ciliated columnar epithelium (see *Figure 12.5*) containing many mucus-producing goblet cells. This lining is continuous with the sinuses (see below). Three conchae or turbinate bones project into the nasal cavity, increasing mucosal surface area and causing air turbulence.

The specialized respiratory mucosa warms and moistens air, and smaller particles of dust carrying micro-organisms adhere to the mucus (which contains an antibacterial enzyme – lysozyme) and are later moved by cilia to the pharynx, where the mucus is swallowed or expectorated (coughed up). An irritation or upper respiratory tract infection can cause swelling of the nasal mucosa, resulting in nasal obstruction. Most of us cope by mouth breathing while this lasts, but for small babies, who normally breathe through the nose, it is important to keep this route open.

It is important to note that air entering the respiratory tract through the mouth during mouth breathing has the disadvantage of bypassing the modification and protective functions of the nose.

Another type of epithelium found in the nasal cavity roof is that concerned with olfaction, which is discussed more fully in Chapter 7.

The paranasal sinuses (see Chapter 18), found in the bones of the face and skull, are air-filled. They function in voice production and lighten the skull. They also produce mucus, which drains into the nasal cavity. This close relationship explains why upper respiratory infections can so easily spread to the sinuses (sinusitis).

Also opening into the nasal cavity are the nasolacrimal ducts, which carry secretions from the lacrimal glands (see Chapter 7). Excess tear production during crying results in a 'runny nose'. At the back of the nasal cavity the posterior nares (*Figure 12.2*) communicate with the pharynx.

The pharynx

The pharynx runs from the base of the skull to the level of the lower cervical vertebrae. It is divided into three parts: the nasopharynx (behind the nose), oropharynx (behind the mouth) and laryngopharynx, which leads into the larynx and oesophagus (*Figure 12.2*). The nasopharynx is exclusively respiratory, but the two lower parts provide a common passageway for air and the food/fluids which enter the oesophagus during swallowing (see page 259 and Chapter 13).

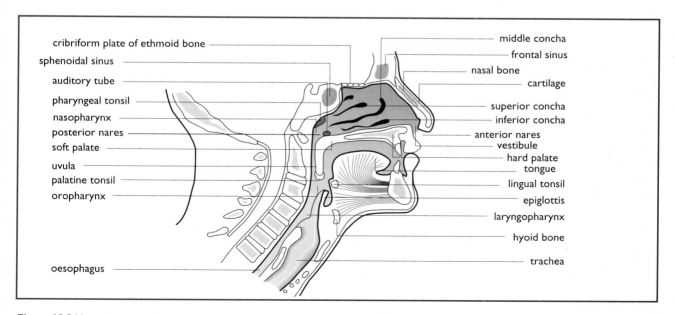

Figure 12.2 Upper respiratory tract.

The pharynx receives blood via several vessels, including the pharyngeal artery and branches from the facial and laryngeal arteries. Venous blood returns to the heart by a pharyngeal plexus and the internal jugular vein.

The pharynx has constrictor muscles concerned with swallowing, which are mostly innervated by the vagus and glossopharyngeal nerves, a fibrous layer and an epithelial lining, which changes along its length. The complexity of the pharynx means that many problems may occur which affect function, e.g. difficult swallowing (dysphagia).

The nasopharyngeal portion is lined with respiratory mucosa, which continues to warm, moisten and filter the air. The oropharynx and laryngopharynx are lined with stratified squamous epithelium (see Chapter 1) continuous with that of the oesophagus. This variation protects the tissues from friction caused by food.

Nasopharynx

The nasopharynx is the uppermost part of the pharynx and lies above the muscular soft palate. The pharyngotympanic (auditory) tubes open into the nasopharynx (see Chapter 7). These communicate with the middle ear and equalize pressure either side of the tympanic membrane during yawning and swallowing. They also provide a route by which respiratory infections spread to the middle ear to cause otitis media. The pharyngeal tonsils (called adenoids when enlarged), which are made up of lymphoid tissue, are located on the posterior wall of the nasopharynx; they provide defence against some micro-organisms entering the respiratory tract (see Chapters 11 and 19). Enlargement of the pharyngeal tonsils (adenoids) caused by to chronic infection leads to obstruction of the nasal airway and mouth breathing. During swallowing the soft palate and uvula (the small fleshy body that hangs down from the soft palate) move upwards to isolate the nasopharynx and stop food entering it.

Oropharynx

The oropharynx lies behind the mouth and extends from the soft palate to the hyoid bone (see *Figures 12.2* and *12.3*). As part of both respiratory and digestive tracts it conveys air and food. Two further paired masses of lymphoid tissue are located within the oropharynx: the palatine tonsils, in folds formed by the soft palate and oropharynx, and the lingual tonsils at the base of the tongue.

Laryngopharynx

The last part of the pharynx extends from the hyoid bone to the level at which the respiratory and digestive tracts separate. The next part of the respiratory tract is the larynx, and the laryngopharynx becomes the oesophagus, which conveys food to the stomach. When we swallow, the larynx is closed off to ensure that food does not 'go the wrong way' and enter the respiratory tract.

Larynx

The larynx lies anterior to the laryngopharynx and opens into the trachea; it extends between the third and sixth cervical vertebrae. Androgens (male hormones) released during puberty cause the male larynx to enlarge. This gives rise to a deeper voice and the 'Adam's apple' prominence on the throat. The larynx provides an open airway between the pharynx and trachea, directs food into the oesophagus during swallowing and allows us to produce sounds.

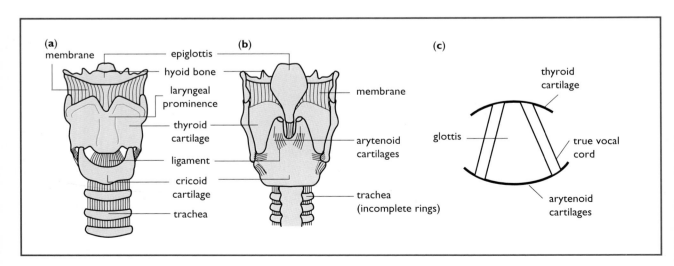

Figure 12.3 Larynx. (**a**) Anterior view; (**b**) posterior view; (**c**) vocal cords.

Arterial blood is supplied by laryngeal branches of the thyroid arteries; venous blood drains through laryngeal veins into the thyroid veins and internal jugular veins.

Innervation of the larynx is through the superior and recurrent laryngeal nerves. These supply parasympathetic sensory and motor fibres from the vagus and accessory nerves to the epithelium and laryngeal muscles. Sympathetic fibres from the cervical ganglion supply the larynx.

The larynx is formed from cartilages joined by ligaments and membranes. The main laryngeal cartilages, which also provide attachment for several muscles, are the epiglottis (elastic cartilage) and the thyroid, cricoid and two arytenoid cartilages, which are hyaline cartilage (*Figure 12.3*). The thyroid cartilage consists of two curved portions which fuse in the midline to form the laryngeal prominence, or Adam's apple. Two small arytenoid cartilages form the lateral and posterior walls and anchor the vocal cords within the interior of the larynx. Below the thyroid cartilage is the complete ring of the cricoid cartilage, which joins the larynx to the trachea.

The leaf-shaped epiglottis, joined to the upper border of the thyroid cartilage, is involved in the mechanism which protects the respiratory tract from food; it contains some taste buds (see Chapter 7).

Swallowing

Food entering the pharynx initiates a series of reflex mechanisms operated by neurones of a swallowing centre in the medulla oblongata: the nasopharynx is closed off by the soft palate, a sphincter closes the inlet into the larynx, breathing stops while swallowing is in progress and an upward movement of the larynx (you can confirm this by feeling your throat while drinking) causes the epiglottis to cover the opening. If these mechanisms fail to operate properly, such as when someone makes you laugh and breathe in while eating, and food does 'go the wrong way' the cough reflex (see page 260) expels the food and usually prevents it from entering the respiratory passages (see Nursing Practice Application – Airway maintenance). Further discussion about swallowing can be found in Chapter 13.

Nursing Practice Application **Airway maintenance**

Obviously, an open airway is vital to life, and we have already discussed ways in which this is achieved, e.g. the epiglottis. In situations which include altered consciousness, with loss of swallowing and cough reflexes, there is risk of airway obstruction if the tongue falls back or food/debris enters the larynx. Patient assessment should include:

- Observing colour and respiration.
- Positioning (*Figure 12.4(a)*) to minimize risk of inhaling vomit – especially in an emergency situation.
- Ensuring that people without the swallowing/cough reflexes are never given anything orally.
- Provision of equipment e.g. plastic airways and suction.

In certain situations the Heimlich manoeuvre, a first-aid measure, can be used to clear the larynx or trachea of a foreign body such as food. Compression over the upper abdomen causes the diaphragm to rise and the resulting expulsion of air from the lungs hopefully dislodges the obstruction (*Figure 12.4(b)*).

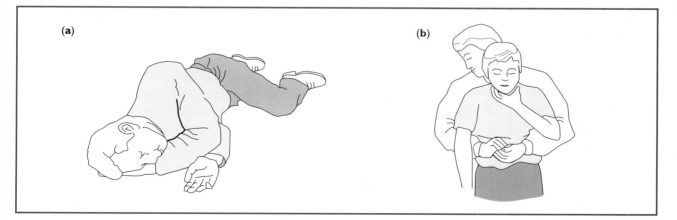

Figure 12.4 Maintaining an airway. (**a**) A position for an unconscious person; (**b**) Heimlich manoeuvre.

Lining and vocal cords

The upper part of the larynx is lined with stratified squamous epithelium (see Chapter 1) and the lower part with ciliated columnar epithelium (*Figure 12.5*), which warms, moistens and filters the air. Mucus and debris are moved upwards by the cilia for expulsion. The two sets of vocal ligaments which join the laryngeal cartilages together are modified to form the vocal cords stretching from front to back inside the larynx. The vestibular folds or false vocal cords close to protect the larynx during swallowing and below these are the vocal folds or true vocal cords, which are concerned with sound production. The true vocal cords are separated by a gap known as the glottis, which allows air to pass through (see *Figure 12.3*).

Voice production

Contraction and relaxation of the laryngeal muscles move the arytenoid cartilages, which alter the position and tension of the true vocal cords, either closer together, narrowing the glottis, or further apart, increasing the opening. Sound is produced as expired air is forced through the larynx to vibrate the vocal cords. The pitch/frequency of the voice changes with the length (tension) of the vocal cords and loudness depends on the force of air moving through the glottis. Males have deeper voices because their vocal cords become longer and thicker during their laryngeal enlargement. Turning sounds into recognizable speech is achieved by the lips, teeth, tongue, soft palate and pharynx (try talking clearly without moving your tongue or lips). The paranasal sinuses, nasal and oral cavities, and pharynx give the voice resonance, which explains why a 'cold' and blocked sinuses make your voice dull and flat. Voice changes result from a variety of causes, including laryngitis, laryngeal tumours and damage to the recurrent laryngeal nerve during thyroid surgery.

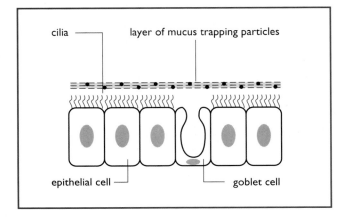

Figure 12.5 Epithelial lining of respiratory passages.

cilia

layer of mucus trapping particles

epithelial cell

goblet cell

Valsalva's manoeuvre

In certain situations, such as straining to defecate when constipated or when lifting heavy weights, air is forced out of the respiratory passages against a closed glottis. This increases pressure in the thorax and abdomen, and reduces venous return to the heart.

Trachea

The trachea (windpipe) extends from the larynx to the level of the fifth thoracic vertebra. Here, it bifurcates (divides) into the right and left main bronchi [*Figure 12.6(a)*]. Around 12 cm in length, the trachea passes through the mediastinum anterior to the oesophagus. The trachea is formed by 15–20 C-shaped rings of hyaline cartilage, which keep it patent, smooth muscle and fibro-elastic tissue. The cartilage rings are open at the back to allow oesophageal distension during swallowing.

The lining mucosa is ciliated columnar epithelium containing numerous mucus-secreting goblet cells. In common with the other respiratory structures, the tracheal mucosa warms, moistens and filters the air. The mucus is moved upwards by the beating cilia, together with any particles it has trapped, to be swallowed or expectorated.

The trachea receives blood from the thyroid arteries and its venous blood drains into the brachiocephalic veins. It is innervated by parasympathetic sensory and motor fibres of the vagus nerve (recurrent laryngeal nerve) and sympathetic fibres from the cervical ganglion.

Cough and sneeze

Coughing and sneezing are protective mechanisms that enable the respiratory tract to expel excess mucus and foreign bodies. Irritation of the tracheal mucosa stimulates a cough, which is a forced **expiration** of air from the mouth. Pressure build-up is achieved by a closed glottis during the start of the expiration. Once released, the air leaves at great speed. Sneezing is similar, but the forced expiration is through the nose and mouth.

Bronchial tree and alveoli

At the level of the fifth thoracic vertebra the trachea divides into the right and left primary (main) bronchi. Each primary bronchus runs through the mediastinum to enter the lung at the hilum. The primary bronchus on the right is shorter, wider and slopes more vertically than the one on the left. This arrangement means that foreign bodies which 'slip past' the elaborate defences already discussed are most often inhaled into the right primary bronchus (see page 262). After entering the lungs the primary bronchi divide into smaller secondary (lobar) bronchi (see *Figure 12.7*) – two on the left and three on the right. These secondary bronchi divide into tertiary (segmental) bronchi, which eventually branch to become tiny airways known as bronchioles. The bronchioles themselves divide to become terminal bronchioles, respiratory bronchioles and the minute alveolar ducts leading into the alveoli.

The larger bronchi are similar in structure to the trachea, with cartilage to keep the airways open, a smooth muscle layer and a ciliated mucous membrane lining, which traps small particles in the mucus (moved upwards by mucociliary clearance – like an escalator in a store) and warms and moistens air. This structural arrangement means that no gaseous exchange occurs here – the bronchi with the nasal cavities, pharynx, larynx and trachea form the conducting airways. This area, with a volume of around 150 ml, constitutes the anatomical dead space, so-called because none of this air takes part in gaseous exchange. The various modifications to structure occurring as the airways divide and become smaller reflect the change in function from conduction to gas exchange:

- Cartilage thins and is absent from the bronchioles. Without the rigid cartilage the diameter of the airways can be altered by changes in smooth muscle tone controlled by the autonomic nerves. Sympathetic stimulation of the β_2 receptors (see Chapter 6) relaxes the muscle to cause bronchodilation. Parasympathetic activity has the opposite effect and causes bronchoconstriction (see *Table 12.1*).
- The ciliated columnar epithelium becomes a single layer of squamous epithelium which forms part of the respiratory membrane found in the respiratory bronchioles, alveolar ducts and alveoli. This area of the bronchial tree, structurally adapted for gaseous exchange, is known as the respiratory zone.

Nursing Practice Application **Tracheostomy**

An opening in the trachea known as a tracheostomy [*Figure 12.6(b)*] may be made for a variety of reasons, including:

- Long-term intermittent positive pressure respiration/ventilation (IPPR/V) using a machine (ventilator) which delivers gases to the patient to inflate the lungs. Assisted ventilation is used in situations where breathing is inadequate or is not occurring spontaneously, e.g. after severe head injury. Assisted ventilation can be achieved by tracheostomy or through an endotracheal tube passed through the mouth.
- To suction copious viscous secretions.
- To improve ventilation by reducing anatomical dead space (see above).
- Following laryngectomy (removal of larynx.
- Where there is upper airway obstruction or vocal cord paralysis.

A plastic or metal tube inserted into the tracheal incision keeps it patent. Tracheostomy does, however, have drawbacks. These include: easy access for micro-organisms, communication difficulties, as speech is affected; and air no longer passes through the upper airways for warming and humidification.

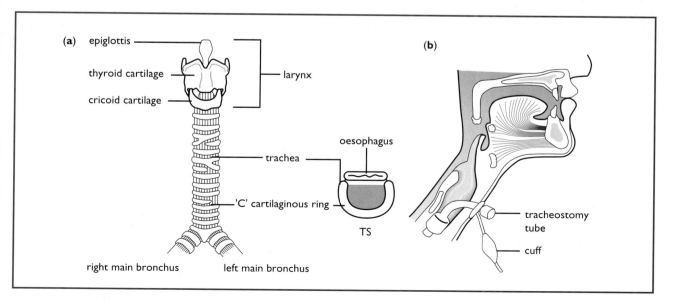

Figure 12.6 (a) Trachea; **(b)** tracheostomy.

Nursing Practice Application **Inhalers and nebulizers (see *Table 12.1*)**

Many people with respiratory conditions such as asthma, causing bronchoconstriction, need bronchodilator drugs, e.g. salbutamol (adrenergic beta $_2$ receptor agonist) or ipratropium bromide (muscarinic (M_1, M_2, M_3) receptor antagonist – anticholinergic). These drugs are most effective when administered via an inhaler or nebulizer because they are delivered to the problem area.

The major nursing responsibility is to ensure that the individual has sufficient knowledge to use both drug and appliance safely and efficiently – proper use of the inhaler/nebulizer is vital for good asthma control. Children and other individuals who find inhaler technique difficult can overcome the problems by using nebulizers or various spacer devices. Gleeson (1995) stresses the need to teach children about inhaler technique directly, rather than through parents.

A programme of drug education should include: how the drug works, use of appliance, correct dosage, associated problems/side-effects, appliance care and drug storage.

Healthier Living **Preventing the inhalation of foreign bodies in young children**

Previously we mentioned that inhaled foreign bodies usually lodge in the right main bronchus (see page 260). Young children are at particular risk – it is very easy for small particles to be aspirated (breathed in). For this reason young children should not be allowed access to food such as peanuts, and toys should be suitable for their age group and meet the most stringent safety standards.

Table 12.1 Factors affecting bronchial muscle tone	
Factor	**Effects**
Bronchodilation	
(i) Sympathetic stimulation of beta$_2$ receptors:	Relaxes bronchial muscle, causes bronchodilation and increased air entry

a. Exercise
   b. Drugs – Salbutamol
      (beta$_2$ agonist)
        – Adrenaline
   c. 'Fight or flight' response	

(ii) Inhibition of parasympathetic nerves by anticholinergics:	Prevents parasympathetic effects of muscle contraction and bronchoconstriction

a. Drugs – Ipratropium
      bromide
      (muscarinic antagonist)	

Bronchoconstriction	

(i) Parasympathetic activity:
   a. During rest
   b. Irritant chemicals, e.g.
     cigarette smoke
   c. Allergic conditions, e.g.
     some types of asthma
   d. Infections
	Contracts bronchial muscle, causes bronchoconstriction and reduces air entry

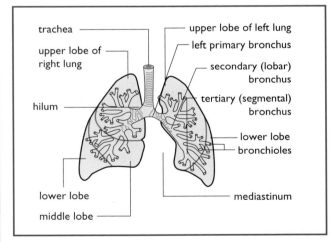

Figure 12.7 Bronchial tree.

Table 12.1 Factors affecting bronchial muscle tone.

Arterial blood reaches the bronchial tree through bronchial arteries, which branch from the aorta to provide a good blood supply. The bronchial veins drain venous blood into the azygos veins, which empty into the superior vena cava.

Alveoli (detail)

The many millions of alveoli which cluster around the respiratory bronchioles and alveolar ducts form air-filled cavities within the lungs [*Figure 12.8(a)*]. The alveoli are in very close contact with the networks of **pulmonary** capillaries (see Chapter 10). The capillary and alveolar walls with their basement membranes form the extremely thin (less than 0.5 μm thick) respiratory membrane [see *Figure 12.8(b)*] which permits the diffusion of gases between alveolar air and blood – external respiration. The branching structure of the respiratory zone and the many clusters of alveoli result in a very large surface area available for gas exchange (in adults the alveolar surface is huge – perhaps as big as a tennis court).

The alveolar wall contains three cell types:
- Phagocytic macrophages (see Chapters 1, 9 and 19) which engulf and destroy micro-organisms and debris reaching the alveoli.

- Squamous epithelial cells (type I), which form the wall.
- Cuboidal epithelial cells (type II), which secrete a phospholipid fluid known as surfactant. Surfactant moistens the respiratory membrane, reduces surface tension and prevents alveolar collapse, and is essential for efficient gaseous exchange (see page 271).

Lungs

The two lungs almost completely fill the thoracic cavity during life. Lying one on each side, they are separated by the mediastinum, a space containing the heart, vessels, trachea, bronchi, oesophagus and other structures (see *Figure 12.9*).

Each cone-shaped lung has:
- A narrow apex level with the clavicle.
- A convex costal surface which comprises the anterior, lateral and posterior surfaces in contact with the ribs, intercostal muscles and costal cartilages.
- The concave base which sits upon the diaphragm.
- A hilum or depression on its medial surface where the primary bronchi, nerves, blood vessels and a very good supply of lymphatics enter or leave.

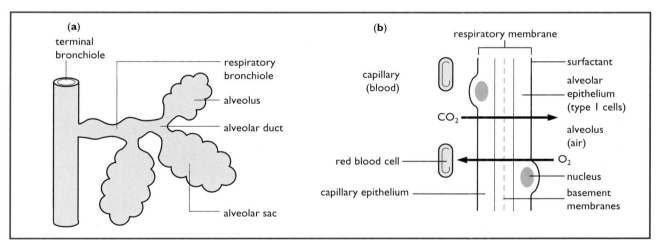

Figure 12.8 (**a**) Alveoli; (**b**) alveolar–capillary membrane. For clarity, cuboidal (type II) cells and macrophages are not shown.

Nursing Practice Application **Surfactant administration**

Preterm infants who have immature lungs and lack surfactant may develop respiratory distress syndrome (hyaline membrane disease) caused by lack of lung compliance – 'stiff lungs' and alveolar collapse. Their management includes assisted ventilation and intratracheal administration of surfactant preparations. Nurses caring for these infants should be aware of the need to readjust administered oxygen levels, as respiratory function improves after treatment with surfactant, to prevent retrolental fibroplasia (fibrosis behind the lens of the eye) – a complication of too much oxygen.

Special Focus **Tuberculosis (TB)**

During the early 1980s TB was thought by many to be a disease of the past or at least under control, but in fact it still affects millions of people and kills more people worldwide than any other single agent. According to the World Health Organization, TB is a 'global emergency'. In developed economies new multidrug-resistant strains have emerged to infect people who are immunocompromised, e.g. those with human immunodeficiency virus, and people enduring poor social conditions, such as those living rough or in night shelters for the homeless.

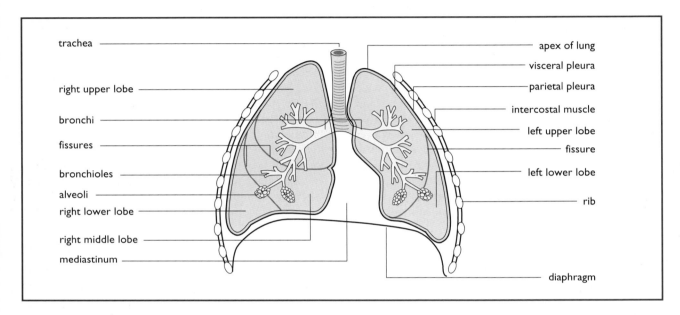

Figure 12.9 Lungs and pleura.

The lungs are divided by fissures into lobes. The left lung, which has to make room for the heart, has two lobes (upper and lower) and the right lung has three (upper, middle and lower lobes). Each lobe is further subdivided into smaller bronchopulmonary segments. As the main bronchus enters the lung it divides to form the smaller branches within the lobes and segments. Lung tissue has a connective framework which helps to prevent the spread of infection, e.g. tuberculosis, and supports the airways, alveoli and pulmonary capillaries. Being filled with air, it is spongy, stretchy (elastic) and weighs very little.

Lung tissue receives its arterial supply from the bronchial arteries and venous blood leaves through bronchial veins (see pages 261 and 263). This, however, is only part of the story; blood for **oxygenation** arrives from the right side of the heart through the pulmonary artery and, after gaseous exchange, returns to the left side of the heart through four pulmonary veins (see Chapter 10).

The lungs are innervated by parasympathetic fibres of the vagus nerves which are concerned with bronchoconstriction and mucus secretion, and sympathetic fibres which initiate bronchodilation (see *Table 12.1*).

Pleura

The pleurae or double serous membranes (see Chapter 1) form three closed compartments, one for each lung and one for the mediastinal contents. The visceral pleura (inside layer) covers the lungs and the parietal pleura (outside layer) lines the thoracic cavity and mediastinum. Between the two layers is a potential space lubricated by pleural fluid, a serous secretion produced by the pleura. Pleural fluid reduces friction as the lungs move during breathing and causes the two layers of the pleura to adhere together by surface tension, helping to create a slight negative pressure within the pleural space (see page 267). Consequently the pleurae hold the lungs to the chest wall. This is vital to lung function as is means that lung inflation and deflation can occur as the chest wall moves.

Nursing Practice Application Cystic fibrosis

Cystic fibrosis (CF) is an autosomal recessive genetic condition affecting 1 in 2000 live Caucasian births. The inheritance of the faulty gene affects chloride transport across the plasma membrane of some secretory cells, resulting in the production of thick mucus/secretions. In the respiratory tract the thick mucus blocks the small airways, leading to infection and eventual respiratory failure. Other secretory cells affected include those in the pancreas which produce digestive enzymes and salivary glands, causing problems with digestion (see Chapter 13); also affected are the sweat glands, which produce sweat containing high levels of sodium and chloride. A screening blood test is available for new-

borns, and with early diagnosis treatment can be started before lung damage occurs. Management includes: antibiotics, vigorous chest physiotherapy, mucolytic preparations via nebulizer to thin the mucus and aid its expulsion from the respiratory tract, pancreatic enzymes, nutritional support and heart–lung transplants where lung changes have caused cardiac failure. About 4–5% of the population carry the defective recessive gene (you need to inherit the faulty gene from both parents to have CF) and testing for carrier status is available. Antenatal testing and diagnosis is also in use (see Chapter 21). Although the availability of testing provides individuals with information, which they can use to make informed

choices about having children or terminating affected pregnancies, it does not offer a cure. Research in progress aimed at a cure includes ways of introducing the normal gene into the lungs ('gene therapy'), e.g. embedded in inactivated 'cold' viruses or in inhaled powders, and ways of improving chloride transport. Without a cure, however, the children, adolescents and young adults affected who now live longer, with newer therapies, must overcome difficulties, including educational problems. An article by Dyer and Morais (1996) stresses that children with CF need support, and specialist nurses can help by providing the education which allows teachers and schools to offer this support.

Abnormal Function Problems with the pleura

Mesothelioma
A rare malignancy of the pleura with a very poor prognosis. It is usually linked with exposure to asbestos and also affects the peritoneum.

Pleurisy
Pleural inflammation, or pleurisy, can reduce pleural fluid, which results in friction between the two layers. A 'pleural rub'

may be heard with a stethoscope when the person is asked to take a deep breath. The affected individual suffers sharp, stabbing pain when breathing, which inevitably leads to a reluctance to breathe normally. Shallow breathing is inefficient (see Table 12.3). Adequate pain relief is essential if the characteristic shallow respirations are to be replaced by breathing of normal depth

which ensures adequate alveolar ventilation (see pages 272–273).

Pleural effusion
Excess pleural fluid production or effusion can prevent normal lung expansion and cause dyspnoea (difficult respiration), and may need to be removed (see Nursing Practice Application).

Nursing Practice Application Pleural/chest aspiration (thoracocentesis)

Pleural effusion may result from a variety of causes, e.g. pulmonary infarction, malignancy, pneumonia or heart failure. Fluid may be removed for diagnosis or to ease dyspnoea and discomfort. The fluid is withdrawn by the medical officer, using a syringe with the needle inserted

between the ribs. When caring for a person requiring this procedure it is important that the nurse provides an explanation and information which meets the patient's needs and reduces anxiety. They should explain what is done, stressing that local anaesthetic is used and that

the nurse will stay throughout. The position (see Figure 12.10) should be explained, and it is important that the person should say if they need to cough or move during the aspiration, as this may cause the needle to penetrate the visceral pleura and lungs.

Environmental and occupational hazards to respiratory health

Dust, fumes and chemicals present in the workplace or environment are implicated in the development of chronic respiratory disease (asthma, bronchial tumours, chronic obstructive pulmonary diseases (COPD, page 267), pneu-

moconioses and fibrosis). Noxious agents include asbestos, coal dust, arsenic, nickel, chromium, vinyl chloride, silica, cadmium, radiation and vegetable matter, e.g. wood dust, dust from mouldy hay or mushroom compost. Atmospheric pollution also has some influence – many chronic respiratory conditions are more common in industrial and urban areas.

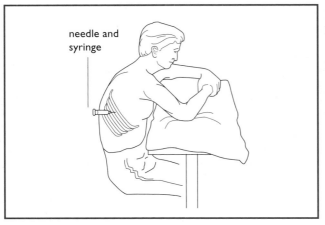

Figure 12.10 Pleural aspiration.

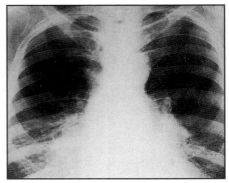

Figure 12.11
Bronchial–alveolar cell carcinoma (Studdy PR, James G (1993) *A Colour Atlas of Respiratory Diseases*, 2nd edn. Wolfe Medical Publications, Ltd. Reprinted with permission.)

Nursing Practice Application Sputum

Sputum (phlegm) is excess mucus produced when respiratory disease affects the goblet cells and mucociliary clearance. People with sputum should be encouraged to expectorate; they need privacy, suitable clean containers and a supply of tissues. Care should also include oral hygiene and a fluid intake sufficient to prevent the sputum becoming thick and sticky. Physiotherapy that assists the person to cough and expectorate is reinforced by the nurse. Change of position and mobilization will help expectoration. If the person has pain on moving or coughing, e.g. after surgery, it is essential that pain relief is adequate. Various inhalations and mucolytic substances may help to loosen the sputum and ease discomfort. When the sputum is infected (purulent) an appropriate antimicrobial drug will be prescribed after microbiological examination of the sputum.

Sputum is an infection risk – both sputum and tissues should be handled with care and disposed of correctly (suitably bagged before placing in the hazardous waste sack), and staff should protect themselves with disposable gloves, plastic aprons and masks as appropriate.

Observations of sputum include: amount, odour, viscosity and colour, which may be white mucoid, yellow/green if purulent, frothy in left heart failure (see Chapter 10), 'rusty' with altered blood in pneumonia, or containing fresh blood with pulmonary embolus or tumour. Blood-stained sputum is known as haemoptysis. Nurses should also assess pain associated with expectoration, type of cough and how tired the person is becoming (see also Breathing assessment, page 270).

Person-Centred Study Sid

Sid lives alone in an inner–city neighbourhood where he rents a ground floor room. Before retiring he worked as a kitchen porter in a large hotel. A heavy smoker for the last 40 years, Sid has always had a cough with sputum but in the last year he has noticed that his cough is more persistent, the sputum is green on occasions and he gets short of breath walking from the shops.

His GP refers him to the chest clinic at a nearby hospital, where a diagnosis of COPD is confirmed.

It is important to note that many people with chronic airways limitation have a combination of conditions, e.g. chronic bronchitis, emphysema (see page 267) and asthma. The following regimen is planned with Sid which aims to improve quality of life, minimize hospital admissions for acute exacerbations and postpone the development of cor pulmonale (see Chapter 10) or respiratory failure:

• Drugs – inhaled salbutamol (see *Table 12.1*) is prescribed and antimicrobial drugs for the infection; he is asked to see his GP whenever his sputum looks infected (see above).
• He is advised to stop smoking (see Healthier Living, page 267).

• The physiotherapist attached to the clinic teaches Sid how to maximize respiratory efforts to improve gaseous exchange and to expectorate sputum to reduce the risk of infection.
• A specialist nurse sees Sid at the clinic and again at home to ensure that he understands his condition and regimen. Respiratory health workers have been found to be effective in improving a person's knowledge of their condition and treatments (Cockcroft *et al.* 1986).
• Social services are asked to assess Sid's needs and to provide long-term community support.

Healthier Living Smoking and the respiratory tract

Smoking is estimated to cause over 111 000 premature deaths in the UK every year (HEA, 1993). Most of these deaths are caused by bronchial tumours (*Figure 12.11*), chronic airways limitation (including COPD) and heart disease (see Chapter 10). Apart from the deaths, there is increased morbidity (disease) from heart, respiratory and peripheral vascular disease. In addition, smoking during pregnancy is associated with low birthweight; exposing infants to cigarette smoke increases the risk for sudden infant death syndrome (SIDS) and later exposure is implicated in the development of childhood asthma and bronchitis.

Carcinogens (see Chapter 1) in tobacco are known to cause malignant changes in the bronchi/lungs. People smoking 25 cigarettes/day are 25 times more likely to develop lung cancer than non-smokers (HEA, 1993). Bronchial cancer is the commonest malignancy in men and is increasingly common in women (commonest cancer death for women in

Scotland and second commonest behind breast cancer in England and Wales).

Unfortunately many bronchial tumours are diagnosed too late for effective surgery and the average life expectancy following diagnosis is less than a year. Cytotoxic drugs and radiotherapy may be used to treat certain tumours and provide palliation in others.

Smoking also causes changes in the respiratory tract, leading to chronic bronchitis and emphysema (over-distension and destruction of alveoli), which are both types of COPD. The chemicals in the smoke cause increased goblet-cell activity, increased mucus and reduction of ciliary action. The excess mucus, inflammation, mucosal oedema and fibrosis results in narrowing and blockage of small airways, disruption of alveoli and eventual reduction in the surface area available for gaseous exchange (see Person-Centred Study – Sid, page 266).

There is no doubt that smoking is a health hazard to those who smoke and

may well threaten the health of people with whom they live or work (passive smoking). Nurses are ideally placed to provide information and advice about smoking. However, this help will only be effective if nurses have a sound knowledge of the pathophysiological effects of smoking and the necessary communication skills to 'sell the idea'. In an evaluation of the Health Education Council (now the Health Education Authority) package (Nurses and Smoking, 1983) it was found that both these aspects were lacking (Haverty *et al.* 1987).

The Health of the Nation (DoH, 1992) sets various targets for the reduction of lung cancer and heart disease, and reducing the prevalence of cigarette smoking features heavily in the strategies for achieving these targets. Various organizations disseminate information about the effects of smoking and offer advise to health professionals and people wanting to give up (see page 286 for addresses).

Breathing/Ventilation

Breathing (ventilation) is the mechanical process by which air moves in and out of the lungs. It consists of inspiration (breathing in), where the lungs expand to fill with air, and expiration (breathing out), where they recoil to expel air. Breathing depends upon pressure changes in the lungs and pleural space, functioning of the diaphragm and intercostal muscles (respiratory muscles – see Chapter 18), the elasticity of the lungs and airway resistance.

Intrathoracic pressures

Air pressure within the lungs/alveoli will always equilibrate (to maintain equilibrium) with atmospheric pressure, which is 101 kPa (760 mmHg) at sea level. As the lung expands during inspiration its volume increases. This causes a pressure drop and air moves into the lungs to equalize the pressure. Movement of air into the lungs depends on Boyle's law, which states that at a constant temperature the pressure of a gas is inversely proportional to its volume.

Intrapleural pressure is 0.5 kPa (4 mmHg) less than alveolar pressure. This negative pressure, produced by opposing forces, ensures that the lungs adhere to the thoracic walls and do not collapse like deflated balloons (see *Figure 12.12*). The negative pressure also creates the 'respiratory' pump which assists venous return to the heart (see Chapter 10).

Loss of the 0.5 kPa difference between intrapleural and alveolar pressure, e.g. if air enters the chest through a wound, results in serious consequences, including lung collapse, impaired gas exchange and in some cases mediastinal shift and cardiovascular problems. This situation, where air is present in the thoracic cavity, is known as a pneumothorax, or haemothorax if there is also blood. It occurs if the chest wall is damaged, e.g stab wounds, during chest surgery and with spontaneous rupture of diseased lung into the pleural space. It is usually treated by the insertion of a drain which allows air and fluid to escape from the thoracic cavity but prevents more air entering (see Nursing Practice Application, page 269).

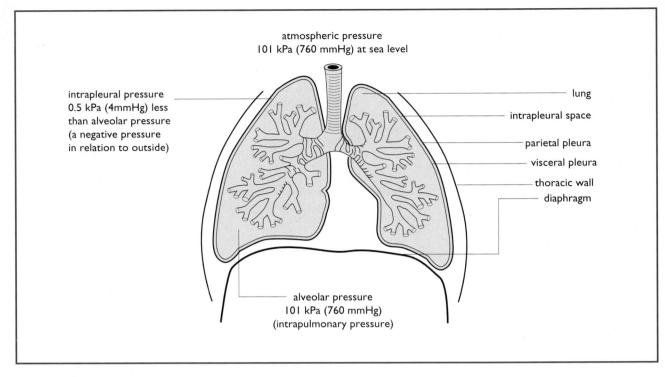

atmospheric pressure
101 kPa (760 mmHg) at sea level

intrapleural pressure
0.5 kPa (4mmHg) less
than alveolar pressure
(a negative pressure
in relation to outside)

lung

intrapleural space

parietal pleura

visceral pleura

thoracic wall

diaphragm

alveolar pressure
101 kPa (760 mmHg)
(intrapulmonary pressure)

Figure 12.12 Intrathoracic pressures.

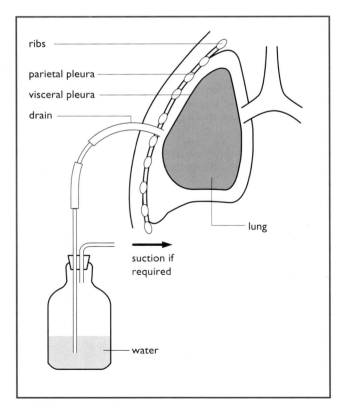

ribs

parietal pleura

visceral pleura

drain

lung

suction if
required

water

Figure 12.13 Underwater seal drainage.

Inspiration

Inspiration is an active process in which the volume of the thorax is increased by the contraction of the respiratory muscles (*Figure 12.14*). As the lungs expand the pressure falls (remember Boyle's law) and air moves in to equalize the alveolar and atmospheric pressures. Intrapleural pressure becomes even more negative as alveolar pressure falls and the elastic lungs expand.

During inspiration the large, dome-shaped diaphragm, which separates the thorax from the abdomen, flattens and moves down. The diaphragm is the most important inspiratory muscle, but the external intercostal muscles also contract to elevate the ribs. Contraction of these muscles increases chest volume laterally, vertically and from front to back.

When inspiration is deep or forced, such as during exertion, we use accessory muscles to lift the ribs and maximize thoracic capacity. Use of accessory muscles, e.g. sternocleidomastoid, scalenes, back muscles and pectorals (see Chapter 18), is seen in people with chronic respiratory disease as they strive to increase their air entry (see Person-Centred Study – Sid, and page 266).

During chest expansion the lungs, which you will remember are attached to the chest wall by the pleurae, stretch by virtue of their elasticity.

Nursing Practice Application **Pneumothorax/haemothorax**

The development of a pneumothorax requires prompt diagnosis and the insertion of a drain (either with a one way valve or a water seal) into the pleural space. This is obviously planned for during chest surgery, but in the case of trauma will be performed as an emergency measure.

Water seal drains – drainage tubes leading from the chest wall – are placed under water to prevent air being sucked into the chest; they are sometimes attached to low-power suction (*Figure 12.13*) and may use one, two or three bottles. Many commercially produced dis-

posable drainage systems are also available. This arrangement allows air/blood/fluid to drain out and the lung to re-expand.

The level of fluid should fluctuate with breathing. If this does not occur it may indicate that the drain is no longer patent, but could be caused by lung re-expansion. Nurses should ensure that chest drain clamps are always available for use if the closed system is breached, e.g. tubing becomes disconnected from drain. This prevents air being sucked in while the system is reconnected.

It is also very important that the water seal bottle is kept below chest level to avoid fluid being 'sucked back' into the pleural space on inspiration.

As well as these factors, the nurse should be alert for changes in condition such as sudden dyspnoea or pain. Assessment will include: respiration, colour, pulse, blood pressure and pain. Frequency of observations will depend upon the reason for chest drainage and the condition of the person.

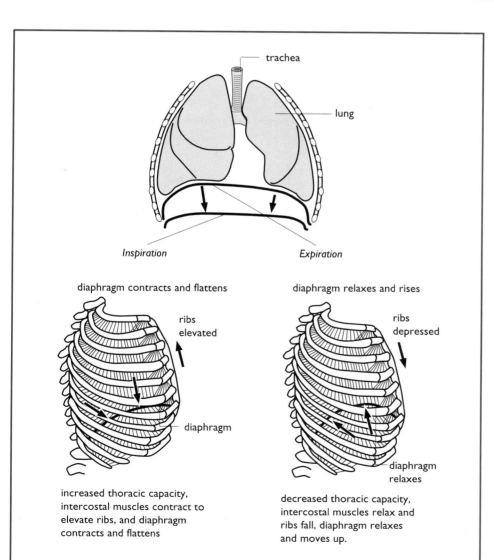

Figure 12.14 Inspiration and expiration.

Nursing Practice Application **Assessment of breathing**

Normally, breathing is quiet, unlaboured and occurs at 12–16 breaths/min in adults at rest. Each breathing cycle consists of inspiration, expiration and a short pause before the next cycle starts. It is important to remember that the rate is much faster in the newborn (40/min), but slows during childhood. Individual variations exist in healthy individuals and factors such as activity affect rate, as does the presence of abnormalities. Apart from rate, other aspects noted during a nursing assessment are:

- The effort required to breathe – the use of accessory muscles, e.g. in COPD or nostril flaring in air hunger.
- Fatigue – individuals putting a 'big effort' into breathing will soon become tired. This can be exacerbated by sleep problems perhaps caused by coughing.
- Depth; for example, shallow breathing may indicate pleural pain (see page 265).
- Regularity: some abnormal patterns, e.g. Cheyne–Stokes, where periods of apnoea (no breathing) are followed by hyperventilation (over-breathing; deep and rapid), may be present in severe respiratory dysfunction.
- Skin colour: blue colour (cyanosis) is caused by the poor oxygenation/saturation of haemoglobin associated with respiratory and other conditions. In Caucasians this is obvious but in Afro-Caribbean or Asian individuals it is easy to miss unless the nail beds and mucous membranes are checked for 'blueness' or dusky colour.
- Noise, such as the wheezing associated with airway obstruction.
- Presence of cough and whether it is productive (with sputum) or non-productive (dry).
- Chest wall movement may be abnormal, e.g. sternal retraction in conditions such as airway obstruction, which increase the respiratory effort required.

Considerable observational skills are required to make an objective assessment as people tend to change breathing rates when being watched. You can try this out on some friends: count their respiratory rate without them knowing, e.g. while they watch television, then repeat the count with their knowledge and compare the results.

Nursing Practice Application **Oxygen administration**

Many people with dyspnoea and poor oxygenation (hypoxia, see page 278) will derive benefit from prescribed oxygen administered both in health-care settings and increasingly at home. Oxygen is usually given via a face mask or nasal cannulae and catheters, but can be administered by endotracheal tube, tracheostomy (see page 261), oxygen tent and at higher than atmospheric pressure in a hyperbaric (high pressure) chamber, e.g. for carbon monoxide poisoning (Figure 12.15).

Oxygen should be prescribed by the medical officer only after careful assessment because for some hypoxic states it is useless (cyanide poisoning) or harmful in high concentration (COPD). Where chronic respiratory diseases such as COPD have existed for many years the central chemoreceptors no longer respond to high carbon dioxide levels in the blood or CSF, and breathing is stimulated by hypoxia (see page 281 – Chemical control). If too much oxygen is given it would cause respiratory depression and further carbon dioxide retention. It is vital that low-concentration oxygen, e.g. 24%, administered through a venturi effect (oxygen flow is diluted by atmospheric air

drawn into the mask) mask is prescribed for these people. Nurses should be sure about what oxygen concentration and delivery method has been prescribed for the individual – a study in one hospital by Bell (1995) showed that in many cases the prescription was not followed, e.g. 26% of patients had oxygen on but no mask was in place, and for 26% of the patients in the sample (62) no prescription existed.

For all its life-saving uses, oxygen therapy is a hazardous business and nurses need to be aware of other potential dangers, including:

- Fire risk as oxygen supports combustion – sparks from electrical appliances are avoided by checking for safety and correct earthing, and the person, their family and friends are asked not to smoke.
- High concentration oxygen can damage the lungs.
- Newborns, given too much oxygen, may be blinded by fibrosis occurring behind the lens of the eye (retrolental fibroplasia).
- If oxygen flow is directed on to the face of infants it can stimulate a diving reflex characterized by a slowing heart rate with peripheral vasocon-

striction and diversion of blood to central areas.

Less dramatic, but still important, are the physical and psychological effects of oxygen therapy. Some people find a mask over their face claustrophobic and may be more comfortable with nasal cannulae. For the already breathless person a face mask presents yet another barrier to effective communication and can lead to fear, anger, frustration and withdrawal. The mask and attachments can cause pressure and soreness – cheeks and nose should be checked regularly. Oxygen has a drying effect upon the mucous membranes and should be humidified before administration. Care will include observations of vital signs and colour (skin and mucous membranes), and appropriate measures to minimize the effects of drying on the mouth and nose, e.g. adequate fluid intake.

Compliance is improved if patients are educated about the benefits of oxygen therapy, encouraged to continue and helped to overcome discomforts (Foss, 1990). People using oxygen at home also need information regarding care of equipment and continuity of supply.

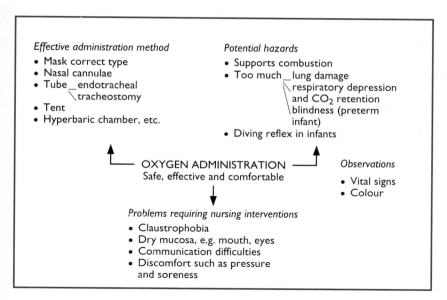

Figure 12.15 Oxygen administration.

Expiration

Normal quiet expiration is a passive process where the inherent elastic recoil of the lungs causes air to be expelled (see *Figure 12.14*). As the diaphragm and external intercostal muscles relax, the thoracic capacity decreases, the alveolar pressure rises and air flows out to once again equilibrate with atmospheric pressure. As the alveolar pressure rises and the lungs recoil, the intrapleural pressure becomes less negative.

Forced expiration, on the other hand, is an active process involving the abdominal muscles and internal intercostals, which contract to reduce thoracic capacity by forcing the abdominal contents up against the diaphragm and depressing the ribs. This may be observed during exercise or where airway obstruction exists.

Breathing: other factors

Earlier we looked at the role of pressure changes and inspiratory muscles in ventilation. A more complete coverage of the factors influencing ventilation includes the following factors.

Airway resistance

The airways produce resistance to air flow, which is subject to the same factors influencing blood flow (see Chapter 10):

$$\text{Air flow} = \frac{\text{Difference in gas pressure along the airway}}{\text{Airway resistance}}$$

Normally airway resistance is very small, but if the bronchial muscle constricts there is more friction and it becomes more difficult for air to reach the alveoli, e.g. in severe asthma. Resistance also increases if the airway is obstructed, e.g. with sputum or when lung volumes change. An extra respiratory effort is then needed to maintain adequate air flow when the airway resistance increases.

Surfactant and surface tension

The phospholipid surfactant reduces surface tension in the alveoli and allows lung expansion. Surfactant normally keeps the alveoli patent (open) between breaths; insufficient surfactant will result in alveolar collapse, which requires considerable energy for reinflation on inspiration (see Nursing Practice Application page 263).

Compliance and elasticity

Compliance is the ability of the lungs and thorax to stretch and distend. Healthy lungs need only a very small inflating pressure of 0.3 kPa (2 mmHg) to move approximately 500 ml of air with each breath (tidal volume). Ventilation becomes more difficult if the lungs lose compliance and become 'stiff', as in respiratory distress syndrome or pulmonary fibrosis.

Overstretching, with loss of elasticity, means that the lungs can no longer recoil to force air out (much like when elastic becomes overstretched and no longer recoils). In this situation, e.g. emphysema (a type of COPD), the lungs are overinflated and the affected person works very hard to move air out of the lungs.

Lung volumes and respiratory function tests

We can now consider the various volumes and derived capacities (the sum of two or more volumes) that exist in the lungs during inspiration and expiration (*Figure 12.16*).

Changes in volume measured by spirometry (an instrument called a spirometer is used to measure lung volume changes) can be used to assess respiratory function, aid diagnosis and give useful insights into progress and response to drug therapy (*Table 12.2*). It is important to realize that they have limitations and, as with all investigations, they should form part of a holistic assessment. This would consist of a full nursing assessment which included breathing (see page 270) and appropriate investigations, e.g. chest radiography.

For most people the thought of having any investigation provokes anxiety, and respiratory function tests are no exception. Nurses should ensure that adequate information is given and that the tests and their purpose are clearly understood. An appropriate explanation reduces anxiety and ensures the relaxation required to produce the best possible results.

Pulmonary ventilation and tidal volume

The amount of air moved in and out of the lungs in 1 minute is termed the pulmonary ventilation, or minute volume. This is about 6000 ml in an 'average' healthy adult at rest. The volume of air moved during one quiet breath is about 500 ml, and is known as the tidal volume. Not all this air is involved in gaseous exchange: some 150 ml is always in the conducting part of the respiratory tract (the anatomical dead space).

Details of other respiratory volumes and capacities can be found in *Figure 12.16* and *Table 12.2*, but readers who require more information are directed to Further Reading, e.g. Kendrick and Smith (1992a, b).

Alveolar ventilation

This is the amount of inspired air reaching the alveoli in one minute available for gaseous exchange. It is tidal volume minus the dead space multiplied by respiratory rate (alveolar ventilation rate = [tidal volume – dead space] × respiratory rate). See example in box.

Table 12.2 Respiratory measurements and function tests		
Test (volume/capacity)	**Definition/Description**	**Average values***
Vital capacity (VC)	Maximum volume expired after greatest inspiratory effort	4600 ml
Total lung capacity (TLC)	Volume of air in lungs following greatest inspiratory effort: TLC = FRC + IC	5800 ml
Inspiratory capacity (IC)	Maximum amount of air inspired after a normal expiratory effort	3500 ml
Functional residual capacity (FRC)	Volume of air in the lungs after a normal expiration: FRC = ERV + RV	2300 ml
Expiratory reserve volume (ERV)	Maximum amount of air that can be forcefully expelled after a normal expiration	1100 ml
Residual volume (RV)	The amount of air remaining in the lungs after a maximal expiratory effort: RV = FRC – ERV	1200 ml
Tidal volume	Amount of air inspired or expired during a normal breath at rest	500 ml
Peak expiratory flow rate (PEFR) uses a peak flow meter with disposable mouthpiece	Measures the greatest flow rate of air during rapid exhalation. This test is commonly performed by nurses when assessing response to bronchodilator drugs. It is vital that everyone understands that this is a flow rate measurement not a volume	400-600 l/min (depends on age, size and gender)
Forced vital capacity (FVC)	Volume of air expired forcefully soon after a maximal inspiratory effort	
Forced expiratory volume in one second (FEV_1)	The volume of air exhaled during the first second of FVC	Normally 80% of the FVC
Forced expiratory ratio (FER)	The ratio between FEV_1 and FVC	Normally 0.8
* *Healthy Adult Male*		

Table 12.2 Respiratory measurements and function tests.

$$[500 \text{ ml} - 150 \text{ ml}] \times 12$$
$$= 4200 \text{ ml (alveolar ventilation rate/min)}$$

These figures represent a healthy adult at rest, but they vary with size, age, health and activity; for example, alveolar ventilation increases greatly during exercise. Slow deep breathing produces an increased alveolar ventilation because the tidal volume increases and the constant anatomical dead space is proportionally smaller. Rapid shallow breathing, on the other hand, decreases alveolar ventilation because the tidal volume is smaller and the anatomical dead space is a proportionally higher percentage (see also hyperventilation and tetany, Chapter 8). The effects of chronic respiratory disease also reduce alveolar ventilation, which leads to dyspnoea and hypoxia. It makes good sense to help an anxious, frightened or breathless person to change to a more efficient breathing pattern (*Table 12.3*) and adopt an upright position to increase lung capacities.

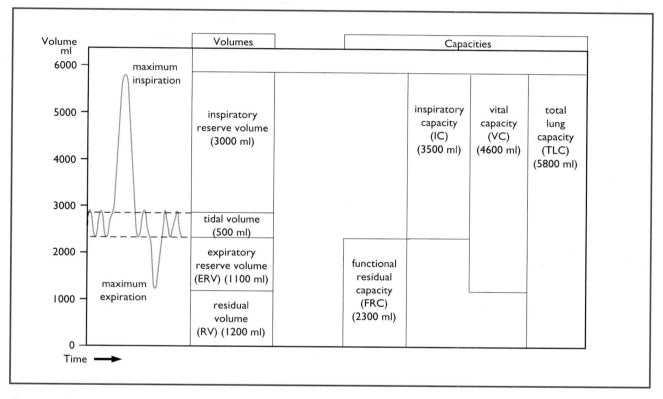

Figure 12.16 Lung volumes and capacities.

Table 12.3 Breathing patterns and alveolar ventilation (hypothetical situations)					
Breathing pattern	**Respiratory rate/min**	**Tidal volume (ml)**	**Pulmonary ventilation Minute volume (ml/min)**	**Alveolar Ventilation (ml/min)**	**% of Tidal volume as dead space***
1. Normal rate and depth	16	500	8000	5600	30%
2. Shallow, rapid	32	250	8000	3200	60%
3. Deep, slow	8	1000	8000	6800	15%
*NB Overall pulmonary ventilation is unchanged. * Assumes the dead space to be a constant 150 ml.*					

Table 12.3 Breathing patterns and alveolar ventilation (hypothetical situations).

Fundamentals of Gaseous Exchange

Before we consider the process of gaseous exchange it is necessary to look at some fundamental principles of gas behaviour. These account for the bulk flow of gases (see page 267 – Boyle's law) and diffusion down pressure gradients in external and internal respiration.

Behaviour of gases and gas laws

Air is a mixture of nitrogen, oxygen, carbon dioxide, water vapour and an insignificant amount of inert gases, e.g. helium (*Figure 12.17*). Each of these gases individually exerts a partial (individual) pressure, measured in kPa or (mmHg), proportional to its percentage concentration in the mixture. Dalton's law (of partial pressures) states that the pressure of a gas mixture is a sum of the partial pressures which each gas would exert if it completely filled the space.

The partial pressure of nitrogen, which forms approximately 79% of air, is approximately 79 kPa (590 mmHg) at sea level, where atmospheric pressure is around 101 kPa (760 mmHg). Partial pressures are calculated thus:

$$\frac{79}{100} \times 101 = 79.79 \text{ kPa}$$

Under the same conditions oxygen, at nearly 21%, has a partial pressure of 21.2 kPa.

We have looked at pressure at sea level, but as altitude increases the atmospheric pressure falls. The consequent fall in the partial pressure of the gases in air, although the proportions remain the same, will lead to problems with gas exchange in the lungs. The opposite also causes difficulties, e.g. working deep under the sea where high pressure can cause decompression sickness (see page 282).

Gases diffuse down partial pressure gradients, i.e. from high to low pressure. These gradients are maintained in the body by the continual use of oxygen and production of carbon dioxide by the cells. The other gas law needed to explain diffusion is Henry's law, which states that the amount of a gas dissolving in a fluid is proportional to its pressure and solubility at a constant temperature. Diffusion rates will depend on the steepness of the pressure gradient, the solubility of the gas (carbon dioxide is the most soluble followed by oxygen and then nitrogen), and the state and surface area of any barrier, e.g. alveolar membrane.

Composition and partial pressures

There are differences in the composition and partial pressures of the gases in atmospheric, alveolar and expired air (*Figure 12.17*). These differences can be explained by:
- Humidification of atmospheric air in the airways.
- The continuous diffusion of gases across the alveolar membrane – oxygen into the blood and carbon dioxide to the alveoli.
- Expired air being a mixture of alveolar air and the air contained in the dead space.

Generally there is little change in alveolar air composition because air remaining after expiration (the functional residual capacity, FRC) is continually mixing with tidal air. The stability of composition prevents marked changes in the blood gases. It is possible, however, to improve oxygen content and remove carbon dioxide more rapidly by increasing alveolar ventilation (see *Table 12.3*).

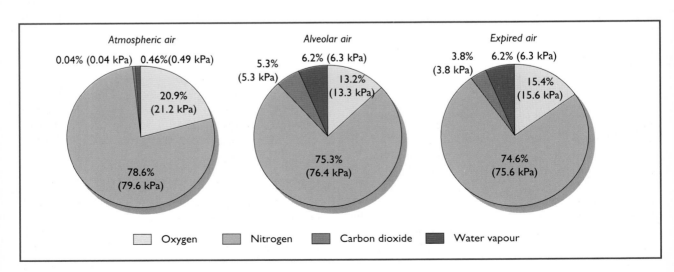

Figure 12.17 Composition (%) and gas partial pressures.

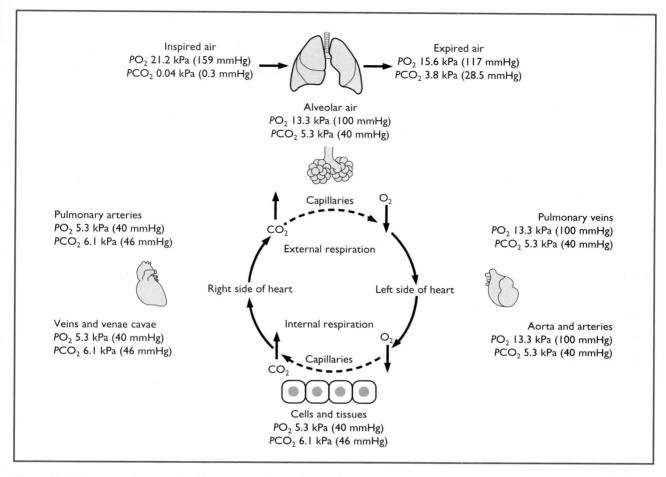

Inspired air
PO_2 21.2 kPa (159 mmHg)
PCO_2 0.04 kPa (0.3 mmHg)

Expired air
PO_2 15.6 kPa (117 mmHg)
PCO_2 3.8 kPa (28.5 mmHg)

Alveolar air
PO_2 13.3 kPa (100 mmHg)
PCO_2 5.3 kPa (40 mmHg)

Capillaries O_2

CO_2 External respiration

Pulmonary arteries
PO_2 5.3 kPa (40 mmHg)
PCO_2 6.1 kPa (46 mmHg)

Pulmonary veins
PO_2 13.3 kPa (100 mmHg)
PCO_2 5.3 kPa (40 mmHg)

Right side of heart   Left side of heart

Veins and venae cavae
PO_2 5.3 kPa (40 mmHg)
PCO_2 6.1 kPa (46 mmHg)

Internal respiration

Aorta and arteries
PO_2 13.3 kPa (100 mmHg)
PCO_2 5.3 kPa (40 mmHg)

CO_2 Capillaries O_2

Cells and tissues
PO_2 5.3 kPa (40 mmHg)
PCO_2 6.1 kPa (46 mmHg)

Figure 12.18 Gaseous exchange and partial pressure gradients – lungs and tissues.

Gaseous exchange in the lungs – external respiration

External respiration is the diffusion of gases between alveolar air and blood in the pulmonary capillaries. It depends upon partial pressure gradients and solubilities, healthy functioning of the alveolar membrane (see *Figure 12.8b*) and the correct ventilation–perfusion ratio.

Partial pressures

The partial pressure of oxygen is 13.3 kPa in the alveoli and 5.3 kPa in the pulmonary capillaries. This means that oxygen passes from the alveolar air into the blood until equilibrium is reached. This takes between 0.2 and 0.3 s; however, the erythrocytes are available in the capillary to pick up oxygen for nearly 1 s (there is time in hand). Oxygen is then transported around the body, mainly by the erythrocytes. Carbon dioxide diffuses in the reverse direction because its partial pressure is 6.1 kPa in the capillary and only 5.3 kPa in the alveoli. The pressure gradient for carbon dioxide is small, but because of its high solubility (20–21 times that of oxygen) it is still able to diffuse into the alveoli for removal during expiration (*Figure 12.18*). The relatively slow blood flow through the pulmonary capillaries allows more than enough time for gas exchange.

Alveolar membrane

Providing a huge surface area for gas exchange (see page 263), the thin, moist alveolar membrane is ideal for the rapid diffusion of gases. Any thickening or severe loss of area caused by disease will impede diffusion and lead to hypoxia.

Ventilation–perfusion relationship

Homeostatic autoregulatory processes operate to maintain an efficient ratio between gases in the alveoli and the blood flow in the capillaries. These include the response of smooth muscle in the walls of the arterioles and the small airways to changes in the partial pressures of carbon dioxide PCO_2 and oxygen PO_2.

Nursing Practice Application Blood gases

The measurement of arterial blood gases (PaO_2, $PaCO_2$, Hb oxygen saturation – SaO_2) and pH is commonly performed in critically ill patients, e.g. with severe asthma or in shock, or in those needing assisted ventilation, and it is used to differentiate between type I (reduced PaO_2 without hypercapnia) and type II or asphyxia (reduced PaO_2 with hypercapnia) respiratory failure. The results provide a guide to alveolar ventilation, gaseous exchange, acid–base balance, and blood and tissue oxygenation.

A sample of arterial blood obtained from a suitable vessel, e.g. the femoral or radial artery, is tested and the results used to diagnose hypoxia/hypercapnia and in decisions regarding treatment, e.g. oxygen therapy. The nursing role includes:

- Patient preparation with explanation.
- Ensuring the sample, which is heparinized, kept cool in an iced container and not exposed to air, arrives at the laboratory quickly and in good condition.
- Prevention of haematoma formation by applying pressure over an arterial puncture for at least 5 min and subsequent checking of puncture site for bleeding or bruising.

It is worth remembering that capillary blood sampling (ear lobes) is less painful than using an artery and gives similar results (Dar et al. 1995).

Capillary oxygen saturation levels can be conveniently measured using cutaneous or pulse oximetry by a sensor/probe placed on the skin of the ear lobe, finger or thumb. The device, which has the advantage of being non-invasive, utilizes light absorption to determine oxygen saturation. There is, however, a downside – it is not reliable in some poorly perfused individuals and there are problems and limitations interpreting results when the person is receiving oxygen. Jones (1995) describes these and suggests that both O_2 saturation and inspired O_2 are recorded.

Normal range of values (reference ranges vary between laboratories)

PaO_2 11–13.3 kPa (82.5–100 mmHg)
Oxygen saturation > 97%
pH 7.35–7.45
Hydrogen ion concentration [H^+] 36–44 nmol/l (40 nmol/l = pH 7.4)
$PaCO_2$ 4.7–6.0 kPa (35–45 mmHg)
Plasma hydrogen carbonate 22–28 mmol/l
See respiratory role in pH regulation (pages 283–284 and Chapter 2).

At rest the ventilation–perfusion ratio is 0.8 if the alveolar ventilation is around 4 l/min and the pulmonary blood flow (i.e. the cardiac output) is 5 l/min:

$$\frac{4}{5} = 0.8$$

For gas exchange to be efficient it is important that the ventilation–perfusion ratio is uniform throughout the lung tissue. While lying down, ratio maintenance is not a problem (pulmonary blood pressure and intrapleural pressures are constant), but the moment we adopt the upright position the effects of gravity on blood pressure means that the lung apex is less well perfused than the base, where an increase in blood pressure causes vessels to expand. In addition, the intrapleural pressure becomes more negative at the apex, which means that the now larger expanded alveoli are not so well ventilated. To help compensate for the increased perfusion at the base the small, less well expanded alveoli in the lung bases expand to increase ventilation. However, differences between apex and base are not fully compensated for even by the autoregulatory processes mentioned earlier.

It is also important to remember that even in the healthiest of lungs there will be areas of lung where ventilated alveoli are not perfused (a physiological dead space) and areas where poorly ventilated alveoli are perfused – here the blood has no chance to exchange gases before returning to the heart (physiological right-to-left shunt) but whatever the reason, the result is less efficient gas exchange.

If a large mismatch occurs, gaseous exchange will be seriously impaired, with the development of hypoxia and possibly hypercapnia (high CO_2 levels in the blood). This may be caused by alveolar underventilation, e.g. with COPD (see page 267), or insufficient blood flowing in the pulmonary capillaries, e.g. after severe haemorrhage and shock (see Chapter 10) or after pulmonary embolus and infarction (see Chapter 9).

Gaseous exchange at the tissues – internal respiration

It seems logical to consider internal respiration at this point, it being the reverse of external respiration in the alveoli. Internal respiration works in exactly the same way, but this time diffusion occurs between the capillaries, the interstitial fluid and the cells (see *Figure 12.18*).

Arterial blood arriving at the tissues has a higher partial pressure of oxygen (13.3 kPa) than the cells (5.3 kPa); this leads to a movement of oxygen into the cells. Cellular carbon dioxide (6.1 kPa) meanwhile moves into the blood, where the partial pressure is only 5.3 kPa. Venous blood drains from the tissues and returns to the lungs to restart the cycle with external respiration. It is important that we remember that gases must be transported between lungs and tissues and *vice versa* before any exchange can occur.

Transport of Gases

Transport of oxygen

Most oxygen is carried to the tissues combined with haemoglobin in erythrocytes and a small amount (1%) is dissolved in the plasma (oxygen has a low solubility). The oxygen in the plasma, although not important for tissue oxygenation, is vital in maintaining oxygen pressure gradients between plasma and tissues.

Haemoglobin

Haemoglobin (see Chapter 9) is the specialized pigment–protein complex found within the erythrocytes. A molecule of haemoglobin (Hb) consists of four haem groups, each containing an atom of ferrous iron, and four globin protein chains. Each molecule of Hb can combine reversibly with four molecules of oxygen. These join with the haem groups to form the bright red oxyhaemoglobin (HbO_2):

$$Hb + O_2 \rightleftharpoons HbO_2$$

Reduced (not saturated with oxygen) haemoglobin (HHb) is a dark purple colour before its oxygenation. One gram of haemoglobin combines with 1.34 ml of oxygen, which means that, given a haemoglobin level of 15 g/dl (150g/l) (normal range 11.5–18 g/dl), each decilitre of blood, when fully saturated (98%), can carry about 20 ml of oxygen. The actual amount depends on the PO_2 of the blood, influenced by the oxygen dissolved in the plasma as well as the Hb content.

Oxygen dissociation curve

In Chapter 9 we discussed how oxygen molecules combine sequentially with haemoglobin. Each of the four haem groups has a different affinity for oxygen, which is illustrated by the sigmoid-shaped dissociation curve (*Figure 12.19*). The first combines with some difficulty, the next two much more easily, but the last has the most

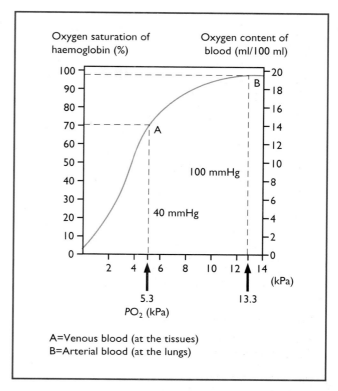

Figure 12.19 Oxygen dissociation curve (at 37°C, pH 7.4, Hb 15g/dl).

difficulty. As the haemoglobin molecule becomes saturated with oxygen its folded globin chains change shape to facilitate the binding of the last oxygen molecule. The interaction between different parts of the haemoglobin molecule during oxygenation increases efficiency.

Once blood reaches the tissues the oxygen molecules are unloaded sequentially, with the release of one molecule assisting the unloading of the next molecule and so on. Under normal conditions only about 5 ml of oxygen is given up at the tissues, which means the haemoglobin molecule is still 75% saturated when it returns to the lungs. If the PO_2 within an actively metabolizing tissue falls very low there is the facility for more oxygen to be released.

Various factors affect the rate at which haemoglobin combines with and unloads oxygen at a given PO_2. These include: temperature, PCO_2, pH and levels of 2,3-diphosphoglycerate (2,3-DPG), a metabolite in erythrocytes (see *Figure 12.20*). An increase in temperature will decrease the affinity of haemoglobin for oxygen, which means that more oxygen is unloaded in the most metabolically active tissues (producing heat). A similar 'shift to the right' of the curve occurs if the PCO_2 or hydrogen ion concentration is raised (fall in pH). Again this ensures that oxygen release is facilitated in metabolically active tissue. The 'right shift' of the oxygen dissociation curve occurring as

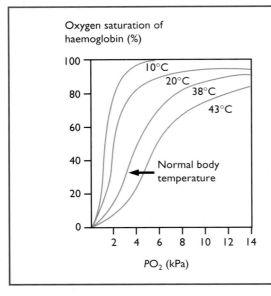
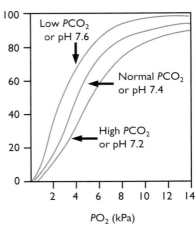

Figure 12.20 Effects of various factors on the oxygen dissociation curve.

Abnormal Function **Problems with oxygen transport**

Hypoxia

Hypoxia is the term used when there is insufficient oxygenation of the tissues or inability to utilize the available oxygen. Causes include:

- Reduced arterial PaO_2 (hypoxic), e.g. COPD affecting gaseous exchange.
- Where haemoglobin levels are reduced or not available for oxygen transport (anaemic), e.g. anaemia, haemorrhage, carbon monoxide poisoning (carbon monoxide is produced in vehicle exhaust gases and by the incomplete combustion of other hydrocarbons such as natural gas). At this point it is worth taking a closer look at carbon monoxide. This colourless, odourless gas causes

problems because it combines more easily with haemoglobin (to form carboxyhaemoglobin) than does oxygen, with which it competes. Carbon monoxide poisoning is managed with oxygen therapy, but a much better idea is prevention (see Healthier Living box).

- Stagnant (ischaemic) hypoxia, where circulation of blood is faulty, e.g. cardiac failure.
- Cellular poisons such as cyanide cause histotoxic hypoxia, where cells are unable to utilize oxygen because their respiratory enzymes are damaged.

Hypoxia usually presents as hyperventilation, nausea, headache, tachycardia and changes in behaviour. If more than 5 g/dl

of Hb is reduced in a person with a normal haemoglobin content, cyanosis will be evident (see page 270). If this were occurring in a person with anaemia, e.g. Hb 8 g/dl, the hypoxia would be severe, with less than 40% of the Hb saturated before cyanosis was observed.

In many types of hypoxia the person would derive benefit from the administration of oxygen (see page 270) after careful assessment, which may include the estimation of blood gases and pH. People who are chronically hypoxic respond physiologically by increasing erythropoiesis, leading to polycythaemia (see Chapter 9), and producing more 2,3-DPG.

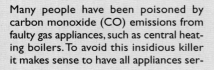

Healthier Living **Preventing carbon monoxide poisoning**

Many people have been poisoned by carbon monoxide (CO) emissions from faulty gas appliances, such as central heating boilers. To avoid this insidious killer it makes sense to have all appliances ser-

viced on a regular basis by approved companies, to use appliances properly having first read the manufacturers instructions, to ensure there is adequate room ventilation and to purchase CO

monitoring devices to give early warning of the presence of the gas. Awareness of pathophysiological effects, e.g. headache and drowsiness, is important in detecting problems at an early stage.

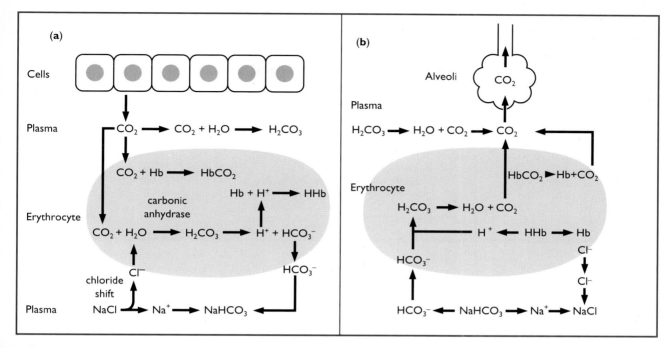

Figure 12.21 Carbon dioxide transport. (**a**) At the tissues; (**b**) in the lungs.

a result of reduced blood pH (becoming more acid as hydrogen ion concentration increases) is also known as the Bohr effect. The substance 2,3-DPG decreases haemoglobin affinity for oxygen and enhances oxygen release to the tissues. Its production by erythrocytes increases where oxygen partial pressures are reduced, e.g. with chronic respiratory disease or at high altitude. It follows that a decrease in temperature, 2,3-DPG and PCO_2 (i.e. rise in pH) will increase the affinity of haemoglobin for oxygen, which makes loading easier (and unloading more difficult).

Transport of carbon dioxide

Carbon dioxide is transported by the blood in three ways: dissolved in plasma, combined with haemoglobin and as hydrogen carbonate ions (*Figure 12.21*). At rest, cellular metabolism produces about 200 ml of carbon dioxide every minute, which must be transported to the lungs for removal by gaseous exchange and expiration (see *Figure 12.18*):

- A small amount of carbon dioxide is transported in simple solution in the plasma as carbonic acid (H_2CO_3):

$$CO_2 + H_2O \rightleftharpoons H_2CO_3$$

This reaction occurs slowly without the help of an enzymic catalyst.

- Some carbon dioxide enters the erythrocyte to combine with amino acid groups in the globin chains of haemoglobin to form the neutral compound carbaminohaemoglobin:

$$Hb + CO_2 \rightleftharpoons HbCO_2$$

The amount of carbon dioxide carried is determined by the PCO_2 and the degree of oxygen saturation. Most carbon dioxide is transported by reduced haemoglobin. Some carbon dioxide forms similar 'carbamino' compounds with the plasma proteins. In the tissues, where the PCO_2 is higher than in the blood, the carbon dioxide moves down the gradient into the blood and combines easily with the haemoglobin. On arrival in the lungs it dissociates because alveolar air PCO_2 is lower than that in the blood.

- The most important method of transport involves a series of chemical reactions, mostly occurring in the erythrocyte, which facilitate the carriage of carbon dioxide as hydrogen carbonate. At the 'tissue end' of the process the carbon dioxide diffuses into the blood and enters the erythrocyte, where it combines with water to form carbonic acid. This time the reversible reaction

Abnormal Function **Problems with carbon dioxide levels**

Hypercapnia

Hypercapnia is the term used to describe an abnormally high arterial $PaCO_2$ (normal range 4.7–6.0 kPa). This happens when there is hypoventilation or where a ventilation–perfusion mismatch exists (see pages 275–276). A high $PaCO_2$ stimulates ventilation in an attempt to flush out excess carbon dioxide. Hypercapnia is always accompanied by hypoxia (see page 278); it can increase blood acidity (acidosis) and at very high levels will affect central nervous system (CNS) function. CNS effects include raised intracranial pressure (see Chapter 4), leading to headaches, confusion, altered consciousness and eventual death if treatment is inadequate. Management is based on increasing ventilation and correcting hypoxia and acidosis.

Hypocapnia

The opposite situation to hypercapnia is hypocapnia, i.e. a reduction in the $PaCO_2$ which is usually caused by hyperventilation. As ventilation increases, excess carbon dioxide is flushed from the body. Some causes of hyperventilation include anxiety, hysteria, pain, high altitude and when the body becomes too acidic, e.g. diabetic ketoacidosis (see Chapter 8). The high carbon dioxide respiratory drive is lost and the blood becomes more alkaline as acid carbon dioxide is lost. This change in pH affects the amount of available calcium in the blood, resulting in tetany (see Chapter 8).

proceeds rapidly because it is catalyzed by the enzyme carbonic anhydrase. The carbonic acid formed within the erythrocyte dissociates into hydrogen carbonate and hydrogen ions.

$$CO_2 + H_2O \rightleftharpoons H_2CO_3 \rightleftharpoons H^+ + HCO_3^-$$

The hydrogen ions combine with haemoglobin (remember the buffering role of haemoglobin), which limits their effect on pH, and most of the hydrogen carbonate diffuses out (the increased concentration of hydrogen carbonate ions in the erythrocyte produces a concentration gradient) of the erythrocyte into the plasma. Hydrogen carbonate ions remaining in the erythrocyte are combined with potassium which, you will remember, is an important intracellular ion (see Chapter 2). As negatively charged hydrogen carbonate ions leave the erythrocyte the electrical balance is restored by the movement of negatively charged chloride ions from the plasma to the erythrocyte – a process known as the chloride shift. The hydrogen carbonate ions combine with sodium ions in the plasma to form sodium hydrogen carbonate.

When the blood arrives in the lungs the reactions go into reverse and carbon dioxide is released into the plasma. From here it diffuses into the alveoli.

Carbon dioxide transport is dependent on the degree of blood oxygenation. Reduced haemoglobin is able to carry more carbon dioxide (known as the Haldane effect), but haemoglobin can carry both gases at the same time because they utilize different sites on the molecule.

By this time you will have realized that the loading and unloading of both gases are closely related processes.

Control of Ventilation

As you can imagine, the vital rhythm, rate and depth of breathing/ventilation requires precise control mechanisms. This control is mostly involuntary, but we have a voluntary override ability in certain situations, e.g. singing.

Respiratory centres

The respiratory control centres, which are situated in the reticular formation of the medulla and pons, receive inputs from chemoreceptors, stretch receptors (airways, pleura and lungs), higher-centre voluntary overrides and the hypothalamus (*Figure 12.22*). Just how the centres in the medulla work is not universally agreed, but one hypothesis is described here.

The respiratory centre consists of inspiratory (dorsal medulla) and expiratory (ventral medulla) neurones, which are mutually inhibitory. Cyclical stimulation of the inspiratory neurones results in impulse transmission to the diaphragm and external intercostal muscles, which contract. Expiratory neurones are possibly only concerned when active expiration is required; expiration is normally passive. The medullary centres produce the basic rhythm of normal breathing.

The frequency of impulse transmission and ventilation is geared to maintaining tissue oxygenation throughout a range of changing physiological needs, e.g. high altitude and exercise. The medullary respiratory centre is depressed by drugs, e.g. opiates, sedatives and ethanol (C_2H_5OH), which if severe will cause apnoea.

Neurones in the pons modulate the medullary inspiratory centre and provide the 'fine tuning' required for a smooth respiratory rhythm. The pneumotaxic centre sends inhibitory impulses to the inspiratory centre to

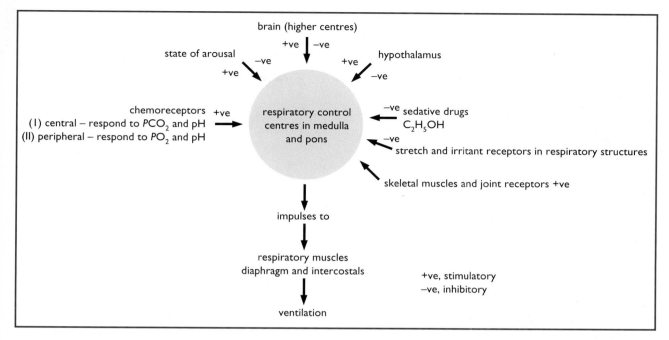

Figure 12.22 Control of respiration (simplified).

prevent jerky changeovers between inspiration and expiration. A hypothetical apneustic centre has been proposed, but it has not been identified. Some authorities postulate that apneustic neurones are responsible for continuous stimulation of the inspiratory centre.

Chemical control

Peripheral chemoreceptor cells situated in the aortic arch and carotid bodies, and some located centrally in the medulla, sample the PCO_2, PO_2 and pH of arterial blood. As we have already discussed, the major influence on the respiratory centre in healthy individuals is a raised PCO_2 and the drive for ventilation is a high carbon dioxide level. This acts through the central chemoreceptors, which are particularly sensitive to chemical changes in the cerebrospinal fluid caused by increasing carbon dioxide and hydrogen ions.

The peripheral chemoreceptors transmit impulses to the medulla through the vagus and glossopharyngeal nerves. They are most sensitive to decreases in PO_2 and pH and less sensitive to increases in PCO_2. The hypoxic drive (low PO_2 is relatively insignificant in healthy people, but a reduction in pH will rapidly stimulate ventilation even when blood gases are normal, as with ketoacidosis.

The hypoxia drive is an important control of ventilation at increased altitude and when chemoreceptor sensitivity to PCO_2 has been lost, e.g. with longstanding COPD (see Oxygen administration, page 270).

Stretch and irritant receptors

Stretch receptors within the airways and pleura send inhibitory impulses through the vagus nerve to the medullary respiratory centres. This mechanism prevents overinflation of the lungs and helps to maintain the rhythm of breathing.

The Hering–Breuer reflex, which operates through the vagus nerve, causes a short period of apnoea if the lungs are overinflated. It may be an important reflex in the newborn, although it appears to be more a protective measure than a control mechanism in adults.

Irritants such as dust stimulate receptors in the airways/lungs and initiate a protective reflex, e.g. coughing or sneezing. These impulses, which modify ventilation patterns, reach the respiratory centres through the vagus nerve.

Higher-centre (voluntary) control

We can all think of situations where it is necessary to override involuntary control of ventilation. Swimming underwater, singing, swallowing, laughing and 'having a good cry' all require some modification to the normal breathing pattern. These changes are for a limited time only: eventually the automatic chemical controls will take over.

The state of arousal/wakefulness also influences the respiratory centre; for example, being 'wide awake' tends to stimulate the respiratory centres. During NREM sleep (stages 3 and 4) the respiratory rate slows, but it increases again with the onset of REM sleep, when the oxygen demands of the brain are greatly increased (see Chapter 4).

Hypothalamic control

Imagine for a moment that you are dozing in the sun (with proper protection) when someone turns a cold hose on you – the sudden inspiratory gasp that follows can be explained by the impulses sent to the respiratory centres from the hypothalamus. Intense emotions, pain and body temperature can all modify the rate and depth of ventilation through hypothalamic/limbic system influences.

Effects of altitude, depth and exercise on ventilation

Altitude

Anyone who has visited a mountainous region will confirm that their breathing pattern was affected. At 18 000 feet (5486 m) above sea level the partial pressure of oxygen is half that at sea level (see page 274) and haemoglobin is not fully saturated. The level of saturation can still be sufficient for tissue oxygenation, if you do not rush about, because the haemoglobin can unload a larger percentage of its oxygen – remember at sea level it goes back to the lungs still 75% saturated, but even the mildest physical activity results in dyspnoea, aching muscles and extreme fatigue. The change in PO_2 will initiate a series of physiological adaptations known as acclimatization. Some of these adaptations occur at once but others take some weeks, which is why climbers spend a period of time acclimatizing at increased altitude rather than rushing at the mountain on the day they arrive. Failure to acclimatize properly leads to the very serious 'acute mountain sickness' caused by hypoxia (see page 278).

Changes with altitude include:

- Hyperventilation, initiated by peripheral chemoreceptors responding to the reduced PaO_2, occurs as the respiratory centre attempts to maintain adequate gaseous exchange. This is an example of the hypoxic drive in operation as opposed to the normal CO_2 drive.
- Reduction in $PaCO_2$ caused by hyperventilation reduces the immediate influence of central chemoreceptors on the respiratory centres and high pH in the CSF is corrected by the choroid plexi, which secrete less hydrogen carbonate ions.
- Increased cardiac output in response to lower PaO_2.
- Increased 2,3-DPG production, which allows easier oxygen unloading from Hb which is carrying less oxygen than usual.

- Increased erythropoiesis over time as the kidneys produce more renal erythropoietic factor in response to hypoxia (see Chapter 9). This increases the packed cell volume and hence the blood viscosity (see Chapter 9).

Depth

The increase in atmospheric pressure below sea level causes problems in the form of decompression sickness, which affects divers and people working deep underground.

At high atmospheric pressure more oxygen and nitrogen dissolve in the blood. During the return to normal pressure the nitrogen (which is poorly soluble; see page 274), which has been dissolved in the blood under increased pressure, can form bubbles in the blood. This is likely to occur if decompression time (return to atmospheric pressure) is too short. The gas bubbles form emboli, which cause pain, abdominal distension and damage to the brain or other vital structures, possibly resulting in death. Decompression sickness or 'the bends' is a serious occupational hazard for divers. In the UK their work, including the use of decompression chambers, is controlled by stringent health, safety and welfare legislation.

Exercise

During strenuous exercise the hardworking skeletal muscles have a huge appetite for oxygen and produce much more carbon dioxide than usual. Obviously, there needs to be considerable respiratory modification to cope with these changes and maintain homeostatic balance. In fit individuals ventilation can increase to 15–20 times the level at rest.

As you would expect, breathing becomes deeper, but the reasons for the particular pattern are not fully understood. Ventilation rises sharply when exercise starts. This rise slows to reach a level stage, which continues while the exercise is in progress. When exercise ceases the ventilation rate falls sharply and then returns to the resting level more slowly. It may be that we consciously prepare for exercise and the cerebral cortex sends appropriate impulses to the respiratory centres, which also receive excitatory impulses from muscle and joint proprioceptors.

Blood gases PO_2 and PCO_2 change very little during moderate exercise, so the pattern cannot be explained solely by normal chemoreceptor mechanisms. While ventilation rates rise, do not forget that cardiac output is also increasing to maintain the ventilation:perfusion ratio.

When contracting muscle fails to increase its oxygen consumption or receive sufficient oxygen because contraction may interfere with blood supply it starts to utilize fuel molecules, e.g. glucose, without oxygen (anaerobic respiration). The muscles are really using credit: their 'oxygen debt' must be repaid eventually, explaining the slow decline in ventilation rate. The slow decline is also linked to the lactic acid produced by anaerobic respiration – its presence lowers blood pH, which stimulates ventilation to correct the pH and makes oxygen easier to unload (see pages 277–279). Lactic acid also accounts for the aching muscles and stiffness felt after unaccustomed or strenuous exercise.

Respiratory role in pH regulation

Respiration has a vital role in the regulation of pH (hydrogen ion concentration) based on the equation (see pages 279–280):

$$CO_2 + H_2O \rightleftharpoons H_2CO_3 \rightleftharpoons H^+ + HCO_3^-$$

The respiratory centre and lungs (through rate and depth of breathing) respond within minutes to changes in pH and PCO_2, and the kidneys (Chapter 15) operate more slowly to initiate processes which maintain pH balance of the body. In the short term, however, it is the buffer systems that prevent any huge swings in pH. Before we continue it would be a good idea for readers to refresh their knowledge regarding the concepts of pH and buffers (especially the hydrogen-carbonate system) with a quick look at Chapter 2. The Henderson–Hasselbalch equation (see below) explains why blood pH is dependent upon the amount of hydrogen carbonate (HCO_3^-) and dissolved carbon dioxide (H_2CO_3), which is determined by the PCO_2. Hypercapnia and/or a fall in blood pH, as you already know, stimulate the medullary respiratory centres through chemoreceptors to increase ventilation.

Henderson–Hasselbalch equation

$$\text{Blood pH} = 6.1 + \log \frac{[HCO_3^-] \text{ Hydrogen carbonate}}{[CO_2] \text{ Carbon dioxide in solution}}$$

The ratio of hydrogen carbonate (base) to carbonic acid (acid) must be 20:1 if blood pH is to remain at 7.4.

How ventilation maintains the 20:1 ratio

If hydrogen carbonate levels fall (as it buffers acid) or the PCO_2 increases, the pH of the blood falls (acidosis), but an increase in ventilation expels more carbon dioxide to restore the ratio.

If hydrogen carbonate levels rise or the PCO_2 decreases, an increase in blood pH (alkalosis) reduces

Table 12.4 Acid–base problems – changes in pH, $PaCO_2$ and [HCO_3^-].

Table 12.4 Acid–base problems – changes in pH, $PaCO_2$ and [HCO_3^-]			
Acid–base problem	pH	$PaCO_2$	[HCO_3^-]
A. Acidosis Respiratory	Falls	Rises	Unchanged
with compensation	Returns to normal as renal compensation occurs	Rises	Rises in renal compensation as HCO_3^- are reabsorbed
Metabolic	Falls	Unchanged	Falls
with compensation	Returns to normal as respiratory compensation occurs	Falls as respiratory compensation occurs	Falls
B. Alkalosis Respiratory	Rises	Falls	Unchanged
with compensation	Returns to normal as renal compensation occurs	Falls	Falls in renal compensation as HCO_3^- are excreted
Metabolic	Rises	Unchanged	Rises
with compensation	Returns to normal as respiratory compensation occurs	Rises as respiratory compensation occurs	Rises

ventilation, more carbon dioxide is retained and again the 20:1 ratio is restored.

These two examples illustrate the respiratory role in changing ventilation to restore and maintain the hydrogen carbonate/carbonic acid buffer system ratio. In each case the regulation of hydrogen carbonate is part of kidney function and takes days, compared with the minutes needed for respiratory regulation of PCO_2.

Abnormal Function **Problems with acid–base balance (see Table 12.4)**

From the examples above you can see that changes in blood pH may have a respiratory or metabolic cause, although some changes have a mixed aetiology. When considering acid–base balance an important feature is the ability of the lungs and kidneys to compensate for disorders in each other, e.g. a high PCO_2 caused by COPD is compensated by renal reabsorption of HCO_3^-.

Acidosis (pH less than 7.35)
Respiratory acidosis is caused by an increase in $PaCO_2$, e.g. respiratory failure. Metabolic acidosis is caused by the production of acids which use up the buffering ability of the hydrogen carbonate, e.g. diabetic ketoacidosis and lactic acid produced during exercise, or by the loss of alkali, e.g. severe diarrhoea.

Alkalosis (pH greater than 7.45)
Respiratory alkalosis results from a decrease in $PaCO_2$ such as that caused by the hyperventilation of severe anxiety. Metabolic alkalosis can be caused by either an increase in the amount of alkali, e.g. taking excessive alkaline indigestion medicine, or acid loss, e.g. vomiting.

Summary/Check List

Introduction.
Respiratory structures – Early development. Nose. Pharynx. Larynx – swallowing, Nursing Practice Application – airway maintenance, lining and vocal cords, voice production, Valsalva's manoeuvre. Trachea – Nursing Practice Application – tracheostomy, cough and sneeze. Bronchial tree, Nursing Practice Application – inhalers and nebulizers. Healthier Living - preventing the inhalation of foreign bodies in young children. Alveoli, Nursing Practice Application – surfactant administration. Lungs, Special Focus – tuberculosis, Nursing Practice Application – cystic fibrosis. Pleura, Nursing Practice Application – pleural aspiration. Healthier Living – smoking. Environmental/occupational hazards, Person-Centred study – Sid, Nursing Practice Application – sputum.
Breathing/ventilation – intrathoracic pressures, Nursing Practice Application – pneumothorax/chest drains. Inspiration.

Expiration. Nursing Practice Application – assessment of breathing, Nursing Practice Application – oxygen administration. Airway resistance, surfactant, compliance/elasticity. Lung volumes/capacities, lung function tests, pulmonary ventilation and tidal volume, alveolar ventilation.
Gaseous exchange – behaviour of gases. Composition/partial pressures. External respiration. Internal respiration. Nursing Practice Application – blood gases.
Transport of gases – oxygen, haemoglobin, oxygen dissociation curve, hypoxia, Healthier Living – preventing carbon-monoxide poisoning. Carbon dioxide, hypercapnia, hypocapnia.
Control of ventilation – respiratory centres. Controls. Effects of altitude/depth/exercise. Respiratory role in pH regulation – acidosis/alkalosis.

Self Test

1 How is air modified on its journey from nose to alveoli?
2 What mechanisms exist to protect the respiratory tract during swallowing?
3 Which of the following statements are true?
   (a) Intrapleural pressure is always greater than alveolar pressure.
   (b) Inspiration is an active process involving the respiratory muscles.
   (c) Expiration depends on the elastic recoil of the lungs.
   (d) Surfactant prevents alveolar collapse.
4 Which of the following should be treated with low concentration oxygen?
   (a) Cyanide poisoning.
   (b) COPD.
   (c) Carbon monoxide poisoning.
5 Why would you encourage Yasim, who is anxious and breathless, to breathe slowly and deeply?

6 Complete the following:
   (a) Atmospheric air has a PO_2 of ___.
   (b) Alveolar air has a PCO_2 of ___.
   (c) Expired air has a PCO_2 of ___.
7 The diffusion of gases between alveoli and blood depends on which factors?
8 Relate the shape of the oxygen dissociation curve to physiological events.
9 Which of the following transports most carbon dioxide:
   (a) Hydrogen carbonate ions in the plasma.
   (b) Dissolved in the plasma.
   (c) Carbaminohaemoglobin.
10 Explain the effects of PCO_2, PO_2 and pH on the respiratory centres.
11 What changes occur in blood pH and PCO_2 in the following situations:
   (a) hyperventilation;
   (b) hypoventilation?

Answers

1 See pages 257–258, 260–261.
2 See pages 258–259.
3 b, c, d.
4 b.
5 See pages 273.
6 (a) 21.2 kPa;
   (b) 5.3 kPa:
   (c) 3.8 kPa.

7 Gas partial pressure gradients, solubilities, state and area of alveolar membrane and ventilation/perfusion relationship.
8 See page 277.
9 a.
10 See page 281.
11 (a) pH increases and PCO_2 falls;
   (b) pH falls and PCO_2 increases.

References

Bell C (1995) Is this what the doctor ordered? Accuracy of oxygen therapy prescribed and delivered in hospital. *Prof Nurs* **10**(5): 297–300.
Cockcroft A, Bagnall P, Heslop A et al. (1986) Controlled trial of a respiratory health worker visiting patients with chronic respiratory disability. *BMJ* **294**: 225–227.
Dar K, Williams T, Aitken R et al. (1995) Arterial versus capillary sampling for analysing blood gas pressures. *BMJ* **310**: 24–25.
DoH (1992) *The Health of the Nation* (Summary). London: HMSO.
Dyer J, Morais A (1996) Supporting children with cystic fibrosis in school. *Prof Nurs* **11**(8): 518–520.

Foss M (1990) Oxygen therapy. *Prof Nurs* **5**(4):188–190.
Gleeson C (1995) Assessing childrens' knowledge of asthma. *Prof Nurs* **10**(8): 517–521.
Haverty S, Macleod Clark J, Elliot K (1987) Helping people to stop smoking. *Nurs Times* **83** (28): (occasional paper **87**(3): 45–9).
Health Education Authority (HEA) (1993) *Cancer: How to Reduce Your Risks*. London: HEA.
Jones SE (1995) Getting the balance right. Pulse oximetry and inspired oxygen concentration. *Prof Nurs* **10**(6): 368–373.

Further Reading

Cross S (1997) The management of acute asthma. *Prof Nurs* **12**(7): 495–7.

Erickson R (1989) Mastering the ins and outs of chest drainage: Part I. *Nursing (USA)* **19**(5): 36–43.

Erickson R (1989) Mastering the ins and outs of chest drainage: Part II. *Nursing (USA)* **19**(6): 46–9.

Kendrick A.H, Smith EC.(1992a) Simple measurements of lung function. *Prof Nurs* **7**(6): 395–404.

Kendrick AH, Smith EC (1992b) Respiratory measurements 2: interpreting simple measurements of lung function. *Prof Nurs* **7**(11): 748–754.

Macleod Clark J, Haverty S, Kendall S (1990) Helping people to stop smoking: a study of the nurse's role. *J Adv Nurs* **15**(3): 357–363.

Sims J (1996) Making sense of pulse oximetry and oxygen dissociation curve. *Nurs Times* **92**(1): 34–35.

Staub NC (1991) *Basic respiratory physiology*. Edinburgh: Churchill Livingstone.

Useful Addresses

Action on Smoking and Health (ASH)
109 Gloucester Place
London W1H 4EJ

Health Education Authority
Hamilton House
Mabledon Place
London WC1H 9TX

National Asthma Campaign
Providence House
Providence Place
London N1 0NT

Digestive System, Metabolism and Nutrition

Overview

- *Digestive tract structure and function.*
- *Metabolism and utilization of nutrients.*
- *Nutrition.*

Learning Outcomes

After studying Chapter 13 you should be able to:

- Describe the gastrointestinal tract and relate the adaptations in general structure to changing function.
- Discuss the role of the accessory digestive structures.
- Describe the location and functions of the peritoneum.
- Explain the processes of ingestion, mastication and swallowing.
- Describe the secretion, composition and functions of saliva.
- Explain food movement through the gastrointestinal tract.
- Outline the neural and hormonal controls of gastric secretion, motility and emptying.
- Describe the composition and functions of gastric juice.
- Discuss the digestive processes occurring in the small intestine, including the role of bile and pancreatic juice.
- Name the enzymes involved in the digestion of carbohydrates, fats and protein, and the products of digestion.
- Describe absorption in the small intestine.
- Describe the functions of the large intestine including defecation.
- Use physiological knowledge in the assessment of bowel function and identification of abnormalities.
- Describe the constituents of a healthy diet.
- Outline briefly the metabolism and utilization of glucose, fatty acids, glycerol and amino acids.
- Describe absorptive and postabsorptive states.
- Outline nutritional assessment.
- Discuss the nutritional requirements of certain special groups, including methods of nutritional support.

Key Words

Absorption – passage of products of digestion, through the gastrointestinal tract epithelium, into the blood or lymph.

Alimentary canal/gastrointestinal tract – the whole digestive tract, a tube extending from mouth to anus.

Aerobic – requiring oxygen or in the presence of oxygen.

Anaerobic – without oxygen.

Colonic – relating to the colon.

Defaecation – the elimination of waste residue (faeces) from the rectum.

Digestion – the catabolism (breakdown) of food into a form that can be absorbed.

Enteric – relating to the intestine.

Enzymes – specific protein catalysts which promote the breakdown of large food molecules into their chemical subunits, facilitating absorption.

Gastric – relating to the stomach.

Gut – the intestine or bowel.

Ingestion – taking in food or other substances into the body.

Peptic – pertaining to digestion.

Peristalsis – the rhythmic, wave-like contractions that convey food/waste through the gastrointestinal tract and other hollow structures.

Introduction

We require raw materials for growth and repair and to produce the energy needed for cellular processes. These are obtained from the food and fluids we consume. Most of this food needs modification before it can be absorbed and utilized. The lunchtime sandwich will need some changes before it can provide energy for the afternoon and raw materials such as amino acids for the synthesis of new proteins. The complex modification process involves: **ingestion**, mastication (chewing), deglutition (swallowing), propulsion, **digestion, absorption,** utilization and elimination (by **defaecation**) of waste residue. The **alimentary canal**, consisting of the mouth, oesophagus, stomach, small intestine, large intestine and anus, is adapted to perform all these functions (*Figure 13.1*), aided by accessory structures which include the teeth, salivary glands, pancreas and liver (see Chapter 14). The alimentary tract measures around 8 m after death, but is shorter (4.5 m) during life because of muscle tone.

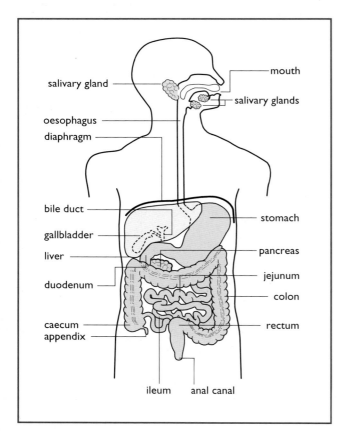

Figure 13.1 Alimentary/gastrointestinal/digestive tract.

Early development

The **gastrointestinal tract** starts to form, by the fourth week of embryonic development, from a simple tube or primitive **gut**. The tube consists of an inner endodermal layer, destined to become epithelium, surrounded by mesoderm, which gives rise to the smooth muscle and connective tissue. The upper part (foregut) develops to form the pharynx and oesophagus and, because development is closely linked with that of the trachea, a failure in oesophageal development can result in a tracheo-oesophageal fistula (abnormal opening between the trachea and oesophagus – see Chapter 12). The stomach forms from a dilation in the primitive foregut and the lower part (midgut and hindgut) grows down to form the small and large intestine and the anal canal. By the eighth week the tube is open at both ends (mouth and anus). The primitive gut dilates and rotates during the following weeks to form the gastrointestinal structures in their final positions. The large intestine eventually rotates to 'frame' the small intestine.

During early development the intestines protrude into the umbilical cord and are outside the abdominal cavity, but by about the tenth week they are enclosed by the abdominal wall. Problems at this stage may result in the congenital abnormality exomphalos, in which the intestines protrude through a gap in the abdominal wall and are covered only by a thin membrane. Surgical repair of the defect is usually undertaken as soon after birth as possible. Other developmental problems include atresia, in which a part of the gastrointestinal tract fails to canalize, i.e. it comes to a full stop and ends as a blind tube. This may happen in the oesophagus, the duodenum or the rectum/anal canal. Whichever site is involved, the result is an obstruction in the gastrointestinal tract, which requires surgery soon after birth.

Later in development the fetal gut contains the thick, sticky black–green substance known as meconium formed from swallowed amniotic fluid and lanugo (see Chapters 20 and 21), gut secretions and bile. Meconium is normally passed as the 'first faeces' soon after birth. Fetal hypoxia, however, can result in premature discharge of meconium into the amniotic fluid – meconium-stained amniotic fluid may indicate fetal distress during labour. The abnormally thick/dry meconium present in babies with cystic fibrosis, where thick mucus is produced (Chapter 12), can cause bowel obstruction (meconium ileus) in newborns.

General structure of the digestive tract

Before we consider the individual digestive structures it is helpful to look at the basic structure common throughout the tract. Along its entire length can be found the same four layers (mucosa, submucosa, muscularis and serosa/adventitia), with local adaptations related to specific function (*Figure 13.2*).

Mucosa: this is the inner mucous membrane lining and is stratified or columnar epithelium containing goblet cells and glands. Depending on location, it is adapted to protect, to secrete mucus and digestive juices or for absorption. Underlying the epithelium is the lamina propria, a layer of connective tissue containing the lymphoid tissue (see Chapter 11) which helps to protect us from the various pathogens (disease-producing organisms) entering the tract. In certain areas a layer of smooth muscle, the muscularis mucosae, produces folding of the mucosa which allows for distension and greatly increases the surface area available for secretion or absorption.

Submucosa: this layer, below the mucosa, consists of areolar connective tissue containing many blood vessels, lymphatics and nerves. The nerves which supply autonomic fibres to the mucosa form the submucosal (Meissner's) plexus.

Muscularis: this layer is smooth involuntary muscle. There are usually two layers – longitudinal and circular fibres – but the stomach has three layers. Running between the layers are blood vessels, lymphatics and the myenteric (Auerbach's) plexus of autonomic nerve fibres. The muscular layer contracts in response to nerve impulses and hormones to propel food along the tract (**peristalsis** see pages 295–296).

Adventitia/serosa: this is the outer protective layer and is either fibrous connective tissue (in the thorax) or, in the abdominal cavity, a serous membrane called the visceral peritoneum (see below). The serosa prevents friction during gut motility.

Nerve supply

The gastrointestinal tract is innervated by the autonomic nervous system (see Chapter 6). Secretion and motility are generally increased by parasympathetic activity and decreased by sympathetic activity.

The most important parasympathetic nerve is the vagus nerve, which innervates the oesophagus, stomach, pancreas, bile ducts and intestine. The salivary glands receive parasympathetic fibres from the facial and glossopharyngeal nerves, and the last part of the colon and rectum/anus are supplied by the sacral outflow of parasympathetic nerves leaving the sacral part of the spinal cord – the nervi erigentes.

Sympathetic fibres from the cervical, coeliac and mesenteric ganglia innervate the digestive structures. Digestive structures have either alpha or beta sympathetic receptors, but in the case of the stomach and intestine both types are present.

As well as these autonomic nerve fibres, the digestive organs are supplied by autonomic nerve plexuses (Meissner's and Auerbach's), which connect different parts of the tract rather like an internal telephone system. This arrangement allows the gastrointestinal tract to function as an integrated unit.

Peritoneum

The peritoneum is the double serous membrane within the abdominal cavity. The outer (parietal) layer lines the abdominal cavity and the inner (visceral) layer covers some of the abdominal and pelvic organs (viscera). Serous fluid is secreted into the potential space between the two layers (normally the two layers are separated by a thin film of serous fluid; there is no actual space).

During embryonic development the organs invaginate into the peritoneal membrane from above, behind and below, resulting in a rather complex arrangement (see *Figure 13.3*). Some organs are nearly enclosed, e.g. the stomach, whereas others, such as the pelvic organs, are only partially covered by peritoneum; to get some idea of this, try pushing objects into a partially inflated balloon.

In the male the peritoneum forms a closed sac in the pelvis, but in females it is open through the uterine tubes (see Chapter 20).

Functions of the peritoneum

The functions of the peritoneum are:

* Allowing the digestive structures/organs to move easily without friction.
* Acting as a fat store.

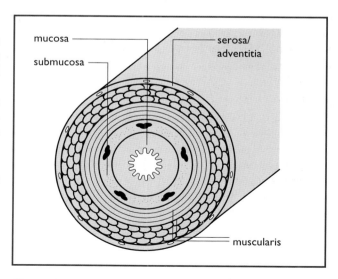

Figure 13.2 Basic structure of the gut wall.

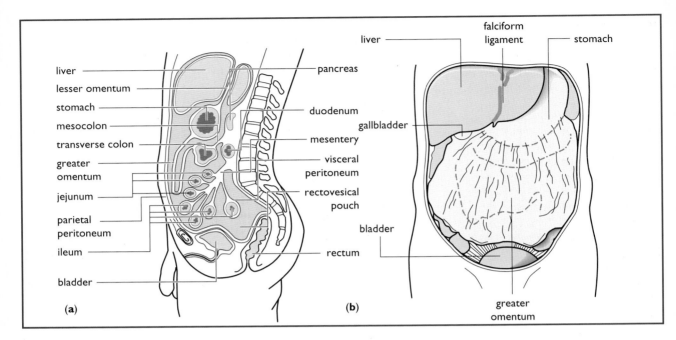

Figure 13.3 (a) The peritoneum (male); **(b)** greater omentum.

Abnormal Function **Problems with the peritoneum**

Malignancy
Mesothelioma is a rare malignancy affecting the peritoneum and also the pleura. It has a very poor prognosis and is usually linked with exposure to asbestos.

Unfortunately, in common with other serous membranes, the peritoneum can act as a route by which malignant cells spread across a cavity (see Chapter 1) and become the site of metastatic spread, e.g. with stomach cancer.

Peritonitis
Peritonitis (inflammation of the peritoneum) may be caused by bacterial infection or chemical irritation. Initially, defence mechanisms attempt to localize the area of inflammation, but failure results in spread and generalized peritonitis. Some causes include: appendicitis, **peptic** ulcer perforation and bowel rupture, e.g. inflammatory bowel disease and biliary perforation, whereby the release of bile causes chemical irritation.

Generalized peritonitis is a life-threatening condition requiring immediate treatment, which includes pain relief, antimicrobial drugs, intravenous fluids to correct fluid and electrolyte imbalance (see Chapter 2), **gastric** emptying through a nasogastric tube and surgery where appropriate. Even with prompt intervention the inflammation produces exudate (fluid) which sticks the inflamed structures together; these adhesions may later obstruct the bowel.

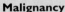

- Anchoring and stabilizing some structures; for example, the mesocolon, a double fold of peritoneum, joins the transverse colon to the posterior abdominal wall.
- Limiting the spread of infection within the cavity – the peritoneum contains many lymph nodes (see Chapter 11). For example, the greater omentum (*Figure 13.3*), which hangs apron-like in front of the small intestine, can move to 'wall off' localized areas of infection (see Peritonitis).
- Supporting blood vessels, lymphatics and nerves; for example, the mesentery, which enfolds part of the small intestine, carries the vessels and nerves supplying the jejunum and ileum.
- Forming the protective outer coat of some organs.

Alimentary Tract – Structure and Function

Before we consider the gastrointestinal tract and the chemical processes involved in the digestion of nutrients, a quick look at the structure of proteins, carbohydrates and fats, discussed in Chapter 1, would be helpful.

Mouth

The mouth (buccal or oral cavity) and accessory structures are concerned with the ingestion, mastication and some chemical digestion of food. The mouth and accessory structures are also important for taste (see Chapter 7) and are vital to our ability to communicate with the world. Without the proper functioning of the tongue and lips it is impossible to speak with clarity or to transmit non-verbal clues about our mood, e.g. smiling.

The mouth is divided into two parts: the vestibule, between the gums/teeth and the lips, and the part more properly called the oral cavity, which lies behind the teeth. It is bounded by the lips anteriorly, the cheek muscles form its lateral walls and posteriorly it is continuous with the oropharynx. Inferiorly there is the tongue and superiorly the hard and soft palates (*Figure 13.4*).

Stratified squamous epithelium lines the mouth and covers the gums as protection against damage during eating. In areas liable to excessive wear and tear, e.g. gums and the external part of the lips, the epithelium is keratinized (see Chapter 1).

The lips and cheeks contain skeletal (voluntary) muscle which assists with ingestion, positioning food for chewing and swallowing and speech.

Tongue

The tongue (*Figure 13.4*) is a highly vascular structure consisting of voluntary muscle. It is attached to the hyoid bone (see *Figure 12.2*) and to the floor of the mouth by a fold of skin called the frenulum. The tongue is supplied with blood from the lingual artery and its venous return drains into the internal jugular vein. The tongue is extremely sensitive and its great mobility is important for speech, mixing food with saliva and the formation of a food bolus (ball of chewed food) for swallowing. Innervation to the tongue is through somatic sensory nerves and three cranial nerves – the facial, glossopharyngeal and hypoglossal.

The upper surface of the tongue, which should be pink and moist, is covered with epithelium that has projections, or papillae, containing the taste buds. Papillae are classified by their shape and may be filiform (filament-shaped), fungiform (mushroom-shaped) or vallate (surrounded by groove or trough); the last are the largest and form a 'V'-shaped pattern on the back of the tongue. Taste, which is discussed more fully in Chapter 7, is linked closely with olfaction to enhance appetite and ensure eating is a safe and enjoyable

process rather than just the intake of nutrients. Different regions of the tongue are concerned with the detection of four basic tastes – bitter, sweet, salt and sour (see *Figure 7.25*). These stimulate the nerve impulses transmitted to the gustatory cortex for interpretation (see Chapters 4 and 7).

Hard and soft palates

The roof of the oral cavity consists of the hard palate anteriorly and the soft palate posteriorly (*Figure 13.4*). The hard palate is formed by the palatine bones and maxilla, which supply the hard surface needed during chewing.

The mobile soft palate is made of voluntary muscle covered with stratified squamous epithelium. From its free edge hangs a projection called the uvula, which can be seen by looking in a mirror and saying 'Ah'. Laterally it is secured to the tongue by the palatoglossal arches and to the oropharynx by the palatopharyngeal arches. It is between these arches that the palatine tonsils are located.

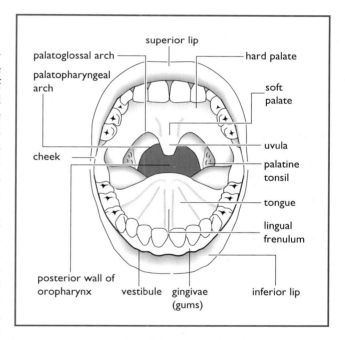

Figure 13.4 The mouth (not all the teeth are shown).

Abnormal Function **Problems with salivary glands – mumps**

Infectious parotitis (mumps) is a viral inflammation of the parotid glands. Apart from pain, swelling and difficulty opening the jaw, it can also cause serious inflammation of the testes (orchitis), which may lead to male sterility, and more rarely of the ovaries (oophoritis). Mumps may also cause inflammation of the pancreas (pancreatitis). Routine immunization against mumps is available during childhood (administered as a combined measles, mumps and rubella vaccine, or MMR). Health professionals should be able to give information regarding this and other infectious disease prophylaxis (see Chapter 19).

During swallowing the soft palate moves upwards to protect the nasopharynx (see Chapter 12).

Salivary glands

Three major pairs of salivary glands – parotid, submaxillary (submandibular) and sublingual – secrete saliva (*Figure 13.5*). The secretion of saliva assists speech, mastication, taste and swallowing; we can all remember how difficult these are with a dry mouth associated with anxiety or fear. Saliva is vital for effective oral hygiene and people with dehydration and a dry mouth will have problems that require nursing interventions (see Nursing Practice Application, page 293). Although saliva contains an enzyme (amylase), it is of very little significance in digestion.

The parotid glands, enclosed in fibrous capsules, are situated just inferior and anterior to the ear. They are the largest salivary glands, but produce only 25% of saliva volume. The saliva leaves by the parotid ducts, which open into the mouth at the level of the second upper molars (teeth). Parasympathetic fibres of the glossopharyngeal nerve stimulate the watery saliva secreted by the parotid glands.

The sublingual glands are situated at the base of the tongue in the floor of the mouth. They produce a small amount of thick, mucous saliva, which enters the mouth through several small ducts. Their nerve supply is from the parasympathetic fibres of the facial nerve.

The submaxillary glands are situated below the maxilla (upper jaw) and have ducts entering the mouth either side of the frenulum. Most saliva is produced by these glands, which are also innervated by the facial nerve.

Saliva

Saliva is mostly water (98–99%) with electrolytes and varying amounts of mucus derived from the glycoprotein mucin. Generally, saliva is slightly acid or neutral (pH 6.8–7.0), but may become alkaline when food is being chewed. The enzyme alpha amylase (previously called ptyalin) is present in saliva and commences the digestion of cooked starch, e.g. bread. Saliva also contains the enzyme lysozyme and immunoglobulin IgA, which protect against micro-organisms (see Chapter 19).

Regulation of salivation

Daily production of saliva is between 1000 and 1500 ml depending on many factors, including level of hydration:

- A conditioned reflex linked to the anticipation, sight or smell of food will stimulate profuse secretion of watery saliva. Certain flavours or personal favourites can produce a more active response, e.g. the smell of a roast lunch, or the sharpness of a lemon drink.
- Salivation occurs in response to the mechanical stimulus of food in the mouth.

Receptors in the mouth send impulses to the salivary nuclei in the medulla and pons (sometimes via the cerebral cortex) which activate the parasympathetic fibres of the facial and glossopharyngeal nerves. These nerve impulses cause vasodilation in the salivary glands, which produce profuse watery secretions. Various drugs, e.g. atropine, block the action of the parasympathetic neurotransmitter acetylcholine (see Chapter 6), resulting in a reduction in salivary, gastric and bronchial secretions. Atropine and similar drugs can be used preoperatively to dry secretions and so

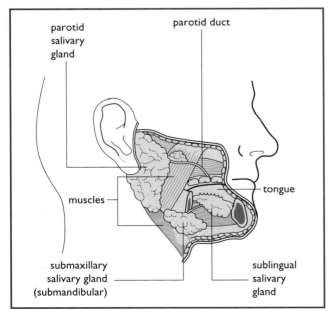

Figure 13.5 Salivary glands.

Nursing Practice Application **Oral hygiene**

An essential part of any nursing assessment is a thorough examination of the person's mouth. The information is obviously needed in planning care, but it can also help in medical diagnosis. The following points should form part of the assessment.

Odour: the mouth should not smell and the presence of halitosis (bad breath) may indicate an abnormality. This may be caused by a reduction in saliva and natural oral cleansing, but will also depend on items ingested, e.g. alcoholic drinks or peppermints. Much more serious are the odours associated with various disease processes, e.g. the 'fruity' smell of diabetic ketoacidosis.

Lips: dryness with cracking may indicate problems with fluid balance (see Chapter 2) or exposure to wind and cold. This problem is overcome by the use of suitable lubricating applications and ensuring an

adequate fluid intake. The presence of 'cold sores' should be noted. These viral (herpes simplex) sores are often seen in debilitated individuals whose reduced resistance allows the dormant virus to be activated.

Tongue: as already discussed, the tongue should be pink and moist, but may become dry and coated in dehydration. Ulcers developing on the tongue feel huge and are extremely painful. They make eating or speaking a trial. Excessive smoothness of the tongue may indicate vitamin-B_{12} deficiency anaemia (see Chapter 9).

Teeth and gums: assessment should include the condition of the teeth (including dentures) and gums, as inflammation and dental problems can cause eating difficulties. The presence of crowns and other appliances should be noted preoperatively to avoid problems connected with anaesthesia.

Candidiasis (thrush): a fungal infection of the mouth and gums that commonly affects very young or old, debilitated individuals, those taking antibiotics and people who are immunosuppressed, e.g. cancer chemotherapy.

Nursing interventions that maintain good oral hygiene are based on stimulating the natural cleansing action of saliva, teeth/gum/mouth brushing and removal of debris or crusts. A vital part of effective 'mouth care' is good general hydration; this ensures comfort and moistens the oral mucosa through normal salivation (Howarth, 1977). The importance of oral care cannot be overstated – the person with a sore, dry mouth has problems with communication, eating and increased vulnerability to infection. Being unable to take in sufficient nutrients will eventually affect weight, skin condition, wound healing and the ability to fight infection.

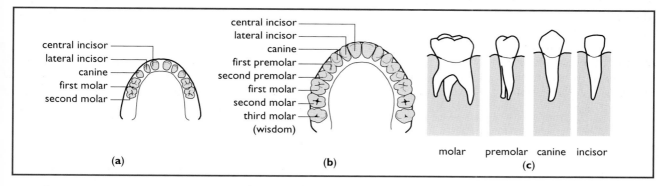

Figure 13.6 (a) First dentition; (b) second dentition; (c) tooth types.

reduce the risk of inhalation while the cough reflex is absent, but since the advent of 'day-case' surgery fewer preoperative drugs are administered.

Sympathetic activity causes vasoconstriction and the production of small amounts of viscous saliva.

Teeth

The teeth are primarily concerned with ingestion and mastication, but they are also important to our appearance and self image. We go to considerable trouble with brushes and braces in our efforts to ensure a dazzling smile.

There are four types of teeth [*Figure 13.6(c)*] embedded within the jaw – incisor (cutting), canine (tearing), premolar and molar (grinding). Each has the same basic

structure (see *Figure 13.7*), but the shape is adapted for the different actions.

Dentition

During a lifetime we have two sets of teeth: the first dentition, of 20 deciduous teeth (milk teeth), which usually erupt between 5–6 months and $2\frac{1}{2}$ years, and the second dentition, of 32 permanent teeth, which starts to replace the deciduous teeth at 5–6 years of age [*Figure 13.6(a),(b)*]. The process of replacement is nearly complete by about 12 years of age but the third molars (wisdom teeth), if they erupt, appear between 18 and 25 years. The wisdom teeth are often impacted in the jaw and their failure to erupt causes problems, such as pain, usually remedied by removing the offending teeth. See Chapter 21 for further coverage.

Structure of a tooth

All teeth consist of a root embedded in the jaw and an exposed part or crown which extends above the gum (gingiva). The constricted region where the crown becomes the root is called the neck. The innermost part of the tooth is the pulp cavity, containing nerves and blood vessels. This is surrounded by a layer of bone-like dentine. Exposed areas, such as the crown, have a further protective layer of extremely hard enamel; if the enamel layer is damaged or breached by decay the inner dentine and eventually the pulp cavity are destroyed by acids. The root is firmly fixed into its socket in the jaw by a substance called cementum and the periodontal membrane or ligament, which together form a type of fibrous joint called a gomphosis (see Chapter 18).

The teeth are innervated by branches of the trigeminal nerve, which can be injected with local anaesthetic to block pain transmission during dental procedures. The abundant arterial blood supply is from the maxillary artery and profuse bleeding can occur after dental extraction.

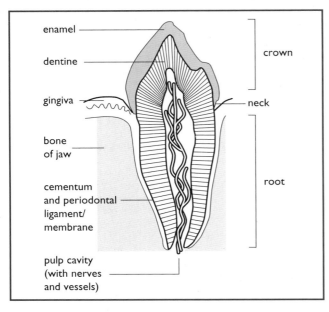

Figure 13.7 Tooth structure.

Pharynx and swallowing

In Chapter 12 we discussed the structure of the pharynx and swallowing in terms of the respiratory tract. You will remember that the oropharynx and laryngopharynx are common channels for food and air, and that various mechanisms normally keep food or fluids out of the larynx.

Abnormal Function **Dental problems — caries and periodontal disease**

Dental caries (decay) is one of the commonest diseases of affluent societies. The problem starts with the formation of plaque – a mixture of bacteria, sugars and food detritus – which collects on the teeth and gums. Bacterial breakdown of the sugar produces acids which damage the enamel and eventually destroy the tooth.

Although dental caries is a serious problem, most teeth are lost because of gum inflammation (gingivitis) and disease.

Periodontal disease, which affects most adults in early midlife, is caused by the calcification of plaque to form tartar. This disturbs the seal between gum and tooth, allowing bacteria to enter the socket with consequent infection and bone destruction.

Prevention of dental caries/gum disease is based on a regimen of dental hygiene which includes careful brushing, cleaning the interdental spaces with tiny brushes or floss, regular dental examination with removal of tartar and avoiding food/fluids that encourage plaque formation, e.g. sugary foods/drinks and 'fizzy drinks' which are acidic and contain sugar.

The use of fluoride supplements or the fluoridation of the water supply have been found to reduce the amount of dental caries. This is especially important during early childhood, when fluoride helps to build decay-resistant teeth.

Healthier Living **Early detection of oral cancers**

We are usually acutely aware of oral problems and the mouth is an easy site for self-examination – all you need is a mirror. Routine dental check-ups are also used to examine the mouth for abnormalities such as cancers. Risk factors for oral cancers include sunlight, smoking, alcohol. Chronic irritation, such as from pipe smoking, poorly fitting dentures or rough teeth, and chewing tobacco or betel leaf/nut also increases the risk. Any persistent ulcers, sore areas that bleed, red or white patches (leukoplakia) and 'lumps and bumps' should be reported to a doctor or dentist. Early detection of oral cancers will increase the efficacy of treatment measures and hopefully lead to a cure.

Nursing Practice Application **Swallowing problems and anxiety**

Dysphagia (difficult swallowing) may have pathophysiological causes, e.g. after a stroke, or sinister causes, such as pharyngeal/oesophageal tumours, but it may be functional (without physical cause).

The affected person complains of a 'lump in the throat' which may be worse when they feel particularly stressed. The condition, which is termed globus hystericus, is caused by spasm of the pharyngeal

muscles. Once pathology has been excluded, nurses can help the person address the underlying problems causing the anxiety and develop ways to minimize the stress effects.

Swallowing has three stages: oral (buccal), pharyngeal and oesophageal. Ingested food is mixed with saliva, chewed and formed into a bolus by the tongue, which moves it to the back of the mouth ready for deglutition (swallowing). As the bolus arrives at the posterior pharyngeal wall it is enclosed by the muscular pharyngeal walls and swallowing ceases to have voluntary control (until this point is reached you decide whether to swallow or not). The involuntary phase now occurs as receptors in the pharynx stimulate the medullary swallowing centre which in turn initiates the swallowing reflex. Impulses from the vagus nerve cause contraction of the pharyngeal constrictor muscles and the food bolus is propelled into the oesophagus, where peristalsis moves it downwards (see below). During the involuntary phase the bolus can go in only one direction because all other routes are blocked: the soft palate blocks the nasopharynx, the larynx rises, the epiglottis covers the trachea, respiration stops and the mouth is closed (try swallowing with your mouth open). If all this fails and food does enter the airways, the cough reflex will operate in a conscious person to clear them.

Oesophagus

The muscular oesophagus only conveys food from the pharynx to the stomach. It plays no part in digestion or absorption. The oesophagus is around 25 cm in length (adults) and runs from the laryngopharynx through the mediastinum and diaphragm to the stomach (*Figure 13.8*).

The oesophagus has the four basic layers of the digestive tract (see page 289), with certain modifications:
- The outer layer is fibrous adventitia.
- The upper third is voluntary muscle, with smooth muscle in the lower two-thirds.
- The mucosa is stratified squamous epithelium containing numerous mucus glands which lubricate the food bolus. At the junction of the oesophagus and stomach the mucosa is columnar.

When no food is being conveyed the oesophageal walls collapse into folds; these distend as food enters.

The food bolus is propelled by a wave of muscular contraction and relaxation, known as peristalsis (see

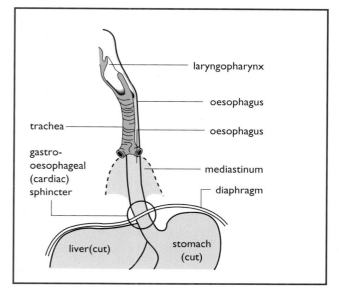

Figure 13.8 Oesophagus (diagrammatic). Lungs, heart and vessels not shown.

Figure 13.9), towards the gastro-oesophageal (cardiac) sphincter or valve. This is a physiological sphincter (the area is anatomically similar to the rest of the oesophagus) where oesophageal muscle contraction keeps the oesophagus closed until a food bolus is swallowed. It functions as a valve and, with the action of the diaphragm, the mechanism usually prevents the reflux of acidic gastric contents into the oesophagus. This mechanism may fail to operate properly if the pressure in the stomach increases, e.g. during pregnancy, abdominal cancers or lying down after an enormous meal. Repeated reflux irritates the mucosa, which leads to oesophagitis and ulcer formation. Reflux may be caused by a structural defect known as hiatus hernia, where the top of the stomach protrudes through the diaphragm into the chest. Congenital forms of hiatus hernia, of varying severity, can also occur. Peristalsis occurs as stretching stimulates the parasympathetic fibres of the vagus nerve and the myenteric nerve plexuses in the muscle layer.

The time taken for a bolus to reach the stomach depends on its consistency (fluids are faster), the body's position (assisted by gravity), and the coordination of the muscular contraction and relaxation (*Figure 13.9*). If you try to eat lying down or too quickly the process is much more difficult.

The oesophagus receives arterial blood from the oesophageal and coeliac arteries, but the venous drainage is more complex. The upper part of the oesophagus drains into the azygos veins, but the lower end drains into the hepatic portal vein and so to the liver (see *Figure 10.45*). There is an anastomosis between the general and hepatic portal systems in the gastrooesophageal region. Varices (dilations) may develop at this site if hepatic portal vein pressure is increased (see Chapters 10 and 14).

Stomach

The stomach is a roughly J-shaped dilatation which in adults can comfortably hold 1.5litres of food and fluids, which it churns and mixes with gastric juices to form the semifluid chyme. Some digestion occurs in the stomach and there is limited absorption. The stomach is situated in the left upper abdomen, usually in the left hypochondriac and epigastric abdominal regions (see *Figure 1.33*).

The stomach can be divided into the cardia (enclosing the cardiac orifice), fundus, body and pylorus. A large lateral convex surface – the greater curvature – and a smaller medial concave surface – the lesser curvature – provide attachments for folds of peritoneum (see *Figure 13.10* and

Figure 13.3). The pyloric portion (antrum), which is continuous with the small intestine, is guarded by the pyloric sphincter, ensuring the coordinated release of gastric contents into the duodenum (first part of small intestine).

The basic four-layer structure, described on page 289, is present in the stomach, with modifications to the muscle and the mucosa. As well as longitudinal and circular muscle fibres, the stomach also has oblique fibres, which make it a highly mobile food mixer. This muscle arrangement allows very efficient mechanical mixing and breakdown of food. The gastric mucosa is columnar epithelium with deep gastric pits containing mucus glands and gastric glands which secrete gastric juice. There is some variation within the stomach, e.g. more mucus glands in the cardia and pylorus. The gastric mucosa is thrown into folds, or rugae, which greatly increase the surface area for secretion and allow for considerable distension following a meal. The stomach receives its arterial blood from several branches of the coeliac artery [see *Figure 10.43(a)*] and the venous return drains through the gastric and splenic veins, which empty into the hepatic portal circulation (see *Figure 10.45*).

Parasympathetic fibres from the vagus nerves stimulate gastric secretion and motility (see below). The opposite effects are achieved by the stimulation of sympathetic fibres from the coeliac ganglion.

Gastric secretions and functions

Gastric secretions include:
- Intrinsic factor.
- Hydrochloric acid (HCl).
- Hormones, e.g. gastrin and paracrine secretions such as histamine.

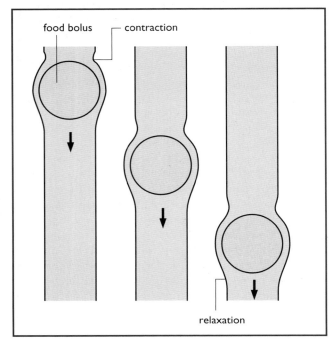

Figure 13.9 Peristalsis.

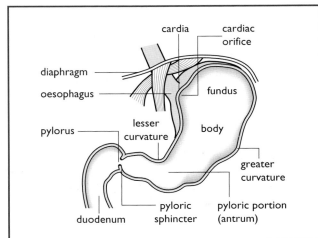

Figure 13.10 The stomach.

- Mucus.
- **Enzymes.**

Parietal (oxyntic) cells situated in the gastric pits produce HCl (*Figure 13.11*) and intrinsic factor, a glycoprotein needed for the absorption of vitamin B$_{12}$ in the small intestine. Where a large part of the stomach has been removed (gastrectomy) the person requires regular injections of vitamin B$_{12}$, lack of which causes megaloblastic anaemia (see Chapter 9) and problems with nerve function (see Chapter 3).

HCl is a strong acid and produces a pH of between 1.5 and 3 in the stomach. The acid is produced by a series of reactions (*Figure 13.11*) involving chloride ions and carbon dioxide from the blood, water and the enzyme carbonic anhydrase (see Chapter 12). Hydrogen and chloride ions are actively secreted, against the gradient, into the stomach lumen, where they combine to form the acid. The hydrogen ions utilize an ATP-powered proton-pump (H$^+$/K$^+$-ATPase) to enter the stomach lumen, with the potassium ions moving into the parietal cell. Meanwhile, hydrogen carbonate ions move from the parietal cell into the blood as the alkaline tide.

The secretion of HCl is stimulated by the hormone gastrin, which is released by the gastric mucosa, the neurotransmitter acetylcholine (vagus nerve) and histamine from mast cells or cells containing histamine (see Chapter 9). All three substances use second-messenger systems (see Chapter 8) to increase HCl secretion. A synthetic gastrin (pentagastrin) is available for use in a rarely performed test which assesses gastric acid secretion using samples obtained through a nasogastric tube.

Histamine stimulates acid secretion by binding to specific sites (H$_2$ receptors) in the cell. This has an important clinical application because drugs which block histamine are used to reduce acid production. These H$_2$ receptor antagonists, e.g. ranitidine and nizatidine, are used in the treatment of reflux oesophagitis and peptic ulceration. Acid secretion can also be reduced by proton pump inhibitors, such as the drug omeprazole.

The functions of gastric acid include destruction of many micro-organisms, inactivation of amylase (from the saliva), chemical breakdown of food, conversion of iron into the easily absorbable ferrous state, conversion of pepsinogen into pepsin and provision of optimal pH for pepsin activity.

Nursing Practice Application **Stomach size and the neonate**

Although an adult can pack 1.5 litres of food and fluids into his or her stomach it is vital to remember that the tiny stomach of a neonate has a capacity of 30–35 millilitres. This has implications for feeding regimens and frequent small volume feeds are required to provide sufficient energy, nutrients and fluid (remember that the infant body is 70–75% water). Gastric capacity, however, increases rapidly and has tripled by the end of the first month. This means that larger feeds can be taken and the time interval between feeds starts to increase naturally, which provides some respite for the exhausted, sleep-deprived new parents.

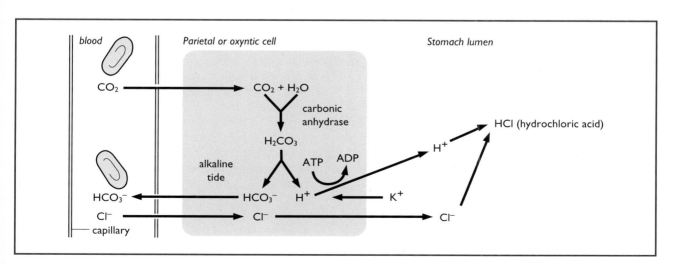

Figure 13.11 Hydrochloric acid production (simplified).

Zymogen (chief) cells, also situated within the gastric pits, secrete the proteolytic enzyme precursor (forerunner) pepsinogen. This is converted by gastric acid to its active form pepsin, which in turn activates more pepsinogen. The pepsin starts the digestion of proteins by breaking them down into polypeptides (long chains of amino acids).

Mucus-secreting cells in the top of the gastric pits produce thick alkaline (contains hydrogen carbonate ions) mucus which adheres to the mucosa of the stomach wall. This protects the stomach wall from digestion by its own proteolytic (protein-digesting) enzyme and damage from HCl. Impairment of mucus production leaves the stomach vulnerable to damage and ulcer formation. Mucus and hydrogen carbonate secretion is stimulated by prostaglandins (see Chapter 8), which also inhibit acid production. This explains why drugs that inhibit prostaglandin synthesis, such as aspirin and other non-steroidal anti-inflammatory drugs (NSAIDs), can reduce the mucus protection and cause gastritis and ulceration.

Hormone-producing cells (enteroendocrine) secrete several hormones, including gastrin, secretin, 5-hydroxytryptamine, histamine and somatostatin (see GHIH, Chapter 8). These hormones are concerned with the regulation of HCl secretion, gastric motility and emptying (see page 297 and below).

Control of gastric secretion and activity

Control of gastric secretions and activity has both neural and hormonal components, and can be divided into three phases – cephalic, gastric and intestinal (*Figure 13.12*). Between 2 and 3 litres of gastric juice are produced by the mucosa each day.

The cephalic phase involves a conditioned reflex in which the vagus nerve is stimulated (via the medulla) by the thought, sight, smell or taste of food. The dramatic increase in gastric secretion of HCl and enzymes is in anticipation of food arriving in the stomach. This reflex ceases to function following vagotomy (surgical division of the gastric branches of the vagus nerve, which may be performed for peptic ulceration not responding to drugs – see page 301).

The gastric phase of secretion is both neural and hormonal. Food entering the stomach stimulates the local nerve plexus (submucosal) through stretch receptors activated by stomach distension. The neural activity (parasympathetic) leads to the release of acetylcholine, which in turn causes the gastric glands to secrete.

During the gastric phase the hormonal influence is also important. Certain foods, protein, caffeine-containing drinks (tea, coffee, colas) and alcohol arriving in the stomach cause the release of the hormone gastrin from the gastric glands of the antrum (see Chapter 8). Gastrin travels in the circulation to the gastric glands, where it stimulates the production of more HCl. The production of gastrin is also linked

to the neural influences already described and to the release of other peptides. As previously mentioned, histamine release, in response to food entering the stomach, is an important stimulator of HCl secretion.

Gastric secretion is inhibited by fear and anxiety (sympathetic nerves) – your appetite disappears instantly if you are upset.

During the intestinal phase small amounts of stimulatory intestinal gastrin are produced by the duodenal mucosa as partially digested acidic food starts to arrive in the small intestine. Eventually, however, the continued arrival of stomach contents distends the duodenum, which initiates an inhibitory enterogastric reflex (see page below) and the release of various intestinal regulatory peptides, e.g. secretin, gastric inhibitory peptide (GIP), vasoactive intestinal peptide (VIP), cholecystokinin (CCK) and somatostatin – all of which inhibit gastric secretion and or motility.

Motility and emptying

The length of time food stays in the stomach depends on its make-up and consistency, but emptying is usually complete within 4–5 hours of eating. As you would expect, fluids soon enter the duodenum, but solid food is first mixed thoroughly with gastric juice by peristaltic contractions. A meal high in carbohydrates passes rapidly into the duodenum, followed by proteins and lastly fats, which may stay in the stomach for 5–6 hours. This has important practice applications when deciding how long to fast a person before surgery (see Further Reading, Hamilton-Smith, 1972).

As acid chyme is squirted through the pyloric sphincter into the duodenum, the enterogastric reflex is initiated by stretch and chemoreceptors. The reflex involves parasympathetic inhibition, which decreases gastric activity, local nerve activity inhibition, sympathetic contraction of the pylorus and the release of regulatory peptides from the duodenal mucosa, e.g secretin, and when chyme is fatty GIP and CCK, which also inhibit gastric secretion, motility and emptying. The neurotransmitter nitric oxide may also influence gastric emptying (see Chapter 3). These controls ensure that the duodenum is not deluged and that there is time for intestinal mixing and digestion before the next batch of chyme arrives. This controlled release of hypertonic (see Chapter 2) gastric contents also prevents the osmotic movement of water from the blood to intestinal lumen, which would result in the development of hypovolaemia (see Chapter 10).

Summary – digestion in the stomach
Mechanical: mixing and churning reduces solid food to liquid chyme.
Chemical: HCl alters the structure of proteins and the enzyme pepsin commences protein digestion.

Gastric absorption

Very little absorption is known to occur through the gastric mucosa, although water and some fat-soluble molecules, e.g. alcohol and some drugs, can be absorbed here. Anyone who has had an alcoholic drink on an empty stomach can vouch for the rapidity of this process: it is always prudent to have something to eat and to drink alcohol within sensible limits (see Chapter 14). Aspirin is one of the drugs absorbed by the stomach and in large doses over long periods it can cause gastritis (irritation of the stomach lining), with bleeding and possible haematemesis (vomiting blood) or melaena (passing altered blood in the stools). For this reason aspirin should not be taken by people with a history of ulcers, by those taking anticoagulants or by those with clotting problems (see Chapter 9).

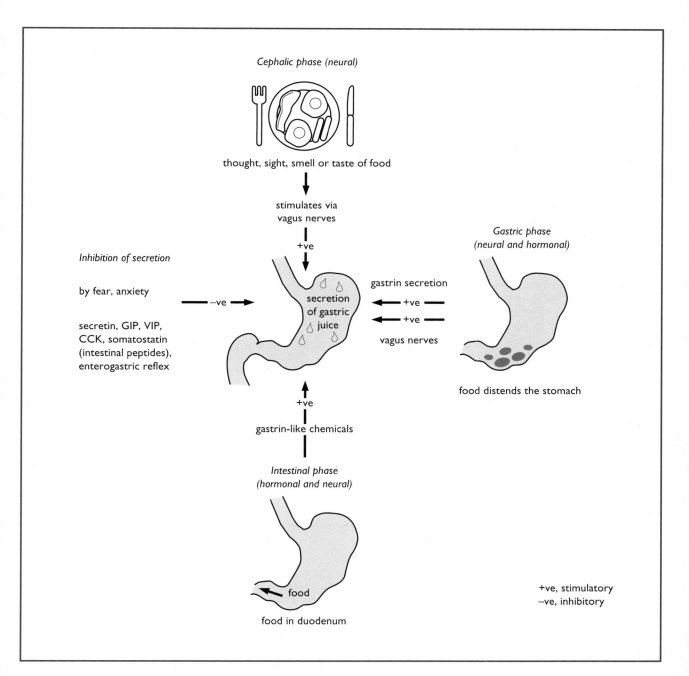

Figure 13.12 Control of gastric secretion.

Nursing Practice Application **Vomiting**

Vomiting is an extremely disagreeable experience that occurs when gastric contents are reflexly expelled through the mouth. It is initiated by two centres in the medulla:

- A chemoreceptor trigger zone (CTZ) [dopamine (D_2) and 5-hydroxytryptamine (5-HT_3) receptors] sensitive to blood-borne chemical stimuli, such as drugs or the abnormal blood chemistry of uraemia (see Chapter 15), and to motion sickness via the inner ear (see Chapter 7) and vestibular nuclei [histamine (H_1) and muscarinic receptors].
- The vomiting centre (muscarinic receptors) which responds to stimuli from the CTZ, higher centres, e.g. pain and emotion (ever been 'sick' before an exam?), and from visceral afferents (5-HT_3 receptors) in the gastrointestinal tract.

The vomiting centre sends impulses which cause the diaphragm and abdominal wall to contract, and with the pylorus closed the increasing gastric pressure forces stomach contents out into the oesophagus and pharynx. The nasopharynx and larynx are normally closed during vomiting to prevent inhalation of vomitus, but if these mechanisms fail to operate, e.g. in an unconscious person, vomitus may enter and block the airway (see Chapter 12).

Before vomiting the person often experiences nausea; they may be pale and sweaty, and their mouth fills with watery saliva. Vomiting may be provoked by gastric/intestinal distension or irritants, e.g. bacterial toxins, alcohol and blood. Other causes of vomiting include motion sickness, drugs such as cytotoxic agents, unpleasant sights or odours, fear, pain, anxiety and raised intracranial pressure (see Chapter 4). In some situations, e.g. after ingestion of mouldy or contaminated food, vomiting may be considered protective.

A person who is vomiting generally needs: privacy and support; a suitable receptacle and a denture container, if appropriate; facilities for teeth cleaning; a mouthwash; and a wash afterwards. Postoperatively people should be encouraged to support wounds with their hands (see wound care, Chapter 19). The vomit and type of vomiting, e.g. projectile, should be observed and accurate records of fluid balance kept. Apart from these simple measures, nurses should ensure that the most appropriate antiemetic drugs (drugs that stop vomiting), e.g. metoclopramide, are administered as prescribed. Kinghorn (1995) identifies the need for proper assessment into the cause of the nausea and vomiting. Antiemetics should always be given in anticipation of expected vomiting such as with cytotoxic drugs.

The following are considered to be important factors in choosing an antiemetic Eburn (1989):

- Whether the drug is for prophylaxis or relief.
- Which route is appropriate.
- Which site of drug action is appropriate.

Antiemetics act in a variety of ways and it is essential to use the most appropriate drug. Types of antiemetics, according to Rang *et al.* (1995), include:

- Central dopamine (D_2) receptor antagonists, e.g. metoclopramide, used in vomiting caused by cytotoxic drugs, radiation, digestive tract problems and migraine, and prochlorperazine (a phenothiazine), which blocks the CTZ.
- Muscarinic-receptor antagonists, e.g. hyosine, used to prevent motion sickness, often transdermally via a skin patch applied behind the ear.
- Histamine receptor (H_1) antagonists, e.g. cyclizine, used in motion sickness, radiation and postoperatively.
- 5–hydroxytryptamine receptor (5-HT_3) antagonists, e.g. ondansetron, used in vomiting caused by cytotoxic drugs and radiation.
- Synthetic cannabinoids, e.g. nabilone, used where other antiemetics fail to control cytotoxic drug induced vomiting. It works by blocking the activation of the CTZ.

The problems of prolonged/excessive vomiting include:

- Fluid and electrolyte imbalance (see Chapter 2).
- Pain and soreness felt in the abdominal muscles, especially after surgery.
- Metabolic alkalosis (see Chapter 12) caused by the loss of HCl. The parietal cells attempt to replace the acid, and the hydrogen carbonate ions entering the blood makes it more alkaline (see *Figure 13.11*). Where vomiting is chronic the person will utilize body fat for energy, which results in the production of ketoacids and metabolic acidosis rather than alkalosis (see Chapter 12).
- Weight loss.
- Damage to teeth.

Small intestine

The small intestine is a coiled tube 5–6 m in length which runs from the pyloric sphincter to the ileocaecal valve. It is divided into three parts – the duodenum (25 cm), jejunum (2 m) and ileum (3 m) – which lie in the abdomen surrounded by large intestine (see *Figure 13.1*). The duodenum (*Figure 13.13*), which loops around the head of the pancreas, receives the duct carrying bile and pancreatic juice. The bile and pancreatic ducts join at a point called the hepato-pancreatic ampulla (previously called ampulla of Vater) to empty through the duodenal papilla, which is controlled by the sphincter of Oddi.

The jejunum is the middle portion of small intestine between the duodenum and ileum. The ileum is the longest

Special Focus **Peptic ulcer**

Peptic ulceration occurs in any area of mucosa exposed to pepsin/gastric acid where the mucosal resistance is impaired. Ulcers are most common in the stomach and duodenum, but can develop in the lower oesophagus, in Meckel's diverticulum (a persistent embryonic yolk sac connection with the umbilical cord) or in the jejunum following its surgical anastomosis to the stomach.

Ulcers may be acute or chronic, and some, but not all, are associated with excess gastric acid. Factors implicated in the aetiology of chronic ulcers include: presence of the bacterium *Helicobacter pylori*, which causes gastritis and is responsible for 70% of gastric and 90% of duodenal ulcers (Edwards *et al.*, 1995), heredity, bile reflux, excess alcohol, drugs such as aspirin, corticosteroids and other anti-inflammatory drugs, and smoking. Stress appears to influence their development; certainly they occur acutely as a result of severe physiological stress such as burns and are linked with stressful situations or occupations.

The presence of a peptic ulcer usually causes a 'gnawing' pain in the upper abdomen which may be associated with food intake or an empty stomach (depends on site), vomiting and chronic health problems such as anaemia caused by slight but persistent bleeding. For most people there is time lost from work and a general reduction in the quality of life. The dangers, however, are massive haemorrhage (haematemesis/melaena), perforation with peritonitis or gastric outlet obstruction due to scar tissue.

A very rare cause of peptic ulcer is Zollinger–Ellison syndrome, where there is an ectopic (outside the normal site) source of gastrin production, usually a pancreatic tumour. As you can imagine, this stimulates excessive gastric acid production, peptic ulcer formation and inactivation of intestinal enzymes, which have an optimum pH of around 7.

part of the small intestine and joins the large intestine at the ileocaecal valve. Both the jejunum and ileum are secured to the posterior abdominal wall by folds of peritoneum (mesentery) which also support its blood vessels, lymphatics and nerves. The small intestine finishes the digestive processes started in the mouth and stomach, using secretions from the intestinal mucosa, pancreas and liver, and is responsible for nearly all the absorption of nutrients and water that occurs. Chyme takes up to 6 hours to move through the small intestine by segmentation. This involves alternate contraction and relaxation of the muscle layer and peristalsis (see *Figure 13.9*). Segmentation also ensures mixing of chyme with intestinal juice. The same four layers (see page 289) are present, but the submucosa and mucosa (columnar epithelium) are highly modified for their role in digestion and absorption (see *Figure 13.14*). There are three adaptations which greatly increase the surface area of the small intestine:

- Circular folding, which remains even when the intestine is distended.
- The mucosa has villi – finger-like projections about 0.5–1.0 mm long (see *Figure 13.16*) – which contain capillaries and a central lymphatic lacteal (see Chapter 11).
- Microvilli (brush border) (see *Figure 13.16*) project from the free edge of the villi. These microvilli increase the area available for absorption and contain some digestive enzymes.

Lymphoid tissue occurs as solitary mucosal nodes in the duodenum and jejunum and as submucosal aggregates known as Peyer's patches in the ileum. These help prevent bacteria from entering the blood.

Alkaline mucus secreted by Brunner's glands situated within the duodenal submucosa helps to neutralize the

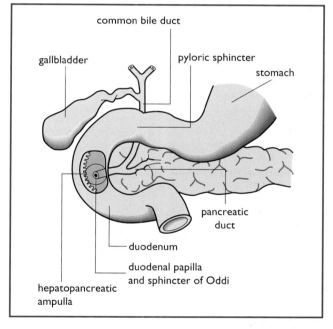

Figure 13.13 Duodenum and related structures.

acidity of the chyme, protects the duodenal mucosa from damage and provides the optimal pH for intestinal enzyme activity. Deep folds, or intestinal crypts (crypts of Lieberkuhn), between the villi form tubular glands containing several cell types, including mucus-secreting goblet cells (see Chapter 12) and columnar cells (enterocytes) which produce intestinal enzymes or are concerned with absorption (*Figure 13.14*).

Cells from the depths of the crypts are continually migrating to the surface of the villi where they replace cells lost through general wear and tear. The surface can be renewed in little more than a day. The small intestine receives arterial blood from the superior mesenteric artery and drains its venous blood through veins which empty into the hepatic portal vein [see *Figures 10.43(b)* and *10.45*].

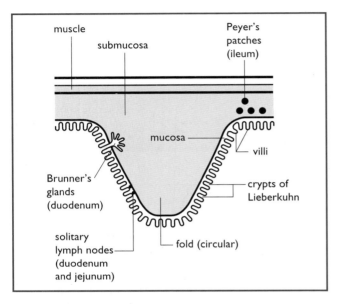

Figure 13.14 Structure of the small intestine (general) – diagrammatic.

Role of the pancreas as an accessory organ of digestion

Earlier we discussed the dual endocrine and exocrine (gland with duct through which its secretions are discharged) roles of the pancreas (see Chapter 8). The pancreas is divided into three: the head, lying within the curve of the duodenum, and the body and tail, which lie behind the stomach and are retroperitoneal [behind the peritoneum (*Figure 13.15*)].

The pancreas, which has a vital role in digestion, produces approximately 1500 ml of alkaline (pH 8.0) pancreatic juice every day. Its exocrine acinar cells (grape-like secretory cells arranged in clusters around a tiny duct system) produce the juice, containing digestive enzymes, hydrogen carbonate ions, which further neutralize acid chyme, electrolytes and mucus. The juice leaves the pancreas in ducts, which join to form the main pancreatic duct. This in turn joins with the bile duct to enter the duodenum. Secretion of pancreatic juice is stimulated by:

- Regulatory peptide hormones – CCK and secretin, which was the first hormone discovered (by Bayliss and Starling in 1902). As chyme enters the duodenum these hormones are produced by the duodenal mucosa – CCK in response to fats and proteins, and secretin in response to acidic chyme. At one time it was thought that there were two separate hormones, CCK and pancreozymin

(PZ), but they are now known to be a single substance (sometimes called CCK-PZ) affecting both pancreatic and gallbladder activity.

- Neural stimulation from the vagus nerve stimulates secretion (during the cephalic and gastric phases; see page 298), but is of much less importance than the hormones.

Pancreatic enzymes

The pancreas produces enzymes concerned with the digestion of proteins, carbohydrates, fats and nucleic acids.

The three proteolytic (protein-digesting) enzymes are secreted as their inactive precursors – trypsinogen, chymotrypsinogen and procarboxypeptidase. These are not activated until they reach the duodenum, to avoid damage to the pancreas by autodigestion. Trypsinogen is converted to the active enzyme trypsin by another enzyme, enterokinase (sometimes called enteropeptidase), produced by the duodenal mucosa. The trypsin, once formed, acts on further trypsinogen and the other precursors, which it activates to form chymotrypsin and carboxypeptidase.

Trypsin and chymotrypsin act upon proteins and polypeptides to form peptides, which are short chains of amino acids. The peptides formed in this way are broken down into individual amino acids by the carboxypeptidase.

Amylase (see page 292) produced by the pancreas converts starch, which is a polysaccharide (composed of many linked monosaccharide units), to the disaccharide (two monosaccharide units) maltose. See Chapter 1 for an explanation of the terms mono-, di- and polysaccharide.

Pancreatic lipase is the enzyme which digests fat. It acts on triglycerides (triacylglycerols), converting them to glycerol and fatty acids (see Chapter 1). Lipase can only operate after the clumps of fat globules have been emulsified by bile salts (see page 304).

Pancreatic juice contains nucleases (ribonuclease, deoxyribonuclease) which convert RNA and DNA to nucleotides (see Chapter 1).

Bile and digestion

We have outlined the formation of bile pigments from haem during erythrocyte breakdown (see Chapter 9) and the details of bile production and excretion by the liver can be found in Chapter 14.

Between 500 and 1000 ml of alkaline (pH 8.0) bile is produced each day by the liver. This is a continuous process and bile not immediately required is stored and concentrated by the gallbladder. Bile is a green–yellow

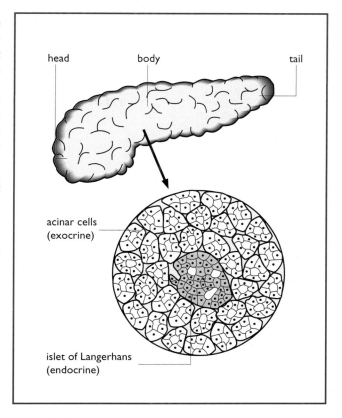

head   body   tail

acinar cells
(exocrine)

islet of Langerhans
(endocrine)

Figure 13.15 Pancreas.

Nursing Practice Application **Starch digestion and the timing of weaning**

The ability to produce starch-digesting enzymes is not present at birth. Secretion does not commence until the infant is aged 12–16 weeks. It is therefore sensible, for this and other reasons, to delay weaning with starch-based foods, e.g. potato or rice, until the ability to deal with starch is reached at 16 weeks. Other reasons for not weaning earlier include: until babies are 12 weeks old swallowing only occurs after suckling and babies reflexly push solid food out of their mouths (extrusion reflex) until 16 weeks of age.

fluid which contains water, bile acids (salts), bile pigments (mainly bilirubin and some biliverdin), cholesterol, phospholipids and electrolytes. It also provides an excretory route for the breakdown products of steroid and other hormones (see Chapter 8) and some drugs which leave the body in the faeces. Bile is both a secretory (secreted by liver cells) and excretory (carries substances for excretion) product.

Bile secretion is stimulated by the intestinal hormone secretin and high levels of bile salts in the blood. Bile salts are reabsorbed in the ileum and returned to the liver by the hepatic portal vein by a recycling process known as the enterohepatic circulation of bile salts. The actual release of bile into the duodenum through the common bile duct, which unites with the pancreatic duct, depends on the simultaneous contraction of the gallbladder and relaxation of the sphincter of Oddi. The main stimulus for this is CCK, already mentioned in connection with pancreatic secretion, which is released in response to fatty and protein-rich chyme entering the duodenum. There is also a neural component via the vagus nerve. After gallbladder emptying the bile flows directly from the liver to duodenum through the bile ducts.

Functions of bile
- Bile acts like a detergent to emulsify fat globules in the partially digested food – much like washing-up liquid works on greasy plates. Bile salts (which have polar and non-polar areas) separate the fat into smaller droplets which can mix with the watery intestinal contents. The smaller droplets have a greater surface area which allows pancreatic lipases to start the chemical breakdown of fat into fatty acids and glycerol.
- Bile salts are also concerned with the absorption of digested fat, cholesterol and fat-soluble vitamins (see pages 306–307). The bile salts form micelles (small 'clumps') with lipids which enhances their 'transport' into the intestinal cells.
- Bile salts deodorize faeces.

It is important to note that bilirubin is oxidized and converted by intestinal bacteria to the substance stercobilinogen. Some of this is reabsorbed into the blood but the remainder becomes stercobilin, which colours the faeces brown. When bile is not present in the intestine, e.g. a gallstone is obstructing the common bile duct, the faeces will be pale (clay coloured) and have a particularly offensive odour caused by the presence of undigested fat.

Intestinal juice
The secreting cells of the intestinal glands produce 1–2 litres of alkaline (pH 8.0) intestinal juice every day.

We might digress here, to remind ourselves just how much fluid is produced by the gastrointestinal tract and accessory organs:

Saliva	1000–1500 ml
Gastric juice	2000–3000 ml
Pancreatic juice	1500 ml
Bile	500–1000 ml
Intestinal juice	1000–2000 ml
TOTAL	6000–9000 ml

Taking the maximum figures, we end up with the staggering total of 9 l of fluid produced per day (enough to fill nearly 16 milk cartons), the majority of which is reabsorbed, along with what you drink. From this it is easy to see why dehydration occurs with severe vomiting and diarrhoea (see Person-Centred Study – Natalie, Chapter 2) and where intestinal obstruction prevents fluid reabsorption. It is important to grasp the concept that fluid in the digestive tract is really 'outside the body'; it is not contributing to cell metabolism, and collection of fluid in the large intestine due to obstruction causes dehydration even though the fluid is not ejected from the intestine.

Intestinal fluid contains water, mucus, electrolytes and enzymes, most of which are present in the brush border of the microvilli (see page 301). Secretion is stimulated by the mechanical and chemical effects of chyme on the intestinal cells and the release of regulatory peptide hormones such as secretin.

Intestinal enzymes
A whole series of intestinal enzymes complete protein and carbohydrate digestion. The duodenal mucosa secretes enterokinase (enteropeptidase), which activates pancreatic trypsinogen. The peptides formed by the pancreatic proteolytic enzymes are reduced to their individual amino acids by the action of aminopeptidases and dipeptidases present in the microvilli (brush border). Aminopeptidases act on the amine (NH_2) end of the peptide chain and dipeptidases cleave the bond between a pair of amino acids (dipeptide).

Carbohydrate digestion is completed by three enzymes which convert disaccharides into monosaccharides, which can then be absorbed: maltase converts maltose to glucose; lactase converts lactose to glucose and galactose; and sucrase converts sucrose to fructose and glucose.

Aminopeptidase acts here   Dipeptidase acts here

▼   ▼

NH_2 – ● – COOH * NH_2 – ● – COOH * NH_2 – ● – COOH * NH_2 – ● – COOH

● = amino acid   * = bond between a pair of amino acids

NH_2 = amine end   COOH = carboxyl end

Enzymes convert:

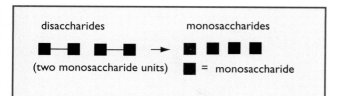

disaccharides   monosaccharides

(two monosaccharide units)   ■ = monosaccharide

Fat digestion is completed by lipases in the microvilli, but you will remember that this is mostly the responsibility of pancreatic lipases and takes place in the duodenum.

Nucleotides produced by the action of pancreatic nucleases on nucleic acids are further broken down. Intestinal enzymes cleave the nucleotides apart to release their component pentose sugar, bases and phosphate.

The digestive processes are now complete. The main products of digestion are the monosaccharides (glucose, fructose and galactose), amino acids, fatty acids and glycerol. The various nutrients are now in a form which can be absorbed and utilized (see charts page 306).

Absorption in the small intestine

As already stated, the small intestine is the major site for the absorption of nutrients and water. To get some idea of the importance of the small intestine in absorption we have only to consider the fate of the 6–9 litres of fluid produced by the gastrointestinal tract and the assorted food and drinks consumed per day. Only about 1 litre of fluid and undigested food reaches the large intestine. This obviously means that something amazing in terms of absorption is occurring in the small intestine. Before we start it will be useful for you to have a quick look at Chapters 1 and 2 to check your understanding of transport mechanisms across plasma membranes.

Some nutrients pass through the cell membrane of the intestinal cells by active transport, which requires metabolic energy (ATP). Active transport occurs against a concentration gradient and requires the presence of carrier molecules. Other nutrients move down gradients by passive transport, which does not use energy. When passive transport requires a protein carrier molecule it is known as facilitated diffusion. Water moves passively by osmosis and is linked to the active and passive movement of water-soluble nutrients.

Nursing Practice Application **Lactose intolerance**

The ability to digest lactose (milk sugar) is obviously important during infancy. Some people continue to produce the enzyme lactase throughout life, and most Caucasians in Europe and North America have this genetic mutation (exposure to dairy products over many generations). They will have no problems digesting milk or milk products; however, those without lactase will have bloating, increased flatus, colic and diarrhoea when they eat foods containing lactose (apart from the obvious foods, many processed foods contain milk products). In the UK lactose intolerance is a problem for many Asian and Afro-Caribbean individuals. Nurses can provide information about which foods should be avoided in a lactose-free/reduced diet and how lactase can be added to food, while ensuring that their advice is culturally sensitive and is sufficient for the person to choose a balanced diet.

Summary of chemical digestion

Gastric juice

PROTEIN
HCl alters protein structure
↓
Pepsin converts proteins ——> polypeptides

Pancreatic
enzymes
↓
Trypsin (activated by enterokinase/enteropeptidase) and chymotrypsin convert polypeptides ——> peptides
Carboxypeptidases convert peptides ——> amino acids

Intestinal enzymes
↓
Aminopeptidases and dipeptidases convert peptides ——> amino acids
↓
AMINO ACIDS

Saliva

CARBOHYDRATES
Salivary amylase converts cooked starch ——> maltose
↓
Pancreatic enzymes
Pancreatic amylase converts starch ——> maltose
↓
Intestinal enzymes
Maltase converts maltose ——> glucose
Lactase converts lactose ——> glucose and galactose
Sucrase converts sucrose ——> glucose and fructose
↓
MONOSACCHARIDES – GLUCOSE, GALACTOSE, FRUCTOSE

Bile

FATS
Emulsification of fat
↓
Pancreatic enzymes
Lipases convert emulsified fats ——> fatty acids and glycerol
↓
Intestinal enzymes
Lipases convert emulsified fats ——> fatty acids and glycerol
↓
FATTY ACIDS and GLYCEROL

The structure of the intestinal mucosa is ideally adapted for absorption – the villi and microvilli provide a huge surface area. Once inside the epithelial cells of the villi, most nutrients enter the capillaries which eventually lead to the hepatic portal vein, but some fatty acids and glycerol are absorbed into the central lymphatic lacteal (*Figure 13.16*).

Absorption details

Amino acids
Amino acid absorption is an active process involving different carrier molecules. Some of the carrier molecules are coupled with sodium transport which appears to increase their activity. Most amino acids are absorbed in the ileum and enter the capillary network of the villus.

Monosaccharides
Monosaccharides are absorbed both actively and passively. Glucose and galactose use the same carrier molecule and their transport is coupled with the active absorption of sodium. Fructose absorption is separate – it uses facilitated diffusion by carrier and is not linked with sodium transport. The monosaccharides enter the capillary network for transport to the liver.

Fats
Fats have an unusual absorption mechanism. They are the only nutrient to enter the lymph as well as the blood. Fatty acids, glycerol and other lipids, such as cholesterol, combine with bile salts (see page 304) to form tiny clusters

or micelles. The micelles transport the fats to the entero-cytes (see page 301) and once there diffuse passively through the lipid component of the plasma membrane into the cells. The bile salts are left in the lumen of the intestine for reuse. Most fat absorption occurs in the duodenum and is completed in the ileum. Once inside the cell most of the fatty acids and glycerol reform as triglycerides/triacylglycerols (three fatty acids and glycerol) within the smooth endoplasmic reticulum:

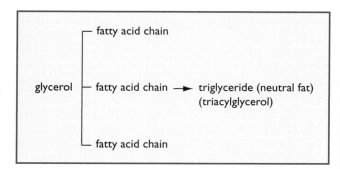

The reconstituted fat is formed into chylomicrons after being coated with other molecules, including lipoproteins and cholesterol, in the Golgi apparatus. The chylomicrons enter the central lacteal to form the creamy chyle, which is transported via the lymph to the blood (see Chapter 11). The remaining fatty acids enter the capillary network. Both routes ensure that eventually the products of fat digestion arrive at the liver for utilization.

Cholesterol is transported in the blood combined with protein, a combination known as lipoprotein. There are various types of lipoprotein, which include very low-density lipoproteins (VLDL), low-density lipoproteins (LDL) and high-density lipoproteins (HDL). The ratio of HDL:VLDL/LDL is very important for health (see Chapter 10). A decreased ratio is associated with arterial disease, whereas an increased ratio appears to have a protective function.

Vitamins

Vitamins are divided into two groups, the water-soluble (B complex and C) and the fat-soluble (A, D, E and K).

Water-soluble vitamins are mostly absorbed passively with water, except vitamin B_{12}, which is absorbed in the terminal part of the ileum and requires intrinsic factor (see page 297). Vitamin B_{12}, a large molecule, needs to form a complex with intrinsic factor before it can be absorbed. The vitamin B_{12}–intrinsic factor complex binds to receptor sites in the mucosa and enters the cell by endocytosis.

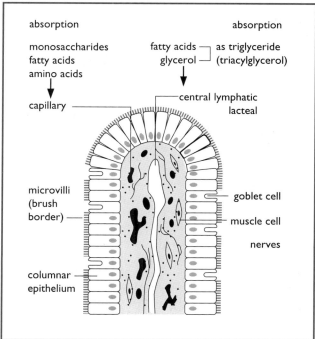

Figure 13.16. Detail of villus and absorption (diagrammatic).

Fat-soluble vitamins are absorbed with fats as part of the micelles. It follows that their efficient absorption is dependent upon the presence of bile in the small intestine and fat in the diet. In situations where the flow of bile is obstructed, such as when a gallstone (see Chapter 14) blocks the duct, there may be inadequate absorption of vitamin K. As you will remember, vitamin K is required for the production of several clotting factors (see Chapter 9). A person having surgery to remove the obstructing gallstone will be given vitamin K by intramuscular injection to ensure that haemostasis operates normally during and after surgery.

Minerals

Minerals are absorbed actively and passively throughout the small intestine and colon (see page 311). Sodium is absorbed actively in the small intestine, where it is linked with the transport of amino acids and monosaccharides, and in the colon. Chloride ions diffuse passively through the intestinal wall or move by active transport in exchange for hydrogen carbonate ions which enter the lumen. Potassium ions are absorbed by passive transport from the ileum and colon. When a person loses water from the bowel he or she will also lose potassium in the watery stool. Loss of potassium leads to hypokalaemia (low levels of potassium in the blood) and may be a feature of severe diarrhoea or ileostomy (a stoma/opening where the ileum discharges onto the abdominal wall).

Before leaving the topic of mineral absorption we should consider how calcium and iron are absorbed. Their absorption rates are linked to demand, helping to ensure that homeostasis for these minerals is maintained. Active calcium absorption from the upper small intestine is linked to the amount of calcium present in the blood. The rate at which calcium is absorbed is controlled by parathyroid hormone and calcitonin (see Chapter 8). The active form of vitamin D (1,25-dihydroxycholecalciferol) facilitates calcium absorption by the intestinal mucosa. The absorption of calcium is inhibited by phytic acid and phosphates present in cereals.

Iron is required for erythropoiesis and details of its metabolism can be found in Chapter 9. Iron is most easily absorbed in the ferrous (bivalent Fe^{2+}) state. Gastric acid and vitamin C facilitate the conversion of ferric (trivalent Fe^{3+}) to ferrous iron, which is absorbed actively in the upper small intestine. Iron can be stored as a complex with a protein (ferritin) within the enterocytes until it is required in the blood. In common with calcium, iron absorption is inhibited by the phytic acid and phosphates present in a high-fibre cereal diet. Iron-deficiency anaemia may be a problem for some vegetarians because absorption is inhibited in this way and because of their avoidance of foods such as red meat which contain high levels of available iron. Those at high risk are teenage girls whose vegetarian diets are inadequate and who also have heavy menstrual losses. Eating disorders in this group, such as anorexia nervosa, exacerbate the problem. Vegetarians can obtain iron from legumes, egg yolk (if eaten), dried fruit, watercress and fortified wholegrain breakfast cereals, but remember that absorption of this iron will, to some extent, be inhibited by the phytic acid also present.

A more comprehensive list of minerals required by the body can be found in *Table 2.1*.

Water

Water is mostly absorbed in the small intestine (80–90%), the remainder being absorbed by the colon. This explains why the discharge from an ileostomy is much more fluid than that from a colostomy (a stoma where the colon discharges onto the abdominal wall). Between 200 and 400 ml of water is absorbed every hour, and of the large volume of fluid (secretions + drinks) passing through the gastrointestinal tract, less than 200 ml/24 hours is lost in the faeces.

The actual amount of water in the faeces depends on the time food residues remain in the intestine. In constipation the food residues spend extra time in the colon and more water is absorbed, which leads to the characteristic small, hard stools. The watery stools of diarrhoea are caused by lack of time for water absorption as the food residue 'rushes' through the intestine. Constipation and diarrhoea are discussed further on page 313. Water also moves in the opposite direction – from cells to intestinal lumen. This occurs if the intestinal contents become hypertonic (see also page 298).

The metabolism and utilization of the main nutrients – amino acids, glucose and fats – is considered later.

Large intestine

The large intestine runs from the ileocaecal valve to end at the anus and measures about 1.5 m in length. It can be divided into: caecum, vermiform (worm-like) appendix, colon (ascending, transverse, descending and sigmoid) and rectum, which opens into the anal canal (*Figure 13.17*). More detail of the different parts can be found below and on page 310.

Nursing Practice Application **Malabsorption**

Malabsorption results from any process which affects the ability of the intestinal mucosa to absorb water and nutrients. This may occur as part of an acute illness, but may be chronic. It is important that nurses are alert to the types of condition where malabsorption is a possibility (see Nutritional assessment, page 323).

We have already mentioned chemicals such as phytic acid that inhibit mineral absorption. Iron or calcium absorption may be inadequate where a high-fibre diet is consumed, e.g. vegetarians.

Intestinal infections which cause diarrhoea lead to dehydration and electrolyte imbalance, particularly of potassium and sodium. These infections include cholera and food poisoning caused by bacterial contamination, e.g. *Campylobacter, Salmonella*.

Inflammatory disease of the intestine, e.g Crohn's disease (regional ileitis), causes malabsorption of nutrients and water.

Some people have an intolerance to a specific nutrient which causes malabsorption; commonly the intolerance is to lactose, gluten (a protein found in some cereals, e.g. wheat) or fats.

Problems also arise if a large area of small intestine is resected (removed) or bypassed by the formation of an ileostomy. These are measures which may be required to alleviate the effects of inflammatory bowel disease.

The major functions of the large intestine (see also page 311) are:

- Absorbs some water, minerals, vitamins and drugs.
- Vitamins (K and some B) are synthesized by **colonic** bacteria.
- Stores food residues until eliminated by defaecation.
- Eliminates waste through defaecation.

The colon forms a frame around the small intestine by making two 90° turns – one under the liver and the other near the spleen, known respectively as the hepatic (right colic) and splenic (left colic) flexures.

Arterial blood reaches the colon from the superior mesenteric and inferior mesenteric arteries, which also supply the proximal part of the rectum [see *Figure 10.43(b)*]. The distal part of the rectum and anus are supplied by branches of the internal iliac arteries. Venous return from the colon and proximal part of the rectum is by mesenteric veins which drain into the hepatic portal vein (see *Figure 10.45*). The rectum is another area where the hepatic portal and systemic circulations anastomose. Varicosities may develop in the rectum when pressure in the hepatic portal vein is raised, such as with cirrhosis. The venous blood from the distal rectum and anus drains into the iliac veins.

The autonomic nervous system innervates the large intestine – the vagus and nervi erigentes are parasympathetic and sympathetic fibres from the coeliac and mesenteric ganglia (see page 289, Chapter 6). The external anal sphincter is, however, under voluntary control and is innervated by the pudendal nerve from the sacral plexus (see Chapter 5).

General structure of the large intestine

Structurally, the large intestine has the usual basic layers (see page 289), but there are differences in the mucosa and muscle layer.

The mucosa is simple columnar epithelium without villi. There are numerous goblet cells within the mucosa of the colon and rectum which produce the mucus required for lubricating the movement of faeces. In the anal canal the mucosa is stratified squamous epithelium, which hangs in vertical folds called the anal columns. This region, which merges with the outside skin, is subjected to considerable friction (see Defaecation, pages 311–312).

Throughout the colon the submucosal layer contains abundant lymphoid tissue which generally prevents the numerous colonic bacteria from entering the bloodstream.

There are several modifications to the muscle layer. Two horizontal folds of the circular muscle layer form the ileocaecal valve, which controls the passage of food residues from small to large intestine. The longitudinal muscle layer

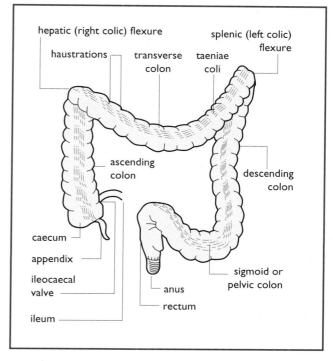

Figure 13.17 Large intestine.

in the colon consists of three bands called the taeniae coli. As these bands are shorter than the colon they produce puckering, or haustrations – much as pulling the thread too tight on some sewing will pucker the material. The circular muscle layer also forms the anal sphincters: the internal, which is smooth muscle (involuntary), and the external, which is skeletal muscle (voluntary).

Detailed structure of the large intestine
Caecum and appendix

The first part of the large intestine or caecum is a blind pouch projecting below the ileocaecal valve, which separates it from the ileum (see *Figure 13.18*). The ileocaecal valve opens when peristalsis brings small bowel contents to the ileum and as a reflex in response to food entering the stomach. This gastrocolic reflex operates through the vagus nerve to initiate peristalsis in the colon, opening of the valve and the urge to defaecate. In grass-eating animals the caecum is a much larger structure which plays a significant part in their digestive processes.

The worm-like vermiform appendix hangs from the lower part of the caecum (see *Figure 13.18*). The appendix is a blind tube which varies greatly in length, but is usually around 5 cm. It is a common site of inflammation (appendicitis), although it contains a great deal of lymphoid tissue.

Colon

The ascending colon runs up the right side of the abdominal cavity to the level of the liver, where it turns at the hepatic flexure to form the transverse colon (see *Figure 13.17*). The transverse colon runs across the abdomen to pass in front of the stomach. It turns at the splenic flexure and runs down the left side of the abdomen as the descending colon. As the colon enters the pelvis it becomes the pelvic or sigmoid colon, so called because of its S-shaped curve.

Level with the mid-sacrum, the sigmoid colon forms the slightly dilated rectum, which curves in front of the sacrum and coccyx. The rectum, which has no taeniae coli, is completely invested (covered, 'clothed') in longitudinal muscle; it also does not have any mesocolon (see page 290). The adult rectum is around 15 cm in length, but only 3 cm in babies. It terminates at the anal canal with two sphincters and stratified squamous epithelium (*Figure 13.19*). The anal canal opens externally at the anus.

Functions of the large intestine
Absorption

The colon absorbs water from food residues. The amount absorbed is related to the time that residues stay in the

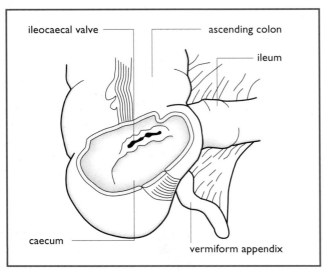

Figure 13.18 Caecum and appendix.

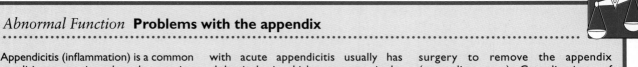

Abnormal Function **Problems with the appendix**

Appendicitis (inflammation) is a common condition occurring when the opening into the appendix is obstructed. This provides ideal conditions for bacterial growth within the appendix, which becomes inflamed and swollen. A person with acute appendicitis usually has abdominal pain which commences in the umbilical region and moves to the right iliac fossa (see *Figure 1.33*), anorexia, nausea and vomiting.

Treatment usually involves immediate surgery to remove the appendix (appendicectomy). Complications of appendicitis include abscess formation or rupture of the appendix, which causes peritonitis (see page 290) and later adhesions.

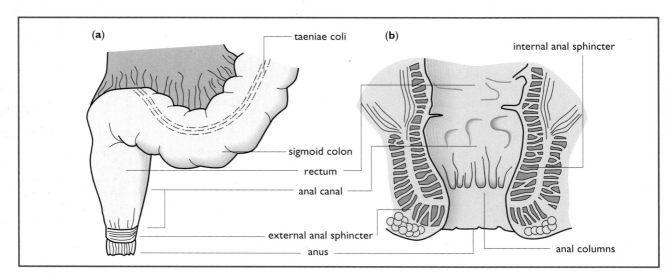

Figure 13.19 (a) Rectum; **(b)** anal canal.

colon, and increases with time. Sodium ions are absorbed actively with chloride ions and water moving passively into the blood.

The colon is able to absorb small amounts of the vitamins (K and B complex) produced by its commensal bacteria (see below). The amounts of vitamins involved are probably of little significance where nutrition is normal.

Mixing of the colonic contents by segmentation (see page 301) aids absorption.

Synthesis

The large intestine is colonized by many commensal (meaning 'to eat at the same table') bacteria. This is a mutually beneficial relationship by which the bacteria are nourished from the food residues and in return synthesize vitamins K and some of the B complex (thiamin, riboflavin, folate and B_{12}). The bacteria involved include *Escherichia coli (E. coli)*, *Enterobacter aerogenes*, *Streptococcus faecalis* and *Clostridium perfringens (C. perfringens)*. These bacteria are commensal in the intestine but can become pathogenic (disease-producing) if they find their way to some other site, e.g. *E. coli* contaminating the bladder or *C. perfringens* in a wound.

The intestinal bacteria also cause the fermentation of undigested food residues with the production of gases (flatus). The gases include methane, carbon dioxide, hydrogen sulphide and hydrogen, some of which contribute to faecal odour. The amount produced (usually 450–700 ml/24 hours) depends on the type of food eaten; individuals vary, but flatus-producing foods include beans, lentils, cabbage, cauliflower and onions. In large amounts flatus can cause considerable distension and discomfort, especially after abdominal surgery.

Storage

Most food residues pass through the large intestine within 12–72 hours, but transit times depend upon many factors, including the amount of indigestible fibre present. The intestine is able to store large amounts of waste, which may take a week or more to travel to the rectum. After eating foods such as sweetcorn or beetroot (red beet) it is easy to establish how long it takes to appear in faeces.

Elimination/defaecation

The large intestine propels the waste towards the rectum by strong peristaltic movements called mass movements. These are linked to the gastrocolic reflex and occur after meals. Mass movement causes the rectum to fill with faeces, which in turn initiates an urge to defaecate. Ordinary peristalsis also helps to move faeces toward the rectum and segmentation ensures that mixing occurs.

As the rectum is stretched by faeces (normally empty), the defaecation reflex is started through the sacral part of the spinal cord. Impulses also travel to the cerebral cortex,

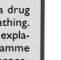

Nursing Practice Application **Absorption of drugs**

The colon is able to absorb several types of drugs, including corticosteroids, antimicrobials, analgesics and bronchodilators. The drugs may be administered as suppositories or a retention enema.

Nurses should ensure that the person and their family understand that the drug is absorbed through the colonic mucosa. Although rectal drug administration is routine in some other European countries, many people in the UK are anxious or confused about the rectal route. They often associate this with enemas used to evacuate the bowel contents and may find incredible the concept that a drug given rectally can help their breathing. There is an obvious need for clear explanations and an education programme which includes administration procedures and the time a preparation should be retained.

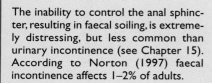

Abnormal Function **Faecal incontinence**

The inability to control the anal sphincter, resulting in faecal soiling, is extremely distressing, but less common than urinary incontinence (see Chapter 15). According to Norton (1997) faecal incontinence affects 1–2% of adults.

Causes:
• Associated with faecal impaction/constipation. It is vital that this is diagnosed correctly and the bowel is evacuated.
• Drugs which cause diarrhoea, e.g. abuse of aperients, antibiotics.
• Rectal prolapse.
• Neurological cause, e.g. spinal cord lesion.
• Dietary indiscretions where anal sphincter control is not adequate to cope with the diarrhoea.

Management includes dealing with the cause if possible, discussion with a continence advisor, establishment of 'good bowel habits', exercise and physiotherapy, adequate fluids and fibre, and protective clothing/bedding only if essential.

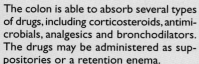

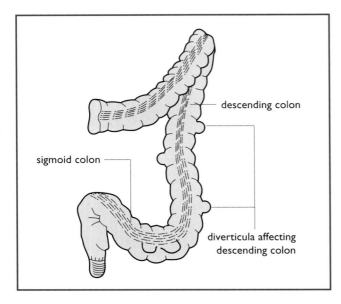

descending colon

sigmoid colon

diverticula affecting
descending colon

Figure 13.20 Diverticular disease.

which can inhibit the reflex until defaecation is convenient. As well as this inhibition we have voluntary control through the pudendal nerve and can keep the external anal sphincter closed. When defaecation is convenient the spinal reflex can proceed. Parasympathetic nerve activity causes the sigmoid colon and rectum to contract and relaxes the internal sphincter, and there is voluntary relaxation of the external sphincter.

Defaecation is aided by voluntary straining which involves Valsalva's manoeuvre (see Chapter 12). The amount of straining required depends on faecal consistency – it is much easier to pass a soft, bulky stool than one that is hard and constipated.

In infants, defaecation occurs as a reflex response to faeces in the rectum – voluntary control of the external anal sphincter is not achieved until the child is 18 months or older. Reflex defaecation also occurs with sacral spinal cord lesions, after cerebrovascular accident or where the pudendal nerve is damaged.

Nursing Practice Application **Irritable bowel syndrome**

Irritable bowel syndrome (IBS) is a commonly occurring functional (without physical cause) bowel disorder. It is characterized by diarrhoea and/or constipation with pain. Affected individuals report that they pass ribbon-like stools or small hard pellets. The cause of this bowel motility dysfunction is unclear, but for some individuals worry and anxiety can precipitate an attack. As with any alterations in function, the presence of organic disease, e.g. inflammatory or malignant bowel disease, must be excluded before a diagnosis of IBS can be made. Nurses can assist people with IBS with careful explanation of their symptoms and drugs prescribed, dietary advice, e.g. increasing fibre intake in constipation, and helping them to develop strategies for coping with stress and anxiety. Drug management may include: antispasmodic drugs, e.g. mebeverine, and antidiarrhoeals such as loperamide; occasionally tranquillizers or antidepressants are prescribed.

Healthier Living **Non-starch polysaccharide (NSP), defaecation and health**

Considerable evidence exists in support of increasing our daily intake of NSP and a report from the Department of Health (DoH, 1991) recommends that fibre intake for adults should be between 12 and 24 g/day (average 18 g/day). This increase should come from a variety of foods such as wholegrain cereals, pulses, fruit and vegetables which contain naturally occurring NSP. The same report also states that children should have a smaller intake and warns that children under 2 years should not have foods containing NSP in place of the high-energy foods they need for growth.

Faecal bulk and transit time through the large intestine depend on the amount of NSP present. Burkitt *et al.* (1972) found that stool weight varied greatly with NSP intake: from 39–223 g on a refined/processed UK diet to 71–488 g on a vegetarian mixed diet; compared with this, rural Ugandans, having an unrefined diet, produced 178–980 g. The increased transit times associated with the refined Western diet leads to the formation of carcinogens (see Chapter 1) in the large intestine. There is a higher incidence of colorectal cancers compared with developing countries, but there may be other aetiological influences such as high fat in Western diets. The risk of developing haemorrhoids may also be reduced by taking enough NSP to ensure that the stool is soft and passed without straining.

Another common condition linked to NSP intake is diverticular disease. This occurs when diverticula – pouches (*Figure 13.20*) which form in the intestinal wall – become inflamed (diverticulitis). The incidence of diverticular disease is higher in meat eaters than vegetarians, who generally have a higher NSP intake. Diverticular disease is also more common in Western countries than in developing countries where the diet contains more NSP and very little meat or processed food.

Last but not least, the intake of sufficient NSP helps to prevent the development of constipation which affects the lives of many older adults (see Special Focus).

Composition of faeces

Faeces contain mainly water with some epithelial cells, mucus, bacteria, fibre or non-starch polysaccharide (NSP) such as undigested cellulose residue, electrolytes, stercobilin (which colours normal stools) and various chemicals, which account for the characteristic odour.

Special Focus '**Normal bowel habit', diarrhoea and constipation**

It is important to remember that 'normal bowel habit' varies from person to person. The study of bowel function in hospital by Wright (1974) found that usual bowel habit before admission was 5–7 stools weekly. Earlier studies of bowel habit in two groups found that 99% of people fell within the range of three stools daily to three stools per week. Any departure from the normal pattern should, however, be noted, as a change may indicate serious disease.

Diarrhoea is frequent loose stools which may, if severe or prolonged, lead to dehydration, hypokalaemia, metabolic acidosis and malabsorption of nutrients.

The causes of diarrhoea include:

- Dietary such as eating too much fruit, change in diet.
- Infection, e.g. food poisoning.
- Inflammatory bowel disease, e.g. Crohn's disease.
- Food allergy or intolerance causing malabsorption.
- Anxiety, e.g. IBS or the morning of an examination.
- Colorectal cancers. Here bowel habit may alternate between diarrhoea and constipation.
- Drugs, e.g. antibiotics and iron or laxative abuse.
- Hyperthyroidism (see Chapter 8).
- After extensive small bowel resection.

It is essential to differentiate between true diarrhoea and the spurious leakage of liquid faeces associated with severe constipation/faecal impaction (see constipation).

After assessment, the nursing interventions should include actions that provide privacy and commode/bedpans whenever required or access to toilet facilities. Simple measures such as perianal hygiene, soft toilet tissue, creams for perianal excoriation and clean linen do much to minimize discomfort. Embarrassment can be eased by providing a side room with toilet or, if this is not possible, ensuring good ventilation and air fresheners to dispel offensive odours. To avoid the possibility of cross-infection all faeces should be disposed of safely and staff should wear disposable gloves and plastic aprons; hand hygiene for all concerned is essential for infection control. Monitoring the frequency of diarrhoea, fluid balance and skin condition are important parts of a continually updated assessment. In addition, the colour, consistency and presence of blood or mucus in the stools should be noted. Nurses will also be involved with the collection of stool specimens for microscopy and culture, the management of oral or intravenous fluid replacement (see Chapter 2) and the administration of antidiarrhoeals.

Constipation is the reverse of diarrhoea, with hard, dry stools which are passed infrequently and with difficulty – the longer the faeces stay in the colon the more water is reabsorbed (see pages 310–311). Often, people feel that they are constipated if they do not defaecate daily. This is especially true in older adults, of whom 20% claim to be constipated, but as many as 50% regularly take aperients (Gupta, 1980).

The causes of constipation include:

- Diet poor in NSP, change in diet.
- Ignoring or being unable to respond to the urge to defaecate. This may be due to the problems of having to use a bedpan in hospital which include lack of privacy, physical difficulties and undue waiting. Wright (1974) found that 44% of people using bedpans/commodes became constipated compared with only 26% of people able to use the toilet. If a person in hospital postponed defaecation because toilet facilities were unavailable they may become constipated.
- Lack of mobility or pain on moving may also be a problem. The thought of having to climb stairs or go into a cold part of the house or outside may cause the person to avoid defaecation.
- Dehydration (see Chapter 2).
- Conditions causing pain on defaecation, such as haemorrhoids or anal fissure (crack), may lead to the person 'putting off' defaecation. This ill-judged action actually exacerbates the problem as the stool becomes even harder and more painful to pass.
- Colorectal cancer may present as alternating constipation and diarrhoea.
- Drugs, e.g. iron, analgesics (such as codeine), anticholinergic drugs and some antidepressants.
- Lack of exercise and immobility.
- Depressive illness.
- Hypothyroidism (see Chapter 8).
- Hypokalaemia.
- Hormones, e.g. progesterone during pregnancy.

At this point we might consider the problems experienced by 'Dorothy', page 314.

Person-Centred Study **Dorothy**

Constipation is a common problem especially for older adults. Since Dorothy, aged 88, moved in with her daughter she is not really 'going properly' and feels bloated. Dorothy mentions this during a visit to the practice nurse, who arranges for her to see the doctor. A change in activity and diet are the most likely explanations, but a rectal examination is performed to check for more sinister pathology. Before leaving, Dorothy has another chat with the nurse, who suggests that she might consider the following:

- Increase NSP intake and visit her dentist if chewing is a problem.
- Drink at least 2.5 litres of fluid daily.
- Respond at once to the urge to defaecate.

- Try to establish a routine for defaecation, e.g. after breakfast.
- Take some gentle exercise, e.g. take their dog Oliver for a walk.

If these measures are unsuccessful Dorothy is asked to make an appointment with the doctor, who may prescribe short-term aperients (dependence can occur) or decide that Dorothy's problem requires further investigation.

Nutrition – Metabolism and Utilization

Following our discussion of digestion and absorption, it would seem sensible if we looked at some aspects of nutrition, metabolism and the uses the body makes of nutrients. By necessity this can only be a brief review and readers are directed to Further Reading, e.g. Garrow and James (1993) and MAFF (1995). The emphasis here will be on carbohydrates, proteins and fats, with only brief mention of the other components of a 'healthy diet'.

Introduction

The intake of the essential nutrients in the correct quantities is essential for health and, ultimately, life. We need a variety of nutrients which provide energy and produce the molecules needed for homeostasis and the materials for cell growth and repair. The nutrients required are macronutrients – carbohydrates, proteins and fats; micronutrients – vitamins (organic) and minerals (inorganic); and water. As you already know, we also need NSP; although this is not absorbed as a nutrient it is important for health (see page 312).

A specific food usually contains several nutrients; for example, 'jacket' potatoes provide carbohydrate, protein, minerals, vitamins, water and NSP before you even consider the filling/dressing. Some nutrients are essential – they are molecules which cannot be synthesized in the body and must be provided by the diet. The body converts the essential nutrients into the many other molecules vital for health.

The metabolism and utilization of nutrients involves a multitude of interrelated, enzyme-facilitated biochemical reactions. These biochemical reactions, many of which occur in the liver, may be:

Catabolic: where fuel molecules are broken down within cells to produce chemical energy in the form of ATP or heat energy. These reactions, in which glucose, fatty acids and amino acids are broken down, are together known as cellular respiration.

Anabolic: where the ATP is used to drive the reactions which build up or synthesize other molecules.

Energy composition of food

Most of the food consumed is oxidized by the body to produce ATP. The energy value of a particular food is measured in the SI unit of kilojoules (kJ) or the widely used

Healthier Living **Eating for health (adults)**

If we make a wide choice from the main food groups – wholegrain cereals, bread, pasta, chapatis and potatoes; fruit and vegetables; meat, fish and eggs or protein alternatives (beans and pulses); and milk and dairy produce – it is very likely that dietary intake will contain all the essential nutrients. Most of our energy should come from unrefined carbohydrates containing sufficient NSP, and fatty foods, such as dairy products, should provide less than 35% of total energy (DoH, 1992). Five portions of fruit and vegetables (excluding potatoes) a day will help to provide the vitamins and minerals required for metabolic processes. Foods high in sugar and salt, and red meat, should be taken sparingly and alcohol intake kept within sensible limits. Overall food intake should keep you at a healthy body weight for age and gender and be a pleasurable experience.

4.2 kJ (approx) = 1 kcal or Calorie

Table 13.1 Energy composition of nutrients	
Nutrient	**Energy yield from 1 g**
Carbohydrate	17 kJ or 4 kcal
Protein	17 kJ or 4 kcal
Fat	37 kJ or 9 kcal

NB Alcohol, which is not a nutrient, yields 29 kJ or 7 kcal/1g.

Table 13.1 Energy composition of nutrients.

kilocalories (kcal), which are also called 'large Calories'.

It is important to note that 1 kcal is the amount of heat required to raise the temperature of 1 kg of water by 1°C.

Our energy requirements vary according to gender, size, activity and health status; for example, raised body temperature increases the energy requirement (1° increase = 7% increase in metabolic rate). The basal metabolic rate (BMR) is the amount of energy needed by the body to drive the vital processes, e.g. respiration, when at complete rest, but awake. BMR is calculated indirectly by measuring the amount of oxygen consumed in a given time (1 litre of oxygen used = 20 kJ of energy released) and is expressed as kJ or kcal per square metre body surface area per hour – kJ or kcal/m^2/hour. Adult males require about 170 kJ or 40 kcal/m^2/hour and females 155 kJ or 37 kcal/m^2/hour.

Example: A man weighing 67 kg, who is 172 cm tall, has a surface area of 1.8 m (calculated from a nomogram). He will need 170 kJ × 1.8 = 306 kJ/hour or 72 kcal/hour. In 24 hours he needs approximately 7344 kJ or 1728 kcal to meet basal metabolic requirements.

If your energy consumption is greater than required, the result is weight gain. Overweight is defined as a body mass index (BMI) between 25 and 30 and obesity as a body mass index greater than 30. Obesity is the most common nutritional disorder of developed countries, where it contributes significantly to ill health and premature death.

$$BMI = \frac{\text{weight in kg}}{\text{height in m}^2}$$

Carbohydrates

Carbohydrate molecules consist of carbon, hydrogen and oxygen. They are obtained mainly from plant sources, with the exception of lactose (milk sugar) and glycogen. Carbohydrates (see pages 304–305 and Chapter 1) are divided into sugars, which may be monosaccharides (glucose, galactose and fructose), disaccharides (maltose, lactose and sucrose) and the more complex polysaccharides (starch, cellulose and glycogen). Monosaccharides are formed from a single sugar unit, disaccharides consist of two linked monosaccharide units and polysaccharides comprise many monosaccharide units.

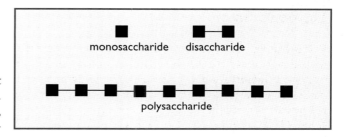

Sugars are obtained from fruit, jam, honey, sugar and milk, and from processed foods, e.g. baked beans. Polysaccharides are found in pulses, root vegetables, e.g. potato, cereals and products made from flour, e.g. bread, pasta, chapatis. During digestion the various carbohydrates are reduced to simple monosaccharides before absorption, but polysaccharides, such as cellulose, remain undigested in humans to provide NSP or fibre.

Monosaccharide metabolism and utilization

The monosaccharides absorbed in the intestine are delivered to the liver, where the fructose and galactose are converted to glucose. It is as glucose that the cells use carbohydrate. Although some cells can use fat as fuel, the erythrocytes and brain cells can only use glucose in the short term. It follows, then, that a fall in blood glucose levels can damage brain cells.

Glucose in excess of immediate energy requirements is converted in the liver to the storage carbohydrate glycogen. This process, known as glycogenesis, requires the presence of insulin and provides around 100 g of storage carbohydrate, which is held in the liver. Skeletal muscles also store glycogen for muscle contraction during exercise. Once energy requirements have been met and glycogen stores replenished the glucose remaining is converted to fat. This fat is stored in the adipose tissue (see Chapter 1).

Most glucose, however, is taken up by the cells under the influence of insulin (see Chapter 8) and oxidized to provide energy ATP (*Figure 13.21*). Initially glucose is broken down (glycolysis) by a series of enzymes, present in the cytosol, to form pyruvic acid. The pyruvic acid is broken down **aerobically** to produce acetyl co-enzyme A (acetyl CoA), which enters the Krebs' (citric acid) cycle (see *Figure 13.24*). The Krebs' cycle is a series of enzyme-controlled reactions occurring inside the mitochondria, where acetyl CoA undergoes changes to produce some

ATP, water and carbon dioxide. Most ATP, however, is harvested from oxidative phosphorylation of ADP. This involves two high-energy electron carrier molecules and an electron transfer chain situated in the inner mitochondrial membrane (see page 320). These reusable high-energy molecules (derived from the B vitamins niacin and riboflavin respectively) – nicotinamide adenine dinucleotide (NADH = reduced form) and flavin adenine dinucleotide ($FADH_2$ = reduced form) – are produced at various stages of glucose metabolism and the Krebs' cycle.

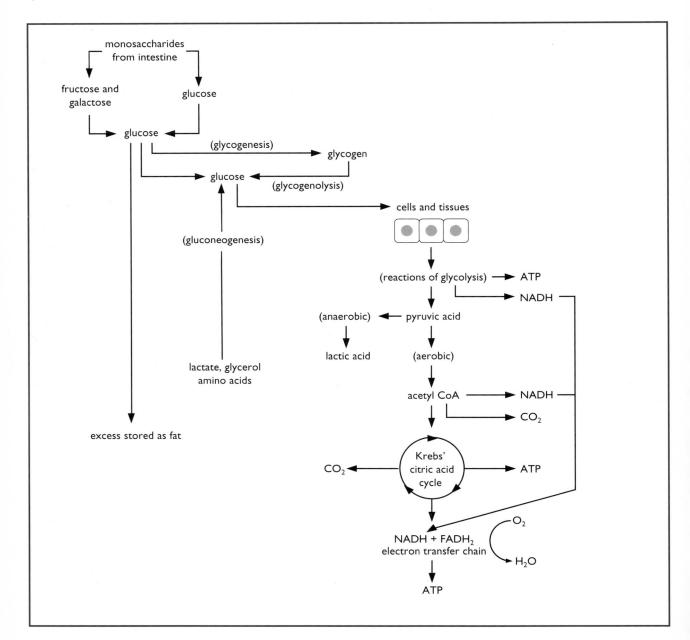

Figure 13.21 Metabolism of monosaccharides.

If the pyruvic acid is broken down **anaerobically**, the waste product lactic acid is produced (see Chapter 12). This occurs in strenuous exercise, but can also result from any hypoxic state. Lactic acid can be converted to glucose for cell use, but only if oxygen is attainable – the conversion occurs in the liver through the reactions of the Cori cycle.

When the amount of glucose in the blood is reduced, the body must correct the deficit to maintain homeostasis. The stored liver glycogen is reconverted to glucose by glycogenolysis, a process regulated by glucagon and adrenaline (see Chapter 8). Where the glycogen stores are low the body is able to produce glucose from non-carbohydrate sources (amino acids, glycerol and lactate) by a process, occurring mainly in the liver, known as gluconeogenesis. After weeks of starvation gluconeogenesis also occurs in the kidneys. Gluconeogenesis will occur when glucose, although in plentiful supply, is unavailable for use, e.g. in diabetes mellitus, where a lack of insulin prevents the transfer of glucose into cells.

Protein

Proteins (see pages 304–305 and Chapter 1) contain carbon, hydrogen, oxygen and nitrogen, and sometimes sulphur and phosphorous. During digestion proteins are broken down into the 20 amino acids which, in different combinations, form every protein (see *Table 1.2*).

Some amino acids are essential/indispensable (must be ingested – cannot be synthesized by the body): isoleucine, leucine, lysine, methionine, phenylalanine, threonine, tryptophan and valine; during childhood histidine is also considered essential. The others are non-essential (can be synthesized): alanine, arginine, asparagine, aspartate (aspartic acid), cysteine, glutamate (glutamic acid), glutamine, glycine, proline, serine and tyrosine.

About 50 g (45–55 g) of protein is required each day by adults to maintain a positive nitrogen balance where protein is being used for repair rather than to produce energy. The reverse, where protein is primarily being used to produce energy, results in the development of a negative nitrogen balance. A negative balance is associated with starvation or following severe physiological stress where protein catabolism increases, e.g. burns, multiple injuries, major surgery and systemic infections (see Nursing Practice Application, page 318).

Although quantity is important, it is vital that the quality of the protein is adequate. Most animal source protein, e.g. meat, eggs, fish and milk, contain the essential/indispensable amino acids, but plant proteins are not complete. Legumes such as beans are deficient in methionine and cereals lack lysine. This can be compensated for by mixing plant proteins, e.g baked beans on toast, lentil curry with rice. Protein is also obtained from nuts and vegetables such as potatoes.

Amino-acid metabolism and utilization

Amino acids are not stored by the body. They circulate in a general pool (free amino acids available for utilization) from where they are 'selected' when required for cell division, growth or repair and to synthesize the functional proteins, e.g. enzymes, some hormones, plasma proteins and haemoglobin (see *Figure 13.22*). As already mentioned, proteins can be oxidized to provide energy, but this is rather wasteful and does not utilize their full potential.

Following absorption, amino acids are transported to the liver. Here the non-essential ones are synthesized by a process called transamination. Various enzymes called aminotransferases (also called transaminases) move amine groups (NH_2) from an amino acid to a keto acid to form different amino acids, e.g. alpha-ketoglutaric acid + NH_2 = glutamate (glutamic acid). Glutamate can then be used in the body to form other non-essential amino acids.

When the body is deficient of stored energy, or amino acids are in excess of anabolic needs, they can be used for energy by a process called oxidative deamination. The amino acid glutamate is deaminated in the liver where the removal of the nitrogenous amine group (NH_2) produces alpha ketoglutaric acid and highly toxic ammonia (NH_3). The keto acid either enters the Krebs' cycle as acetyl CoA or another intermediate and the NADH generated is used to produce ATP via the electron-transfer chain, or the keto acid is converted to glucose (gluconeogenesis). Keto acids also form pyruvic acid and, because most of the reactions of glycolysis are reversible, can form glucose.

Meanwhile the NH_3 is combined with carbon dioxide to form urea by the reactions of the Krebs' urea cycle. These reactions convert highly toxic ammonia to less toxic urea, which travels in the blood to the kidneys to be excreted in the urine (see Chapters 14 and 15). Deamination reactions may be coupled chemically with those involving transamination.

Amino acids can also provide energy by their conversion to lipids (lipogenesis) – again through the important molecule acetyl CoA.

Fats

Fats (see page 307 and Chapter 1) consist of carbon, hydrogen and oxygen, but in different proportions to carbohydrates. Our consumption of fat is mostly as triglycerides (triacylglycerol) (glycerol + three fatty acids), but we also ingest other fatty substances, e.g. cholesterol found in offal and egg yolk.

When fat is oxidized it yields over twice the amount of energy as carbohydrate or protein. It is therefore a valuable fuel when energy requirements are high, but in sedentary individuals excess intake results in obesity.

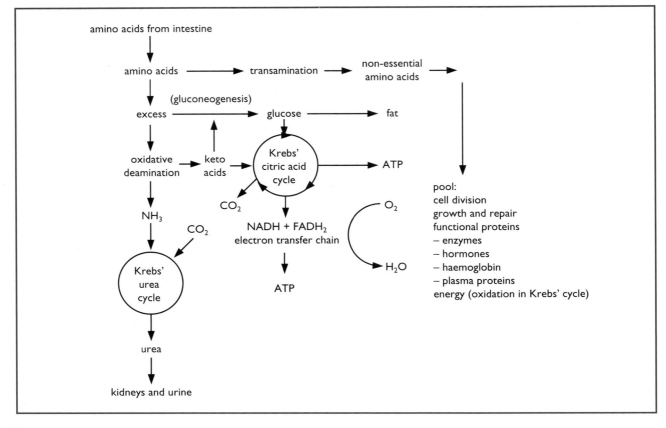

Figure 13.22 Metabolism of amino acids.

Nursing Practice Application Meals in hospital and protein energy malnutrition (PEM)

Situations where the hospital patient receives inadequate protein and energy are unfortunately common and malnutrition may affect up to 50% of adults (Goodinson, 1987a). PEM may contribute to delayed recovery and complications such as poor wound healing, infection and depression.

Obviously any physical, psychological or social factor that affected intake or absorption of food before admission must be considered, e.g. anorexia, immobility or low income, but the problem may well start within the hospital setting. Dickerson (1995) identifies the following as being at particular risk for PEM — emergencies, some elderly, cancer patients and those with chronic bowel problems.

In recent years the serving and supervision of meals have been regarded by many as a non-nursing duty. This has led to confusion regarding responsibility for ensuring that diet is eaten. As with most aspects of care, the team approach is essential, with the patient/family, nurse, doctor, catering staff, dietitian and biochemist all involved in preventing and recognizing malnutrition (see nutritional assessment, page 323). Where they exist, the nutrition team and specialist nurse should be consulted.

Well over a century ago Florence Nightingale thought nurses had a central role: 'If the nurse is an intelligent being, and not a mere carrier of diets to and from the patient, let her exercise her intelligence in these things' (Nightingale, 1859). It is important to ensure that the mealtime environment is quiet and free from activities such as treatments. Nurses should help the patient to select appropriately from the menu, adopt suitable positions, provide special utensils or skilled help with feeding if required and assess what has been eaten.

The nutritional education of nursing/medical staff has been a neglected area, with a low priority in basic courses. The case for nutrition education is reinforced in a review of undernutrition in elderly patients by Tierney (1996), who found that training improves the skills of nurses and medical staff to detect undernutrition.

Nursing Practice Application **Phenylketonuria (PKU)**

PKU is an inborn error of metabolism where the enzyme (phenylalanine hydoxylase) required to convert the amino acid phenylalanine to tyrosine is absent. Untreated, this leads to an accumulation of phenylalanine and its toxic metabolites which cause brain damage and varying degrees of learning disability.

A routine test (blood or urine) performed on all babies during the first days of life can detect the condition, which is managed with a diet low in phenylalanine. As phenylalanine is an essential amino acid (not synthesized) it must be included in the diet, but amounts given are carefully controlled by regular blood tests to measure the level of toxic metabolites.

The phenylalanine-restricted diet is continued throughout childhood with its growth periods and, in the case of female sufferers, is restarted if they decide to have a baby, to protect the fetus. Affected individuals have unusually pale colouring with fair hair and blue eyes because the tyrosine required for pigment production (melanin) is not synthesized.

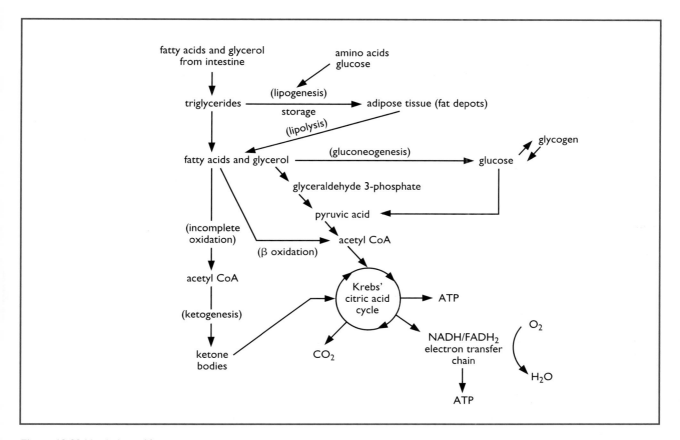

Figure 13.23 Metabolism of fats.

A great deal is heard about whether a fat is saturated or not. This is simply a way of describing its particular chemical bond structure (see Chapter 1). Saturated fats are generally found in animal products, e.g. fat around meat, lard, dairy products, and are solid at room temperature. Unsaturated fats may be monounsaturated or polyunsaturated. They are found in nuts, seeds, some fish oils (omega-3 fatty acids) and most vegetable oils, e.g. sunflower oil, and most are liquid at room temperature. Some unsaturated fatty acids are essential and cannot be synthesized in the body – linoleic acid, linolenic acid. Others, such as arachidonic acid, can be made in small amounts only and so are also considered essential. These essential fatty acids (EFAs) form the basis of structural phospholipids, and prostaglandins – the important control molecules (see Chapter 8) are derived from arachidonic acid.

Fat metabolism and utilization

Fatty acids and glycerol absorbed in the intestine are reformed into triglycerides (triacylglycerols). Any not needed for immediate energy production are stored in the adipose tissue of the fat depots, e.g. under the skin. A process stimulated by insulin, by which glucose and amino acids are converted to glycerol and fatty acids prior to storage as triglycerides (triacylglycerols) in adipose tissue, is termed lipogenesis. The stored fat provides insulation, an energy source and protection for some organs, e.g. kidneys. Fat taken in the diet is also required for the absorption of fat-soluble vitamins (see page 307).

Stored fat is released from the adipose tissue by various hormones, e.g. cortisol, in a process called lipolysis. The triglycerides (triacylglycerols) travel in the blood to the liver, where they are again converted into fatty acids and glycerol which can be used by the cells for energy.

Glycerol is transformed into an intermediate of glycolysis (glyceraldehyde 3-phosphate). It is then converted to pyruvic acid and acetyl CoA, which enters the Krebs' cycle to produce ATP, or to glucose (remember glycolytic reactions are reversible).

Fatty acids are transformed to acetyl CoA by β-oxidation, a mitochondrial process requiring oxygen and glucose. The resultant acetyl CoA enters the Krebs' cycle to produce ATP, carbon dioxide and water. When fatty acids are broken down in the absence of glucose the incomplete oxidation produces too much acetyl CoA, which forms ketone bodies (acetoacetic acid, β-hydroxybutyric acid and acetone) by a process called ketogenesis (see *Figure 13.23*).

Small amounts of ketone bodies can be used as a fuel molecule in the Krebs' cycle; however, an excess causes a life-threatening condition known as ketoacidosis. This occurs when glucose is either in short supply during starvation or unavailable in uncontrolled diabetes mellitus (see Chapter 8). High levels of the acidic ketone bodies leads to metabolic acidosis and dehydration (see *Figure 8.19*).

Fats, in the form of triglycerides (triacylglycerols), are extremely versatile in metabolism.

Summary – the final common pathway

The metabolites of the energy-producing nutrients – glucose, fatty acids, glycerol and amino acids – are all eventually oxidized to produce energy (ATP). Some is generated by the reactions of the Krebs' cycle, but most is produced by the addition of a phosphate group to ADP in a process, called oxidative phosphorylation, which occurs as the H^+ released from NADH and $FADH_2$ moves between electron carriers of the electron transfer chain in a series of oxidation–reduction reactions (*Figure 13.24*). Electron carriers are flavins (formed from riboflavin) or cytochromes, such as cytochrome *c*, which are highly coloured protein–iron (haem) complexes.

The interconversion of the main nutrient molecules by processes such as lipogenesis and gluconeogenesis is vital to homeostasis, and by now you will have realised the importance of this ability to change some nutrients into others and the flexibility it provides.

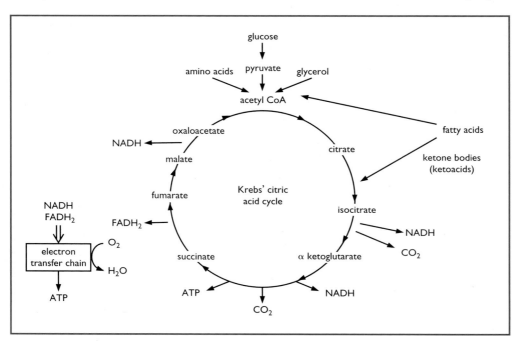

Figure 13.24 Final common pathway (simplified).

Body states – absorptive and postabsorptive

The metabolic state of the body is either absorptive (fed) after a meal or postabsorptive (fasted) between meals (*Figure 13.25*).

An absorptive state exists immediately after a meal and lasts for about 4 hours. During this time the nutrients taken in the meal are absorbed and used to provide instant energy or in anabolic processes such as glycogenesis or lipogenesis (excess stored as fat).

Between meals – during the night, late morning and late afternoon – the metabolic state is postabsorptive. Now the fuel molecules are in short supply and catabolic processes predominate as the body strives to maintain blood glucose levels by glycogenolysis, lipolysis (fatty acids converted to acetyl CoA and glycerol used for gluconeogenesis) and later the catabolism of body protein. The body must ensure that the brain and erythrocytes receive enough glucose, but some tissues can use small amounts of ketones for energy (see page 320). The current advice to have breakfast is very sensible if you consider that the overnight postabsorptive state may already be some 9 hours if your evening meal is at 6 pm

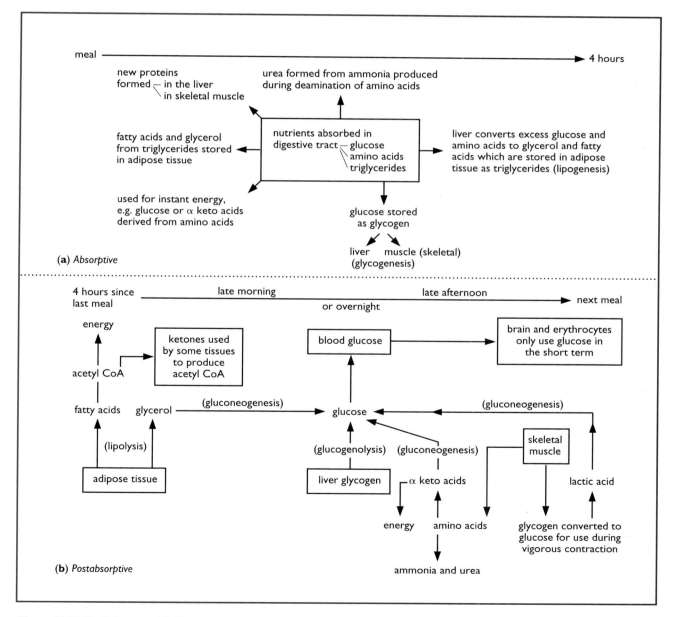

Figure 13.25 Metabolic states. (**a**) Absorptive; (**b**) postabsorptive.

(absorptive until 10 p.m.) and breakfast is 7 a.m. – it will come as no surprise to hear that those who go without breakfast function less well during the morning.

During prolonged fasting the body will consume its own muscle tissue to maintain blood glucose (see PEM, page 318).

Vitamins

Vitamins are organic molecules required in minute quantities for all metabolic processes. They do not produce energy, but are vital to its release from the fuel molecules and the regulation of anabolic processes. Many vitamins act as coenzymes, functioning with enzymes to facilitate reactions involving the metabolism and utilization of carbohydrates, proteins and fats. An example of this is vitamin B_1 thiamin, which is required for the conversion of pyruvic acid to acetyl CoA in carbohydrate metabolism and for a reaction of the Krebs' cycle (alpha ketoglutarate to succinate); and earlier we mentioned riboflavin and niacin and the production of NADH and $FADH_2$. Without the intake and absorption (see page 307) of the correct vitamins the body is unable to use the other nutrients.

Most vitamins must be ingested, but vitamins D, K and some of the B complex can be synthesized in the body.

Vitamin D is produced by the action of ultraviolet light upon 7-dehydrocholesterol, a cholesterol-based substance found in the skin. Vitamin D may be deficient where an inadequate intake is combined with limited exposure to sunlight. This situation may lead to the development of rickets or osteomalacia (see Chapter 16). People at risk may belong to groups whose culture limits exposure to sunlight, or people in lower socioeconomic groups. Iqbal *et al.* (1994) state that more needs to be done to address the problems of vitamin D deficiency and describe symptoms experienced by 26 Asian patients, ranging from pain to walking difficulties.

The commensal bacteria of the intestine produce vitamin K which, in common with the other fat-soluble vitamins, requires the presence of bile for its absorption (see page 307). B-complex vitamins are also produced by the gut bacteria, but in fairly insignificant amounts.

The body is also able to convert certain provitamins, such as the yellow colouring carotene found in carrots and dark green vegetables, into active vitamin A.

Vitamins can be classified into two main groups:

Water-soluble vitamins:
- Vitamin C – ascorbic acid.
- Vitamin B complex – B_1 thiamin, B_2 riboflavin, niacin (nicotinic acid and nicotinamide), B_6 pyridoxine, biotin, folate (folic acid), B_{12} cobalamins and pantothenic acid.

Table 13.2 Nutritional needs of selected special groups.

Table 13.2 Nutritional needs of selected special groups	
Special group	**Additional nutritional needs**
Infants and children	The requirement for energy and other nutrients, e.g. protein, calcium, is high in relation to body area. Extra vitamins A and D[a] may be required, e.g. in breast-fed infants. NB Children, adolescents and women living in communities where cases of rickets are likely to occur should have vitamin D supplements.
Pregnancy	Energy, protein, iron, folate[b], vitamins B, C, A and D, calcium, zinc and iodine. NB High levels of retinol may be associated with birth defects. Excessive vitamin A intake, in the form of supplements or liver, should be avoided as a precautionary measure in pregnant women and those intending to become pregnant.
Lactation	Energy, protein, calcium, folate, vitamins C, D, and A and extra fluid needed.
Older people	Reduction in energy requirements if they become less active. Important that diet provides adequate iron, calcium, and vitamins, especially B-complex, C and D. With inactivity may need more NSP.

a A supplement may be recommended DoH (1994).
b Results from a study Wald et al. (MRC, 1991) confirm that folate supplements should be taken by women planning to conceive and continued during early pregnancy where a previous pregnancy was affected by a neural tube defect, e.g. spina bifida. The same report also states that all women of childbearing age should have a diet containing adequate folic acid (see Chapter 4).

Fat-soluble vitamins:

- Vitamin A – retinol found in animal products, but is also synthesized from the provitamin carotene.
- Vitamin D – cholecalciferol.
- Vitamin E – tocopherols.
- Vitamin K – phylloquinone (plants) and menaquinones made in the intestine.

Probably the most efficient way to take vitamins is as part of a 'healthy' balanced diet which includes items selected from all the food groups. It is important to remember that vitamin content of some foods may vary seasonally, e.g. old potatoes have less vitamin C than new, and that cooking and exposure to light can decrease vitamin levels. The

practice of adding sodium hydrogen carbonate to greens which are then boiled destroys much of the vitamin C. Milk left on the doorstep in the sunlight will lose riboflavin as well as turn sour; it makes good sense to store it in a cool place until needed.

The habit of supplementing vitamin intake with 'pills and potions' is not necessary for most healthy individuals taking a balanced diet. Water-soluble vitamins cannot be stored and are 'thrown away' via the urine. If fat-soluble vitamins are consumed in excess they accumulate in the body to cause hypervitaminosis with toxic effects. For certain special groups, which are discussed in *Table 13.2*, it may be beneficial to consume vitamin supplements.

Nursing Practice Application **Nutritional assessment and support**

Nutritional assessment

Nutritional status is important to many aspects of practice, e.g. wound care and healing, mobility and preventing pressure sores. It is essential to recognize those individuals who may be malnourished and assess nutritional status as part of nursing assessments. Nutritional assessment is rather more than recording weight or asking about food preferences and involves the whole care team (see PEM, page 318). In a series of articles, Goodinson (1987a, b, c, d) describes nutritional assessment and identifies the following methods:

- Biochemical tests, e.g. serum proteins, muscle breakdown products.
- Anthropometric, e.g. weight, body mass index (BMI – weight in kg divided by height in m²), skin fold thickness.
- Subjective methods, e.g. dietary history, physical examination.

To ensure accuracy no method should be used in isolation as factors other than nutrition may influence the data obtained. Serial tests over a period of time are required to monitor changes which denote improvement or deterioration. Watson (1994) advocates weekly weighing and BMI to screen elderly hospitalized people for nutritional deficiencies.

Nutritional support

When the intake of nutrients is inadequate or impossible the individual will need some form of nutritional support. This may take the form of extra energy and protein or it may be necessary to give all the nutrients as total parenteral nutrition (TPN).

As already mentioned, the people involved in maintaining nutrition include the patient/family, nurses, doctors, dietitian, catering staff and biochemist, but the provision of extra support will also involve the pharmacist.

Oral supplements/sip feeding should be used where possible because the oral route has many advantages. It maintains independence and normality as the person is still taking nourishment via the 'normal' route. The physiological mechanisms for oral cleansing still operate, although their effectiveness may be reduced by other factors (page 293).

Enteral tube feeding involves the use of the gastrointestinal tract. It may be achieved by a nasogastric tube or by tubes situated in the stomach (often by percutaneous endoscopic gastrostomy) or jejunum (jejunostomy) which exit through the abdominal wall. If the nasogastric route is used the fine-bore enteral tube is usually well tolerated and does not preclude oral nourishment, so the two methods may be used together.

Enteral tube feeding is used in situations where oral intake is inadequate or impossible but the gut is still functioning, e.g. altered consciousness, facial trauma/burns, hypercatabolic states. Complete nutritional needs, including that for water, can be met by this route and it is cheaper and involves fewer hazards than parenteral feeding (Taylor, 1989). The benefits of enteral feeding, according to Raper and Maynard (1992), include: possible improvement in outcomes, less time in hospital with certain supplements, maintenance of intestinal mucosa (remember cells have a high turnover) which prevents the passage of bacteria, improved blood flow regulation and a reduction in sepsis. The use of commercially prepared feeds reduces the risk of bacterial contamination.

Parenteral feeding through a central vein may be used to provide TPN or to supplement oral and enteral feeding. Use of a central vein is essential for prolonged access and when hypertonic solutions are administered. Phlebitis (inflammation of a vein) results if hypertonic solutions are administered into a peripheral vein.

The intravenous route should only be chosen in the absence of gastrointestinal function or when it is impossible to provide sufficient nourishment by other methods. Finlay (1997) states that people with some gut function should be fed enterally. The indications for TPN may include: after gastrointestinal surgery where gut function is absent, extreme hypercatabolic states, severe malabsorption or loss through gastrointestinal fistulae. TPN has serious disadvantages, including problems with the insertion of the line, e.g. pneumothorax, infection, metabolic disturbances such as hyperglycaemia, immunosuppression, and expense.

The DoH (1991) provides information regarding dietary reference values for the UK, and further details of vitamins, their sources, uses, excesses and deficiencies can be found in Further Reading, e.g. MAFF (1995).

Minerals

Minerals are vital to homeostasis and have a role in all metabolic processes. The major elements required by the body are: calcium, chlorine, iodine, iron, magnesium, phosphorus, potassium, sodium and sulphur. Other minerals, needed only in minute quantities (trace elements), include: chromium, cobalt, copper, fluorine, manganese, molybdenum, selenium and zinc. Minerals are needed for:

- Utilization of nutrients.
- Enzymes, e.g. zinc required for carboxypeptidase (see page 303).
- Hormones, e.g. iodine required for thyroid hormones (see Chapter 8).
- Formation of functional proteins, e.g. iron and haemoglobin (see Chapter 9).
- Maintenance of fluid compartments, e.g. sodium, chlorine and potassium (see Chapter 2).
- Nerve and muscle function, e.g. sodium, potassium and calcium (see Chapters 3 and 17).
- Structural strength, e.g. calcium, magnesium and phosphorus in bone (see Chapter 16).

Further information is given in Chapter 2 (*Table 2.1*).

Again the dietary reference values are found in DoH (1991) and other information in MAFF (1995).

Water

In health, water forms 45–75% of the body mass depending on age (see Chapter 2). It is required for every metabolic process and is vital to all homeostatic mechanisms. Our requirement for water intake varies according to activity, climate and losses, e.g. in urine and faeces, but generally an adult needs to consume around 2.5 litres daily (remember that most foods also contain water).

Non-starch polysaccharide/fibre

NSP, which forms an important component of a healthy diet, consists of indigestible plant polysaccharides such as cellulose. It adds bulk to the faeces, decreases transit times for food residues and gives a feeling of fullness without excessive energy consumption (see page 312). The recommended average daily intake of 18 g (DoH, 1991) is easily obtained from wholegrain cereals, pulses, fruit and unpeeled vegetables. There are, however, some drawbacks of a high-fibre diet:

- Increased flatulence, which may be socially inconvenient or more seriously causes distension and pain.
- Inhibited absorption of minerals, e.g. calcium, iron and zinc (see page 308).

Summary/Check List

Introduction – early development. General structure of digestive tract. Nerve supply. Peritoneum – peritonitis.
Alimentary tract – mouth. Tongue. Palate, Nursing Practice Application – cleft palate/lip. Salivary glands – mumps, composition of saliva, regulation of salivation, Nursing Practice Application – oral hygiene. Teeth – dentition, dental caries/periodontal disease. Healthier Living – early detection of oral cancers. Pharynx, swallowing, Nursing Practice Application – swallowing problems and anxiety. Oesophagus – peristalsis. Stomach structure. Nursing Practice Application – stomach size and the neonate. Gastric secretions/functions – control, activity, motility, emptying, absorption, Nursing Practice Application – vomiting, Special Focus – peptic ulceration, Person-centred Study – Ken. Small intestine – structure. Pancreas and pancreatic enzymes. Nursing Practice Application – starch digestion and the timing of weaning. Bile and digestion – functions of bile. Intestinal juice and enzymes. Nursing Practice Application – lactose intolerance. Summary – chemical digestion. Absorption in the small intestine – amino acids, monosaccharides, fats, vitamins, minerals, water,

Nursing Practice Application – malabsorption. Large intestine – caecum/appendix, appendicitis, colon, rectum and anal canal. Functions of large intestine – absorption, Nursing Practice Application – absorption of drugs, synthesis, storage, elimination (defecation). Nursing Practice Application – irritable bowel syndrome. Composition of faeces. Healthier Living – NSP, defecation and health, faecal incontinence, Special Focus – normal bowel habit, diarrhoea, constipation, Person-centred Study – Dorothy.
Nutrition, metabolism and utilization – introduction. Healthier Living – eating for health (adults). Energy composition of food. Carbohydrates – metabolism and utilization of monosaccharides. Protein, Nursing Practice Application – PEM and meals in hospital, metabolism and utilization of amino acids, Nursing Practice Application – phenylketonuria. Fats – metabolism and utilization of fatty acids/glycerol. Final common pathway. Absorptive and postabsorptive states. Vitamins, minerals, water, NSP. Nursing Practice Application – nutritional assessment and support.

Self Test

1 Put the following in their correct order:
   (a) stomach;
   (b) jejunum;
   (c) oesophagus;
   (d) pharynx;
   (e) ileum;
   (f) rectum;
   (g) duodenum;
   (h) colon;
   (i) mouth;
   (j) anus.
2 Which of these statements are true?
   (a) Enzymes in saliva are important in the digestion of starch.
   (b) 1000–1500 ml of saliva is produced daily.
   (c) The first dentition consists of 20 teeth.
   (d) Periodontal disease is common from midlife.
3 What does gastric juice contain and how is its secretion controlled?
4 Explain how vomiting may cause:
   (a) metabolic alkalosis;
   (b) metabolic acidosis.
5 Complete the following:
   (a) Pancreatic secretion is stimulated by the regulatory peptides _ _ _ _ _ _ _ _ _ _ _ _ _ _ _ and _ _ _ _ _ _ _.
   (b) Trypsinogen is activated by _ _ _ _ _ _ _ _ _ _ _.

(c) Bile _ _ _ _ _ _ _ _ _ _ fat globules prior to their chemical breakdown by _ _ _ _ _ _ _.
6 What are the products of protein, fat and carbohydrate digestion, and how are they absorbed?
7 Describe the following:
   (a) gastrocolic reflex;
   (b) mass movements;
   (c) defaecation reflex.
8 Match the pairs correctly:
   (a) calcium;
   (b) monosaccharide;
   (c) EFA;
   (d) carotene;
   (e) phenylalanine;
   (f) mineral;
   (g) fructose;
   (h) linoleic acid;
   (i) vitamin A;
   (j) amino acid.
9 What would you say to Winnie who asks you about the plus and minus points of fibre (NSP) in the diet?
10 Which of the following statements are true:
   (a) Amino acids are a major energy source.
   (b) Pyruvic acid is converted aerobically into acetyl CoA.
   (c) Ketone bodies are produced by the incomplete oxidation of fatty acids.
   (d) Fat is stored as triglycerides (triacylglycerols).

Answers

1 i, d, c, a, g, b, e, h, f, j.
2 b, c, d.
3 See pages 296–8.
4 See page 300.
5 (a) Cholecystokinin, secretin;
   (b) enterokinase;
   (c) emulsifies, lipases.
6 See pages 306–7.
7 See pages 309 and 311.
8 a–f, b–g, c–h, d–i and e–j.
9 See pages 312 and 324.
10 b, c, d.

References

Burkitt D, Walker A, Painter N (1972) Effect of dietary fibre on stools and transit times and its role in the causation of disease. *Lancet* ii: 1408–12.

de Boer W, Driessen W, Jansz A *et al.* (1995) Effects of acid suppression on efficacy of treatment for *Helicobacter pylori* infection. *Lancet* 345: 817–20.

DoH (1991) *Dietary Reference Values for Food Energy and Nutrients for the United Kingdom*. Report on Health and Social Subjects, no. 41. London: HMSO.

DoH (1992) *The Health of the Nation* (Summary). London: HMSO.

DoH (1994) *Weaning and the Weaning Diet*. Report on Health and Social Subjects, no. 45. London: HMSO.

Dickerson J (1995) The problem of hospital-induced malnutrition. *Nurs Times* 91(4): 44–5.

Eburn E (1989) Choosing the right antiemetic. *Nurs Times* 85(24): 36–8.

Edwards CRW, Bouchier IAD, Haslett C, Eds, et al. (1995) *Davidson's Principles and Practice of Medicine*, 17th edn. Edinburgh: Churchill Livingstone.

Finlay T (1997) Making sense of .... parenteral nutrition in adult patients. *Nurs Times* **93**(2): 35–6.

Goodinson SM (1987a) Assessment of nutritional status. *Prof Nurs* **2**(11): 367–9.

Goodinson SM (1987b) Anthropometric assessment of nutritional status. *Prof Nurs* **2**(12): 388–93.

Goodinson SM (1987c) Biochemical assessment of nutritional status. *Prof Nurs* **3**(1): 8–12.

Goodinson SM (1987d) Assessing nutritional status: subjective methods. *Prof Nurs* **3**(2): 48–51.

Gupta K (1980) Constipation. *Geriatr Med* **10**(12): 45.

Howarth H (1977) Mouth care procedures for the very ill. *Nurs Times* **73**(10): 354–355.

Iqbal S, Kaddam I, Wassif W et al. (1994) Continuing clinically severe vitamin D deficiency in Asians in the UK (Leicester). *Postgrad Med J* **70**(828): 708–14.

Kinghorn S (1995) Easing patient discomfort. *Nurs Times* **91**(34):57–9.

Nightingale F (1859) *Notes on Nursing*. London: Duckworth (1970).

Norton C (1997) Faecal incontinence in adults 2: treatment and management. *Br J Nurs* **6**(1): 23–6.

Rang HP, Dale MM, Ritter JM (1995) *Pharmacology*, 3rd edn. Edinburgh: Churchill Livingstone.

Raper S, Maynard N (1992) Feeding the critically ill patient. *Br J Nurs* **1**(6):273–80.

Taylor SJ (1989) A guide to enteral feeding. *Prof Nurs* **4**(4):195–200.

Tierney AJ (1996) Undernutrition and elderly hospital patients: a review. *J Adv Nurs*, **23**(2):228–36.

Watson R (1994) Guest editorial: nutritional standards and the older adult. *J Adv Nurs* **20**(2):205–6.

Wright L (1974) *Bowel Function in Hospital Patients*. Royal College of Nursing (RCN) Research Project, Series 1, no. 4. London: RCN.

Further Reading

Finnegan S, Oldfield K (1989) When eating is impossible: TPN in maintaining nutritional status. *Prof Nurs* **4**(6):271–275.

Garrow J, James W, Eds (1993) *Human Nutrition and Dietetics*, 9th edn. Edinburgh: Churchill Livingstone.

Hamilton-Smith S (1972) *Nil by mouth?* London: Royal College of Nursing.

MAFF (1995) *Manual of Nutrition*, 10th edn. London: HMSO.

Montgomary SM, Pounder RE, Wakefield AJ (1997) Infant mortality and the incidence of Inflammatory bowel disease. *Lancet* **349**: 472–473

Royal College of Nursing (1993) *Nutritional standards and the older adult*. RCN Dynamic Quality Improvement Programme. London: RCN.

Shearman D, Finlayson N, Carter D et al. (1997) *Diseases of the Gastrointestinal Tract and Liver*, 3rd edn. Edinburgh: Churchill Livingstone.

Trivedy C, Baldwin D, Warnakulasuriya S et al. (1997) Copper content in Areca catechu (betel nut) products and oral submucous fibrosis. *Lancet* **349**: (9063) 1447.

Useful Addresses

British Association for Parenteral and Enteral Nutrition (BAPEN)
PO Box 922
Maidenhead
Berkshire SL6 4SH

Ileostomy Association of Britain and Ireland
PO Box 23
Mansfield
Nottinghamshire NG18 4TT

Liver and Biliary Tract

Overview

- *Structure and functions of the liver and biliary tract.*

Learning Outcomes

After studying Chapter 14 you should be able to:

- Describe the gross structure and position of the liver.
- Describe blood flow through the liver.
- Describe the histology of the liver lobules.
- Discuss the formation and secretion of bile.
- Describe the biliary tract and explain how bile reaches the duodenum.
- Discuss the types and causes of jaundice.
- Outline synthesis in the liver.
- Discuss the importance of hepatic detoxification.
- Discuss the effects of excess alcohol on liver function.
- Describe storage in the liver.
- Outline the metabolic role of the liver.
- Describe how liver function is investigated.
- Discuss the consequences of failing liver function.

Key Words

Biliary tract – the ducts that transport bile from the liver to the gallbladder and duodenum.

Bilirubin/biliverdin – the bile pigments derived from haem.

Cholelithiasis – formation of gallstones.

Conjugation – 'joining together'. Bilirubin is conjugated with glucuronic acid within the liver.

Gluconeogenesis – the formation of glucose from non-carbohydrate sources, e.g. lactate, glycerol and amino acids. Used when glycogen stores are low.

Glycogenesis – process by which glucose, in excess of immediate energy needs, is converted to glycogen (storage carbohydrate) in the liver.

Glycogenolysis – process by which liver glycogen is converted to glucose to restore homeostasis.

Glycolysis – series of reversible reactions where glucose is broken down to form pyruvic acid.

Hepatic – pertaining to the liver.

Hepatocytes – the parenchymal (functional) cells of the liver.

Hyperbilirubinaemia – elevated levels of bilirubin in the blood.

Ketogenesis – the formation of ketone bodies from the acetyl CoA formed from the incomplete oxidation of fats.

Lipogenesis – the deposition of excess triglycerides [triacylglycerols (formed from non-lipid sources)] in adipose tissue.

Lipolysis – the release of stored triglycerides (triacylglycerols) from adipose tissue for use as energy.

Introduction

The liver, with its many essential functions, is vital to life. Some of these functions have already been mentioned – erythrocyte breakdown (Chapter 9), role of bile in the digestion and absorption of fats and the metabolism of nutrients (Chapter 13). The liver also synthesizes proteins, stores vitamins and minerals, and is involved in the detoxification of many of the molecules produced by or taken into the body. With all these processes occurring, the high metabolic rate of the liver is responsible for the production of a considerable amount of heat.

Luckily for us the liver has huge functional reserves, which is illustrated by the fact that people with serious liver disease may exhibit no ill effects until considerable damage has occurred. Liver cells can regenerate if damage is not too severe, e.g. when part of the liver is removed after trauma or in transplant surgery of the liver when liver tissue from a living donor is used (unusual). What the liver cannot cope with is continuous damage from a toxic agent, e.g. alcohol. In this situation liver cells are destroyed and fibrosis occurs.

The Liver and Biliary Tract

Early development

During week 4 of embryonic development the liver, gallbladder and bile ducts, in common with the other accessory digestive structures, start to form from endodermal 'offshoots' of the primitive foregut. Endodermal cells form columns of liver cells around blood channels (sinu-

soids) in a mesodermal mass from which the haemopoietic tissue, Kupffer cells and fibrous capsule form. Haemopoiesis occurs in the developing liver from week 6, but stops before birth. Bile production starts by week 16 and the bile pigments colour the meconium (see Chapter 13). The liver develops very rapidly during fetal life. It is proportionally very large in the newborn infant and contains vast carbohydrate stores for use in the first few days of life before feeding is well established.

Gross structure of the liver

The liver, which weighs 1.2–1.5 kg, is the largest gland in the body. Located in the right upper abdomen, it fills most of the right hypochondriac region and extends into the epigastric and left hypochondriac regions (see *Figure 1.33*). The smooth superior and anterior surfaces of the liver are situated under the diaphragm and are well protected by the rib cage. The liver cannot normally be felt below the costal margin. Liver bulk displaces the right kidney downwards.

The liver consists of four lobes: the right and left lobes, and two small lobes – the caudate and quadrate – which are situated on its irregular posterior surface (*Figure 14.1*). The gallbladder can be found in a depression on this posterior surface. The liver is enclosed within a thin connective-tissue capsule and partially covered by peritoneum. It is attached to the diaphragm and abdominal wall by ligaments formed from folds of peritoneum, e.g. the falciform ligament, which also divides the right and left lobes. Within the falciform ligament is the fibrous remnant of the fetal umbilical vein (see Chapter 21) known as the ligamentum teres. A more

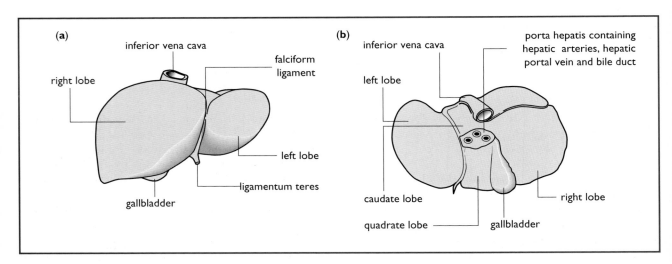

Figure 14.1 The liver. (a) Anterior surface; (b) posterior surface.

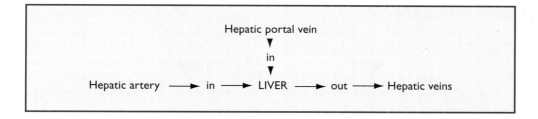

recent trend, however, is to describe the liver as having two halves (right and left) defined by a dividing line along the plane of the gallbladder depression and inferior vena cava. Each half is drained by the right and left **hepatic** ducts respectively (see page 332).

The porta hepatis (portal fissure) is the area on the posterior surface where blood vessels (hepatic artery and hepatic portal vein), nerves, lymphatic vessels and bile ducts enter and leave the liver.

Blood supply of the liver

As you will remember, the liver has a special arrangement of blood vessels. The blood flow through the liver will be covered in more detail when we consider the liver lobule (see below and page 330).

To facilitate its metabolic role the liver receives an abundant supply of oxygenated blood from the hepatic artery. In addition, venous blood from the digestive organs is conveyed to the liver by the hepatic portal vein (see Chapters 10 and 13). The advantages of this arrangement are obvious when you consider the role of the liver in the metabolism and utilization of nutrients. All the venous blood eventually leaves the liver by three main hepatic veins.

Liver blood flow is autoregulated by vascular sphincters which control the amount of blood entering from the hepatic artery. This allows for variations in flow through the hepatic portal vein and keeps total hepatic blood flow fairly constant.

Nerve supply

The liver is innervated by some parasympathetic fibres of the vagus nerve, and sympathetic fibres from the coeliac ganglia (see Chapter 6) which stimulate **glycogenolysis.**

Microscopic structure of the liver

The liver consists of many hexagonal functional units called lobules (*Figure 14.2*). A lobule, which measures less than 2 mm in diameter, contains **hepatocytes** (parenchymal or functional cells of the liver), blood vessels, bile ducts and phagocytic Kupffer cells (see page 330).

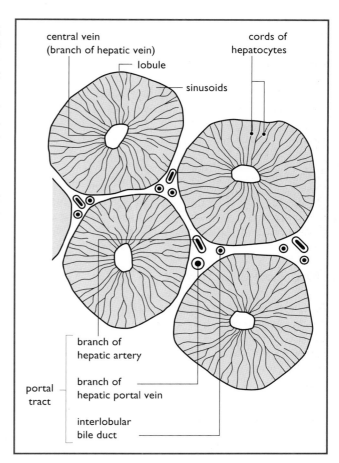

Figure 14.2 Liver lobules.

Each lobule has a central vein (branch of hepatic vein) and cords of hepatocytes which radiate like the spokes of a wheel (*Figure 14.2*). Blood-filled channels called sinusoids (see Chapter 10) permeate the cords of hepatocytes, which allows for slow blood flow and very close contact between hepatocytes and blood.

At each corner of the hexagonal lobule is a portal tract, which contains a branch of both the hepatic artery and hepatic portal vein and a bile duct. Blood from the hepatic artery and hepatic portal vein flows through the sinusoids to drain by the central vein to eventually reach the hepatic veins and inferior vena cava. The direction of blood flow is therefore away from the portal tract whereas bile secreted by the hepatocytes flows in the opposite direction (*Figure 14.3*).

The secreted bile is collected in a network of tiny tubes called bile canaliculi, which are situated between the hepatocytes. The canaliculi unite to form the interlobular bile ducts of the portal tracts, which eventually become the right and left hepatic ducts carrying bile from the liver. The special Kupffer cells lining the sinusoids are phagocytic macrophages (see Chapters 1 and 9), which are part of the more widespread mononuclear phagocytic system. Kupffer cells are concerned with the phagocytosis of bacteria and 'spent' erythrocytes.

Abnormal Function
Liver problems – acute hepatitis (acute parenchymal disease of the liver)

Acute inflammation of hepatocytes may be caused by infections, toxic substances, circulatory problems or metabolic abnormalities.

Infections
- Viruses – hepatitis A (HAV), hepatitis B (HBV) (see Chapter 9), hepatitis C (HCV), hepatitis D (HDV), hepatitis E (HEV), other viruses (previously known as non-A non-B hepatitis), Epstein–Barr virus (glandular fever) and cytomegalovirus (CMV).
- Reye's syndrome, which occurs mainly in children following a viral infection treated with aspirin. This is why the use of aspirin is contraindicated in children aged under 12 years (except

to treat rheumatoid arthritis).
- Other micro-organisms, e.g. *Leptospira icterohaemorrhagiae* – a spirochaete that causes Weil's disease.

Toxic substances
- Alcohol (see pages 335 and 336).
- Drugs, e.g. paracetamol – commonly chosen for self-poisoning, antidepressants, halothane, antituberculous drugs, chlorpromazine, and many more.
- Chemicals, e.g. carbon tetrachloride used in dry cleaning, antifreeze and toxins present in certain poisonous fungi.

Circulatory problems
Damage will occur if the very active

hepatocytes are deprived of an adequate blood supply, e.g. shock or right-sided cardiac failure (see Chapter 10).

Metabolic abnormalites
An example of a metabolic abnormality is Wilson's disease, where copper accumulates in the liver and basal nuclei.

The outcome of acute hepatitis depends on the cause and the extent of hepatocyte loss by necrosis (tissue death). Complete recovery is possible, e.g. after hepatitis A, and hepatitis B in some cases, but in other conditions the individual develops a chronic progressive disorder which may eventually lead to complications, hepatic failure and death.

Nursing Practice Application Injuries to the liver

Traumatic damage to the liver may be caused by a road traffic accident, crush injuries and penetrating wounds, e.g. stabbing. As you can imagine, the highly vascular liver bleeds profusely; if uncontrolled,

this very quickly leads to hypovolaemic shock (see Chapter 10). People with a history of abdominal injury need careful monitoring of vital signs to detect the changes indicative of internal haemorrhage at an

early stage. This allows the diagnosis of liver trauma to be made quickly and, after stabilization of their condition, e.g. blood transfusion (see Chapter 9), surgical repair is undertaken.

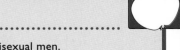

Healthier Living Hepatitis B – immunization

High levels of protection against HBV can be achieved by use of a recombinant vaccine in those at high risk for the infection. The groups who should be

offered immunization include: healthcare staff, laboratory staff, intravenous drug users, infants of infected mothers, people having haemodialysis and homo-

sexual/bisexual men.

Many authorities, including the WHO, recommend that HBV immunization is offered routinely during childhood.

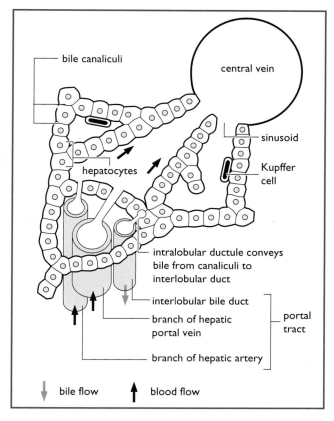

Figure 14.3 Detail of lobule to show blood and bile flow.

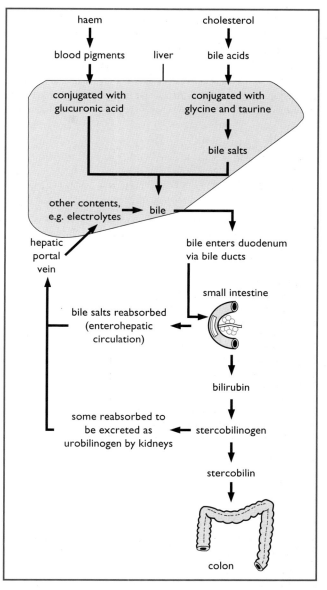

Figure 14.4 Production of bile and reabsorption of bile salts.

Liver Functions

As we have already mentioned, the liver plays a vital part in homeostatic regulation and the healthy functioning of every body system. In an attempt to clarify the diversity of hepatocyte function, the list that follows will be developed by more detailed discussion where appropriate:

• Bile production.
• Synthesis – proteins and other molecules.
• Detoxification of alcohol, drugs and hormones.
• Storage.
• Metabolism of carbohydrates, protein, fats and vitamins. With this list in mind it is easy to see why a person with failing hepatic function (see page 339) is so very ill and why the medical management is extremely complex and difficult.

Bile production

The hepatocytes produce about 500–1000 ml of alkaline (pH 8.0) bile daily. Bile is a viscous green–yellow fluid that contains: water, bile acids (salts), bile pigments, cholesterol, phospholipids, electrolytes, enzymes produced by the liver, e.g. alkaline phosphatase, and various molecules for excretion, such as hormones.

The bile acids, e.g. cholic and chenodeoxycholic acids, are derived from cholesterol. Conjugation (joining) of the bile acids with glycine and taurine occurs in the liver and the conjugated acids form bile salts with sodium – sodium glycocholate and sodium taurocholate. The bile salts are secreted into the bile ducts and enter the intestine, where most are reabsorbed. In a recycling process known as enterohepatic circulation the bile salts return to the liver through the hepatic portal vein. Returning bile salts stimulate further bile and bile-acid production (*Figure 14.4*).

The bile pigments, **bilirubin** and **biliverdin**, are formed from the haem molecule produced mainly from the breakdown of erythrocytes. The unconjugated fat-soluble bilirubin, which is toxic to cells, is transported in the plasma bound to albumin. It is conjugated (joined) with glucuronic acid within the liver cells in reactions requiring microsomal enzymes (present on the smooth endoplasmic reticulum) such as glucuronyl transferase, and the less toxic water-soluble product passes with the bile into the duodenum. These microsomal enzymes are not fully active until the third month of life, which accounts for the 'physiological jaundice' seen in many newborns. Neonatal ability to bind and conjugate bilirubin is further reduced by certain drugs (see below). At the other end of the lifespan the decline in enzyme activity leads to problems dealing with drugs (see Nursing Practice Application – Liver function and ageing).

Microbial activity in the bowel converts bilirubin to stercobilinogen. Some is reabsorbed and passes through the liver into the general circulation to be excreted as urobilinogen by the kidney (see Chapter 15). The remaining stercobilinogen is converted in the bowel to stercobilin, which is excreted in the faeces.

Many drugs interfere with the complex, enzyme-catalyzed reactions involved with bilirubin binding, transport and **conjugation**. Drugs such as salicylates interfere with the binding and transport of unconjugated bilirubin, and so should not be given late in pregnancy or to infants under 4 weeks of age suffering from jaundice (see page 334). The presence in the serum of unbound unconjugated (lipid soluble) bilirubin can cause kernicterus (staining of brain cells, especially those of the basal nuclei, with bilirubin), which results in brain damage and learning disabilities. Remember that the blood–brain barrier is not well developed in babies (and young children) and the lipid-soluble bilirubin is able to 'home in' on nerve cells.

Those drugs that stimulate liver (microsomal) enzymes, e.g. primidone, barbiturates, corticosteroids and rifampicin, are termed enzyme inducers. These enzyme inducers may increase the metabolism of other drugs, e.g. oral contraceptives, causing lower blood levels and reduced effectiveness. Some drugs, such as cimetidine (H_2 antagonist), can decrease microsomal enzyme activity and slow the metabolism of other drugs, e.g. tricyclic antidepressants, which increases the risk of toxicity.

Bile also provides a route for the excretion of cholesterol, phospholipids, and drug and hormone metabolites, which leave the body in the faeces.

Secretion of bile is stimulated by returning bile salts and the intestinal hormone secretin (see Chapter 13).

The actual release of bile into the duodenum depends on the hormone cholecystokinin and to a lesser extent vagal activity. The role of bile in digestion is discussed in Chapter 13.

Biliary tract, gallbladder and the excretion of bile

Bile drains from the main lobes (or halves) of the liver into the right and left hepatic ducts, which drain their respective lobes. The two ducts unite to form the common hepatic duct, which leaves the liver at the porta hepatis [see *Figure 14.1(b)*]. The cystic duct leads from the common hepatic duct to the gallbladder, where bile not needed immediately is stored and concentrated.

The gallbladder is a pear-shaped sac, about 10 cm long, which lies in a fossa on the posterior surface of the liver. It has a muscular layer and a mucosal lining of columnar epithelium thrown up into rugae very similar to those in the stomach. The rugae allow the gallbladder to distend when storing bile. When bile is required for digestion the muscle layer contracts and bile is expelled into the cystic duct. The cystic duct forms the common bile duct, which joins with the pancreatic duct to enter the duodenum at the hepatopancreatic ampulla (see Chapter 13). The opening into the duodenum is guarded by the sphincter of Oddi, which regulates the flow of bile. Sphincter opening is controlled by the release of cholecystokinin, which simultaneously contracts the gallbladder (*Figure 14.5*).

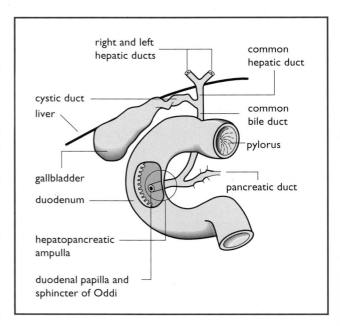

Figure 14.5 Bile ducts and gallbladder (diagrammatic).

Abnormal Function Gallbladder problems – gallstones (cholelithiasis)

Gallstones are common in developed countries. In the UK they are known to affect 10–15% of adults, with many more being asymptomatic. The incidence is higher in women and is becoming increasingly common in younger adults (under 40).

In the UK the most common type of gallstones are those containing mostly cholesterol. They are formed by the crystallization of cholesterol in the gallbladder, which occurs when the cholesterol level is high or the level of bile salts is reduced. The factors which predispose to the formation of cholesterol gallstones include multiparity, obesity, oral contraceptives, total parenteral nutrition, drugs that reduce serum lipid levels and problems with the reabsorption of bile salts.

The other type of gallstone, which consists of bile pigments, is much less common and is associated with conditions where excess bilirubin is produced, e.g. haemolysis (see Chapter 9).

Although many people with gallstones are asymptomatic, the stones can cause various problems, including cholecystitis (inflammation), which may be acute (see Person-Centred Study – Daphne) or chronic; biliary colic, characterized by extremely intense pain caused by a stone moving along the ducts; obstruction of the common bile duct with jaundice; and the remote possibility of perforation of the gallbladder with peritonitis (see Chapter 13).

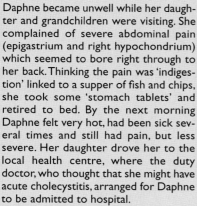

Person-Centred Study Daphne

Daphne became unwell while her daughter and grandchildren were visiting. She complained of severe abdominal pain (epigastrium and right hypochondrium) which seemed to bore right through to her back. Thinking the pain was 'indigestion' linked to a supper of fish and chips, she took some 'stomach tablets' and retired to bed. By the next morning Daphne felt very hot, had been sick several times and still had pain, but less severe. Her daughter drove her to the local health centre, where the duty doctor, who thought that she might have acute cholecystitis, arranged for Daphne to be admitted to hospital.

Once in hospital, where the provisional diagnosis of acute cholecystitis is confirmed, Daphne is given intramuscular analgesia (pentazocine), an antiemetic (metoclopramide) and, because infection is present, an antimicrobial (a cephalosporin). The management regimen consists of intravenous fluid replacement and careful monitoring of pain, vital signs and fluid balance.

Daphne will have investigations to confirm the presence of gallstones, which are found to obstruct the cystic duct in 96% of people with acute cholecystitis (Sherlock, 1989). The possible investigations include ultrasonography, computed tomography (CT scan), radionuclide scan and possibly cholecystography. If the diagnosis of gallstones/inflammation is confirmed it is likely that Daphne will be offered surgical treatment to remove the gallbladder (cholecystectomy). This can be done within 2–3 days of the acute attack or delayed for 2–3 months. The first option has the advantage of reducing the chance of further attacks while waiting. Surgical treatment may be open cholecystectomy or increasingly a laporoscopic minimal access approach. Minimal access surgery (MAS) has some obvious advantages, including less pain, shorter in-patient stay and quicker return to full activity. There are problems, however, and an article by White and Cartheus (1995) outlines the numerous hazards associated with MAS. Other treatments for gallstones include: removal of stones located within the bile ducts by endoscopic retrograde cholangiopancreatography (ERCP); the lithotripter, a machine which produces shockwaves to disintegrate the gallstones (being noninvasive, lithotripsy has some important plus points, such as reduced discomfort and safety); and (rarely) chemical dispersal of the gallstones with oral bile acids.

Non-surgical treatments have one big drawback – the gallbladder is still there and stones can recur, especially if the same pathophysiological conditions pertain.

Synthesis in the liver

The liver can synthesize many different molecules, ranging from clotting factors to active vitamins.

The plasma proteins (see Chapter 9) albumin, α- and β-globulins and fibrinogen are made in the liver from amino acids. The γ-globulins are made elsewhere in the mononuclear phagocytic system. A useful test of liver function is to measure plasma proteins and the albumin:globulin ratio; a fall in albumin may indicate liver malfunction or protein malnutrition.

As well as fibrinogen, the liver also manufactures other clotting factors, which include prothrombin and factors V, VII, VIII, IX, X, XI, XII and XIII (see *Table 9.3*). The liver is responsible for the production of heparin, a natural anticoagulant, which is involved with other substances in the prevention of excess coagulation.

During embryonic life the liver is a site of haemopoiesis and this function can be revived if the demand for blood cells exceeds supply. Transport proteins such as transferrin (iron carriage) are made in the liver, as are the proteins of the 'complement' defence system (see Chapter 19).

Nursing Practice Application **Biliary surgery**

It is understandable for people to feel anxious about losing a part of their anatomy. It is therefore important that before a person undergoes cholecystectomy the nurse explains that digestion functions without the gallbladder, as bile will trickle continuously into the duodenum.

Where the common bile duct has been explored to remove a stone it may be necessary for the bile to be drained externally through a T tube until the swelling subsides and the duct is again patent (open). Considerable fluid and electrolyte losses occur, and nurses should ensure that accurate records of drainage are kept and that replacement fluid/electrolyte is administered as prescribed.

Special Focus **Jaundice**

Jaundice (yellow discoloration of skin, mucous membranes and sclera) is not a disease but a sign of some malfunction of bile production, transport or excretion. Apart from the yellow discoloration, which becomes apparent when the serum bilirubin reaches 35–50 μmol/litre (normal 2–17 μmol/litre), the affected person may also complain of intense skin irritation (pruritus).

A very simple classification of jaundice considers the three types: prehepatic; hepatocellular; and obstructive (*Figure 14.6*). Many other classifications exist.

Prehepatic or haemolytic jaundice
The hyperbilirubinaemia (elevated levels of bilirubin in the blood) is usually caused by excessive breakdown of erythrocytes. This occurs in haemolytic disease of the newborn (see Chapter 9) where the unconjugated bilirubin crosses the blood–brain barrier to cause kernicterus (see page 332).

Other causes of prehepatic jaundice include excessive haemolysis by the spleen, drugs (e.g. sulphonamides), incompatible ABO blood transfusion, severe infections and erythrocyte abnormality, e.g. thalassaemia.

Prehepatic jaundice is usually mild and is accompanied by an increase in urobilinogen excretion in the urine and excess stercobilin in the faeces, which may be very dark. Levels of unconjugated bilirubin in the serum are increased. This type of jaundice is sometimes termed acholuric because unconjugated bilirubin does not pass through the kidney and is consequently absent from the urine. The affected person usually has some degree of anaemia (see Chapter 9).

Hepatocellular jaundice
This type of jaundice is caused by some defect in the transport of bilirubin within the liver. It may be due to the hepatitis caused by agents such as viruses, alcohol or drugs. Hepatocellular jaundice also occurs in newborns because their immature livers lack the enzyme activity required for bilirubin conjugation. As with haemolytic disease, the unconjugated bilirubin levels present in severe 'physiological' jaundice, can cross into the brain tissue, especially the basal nuclei, to cause kernicterus and damage which may lead to learning disabilities. Another problem for some breast-fed babies is the inhibition of transferase enzyme activity caused by hormonal substances in breast milk.

A more unusual cause of jaundice is the inherited Gilbert's syndrome, where a deficiency of conjugation enzymes leads to a mild but fluctuating jaundice.

Hepatocellular jaundice varies in severity, and associated features depend upon the cause; for example, bilirubin may appear in the urine in hepatitis but not with Gilbert's syndrome. The hyperbilirubinaemia is unconjugated if the required enzymes are deficient, but where hepatocyte damage is present it is a conjugated hyperbilirubinaemia.

Obstructive or cholestatic jaundice
Obstructive or cholestatic jaundice (cholestasis – an obstruction to the flow of bile) may be caused by intrahepatic obstruction to the flow of bile or the extrahepatic blockage of a large bile duct.

Intrahepatic causes, where the tiny bile ducts are affected, include: cirrhosis, hepatitis, drugs, e.g. oral contraceptives and androgenic anabolic steroids (see Healthier Living), and widespread metastatic malignancy.

Extrahepatic obstruction is commonly caused by a gallstone occluding the common bile duct, but other causes include carcinoma of the head of the pancreas, other tumours, bile-duct strictures (narrowing) and even parasitic worms migrating from the gut.

When bile flow to the duodenum is obstructed the affected person will have dark urine, which contains bilirubin but no urobilinogen, and pale faeces, caused by the absence of stercobilin. The jaundice is usually severe, and may produce a greenish tinge to the skin and a metallic taste in the mouth. There is an increase in both unconjugated and conjugated bilirubin in the serum, but in practice usually only the total bilirubin is measured. If unrelieved, it will lead to hepatocyte damage, malabsorption and coagulation problems because of lack of vitamin K and prothrombin (see Chapters 9 and 13).

The liver is concerned with the production and activation of certain vitamins; it can convert the provitamin β-carotene to vitamin A (retinol) and the amino acid tryptophan to nicotinic acid (see niacin). The inactive vitamin D (cholecalciferol) is converted by the liver to a storage form (25-hydroxycholecalciferol) which is converted to the active vitamin by the kidney.

Some of the other molecules produced by the liver are covered under Metabolism of nutrients (see pages 337, 338 and 340).

Prehepatic or haemolytic	Hepatocellular	Obstructive (cholestatic)
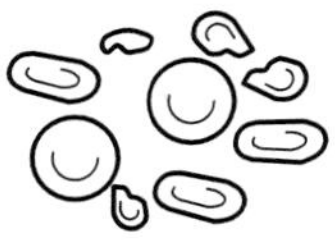 haemolysis and release of haem	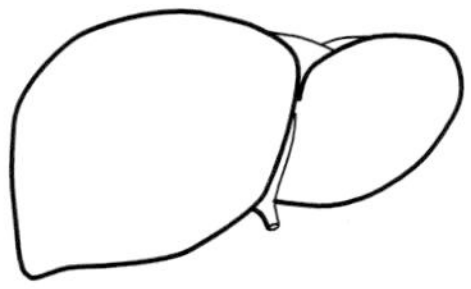	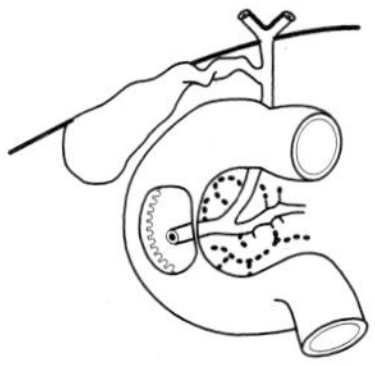

Causes:
Overactive spleen
Rhesus incompatibility
ABO mismatch
Abnormal RBCs
Drugs
Infections
	Causes:
	Hepatitis
	  drugs
	  alcohol
	  viruses
	Conjugation problems in the newborn
	Gilbert's syndrome
		Causes:
		A Intrahepatic
		   Cirrhosis
		   Drugs
		   Metastatic cancer
		   Hepatitis
		
		B Extrahepatic
		   Gallstones in CBD
		   Cancer in head of pancreas
		   Other tumours, etc.

Results: Mild jaundice (lemon) 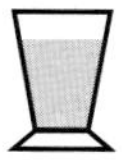 Urine contains increased urobilinogen but no bilirubin (acholuric) Stools Dark due to increased stercobilin	Results: Jaundice variable 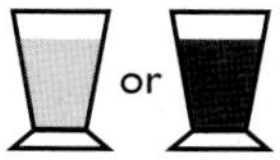 or Urine may have bilirubin and urobilinogen varies Stools Normal or paler	Results: Jaundice severe (green) 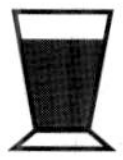 Urine contains bilirubin but no urobilinogen Stools Pale (clay coloured)

Figure 14.6 Types and causes of jaundice.

Detoxification

The liver is the all-important organ in the modification of alcohol, drugs (see also Enzyme inducers/inhibitors, page 332) and some hormones before their elimination from the body. The metabolites produced by the liver are excreted by the kidneys (small molecules) or leave in the bile (large molecules).

Alcohol (see Nursing Practice Application – Alcohol and the liver and Healthier Living – How much alcohol?)

The alcohol in alcoholic drinks is ethanol. This is oxidized in the mitochondria of the hepatocytes, mainly by an enzyme called alcohol dehydrogenase, which produces a toxic intermediate called acetaldehyde. The acetaldehyde

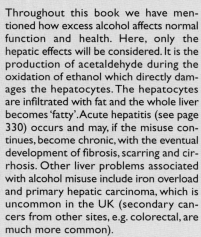

Healthier Living **How much alcohol?**

The level at which alcohol intake will cause harm is difficult to determine for the whole population, but information regarding levels below which harm is unlikely can offer guidelines to sensible drinking. In the UK, until late 1995, the advice offered by the Health Education Authority was up to 14 units of alcohol/week for non-pregnant women and 21 units of alcohol/week for men. Currently the advice offered is that an intake of 2–3 standard units of alcohol/day for non-pregnant women and 3–4 standard units of alcohol/day for men (Health Education Authority, 1996) is unlikely to cause harm. Additionally there should be alcohol-free days, and drinking 'binges' should be avoided. Regularly drinking 4 units/day or more for men or 3 units/day or more for women is not advised as the risks to health increase at this level. Other sensible measures include not drinking alcohol when driving, working with electricity or operating machinery, and when taking certain drugs which may interact with alcohol.

Advice to pregnant women or those planning to conceive is generally that they limit their alcohol intake to 1–2 units once or twice a week. Some authorities go further than this and suggest that only total abstinence from alcohol can be considered safe (see Chapter 20).

One plus point is the recent research finding which indicates that a moderate alcohol intake (1–2 units/day) reduces the risk of coronary heart disease in post-menopausal women and men over 40.

Nursing Practice Application **Alcohol and the liver**

Throughout this book we have mentioned how excess alcohol affects normal function and health. Here, only the hepatic effects will be considered. It is the production of acetaldehyde during the oxidation of ethanol which directly damages the hepatocytes. The hepatocytes are infiltrated with fat and the whole liver becomes 'fatty'. Acute hepatitis (see page 330) occurs and may, if the misuse continues, become chronic, with the eventual development of fibrosis, scarring and cirrhosis. Other liver problems associated with alcohol misuse include iron overload and primary hepatic carcinoma, which is uncommon in the UK (secondary cancers from other sites, e.g. colorectal, are much more common).

Individual response to alcohol varies for reasons not fully understood, but it is known that women suffer liver damage with smaller amounts of alcohol than men. This is caused in part by the amount of water present in the body – women have a lower percentage of water and consequently the alcohol they consume is less diluted. There are also factors concerned with the actual metabolism of alcohol within the liver that make women more susceptible to damage.

Although alcohol consumption has increased generally in the UK, it is in women and young people that the rise is most marked. In their study of at-risk drinkers in a health visitor's case load Robinson and Gaskell (1989) identified various factors associated with alcohol use, e.g. marital status, number and age of children, and whether employed. They found that the group with the highest alcohol intake were single, unemployed mothers with more than two children.

Questioning of young people aged 16–18 revealed that 97% had tried alcohol and that 71% felt that they had associated physical or social problems (Smith and Collins, 1989).

However, we should not forget other groups in relation to problems associated with alcohol consumption. Mudd *et al.* (1994) state that nurses in most practice areas can expect to have contact with older adults who have alcohol-related problems.

There is a great need for information about the results of excess alcohol intake and for the early identification of problem drinking. According to Roberts (1996), nurses can motivate some people to decrease their alcohol consumption to a safer limit if the problem is identified at an early stage. This is especially important in the case of alcohol-induced liver disease, e.g. cirrhosis, which is occurring more frequently – in the USA it is the fourth most common cause of death (Sherlock, 1989). In developed countries the misuse of alcohol is the commonest cause of liver disease (Edwards *et al.* 1995).

Support and information for those with an alcohol-associated problem (the drinker, family/friends and employer) is available from various organizations, e.g. Alcoholics Anonymous – a selection of addresses can be found on page 342.

is further oxidized to acetyl CoA, which can then be used to produce ATP (plus CO_2 and H_2O) through the Krebs' (citric acid) cycle and the electron-transfer chain.

Other oxidase enzyme systems, situated in the smooth endoplasmic reticulum, are also concerned with the oxidation of ethanol. These enzymes are actually stimulated by the intake of alcohol (an enzyme inducer), which may explain why heavy drinkers develop some tolerance to alcohol in the short term.

Drugs (see Nursing Practice Application – Liver function and ageing)

The liver metabolizes drugs by either modifying their activity or converting fat-soluble (nonpolar) drugs to

$$\text{Ethanol} \longrightarrow \text{Acetaldehyde} \longrightarrow \text{Acetyl CoA} \longrightarrow \text{ATP} + CO_2 + H_2O$$

inactive water-soluble (polar) molecules before excretion in the urine or bile. Many oxidase enzymes, such as cytochrome P_{450}, are involved in these processes. Various drugs are altered chemically before conjugation with substances such as glucuronic acid, glutathione (see Person-Centred Study – Steve) and amino acids to produce highly polar molecules. The ability of the liver to deal with drugs depends on factors which include:

- Age.
- Genetic make-up.
- Drug levels.
- Number and type of drugs (enzyme inducers/inhibitors).
- Drug administration route – those absorbed from the intestine are taken directly to the liver by the hepatic portal vein and are cleared on the first pass.
- Healthy liver function.
- Nutritional status.

Drugs that are already water-soluble (polar) need little processing by the liver.

Hormones

Several hormones are broken down in the liver before their excretion in the bile. These include those from the thyroid gland, growth hormone, insulin, glucagon, glucocorticoids (see Chapter 8) and other steroid hormones such as oestrogens. In health the liver is able to prevent an accumulation of hormones in the blood and tissues. The failure of the liver to metabolize oestrogen may account for the gynaecomastia (male breast development) seen when hepatic function is seriously impaired.

Storage

The liver stores iron, vitamin B_{12}, folic acid and the fat-soluble vitamins A, D, E and K.

Iron derived from erythrocyte destruction is stored as ferritin and haemosiderin (see Chapter 9) until needed for the synthesis of new haem. Deposition of excess iron in the liver is known as haemochromatosis. This may be primary, caused by an inability to control iron absorption, or may result from excess iron intake, e.g. dietary overload or repeated blood transfusion.

Large reserves of vitamin B_{12} are held in the liver and conditions associated with its deficiency, e.g. megaloblastic anaemia, may take several years to become apparent. There are much smaller stocks (few weeks) of folic acid which must regularly be replenished by dietary intake.

The liver stores large quantities of the vitamin A and D reserves and small amounts of E and K. It is worth remembering that hypervitaminosis A or D, which results from an excessive intake (see Chapter 13), can cause serious problems, e.g. liver damage and hepatomegaly (enlarged liver) with vitamin A.

Metabolism of nutrients

In Chapter 13 we discussed in some detail the metabolism of carbohydrates, protein and fats, so here we need only restate the main points and put them all together in terms of liver function.

Nursing Practice Application **Liver function and ageing**

Liver size and function declines with normal ageing, and in people over 70 there may be a significant loss of hepatocytes and reduced blood flow. As we have discussed, the liver plays a vital part in the detoxification of drugs prior to their excretion. These functions may be seriously, but very variably, impaired in older people as enzyme activity declines, and nurses should be particularly vigilant in observing for side-effects which may indicate that fat-soluble drug metabolism is abnormal, e.g. confusion and ataxia with benzodiazepines. The half-life of fat-soluble drugs increases and they tend to accumulate in the body. Another factor to be considered is the possibility of drug interactions, as the use of drugs tends to increase with ageing. Nurses can also help by checking that only essential drugs are prescribed or self-administered and that doses have been adjusted for increasing age, and by providing effective drug education for the person, family/friends and carers. Drug metabolism and activity in older adults is also influenced by factors such as body fat/water content, reduced temperature and cardiovascular changes.

Nursing Practice Application Liver biopsy

Liver biopsy (*Figure 14.7*) is useful in the diagnosis of certain conditions, e.g. cirrhosis, but is contraindicated where coagulation is seriously impaired. As with all investigations, the person concerned needs adequate information about what is going to happen and their care will include measures which ensure safety and comfort. It is likely that the person already has serious hepatic malfunction, and this increases the risks associated with the procedure. Before the biopsy, blood is taken to measure platelet numbers and prothrombin time. Obviously the risk of bleeding is increased where these are abnormal, and compatible blood should be available for transfusion, if required. Where the prothrombin time is extended it might be necessary to administer vitamin K to minimize any tendency to bleed.

The biopsy is performed after local anaesthesia of the tissues, and in some cases sedation may also be given to relieve anxiety. A special needle is introduced by the intercostal route and a sample of liver tissue is obtained when the person has exhaled and is holding his or her breath to avoid lung damage.

Following the procedure, the person rests in bed for 24 hours and the nurse monitors blood pressure, pulse, temperature, respiration, leakage from puncture site and pain, so that bleeding, haematoma, biliary peritonitis, pleural problems and infection may be detected.

Table 14.1 Liver function tests	
Blood test	**Normal range (adults)**
Bilirubin (total)	2–17 µmol/litre
Enzymes	
alkaline phosphatase	35–125 i.u./litre
aminotransferases	
ALT	10–40 i.u./litre
AST	10–35 i.u./litre
gamma glutamyl transferase	10–55 i.u./litre (males)
(GGT)	5–35 i.u./litre (females)
Plasma proteins	
albumin	35–50 g/litre
globulins	23–35 g/litre
Coagulation ability	
prothrombin time	11–15 s

Reference ranges vary between centres and depend upon the type of analytical equipment and temperature used. i.u. = international unit.

Table 14.1 Liver function tests.

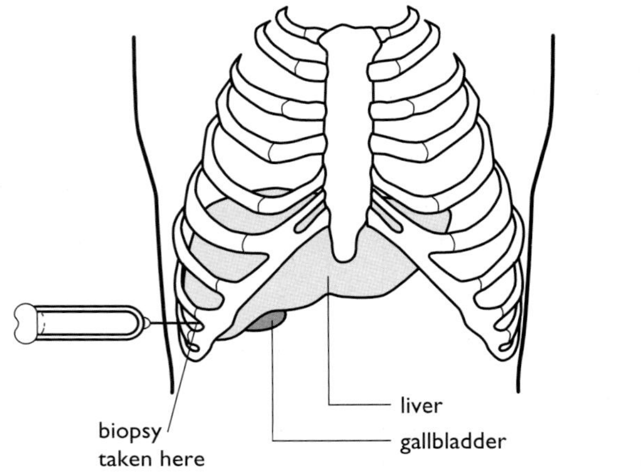

Figure 14.7 Liver biopsy.

Carbohydrates

The liver has a central role in blood glucose homeostasis (see *Figure 8.18*):

- Converts fructose and galactose to glucose.
- Stores glucose as glycogen (**glycogenesis**), which can be broken down when required to provide glucose (glycogenolysis).
- Utilizes glucose to produce the energy required for its considerable metabolic activity.
- Converts excess glucose to triglycerides (triacylglycerols) for storage in the fat depots.
- Produces glucose from amino acids, glycerol and lactate by **gluconeogenesis**.

Protein

The liver is important in metabolism of amino acids, their conversion to structural and functional proteins (see Synthesis, page 333), and the safe disposal of the waste ammonia.

- Produces non-essential amino acids by the process of transamination, which is facilitated by enzymes known as aminotransferases (previously transaminases). The two main enzymes are alanine aminotransferase (ALT) and aspartate aminotransferase (AST), both of which are produced in the liver. Measurement of AST and ALT in the serum can be used in the diagnosis and assessment of liver disease

Abnormal Function **Chronic liver diseases and failing hepatic function**

A detailed classification of chronic parenchymal disease of the liver does not really concern us here; readers are directed to the reading list for more specific information.

Chronic parenchymal disease of the liver includes various types of chronic hepatitis and cirrhosis, where the liver may show areas of inflammation, and fibrosis with hepatocyte or portal tract destruction. The common causes of chronic liver disease, in developed countries, are alcohol misuse, cirrhosis, HBV and HCV, but other factors, including those listed for acute hepatitis (see page 330), are possible causes.

Manifestations of failing hepatic function

Failure of liver function may result from many of the conditions already discussed, e.g. HBV, alcoholic hepatitis, cirrhosis and drug toxicity (see Person-Centred Study – Steve).

There is considerable variation in clinical presentation, depending upon the cause. Linking commonly occurring problems with the failure of normal function emphasizes just how much we depend on a healthy liver. The most commonly occurring problems are:

- Hepatomegaly: the liver may enlarge and cause abdominal discomfort, but later it becomes smaller as fibrosis and hepatocyte destruction occurs.
- Jaundice (see page 334): caused by hepatocellular failure and intrahepatic obstruction.
- Ascites (fluid in the peritoneal cavity): caused by portal hypertension, sodium and water retention and possibly hypoalbuminaemia (remember the liver makes albumin).
- Portal hypertension and varices (see Chapter 10): caused by liver fibrosis and structural disorganization. This may result in haematemesis, which, if severe, will cause hypovolaemia (see Chapter 10); and the blood (which, remember, contains protein) digested in the gastrointestinal tract adds further to the problems of protein metabolism and hepatic encephalopathy (brain disease caused as toxins accumulate – see below). The management of portal hypertension includes:

  (a) Measures to control haematemesis, e.g. compression with a Sengstaken–Blakemore tube or procedures such as endoscopic sclerotherapy, putting bands around the varices or introducing stents (via the venous system) between the hepatic portal vein and hepatic vein, stapling the varices and shunt surgery. which ensures that some blood bypasses the liver.

  (b) Drugs administered to reduce portal pressure, e.g. vasopressin (see Chapter 8), which also stimulates bowel emptying and the evacuation of blood that has entered the intestine.

  (c) Blood transfusion.

  (d) Administration of neomycin (antimicrobial drug) to reduce bacterial action in the gut.

Other features of portal hypertension include splenomegaly (enlarged spleen), collateral vessels seen around the umbilicus – a caput medusae (named for the mythological Medusa whose hair was made of snakes) – and rectal varices.

- Cerebral oedema: this occurs in hepatic failure and may present with confusion and disorientation, progressing to altered consciousness, fits and death.
- Coagulation problems: due to thrombocytopenia and the inability of the liver to produce prothrombin and other clotting factors, which results in gastrointestinal bleeding, bruising (intramuscular injections best avoided) and purpura (red/purple spots or patches caused by bleeding into the skin).
- Abnormal reaction to drugs: metabolism and conjugation fail to occur. This results in accumulation of the drug and side-effects (see also Ageing and liver function, page 337).
- Hormonal effects: gynaecomastia (male breast development) occurs because hormones are not being degraded by the liver, which allows the build-up of oestrogens and other molecules. Other problems associated with abnormal hormone metabolism include amenorrhoea (absent menstruation), testicular atrophy and loss of libido.
- Hypoglycaemia: this occurs because blood glucose homeostasis is seriously impaired.
- Hepatic (portasystemic) encephalopathy and coma: these occur when blood is shunted from the hepatic portal vein to the systemic circulation without going to the liver. The brain changes are thought to be caused by nitrogenous metabolites produced in the intestine, and ammonia from amino acid metabolism as urea (levels normal or low) production is impaired. Many other molecules are thought to be involved, e.g. fatty acids, and drugs such as sedatives and electrolyte disturbances can precipitate encephalopathy in a person with severe liver disease. Abnormal metabolites of amino acids excreted by the lungs (caused by shunting of blood) account for the characteristic musty, sweet odour of the breath known as fetor hepaticus.

Energy requirements during hepatic failure are met with a high carbohydrate intake and protein intake may be restricted to minimize the toxic effects of the metabolites produced. Laxatives such as lactulose may be given to produce adequate evacuation, which reduces the absorption of nitrogenous material from the gut.

- Flapping tremor of the hands.
- Circulatory changes: e.g. red palms and spider naevi.
- Associated renal failure (hepatorenal syndrome).
- Abnormal skin pigmentation ('bronze diabetes'): seen in the abnormal iron metabolism associated with cirrhosis.
- Systemic effects: e.g. nausea and pruritus.

Person-Centred Study **Steve**

Steve, aged 17, has been very depressed about finding work; although he has been offered a training place at the local garage, he wanted a job with more money to start. One evening it was all too much, and after drinking two cans of strong lager he took 15 (500 mg) paracetamol tablets. After an hour Steve became very frightened and told his parents, who took him immediately to the nearest accident and emergency department.

His emergency management consisted of a gastric lavage (stomach washout),

oral activated charcoal, estimation of plasma paracetamol levels and intravenous acetylcysteine, which restores glutathione levels in the liver. Glutathione protects against liver/kidney damage by conjugating the paracetamol and so preventing the formation of a toxic metabolite. Steve is admitted for observation and monitoring of liver function, which luckily remains unaffected. While in hospital Steve is able to talk about his feelings (depressed about job prospects, but not really wanting to die) and money

worries with his parents and the nurses. Eventually he decides to take up the training vacancy and accept financial support from his parents for a few months.

Methionine might be given orally as a protective agent instead of acetylcysteine. If Steve had delayed (approximately 10–12 hours) getting help these antidotes would have been of no value, but haemoperfusion could have been used in an attempt to remove the paracetamol from his blood.

Healthier Living **Safer use of paracetamol**

One of the targets of the Health of the Nation document (DoH, 1992) is to reduce the overall suicide rate by 15% by the year 2000. Making the dangers of paracetamol overdose more widely known could help to achieve this target. Paracetamol overdose is particularly

dangerous when combined with dextropropoxyphene as co-proxamol, and when taken with alcohol. As with all drugs, paracetamol should be kept away from children. Doses should be kept within those recommended by the manufacturer and should not be taken with preparations contain-

ing dextropropoxyphene or with alcohol. The possibility of producing paracetamol combined with an agent which protects against hepatotoxicity is being considered and a limitiation on sales is to be implemented.

(see below). The enzymes are also produced by other tissues, e.g. myocardium and skeletal muscle; estimation of AST levels can be useful in the diagnosis of myocardial damage (see Chapter 10). NB AST was previously called glutamic–oxaloacetic transaminase (GOT) and ALT was called glutamic–pyruvic transaminase (GPT).

- Deaminates amino acids before their oxidation or conversion to glucose.
- Combines the toxic ammonia formed in deamination with carbon dioxide to produce urea. The high level of ammonia in the blood, resulting from serious hepatic malfunction, is partly responsible for hepatic encephalopathy/coma.
- Converts amino acids into the purines and pyrimidines required for nucleic acid synthesis.

Fats

Many cells use fats, but a considerable part of fat metabolism occurs within the liver.

- It is an important area for the β-oxidation (see Chapter 13) of fats for energy.
- Ketone bodies are produced from excess acetyl CoA and used in small amounts by body cells (**ketogenesis**).
- Stores fat and forms triglycerides (triacylglycerols) which are stored in the fat depots (**lipogenesis**) and releases stored fats for energy use (**lipolysis**).
- Produces other lipids, e.g. lipoproteins such as very low density lipoproteins for lipid transport, cholesterol (for steroid hormones and bile acids) and phospholipids.

Liver function tests

As you would expect, the investigation of liver function requires a whole battery of biochemical tests. Samples of venous blood are obtained and various constituents in the serum are measured (see *Table 14.1*). The results assist in the diagnosis of parenchymal disease, biliary obstruction and the progress of established disease.

Paracetamol poisoning

The painkiller paracetamol is one of the most common drugs used in accidental or intentional self-poisoning. It is freely available without prescription and its accessibility in most homes makes it a favourite choice for both planned and impulse suicide attempts (see Person-Centred Study – Steve and Healthier Living – Safer use of paracetamol).

What is not generally known is that it damages the liver and kidneys in quite moderate overdoses. The paraceta-mol overwhelms the conjugating enzymes and this allows oxidase enzymes (cytochrome P_{450}) to convert it to the toxic metabolite (N-acetyl-p-benzoquinone imine), which eventually destroys the hepatocytes. The person concerned recovers from the suicide attempt only to succumb to hepatic or renal failure (less common) 3–5 days later. A liver transplant may be a treatment option where the liver is severely damaged. Paracetamol is the most common cause of hepatic necrosis in the UK and accounts for 200 deaths/year (Henry and Volans, 1984).

Summary/Check List

Introduction.
Liver structure – early development, gross structure, blood supply, Nursing Practice Application – liver injuries, nerve supply. Microscopic structure. Acute hepatitis. Healthier Living – hepatitis B immunization.
Liver functions – bile production, biliary tract, gallbladder and bile excretion. Gallstones, Person-centred Study – Daphne, Nursing Practice Application – biliary surgery. Special

Focus – jaundice. Healthier Living - androgenic anabolic steroid misuse. Synthesis. Detoxification, Nursing Practice Application – alcohol and the liver, Healthier Living – how much alcohol? Nursing Practice Application – liver function and ageing. Storage. Metabolism of nutrients. Liver function tests, Nursing Practice Application – liver biopsy. Failing hepatic function. Poisoning – paracetamol, Person-centred Study – Steve, Healthy Living – safer use of paracetamol.

Self Test

1 Which of the following statements about the liver are true?
  (a) The adult liver weighs about 1.5 lbs.
  (b) Vessels and ducts leave at the porta hepatis.
  (c) The caudate and quadrate are the smallest lobes.
  (d) All its venous blood leaves via the hepatic veins.
2 Draw and label a liver lobule.
3 Complete the following:
  (a) The daily production of bile is _ _ _ _ _ _ _ _ ml.
  (b) Bile has a pH of _ _ _.
  (c) Bilirubin is the major bile _ _ _ _ _ _ _.
4 Which of the following would cause jaundice and what type would it be?
  (a) Transfusion of group A blood to a group B recipient.
  (b) Gallstone in the cystic duct.
  (c) Acute hepatitis.
  (d) Carcinoma in the head of the pancreas.
5 Why is measuring the albumin:globulin ratio a good test of liver function?

6 Explain the following:
  (a) Development of alcohol tolerance in heavy drinkers.
  (b) Increased drug toxicity in older adults.
7 Name six substances stored in the liver.
8 Put the following in their logical pairs:
  (a) Urea;
  (b) Ferritin;
  (c) Ethanol;
  (d) Retinol;
  (e) Vitamin K;
  (f) Prothrombin;
  (g) Carotene;
  (h) Acetaldehyde;
  (i) Iron;
  (j) Ammonia.
9 Describe the role of the liver in blood glucose homeostasis.
10 Explain the following features of failing hepatic function: ascites, bruising, encephalopathy and jaundice.

Answers

1 b, c, d.
2 See pages 329–330.
3 (a) 500–1000 ml;
   (b) 8.0;
   (c) Pigment.
4 (a) Prehepatic;
   (c) Hepatocellular;
   (d) Obstructive.

5 See page 333.
6 See pages 335–337.
7 Iron, vitamin B_{12}, folic acid, vitamins A, D, E and K, and glucose as glycogen.
8 a–j, b–i, c–h, d–g and e–f.
9 See pages 337–338.
10 See page 339.

References

DoH (1992) *The Health of the Nation. A Summary of the Strategy for Health in England.* London: HMSO.

Edwards CRW, Bouchier IAD, Haslett C, Eds, *et al.* (1995) *Davidson's Principles and Practice of Medicine*, 17th edn. Edinburgh: Churchill Livingstone.

Health Education Authority (HEA) (1996) *Think About Drink.* London: HEA.

Henry J, Volans G (1984) *ABC of Poisoning – Part I.* London: British Medical Association.

Mudd S, Boyd C, Brower K *et al.* (1994) Alcohol withdrawal and related nursing care in older adults. *J Gerontol Nurs* **20**(10): 17–27.

Roberts C (1996) The physiological effects of alcohol misuse. *Prof Nurs* **11**(10): 646–648.

Robinson B, Gaskell K (1989) Prevalence and characteristics of at-risk drinkers among a health visitor's case load. *Health Visitor*, **62**: 242–243.

Sherlock S (1989) *Diseases of the Liver and Biliary System*, 8th edn. Oxford: Blackwell Scientific Publications.

Smith I, Collins F (1989) Patterns of drug abuse. *Nurs Times* **85** (10):55.

White J, Cartheus L (1995) The Hazards of Minimal Access Surgery. *Surg Nurs* **8**(3):9–12.

Further Reading

Budden L, Vink R (1996) Paracetamol overdose: pathophysiology and nursing management. *Br J Nurs* **5**(3):145–52.

Plant M (1990) Advising on alcohol. *Nurs Times (Midwives Journal)*, **86**(12):64–65.

Shearman DJC, Finlayson NDC, Carter D *et al.* (1997) *Diseases of the Gastrointestinal Tract and Liver*, 3rd edn. Edinburgh: Churchill Livingstone.

Useful Addresses

Alcohol Concern
Waterbridge House
Loman Street
London SE1 0EE

Alcoholics Anonymous
PO Box 1
Stonebow House
Stonebow
York YO1 2NJ

Alcoholics Anonymous
(Scotland)
50 Wellington Street
Glasgow G2 6HJ.

Al Anon Family Groups
61 Great Dover Street
London SE1 4YF

Urinary System

Overview

- *Urinary system structure and function.*
- *The role of the kidneys in maintaining homeostasis.*
- *Micturition.*

Learning Outcomes

After studying Chapter 15 you should be able to:

- Describe the gross structure and position of the kidneys.
- Describe renal blood flow.
- Describe the structure of a nephron.
- Discuss the homeostatic role of the kidneys.
- List the normal constituents of urine.
- Describe the formation of urine.
- Outline mechanisms by which the kidney varies the volume and concentration of urine.
- List some abnormal constituents of urine and discuss their possible significance.
- Discuss the causes and consequences of renal failure.
- Describe the structure of the ureters, bladder and urethra.
- Describe the process of normal micturition.
- Use physiological knowledge in the assessment of micturition and the identification of abnormalities.

Key Words

Anuria – cessation of urine production by the kidneys.

Dysuria – difficult or painful micturition.

Glomerular filtration rate (GFR) – the amount of plasma filtered by the kidneys in 1 min.

Micturition – passing or voiding urine. Urination.

Nephron – the functional unit of the kidney.

Oliguria – diminished volume of urine produced by the kidneys.

Polyuria – increased volume of urine produced by the kidneys.

Renal – relating to the kidney.

Renin – proteolytic enzyme produced by the kidney that activates angiotensin, in turn causing the release of aldosterone.

Introduction

The kidneys are central to homeostatic regulation. They excrete soluble waste, help to maintain the water and electrolyte composition of body fluids and regulate pH in conjunction with the lungs and other buffer systems. Without the complex **renal** processes, the body's 'waste' builds up, pollution occurs and the delicate balance of the internal environment is lost (see Chapter 2).

Other functions of the kidney include the secretion of erythropoietin, which stimulates erythropoiesis (see Chapter 9), and the proteolytic enzyme **renin**, which activates the angiotensin–aldosterone system that helps to regulate blood pressure. The kidney also converts vitamin D to 1,25-dihydroxycholecalciferol, its most active form (see Chapter 8).

The Urinary System

Apart from two kidneys, which produce urine, the structures of the urinary system are two ureters, which transport urine; the bladder, which acts as a temporary reservoir for urine; and the urethra, which conveys urine to the exterior during **micturition** (*Figure 15.1*).

Early development

During the fourth week of embryonic life the primitive kidneys start to develop from mesodermal ridges. Initially, they form within the pelvis and later, after many changes, they migrate upwards to the adult position in the abdomen. The embryonic 'kidney' develops through three stages: the pronephros (never functional), the mesonephros and the metanephros, destined to become the 'final version' of the adult kidney. One part of the early lobulated kidney will become the renal pelvis, calyces, collecting ducts and a ureter, which by the eighth week is connected to a bladder that develops from the cloaca (embryonic gut structure) and urogenital sinus. The other part of the developing kidney is destined to form the **nephrons**. At this early stage of development there is a close link between the urinary tract, external genitalia and the internal reproductive structures which develop from the Mullerian and Wolffian ducts (see Chapter 20). The fetal kidneys are structurally complete, but remain functionally immature (although they do produce urine as early as week 8 of development) until some weeks after birth, when they become capable of producing concentrated urine. The lobulation of the neonatal kidney disappears around 4–5 years of age.

Problems occurring during the early weeks of development may result in:
- The formation of only one kidney.
- Polycystic disease, where normal fusion of the two kidney components fails to occur.
- A single horseshoe kidney which results from an abnormal fusion between both kidneys.

Figure 15.1 The urinary system.

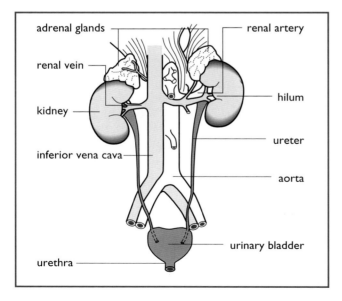

adrenal glands
renal artery
renal vein
hilum
kidney
ureter
inferior vena cava
aorta
urinary bladder
urethra

The Kidney

Gross structure of the kidney

The paired kidneys are situated behind the peritoneum (retroperitoneal) and are attached to the posterior abdominal wall by adipose and fibrous tissue. The kidneys lie, one either side of the spine, at a level extending from the last thoracic vertebra to the third lumbar vertebra, with the right kidney slightly lower to accommodate the liver (see Chapter 14). Each bean-shaped kidney carries on its superior surface an adrenal (suprarenal) gland, which we discussed in Chapter 8.

In adults each kidney weighs around 140 g and is about 12 cm long, 7 cm wide and 3 cm thick. On its concave medial surface there is a depression, known as the hilum, where blood vessels, lymphatics, nerves and a ureter enter or leave the kidney.

The kidney is enclosed within several layers of supporting tissue: an outer fibrous connective layer; a middle adipose layer, which helps to cushion the kidney; and, around the kidney itself, a transparent fibrous renal capsule.

If we look at a cut kidney (coronal section) several separate regions can be recognized (*Figure 15.2*). There is an outer cortex forming a pale red–brown layer under the capsule. Below the cortex is the darker medulla containing the cone-shaped striations called renal pyramids. At the apex of each pyramid a papilla opens into a minor calyx. This communicates with major calyces and the funnel-shaped renal pelvis, which distends to receive urine. Contraction of smooth muscle in the walls of the calyces and renal pelvis conveys the urine into the ureter.

Blood and nerve supply of the kidney

The kidneys receive around 1200 ml of blood per minute – 25% of the resting cardiac output – from renal arteries which branch directly from the abdominal aorta (see Chapter 10). The continuity of this supply is vital to effective renal function and later we will discuss how the kidney autoregulates blood flow (see page 350). Venous blood leaves the kidney via renal veins which empty into the inferior vena cava. The smaller vessels and the two-capillary system of the kidney are covered in more detail when we consider the nephron (see below).

The kidney is well supplied with sympathetic nerve fibres (see Chapter 6) from the coeliac plexus, which when stimulated cause renal vasoconstriction, secretion of renin and decreased urine production. A few parasympathetic fibres derived from the vagus are present, but their role is unknown. Sensory fibres also leave the kidney and are responsible for the transmission of pain.

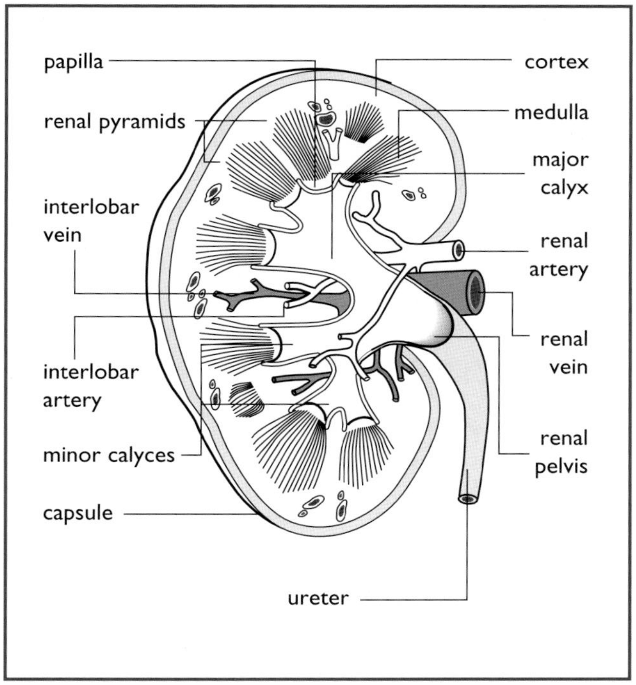

Figure 15.2 Section through a kidney.

papilla

renal pyramids

interlobar vein

interlobar artery

minor calyces

capsule

ureter

cortex

medulla

major calyx

renal artery

renal vein

renal pelvis

Nursing Practice Application **Renal calculi (kidney stones)**

Renal calculi are often associated with recurrent infections of the urinary tract (see page 365). Other causes include disturbances of calcium and phosphate homeostasis, such as may occur in immobility, or hyperparathyroidism (see Chapter 8), where excess calcium salts excreted in the urine (hypercalciuria) are deposited as stones.

Renal calculi may be large enough to fill the renal pelvis and calyces (staghorn calculus); they may obstruct the outflow of urine, which leads to hydronephrosis (water in the kidney), chronic infection and possibly renal failure (see page 359). If the stone moves into and obstructs the narrow lumen of the ureter it causes renal colic, which is characterized by excruciating loin pain, nausea and haematuria (blood in the urine). Nursing interventions should include adequate pain relief, a fluid intake of at least 2–3 litres/day, testing urine for blood (see page 358) and straining all urine passed for small stones/debris.

Treatment of renal calculi has undergone great changes in recent years. Non-invasive techniques such as lithotripsy (shockwaves) may be used to disintegrate the stone, but where a stone is impacted in the ureter with distal obstruction a percutaneous nephrolithotomy is performed. Here a nephroscope (instrument with a light source used to view inside the kidney) is passed through a small skin incision and used to locate the stone in the renal pelvis, which is then removed through the nephroscope without the need for a large incision. When available, these developments can replace major surgical intervention, which reduces pain and inconvenience, in-patient stay and complications associated with traditional operations (pyelolithotomy). Obviously, the underlying cause of the calculus formation is treated, e.g. antimicrobial drugs for infection.

Nephron

One kidney contains about one million microscopic nephrons of two types: 85% are cortical (located mainly in the cortex, though some may extend into the medulla) and 15% are juxtamedullary (located close to the junction between the cortex and the medulla, they extend well into the medulla). The number of nephrons is more than we actually need and forms a useful reserve. It is entirely possible to function with only one kidney (see page 344), e.g. congenital absence of a kidney is a frequent anomaly occurring in about 1 in 500 infants or after nephrectomy (removal of a kidney).

A nephron comprises a renal tubule and the glomerulus, a knot of capillaries which lies within the invaginated blind end of the tubule. The tubule, which is lined with cuboidal epithelium, is divided into Bowman's capsule, which encloses the glomerulus; the proximal convoluted tubule (PCT); the loop of Henle; the distal convoluted tubule (DCT); and the collecting ducts/tubules which drain urine from several nephrons (*Figure 15.3*).

Within the cortex of the kidney the glomerulus is formed from a wide-bore afferent arteriole. This supplies blood at a rate that ensures that the pressure of blood in the capillaries is sufficient to force fluid out into the tubule. The epithelium of the capillaries, which have fenestrations (pores), and Bowman's capsule is highly permeable and adapted for filtration. These two epithelial layers, divided by a basement membrane (see Chapter 1), form an efficient filtration membrane which allows the passage of water and molecules with a molecular weight of 69 000 or less. Selectivity based on size is important as it means that blood cells and plasma proteins do not normally cross into the filtrate (fluid within the tubule derived from blood).

Most unusually, the glomerulus is drained by a smaller-bore efferent arteriole, which forms a second, low-pressure peritubular capillary network. The lower pressure in these capillaries is a feature which allows reabsorption of filtrate from the tubule.

Leading from Bowman's capsule is the much coiled PCT. With its specialized epithelial lining containing microvilli, and thus a greatly increased surface area, the PCT is well adapted for reabsorption.

The loop of Henle, which consists of a descending (thin) and an ascending (thick) limb, is a simple loop. The epithelium lining the loop of Henle consists of flattened cells containing few microvilli – it is highly permeable to water in the thin segment of the descending limb. In certain nephrons (the juxtamedullary nephrons) the loop of Henle is surrounded by looped capillaries known as the vasa recta, in addition to the peritubular capillary network. The juxtamedullary nephrons have a long loop of Henle which extends into the medulla (in contrast to the shorter cortical nephrons, which are mostly confined to the cortex). The advantage of having two types of nephron is that the kidney is able to adjust the concentration of urine and the amount of sodium excreted to maintain homeostasis under differing conditions.

From the ascending limb of the loop of Henle the DCT twists and coils so as to have contact with the afferent arteriole. The area in contact with the arteriole is known as the macula densa; it contains special cells which form part of the juxtaglomerular apparatus (JGA). The cuboid epithelium lining the DCT is adapted for secretion rather than absorption – it is thin and has no microvilli.

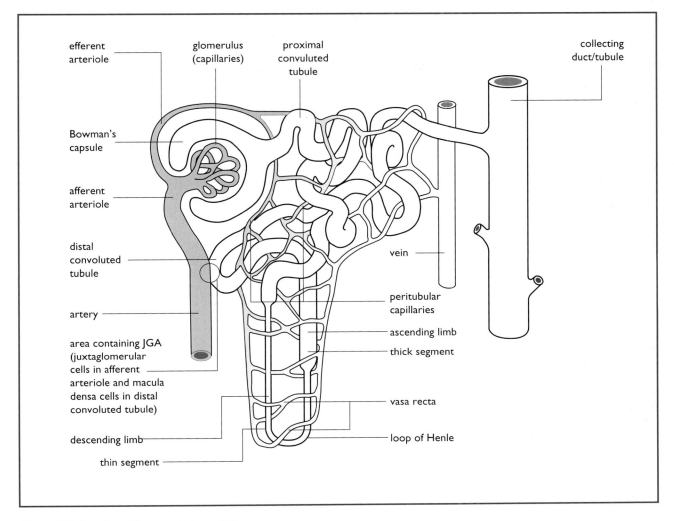

Figure 15.3 A nephron (diagrammatic for clarity).

The DCT leads into a collecting tubule. These unite to form larger ducts that eventually empty into the minor calyces.

Juxtaglomerular apparatus

The JGA is a region formed from modified cells of the DCT and the afferent arteriole. The osmoreceptor/chemoreceptor cells of the macula densa monitor the levels of sodium and chloride in the filtrate. Modified muscle cells in the arteriole (granular juxtaglomerular cells) which contain renin granules are mechanoreceptors sensitive to blood pressure in the afferent arteriole. The JGA plays an important part in renal autoregulation of blood pressure and filtration, and will be discussed further (see page 350).

Renal blood flow

As the renal arteries enter at the hilum they divide to form interlobar arteries (see *Figure 15.2*) that pass between the pyramids. Further subdivision gives rise to smaller arcuate and cortical interlobular arteries, which eventually become the afferent arterioles supplying the capillary bed of the glomerulus. The efferent arteriole draining the glomerulus forms a second capillary bed around the tubule (peritubular). Most of the filtrate, which is reabsorbed in the tubule, returns to the circulation in the peritubular capillaries (*Figure 15.3*). The peritubular capillary bed drains into venous plexi, which become larger veins corresponding to the arteries. Eventually the venous blood leaves the kidney by the renal vein to empty into the inferior vena cava.

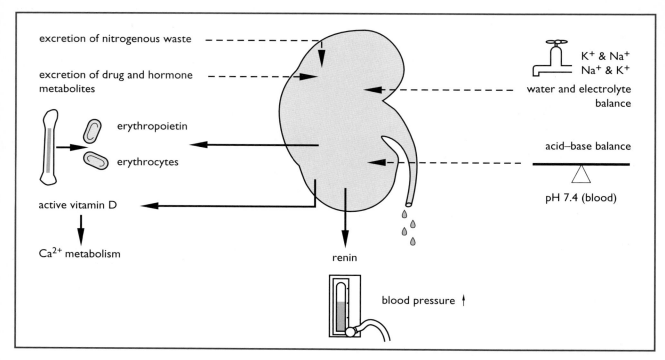

Figure 15.4 Functions of the kidney.

Functions of the kidney

- Maintains water and electrolyte balance.
- Regulates acid–base balance.
- Excretes nitrogenous waste.
- Excretes the metabolites of many drugs and some hormones.
- Haemopoietic role – secretion of erythropoietin, which stimulates red bone marrow (see Chapter 9).
- Regulation of arterial blood pressure and renal function through renin secretion.
- Production of active vitamin D (see Chapters 8 and 16).

Figure 15.4 illustrates the functions of the kidney. The kidney accomplishes the first four functions listed above through the formation of urine. This involves the processes of filtration, reabsorption and secretion, which occur exclusively within the nephrons.

Composition and characteristics of urine

Normal physical characteristics

In adults between 1 and 1.5 litres of urine is produced each day, but infants pass a much greater volume in proportion to their small body size, e.g. an infant weighing 6–8 kg produces around 0.5 litres/day (Heath, 1995), because the nephrons do not become efficient in concentrating urine for some months. The volume and composition depend upon many factors apart from age, including fluid intake, diet, climate, activity and health.

Urine is normally clear straw-yellow to amber in colour, the colour being produced by the presence of urochrome, a pigment derived from haemoglobin breakdown. Concentrated urine is darker in colour than dilute urine, which may resemble water. Drugs such as rifampicin colour the urine orange and eating beetroot (red beet) causes red urine, which may lead to some alarm until you remember what you have eaten.

The normal pH of urine is around 6.0, but a range of 4.5–8.0 is possible; a vegetarian (alkaline–ash) diet tends to produce alkaline urine and a diet containing high levels of animal protein and wholewheat (acid–ash diet) will make the urine more acidic.

The specific gravity (SG) is usually in the range 1.010–1.030 and depends upon the amount of solid material or solute present; the SG of urine measures its density compared with that of distilled water, which has a SG of 1.000.

Urine has a characteristic aromatic odour when fresh; the ammoniacal odour only develops on standing or when infection is present. Other odours are associated with certain foods, e.g. asparagus, or conditions where abnormal substances are excreted, such as diabetes mellitus (see Chapter 8) and maple syrup disease, when amino acids passed in the urine cause an odour of maple syrup.

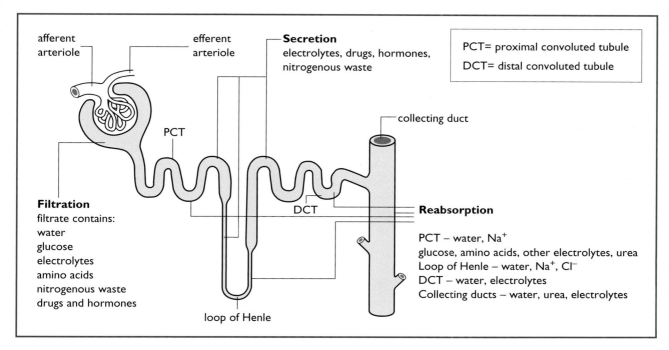

Figure 15.5 Formation of urine – filtration, reabsorption and secretion.

Composition of urine

Urine is 96% water and 4% solids. The solids comprise:

- Nitrogenous waste, which includes urea (see Chapter 14), uric acid (from nucleic acid metabolism) and creatinine derived from voluntary muscle.
- Sodium, potassium, calcium, magnesium, phosphates, sulphates, nitrates, chlorides and hydrogen carbonate.
- Organic acids, ammonia as ammonium salts.
- Drug and hormone metabolites.

Urine formation

To produce the 1–1.5 litres of urine daily the kidneys filter about 180 litres of plasma, which means that reabsorption in the tubule must be a very efficient process or you would soon become dehydrated. The cells of the tubule put the finishing touches to the filtrate by secreting electrolytes, drugs and hydrogen ions into the lumen of the tubule, much as you might add seasoning to a meal (*Figure 15.5*).

When you think about this mighty undertaking it becomes obvious why the kidneys need 25% of the resting cardiac output to provide the necessary oxygenated blood. We shall now consider the three stages of filtration, reabsorption and tubular secretion in more detail.

Filtration

Every minute about 125 ml of plasma is forced through the porous glomerular filtration membrane (which consists of three layers – the glomerular capillary epithelium, basement membrane and epithelium of Bowman's capsule) into the tubule by the hydrostatic pressure within the glomerulus. This is known as the **glomerular filtration rate** (GFR). This rate is much less at the extremes of the normal lifespan and accounts for the inability of small infants to cope with extra fluid and problems associated with drug excretion in older adults. Generally, in people aged over 70 years the GFR has fallen by one-half, which may lead to the accumulation of drugs within the body and toxic side-effects, e.g. anorexia and nausea with digoxin (see Chapter 10). Others with impaired renal function are similarly affected and great care is required in the prescribing and subsequent management of drug therapy.

Water and small molecules pass passively down the pressure gradient, as they do in other capillary beds, but this time, because of the specialized structure of the filtration barrier, this occurs more efficiently. Normally, the filtration barrier prevents loss of larger proteins and blood cells (see page 346), but when the membrane is damaged, e.g. by inflammation in glomerulonephritis, the pores enlarge, making the membrane 'leaky', and albumin (molecular weight 69 000) appears in the urine (see page 358).

The hydrostatic pressure (see Chapter 10) within the glomerulus, at around 7.3 kPa (55 mmHg), is greater than in other capillaries because the afferent arteriole has a larger calibre than the efferent arteriole. We are left, however, with a net filtration pressure of around 1.3 kPa (10 mmHg) after the pressures which oppose the movement

Glomerular hydrostatic pressure – (osmotic pressure + Bowman's capsule pressure) = net filtration pressure

$$7.3 \text{ kPa} - (4 \text{ kPa} + 2 \text{ kPa}) = 1.3 \text{ kPa}$$
or
$$55 \text{ mmHg} - (30 \text{ mmHg} + 15 \text{ mmHg}) = 10 \text{ mmHg}$$

of fluid from the blood to the tubule, the osmotic pressure of the plasma proteins in the capillaries (see Chapter 10) and the hydrostatic pressure exerted by fluid in Bowman's capsule have been taken into account.

The small molecules that pass with the water into the filtrate in the tubule include glucose, amino acids, electrolytes, drug and hormone metabolites, urea, uric acid and creatinine (see *Figure 15.5*). Many of these, which are needed by the body, are later reabsorbed, e.g. glucose, which does not normally appear in the urine.

By the time blood reaches the end of the glomerulus, filtration has all but stopped. This is because the movement of fluid from blood to filtrate increases the osmotic pressure to a point where it equals the glomerular hydrostatic pressure.

Glomerular filtration rate and regulation

The glomerular filtration rate of about 125 ml/min in healthy adults is dependent upon the pressure gradients produced by sufficient blood reaching the glomerulus. Although the kidneys already receive 25% of the cardiac output there are intrinsic (autoregulatory) mechanisms which operate to ensure that enough blood at the correct pressure reaches the nephrons.

There are also extrinsic neural controls which modify blood flow in stress situations. In Chapter 10 we discussed shock caused by hypovolaemia, which leads to a marked or sustained fall in systemic blood pressure. This reduces renal perfusion and filtration, which explains the **oliguria** (reduced volume of urine) associated with shock.

Autoregulation

Possible autoregulatory mechanisms which operate under everyday conditions include a mechanism where smooth muscle in the afferent arterioles constrict when systemic blood pressure is high and dilate when pressure is low. The other is the tubuglomerular feedback loop that operates through the macula densa which responds to the amount of fluid and sodium arriving at the tubule by altering the size of afferent arterioles. In these ways the GFR remains matched with reabsorption and the nephron is protected from changes in blood flow as systemic blood pressure fluctuates within a range (80–180 mmHg). Changes in arteriolar diameter due

to the tubuglomerular feedback are probably caused by the release of a paracrine agent such as a prostaglandin (see Chapter 8) by renal cells. Autoregulatory mechanisms are not, however, able to maintain the GFR during shock – if systolic blood pressure falls well below 80 mmHg filtration will stop.

The other autoregulatory mechanism involves the cells of the juxtaglomerular apparatus (see page 347). Juxtaglomerular cells in the afferent arteriole, which are sensitive to changes in pressure, release the enzyme renin into the blood if blood pressure falls. Renin acts upon the plasma protein angiotensinogen, which it converts to angiotensin I.

Angiotensin-converting enzyme (ACE), situated in the endothelium of blood vessels (mainly in the lungs), converts angiotensin I to angiotensin II, which causes vasoconstriction and a rise in systemic blood pressure (*Figure 15.6* and Chapter 10). Cells of the macula densa (which you will remember monitor sodium content of the filtrate) can, if sodium levels are low or blood flow is slow, trigger a release of renin. Apart from being a powerful vasoconstrictor, the angiotensin II formed stimulates the adrenal cortex to release aldosterone (see Chapter 8), which causes more sodium to be reabsorbed in the DCT (*Figure 15.6*). As the sodium ions move back into the blood they are accompanied by water, which increases blood volume and hence pressure. We shall discuss renin–angiotensin–aldosterone again in the consideration of water/electrolyte homeostasis.

Many chemicals released by the renal cells are known to act as local messengers, or paracrine agents, which modulate processes within the kidney, e.g. prostaglandins, endothelin, kallikrein – which causes bradykinin release – and the ubiquitous nitric oxide functioning as endothelium-derived/dependent relaxing factor. These function as vasodilators or vasoconstrictors, but as yet their exact functions are not well understood, and some paracrine agents await identification – such as the chemical mediator of the tubuglomerular feedback loop.

Extrinsic mechanisms

Whereas autoregulation deals with everyday needs, the extrinsic mechanisms come into play during stress, exercise, pain and abnormal situations, such as severe hypovolaemic shock. Sympathetic nerve stimulation and the release of adrenaline cause renal vasoconstriction as blood is diverted to the heart and brain, which reduces GFR and urinary output. In addition, the JGA is stimulated directly by sympathetic activity and the renin released assists by causing general vasoconstriction and reabsorption of fluid in an attempt to maintain blood volume and pressure.

It must be clear by now just how important the renal mechanisms are in regulating local renal blood pressure and flow. However, that is not all – the kidney is a 'major player'

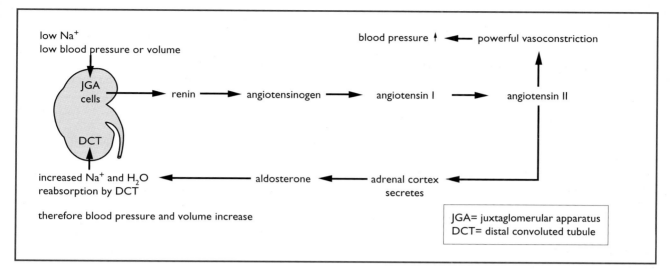

Figure 15.6 Renin–angiotensin–aldosterone system.

Nursing Practice Application **Renal clearance**

Renal clearance is a way of measuring the GFR (see page 349) and assessing renal function. This is done by calculating how well the kidneys can clear a particular substance from the blood in a given time, usually a minute. For a marker substance, which is filtered but not significantly reabsorbed or secreted, such as creatinine or the polysaccharide inulin, the amount of blood cleared in 1 min will equal the GFR. It is calculated using the formula below, used here to illustrate creatinine clearance.

Normally the creatinine clearance is between 120 and 125 ml/min (depends on body area). For the laboratory to ascertain the values it is necessary to have an accurate 24-hour urine collec-

$$GFR\ ml/min = \frac{(U \times V)}{P}$$

where U = urinary concentration of creatinine (mg/ml),
P = plasma creatinine concentration (mg/ml) and
V = urine volume per minute.

tion and a sample of venous blood taken during this time. Collecting urine is usually the responsibility of the nurse, who should ensure that:

• The collection is timed to finish during a weekday morning.

• The person concerned understands that all urine passed must be saved (after first emptying the bladder).
• The correct receptacle is available.
• Adequate privacy is provided.
• All staff are aware of the collection.
• The sample, properly labelled, arrives in the laboratory as soon after completion as possible for testing.

Renal clearance estimation is used in the diagnosis of renal impairment and to monitor progress in existing disease. It is straightforward to execute and causes minimal inconvenience and discomfort; however, as with all investigations, the nurse should offer clear explanations to the patient and support workers.

---

in the control of arterial blood pressure generally (see Chapter 10), with mechanisms involving renin–angiotensin–aldosterone and antidiuretic hormone (ADH) (see pages 352–353).

Reabsorption

Reabsorption of water and molecules from the filtrate is a vital activity in the production of 1–1.5 litres of urine from 180 litres of filtrate. Of the 125 ml of filtrate formed per minute, only 1 ml becomes urine. Filtrate, which is very similar to plasma but without the proteins, needs considerable modification in the tubule before it conforms with the composition of urine (see pages 348–349).

The renal tubules provide a large surface area for the reabsorption of water and other molecules from the filtrate. Reabsorbed substances cross the epithelial layer and basement membrane of the tubule cells and return to the blood through the endothelium of the peritubular capillaries (see *Figure 15.7*).

The cells of the PCT, with their microvilli, are particularly well adapted for reabsorption and this part of the

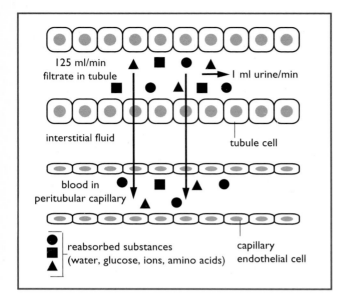

125 ml/min
filtrate in tubule

1 ml urine/min

interstitial fluid

tubule cell

blood in
peritubular capillary

capillary
endothelial cell

● ■ ▲ reabsorbed substances
(water, glucose, ions, amino acids)

Figure 15.7 Reabsorption.

tubule is responsible for reclaiming around two-thirds of the filtered water and sodium ions. The PCT reabsorbs the nutrients, amino acids and glucose along with water and electrolytes, which are also reabsorbed in the loop of Henle, DCT and collecting ducts (see *Figure 15.5*).

In Chapters 1 and 2 we looked at the transport of water and other molecules across plasma membranes, and you might care to revise the main points, which are highly relevant to our consideration of tubular reabsorption.

Passive transport mechanisms, which include osmosis, diffusion and facilitated diffusion with a carrier molecule, are all used for reabsorption. Water moves passively down osmotic gradients and certain solutes diffuse down chemical concentration or electrical gradients (potential difference; see Chapter 3) without the use of energy. Water, some urea, chloride and hydrogen carbonate ions are absorbed in this way.

The other form of transport is active and requires ATP to move substances against electrochemical gradients. Molecules usually diffuse into the tubule cell from the filtrate, but ATP carriers are needed to move molecules into the interstitial fluid, from where they enter the capillary passively. Actively transported molecules include glucose, amino acids, vitamins and sodium, calcium, potassium, phosphate and chloride ions. This type of reabsorption is often interdependent; for example, glucose depends on the active reabsorption of sodium in a process called co-transfer. The active transport mechanisms only work up to a maximum level, known as the transport maximum (T_m), for any substance. When all the carrier molecules are occupied, it is not possible for any more molecules of that substance to be reabsorbed and it will appear in the urine (remember the

revolving door analogy in Chapter 1). This occurs in diabetic hyperglycaemia, when the amount of glucose filtered exceeds its T_m value, which results in glycosuria (see Chapter 8). The amount of a substance, such as glucose, that can be reabsorbed is also termed the renal threshold. If the level of a substance rises beyond its threshold it will appear in the urine. It is worth remembering that glycosuria does not always mean that the person has diabetes mellitus.

Substances which are too large or not lipid-soluble, such as urea, creatinine and uric acid (nitrogenous waste), are either not reabsorbed or in the case of urea only partially so. This inability to reabsorb all filtered molecules means that unwanted waste can be excreted in the urine.

Further considerations of reabsorption

Details of molecules reabsorbed can be found in *Figure 15.5*, but we should note certain other important aspects – especially the conservation of sodium through reabsorption and its importance in the homeostasis of other molecules.

Ions such as sodium and chloride are reabsorbed both passively and actively depending upon the location. Active transport produces the gradients required for some passive transport and osmosis; for example, active sodium reabsorption is accompanied by the osmotic movement of water (obligatory water absorption) and the passive absorption of chloride ions, which maintains electrical neutrality.

As we have already said, most reabsorption takes place in the PCT. The reabsorption which occurs in the remainder of the tubule depends on homeostatic needs and is often regulated by hormones:

- The permeability of the distal tubule and collecting ducts to water is influenced by ADH from the posterior pituitary gland. This change in permeability, which allows the kidney to produce dilute and concentrated urine, is discussed more fully on pages 353–354.
- Calcium and phosphate reabsorption is regulated by active vitamin D, parathyroid hormone and calcitonin (see Chapter 8).
- From our discussion of renal autoregulation you already know that sodium reabsorption in the distal tubule is influenced by secretion of aldosterone (see *Figure 15.6*). The adrenal cortex secretes aldosterone in response to renin–angiotensin release stimulated by low plasma sodium levels (hyponatraemia), a reduction in blood volume and or blood pressure, and sympathetic nerve stimulation. Direct aldosterone release occurs when potassium is high (hyperkalaemia). Here potassium ions are secreted in exchange for the reabsorption of sodium in the distal tubule. Atrial natriuretic peptide hormones (see Chapter 10) have the reverse effect of reducing sodium and water reabsorption by blocking renin–aldosterone secretion and inhibiting ADH.

Reabsorption is also important in regulating the pH of the blood; further discussion can be found on pages 354–357.

Secretion

Tubular secretion is the passage of molecules from the blood in the peritubular capillaries, through the tubule cell, and into the filtrate. As with reabsorption the molecules are moved either actively or passively and secretion occurs throughout the tubule.

The molecules secreted may be those not wanted by the body, e.g. drug and hormone metabolites, or those present in excess amounts, e.g. potassium or hydrogen. Either potassium or hydrogen ions are secreted into the filtrate in exchange for the reabsorption of sodium, which we discussed earlier. It follows that increased levels of hydrogen or potassium ions will affect the level of the other; for example, in acidosis, hydrogen ions are secreted and potassium is retained. Other molecules that find their way into the filtrate by tubular secretion include urea, creatinine and ammonia.

The much-modified filtrate is now urine, which travels in the collecting ducts (see *Figure 15.3*) and through the calyces to the renal pelvis and ureter (see *Figures 15.1* and *15.2*).

Further consideration of urine concentration and volume

The kidneys can respond to changes in body fluid solute concentration (osmolarity/osmolality; see Chapter 2) by producing either dilute or concentrated urine (*Figure 15.8*). The mechanisms by which this is achieved involve osmoreceptors, the secretion of ADH, permeability of the tubule to water and countercurrent multiplication theory, a hypothesis used to explain the production of osmolarity gradients within the medullary interstitial fluid (see *Figure 15.9*).

For our purposes it might be easier to consider the production of concentrated and dilute urine separately.

Concentrated urine

Osmoreceptors in the hypothalamus monitor the osmolarity of the blood and, when this is too high (in dehydration), stored ADH is released by the posterior pituitary gland (see Chapter 8). ADH affects the distal tubule and collecting duct by making the cells more permeable to water. This, however, is only part of the story because the hypothetical countercurrent movement of water and sodium and chloride ions between the loop of Henle, the medullary interstitial fluid and the vasa recta produces osmolarity gradients in the medulla, which ensure that dilute filtrate reaches the distal tubule (see *Figure 15.9*).

Water moves passively, by osmosis, from the descending limb of the loop of Henle, thereby increasing filtrate concentration. The ascending limb is imper-

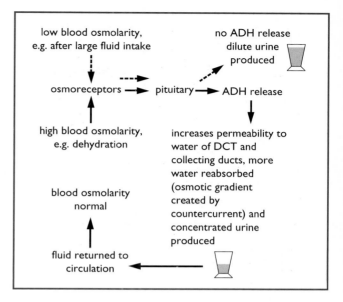

Figure 15.8 Antidiuretic hormone and urine concentration

meable to water, but sodium and chloride ions move actively out into the medullary interstitial fluid. The sodium and chloride ions, with the urea absorbed in the collecting ducts, diffuse into the descending limb to maximize filtrate concentration at the bottom of the loop. It is this movement of solutes without water that sets up the multiplier system which further increases the osmotic gradients.

The vasa recta, associated with juxtamedullary nephrons, act with the loop of Henle as part of the countercurrent exchange to maintain the osmotic gradients. The descending portion of the vasa recta gains sodium chloride and loses water; in contrast the ascending portion loses sodium chloride and reclaims water, which is returned to the circulation.

Thus, the filtrate entering the distal tubule, having lost both water and solutes, is dilute. The difference in osmolarity between the filtrate in the distal tubule and the medullary region produces the osmotic movement of water through the highly permeable tubule, which results in concentrated urine. The water returns to the circulation via the peritubular capillaries, which results in fluid conservation, the production of a smaller volume of concentrated urine and a fall in blood osmolarity – thus restoring homeostasis.

Our ability to form concentrated urine and conserve water is vital to life. Although the secretion of ADH is of prime importance, it is the osmotic gradients set up by the movement of sodium and urea that are crucial in producing concentrated urine – yet another example of the importance of sodium in maintaining homeostasis.

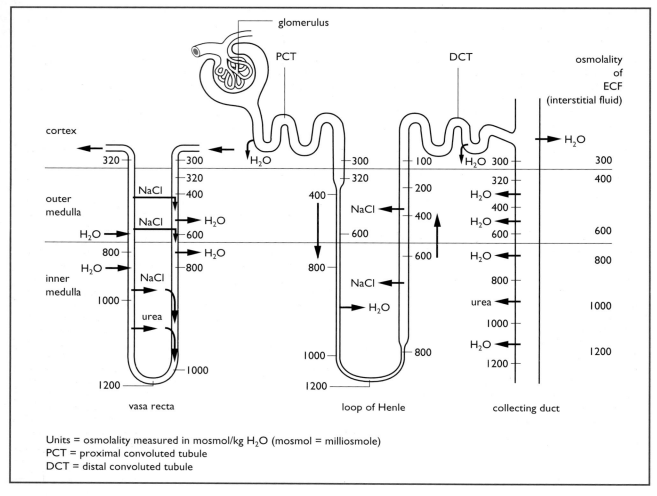

Figure 15.9 Hypothetical countercurrent multiplier system.

Nursing Practice Application **Age and the ability to produce concentrated urine**

Increasing age reduces the kidneys' ability to concentrate urine – by 70 years of age GFR has decreased by 50% and ADH secretion is diminished. The reduction in ADH means that the volume of urine produced shows no circadian variation, the same amount being passed day and night (Armstrong-Ester and Hawkins, 1982). The production of more dilute urine combined with a smaller, less elastic bladder accounts for the nocturia (voiding at night) experienced by many older adults. Apart from sleep disturbances, there are also implications for practice in terms of maintaining hydration and fluid homeostasis.

Dilute urine

If the blood reaching the osmoreceptors has a low osmolarity, such as following a large fluid intake, no ADH is released and the distal tubule and collecting ducts remain impermeable to water. Consequently, the dilute filtrate produced by the countercurrent mechanisms is excreted as dilute urine, which ensures the loss of excess water and a return to homeostatic balance.

Role of the kidneys in the regulation of pH

The kidneys provide the long-term means of maintaining the normal blood pH in the range 7.35–7.45. They function in conjunction with the more immediate effects of the blood buffer systems and lungs (see Chapters 2 and 12). Every day we ingest acids and the body produces acidic substances during metabolism: carbon dioxide, lactic acid,

Nursing Practice Application **Diuretics**

Drugs which increase urine production are known as diuretics. They act in a variety of ways, but all rid the body of excess fluid. Many everyday substances, including tea, coffee and alcohol, have a similar diuretic effect. One of the more unpleasant effects of a 'hangover' is the dehydration which results from the alcohol-induced diuresis caused by ADH inhibition.

Different types of diuretic drugs include:

Thiazides, e.g. bendrofluazide: used to control the oedema of cardiac failure (see Chapter 10). They act on the early distal tubule, where they reduce sodium and chloride reabsorption by inhibition of their shared carrier; this increases the excretion of water, sodium and chloride, and in addition potassium is lost and calcium conserved.

Loop diuretics, e.g. frusemide and bumetanide: these are more powerful drugs used for oedema and oliguria caused by renal failure. They act by preventing reabsorption of sodium, chloride and potassium in the thick segment of the ascending limb of the loop of Henle by carrier inhibition.

Potassium sparing, e.g. spironolactone: used for the oedema of hepatic and cardiac disease. Spironolactone is an aldosterone antagonist and competes with its tubular receptor sites, which results in retention of potassium and increased excretion of water and sodium. It also potentiates the action of thiazide and loop diuretics. Other potassium sparing diuretics include amiloride, which acts on the collecting ducts to reduce sodium reabsorption and potassium excretion by blocking the sodium channels through which aldosterone operates.

Osmotic diuretics, e.g. mannitol (a sugar): these are given intravenously to reduce cerebral oedema or produce a diuresis after a drug overdose. The diuresis is achieved by the osmotic 'pull' created by the inert sugar (which is filtered, but not reabsorbed) during its excretion.

Carbonic anhydrase inhibitors, e.g. acetazolamide: used to reduce intraocular pressure in glaucoma (see Chapter 7) by limiting the production of aqueous humor, rather than as diuretics. They also act at the proximal tubule by preventing the reabsorption of hydrogen carbonate (see page 356), sodium, water and potassium – all of which increase urine output.

You will have noticed that many diuretics work by preventing sodium reabsorption and because the movement of water and sodium are linked, the excess water stays with the sodium in the filtrate and is excreted as urine. Sometimes, ACE inhibiting drugs, such as captopril (used for hypertension), are given with diuretics because they block the enzymic conversion of angiotensin I to angiotensin II, which prevents the secretion of aldosterone.

During diuretic therapy drug effectiveness can be assessed by monitoring fluid balance, extent of oedema, weight, blood pressure and serum electrolyte levels (see Chapter 2).

Nursing observations for side-effects should include hypokalaemia – which may present as cardiac arrhythmias, leg cramps and muscle weakness, dehydration and hypotension. It is important that diuretics are given early enough in the day to avoid nocturia and that potassium supplements are given as prescribed. The person is advised to maintain an adequate (2–3 l) fluid intake unless this is contraindicated, e.g. renal failure. For those affected by postural hypotension changing position slowly will help to avoid dizziness or fainting. Compliance can be increased by ensuring that the person and his/her family have adequate information about the drug; this should include details of side-effects and the need to report any adverse reactions such as rashes or nausea.

---

ketone bodies and acids, such as sulphuric and phosphoric acids, produced from the breakdown of proteins and lipids. Sulphuric and phosphoric acids are termed the metabolic or 'fixed acids' – because they cannot be converted to CO_2. The buffer systems 'mop up' or counteract the effects of the acids as a temporary solution, but it is the lungs and kidneys which operate to remove or retain the acids and prevent pH changes.

Depending upon body chemistry, the kidneys are able to produce urine within a range pH 4.5–8.0 to maintain homeostasis. Renal mechanisms for preventing pH changes, which take place over several hours, are responsible for excreting fixed acids (see pages 356–357) as required and for conserving or eliminating hydrogencarbonate ions.

If either one of the main (renal or respiratory) pH regulation systems is impaired the other will attempt to compensate; for example, if ventilation decreases, causing PCO_2 to rise, the kidneys conserve more hydrogen carbonate ions to restore blood pH to normal.

The kidneys help to maintain acid–base balance with a variety of complex mechanisms which we outline only (*Figure 15.10* and *Flowcharts 15.1–15.3*). Readers requiring more information are directed to Further Reading (e.g. Robinson, 1975).

Secretion of hydrogen ions into the filtrate

Hydrogen ions are released into the filtrate by the dissociation of carbonic acid formed in the tubule cells. Carbonic acid, you will remember, is produced from water and carbon dioxide in the presence of the enzyme carbonic anhydrase. Hydrogen ion secretion is closely linked to sodium and potassium balance (see page 353). For every hydrogen or potassium ion secreted and subsequently excreted a sodium ion is reabsorbed to maintain the electrochemical balance.

Problems arise in hyperkalaemia (some causes) where the increased potassium excretion results in the retention of hydrogen ions and metabolic acidosis.

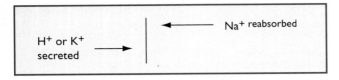

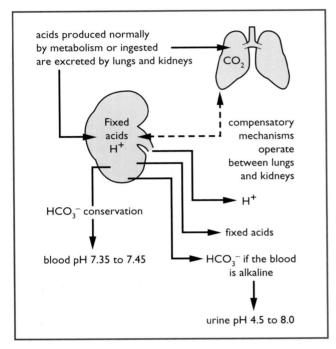

Figure 15.10 Role of the kidneys in pH regulation.

Regulation and replenishment of alkali reserve in the blood

The alkali reserve in the blood is replenished by the conservation and reabsorption of hydrogen carbonate ions, which are produced as hydrogen ions are secreted or buffered. The return of hydrogen carbonate ions to the blood is dependent upon the presence of hydrogen ions in the filtrate and, with this mechanism, the kidneys provide a second means of reducing acidity. In a situation where the alkali reserve is high and few hydrogen ions are being secreted, e.g. respiratory alkalosis, the tubule cells will produce an alkaline urine containing hydrogen carbonate ions (*Flowchart 15.1*).

Excretion of the hydrogen ions and anions

Excretion of hydrogen ions and anions is achieved through the two buffer systems, the ammonia–ammonium and hydrogen phosphate systems, present in the kidney (see *Flowcharts 15.2* and *15.3*). Hydrogen ions secreted into the filtrate are buffered to prevent the urine becoming too acidic, and anions, such as sulphates and chlorides, combine with ammonia produced in the tubule cells to form ammonium salts, e.g. ammonium sulphate and ammonium chloride, which are excreted in the urine.

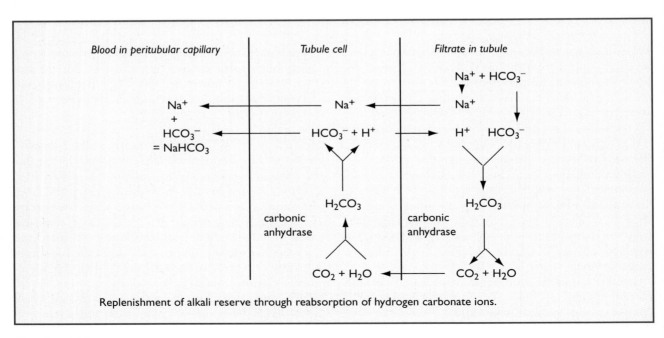

Replenishment of alkali reserve through reabsorption of hydrogen carbonate ions.

Flowchart 15.1

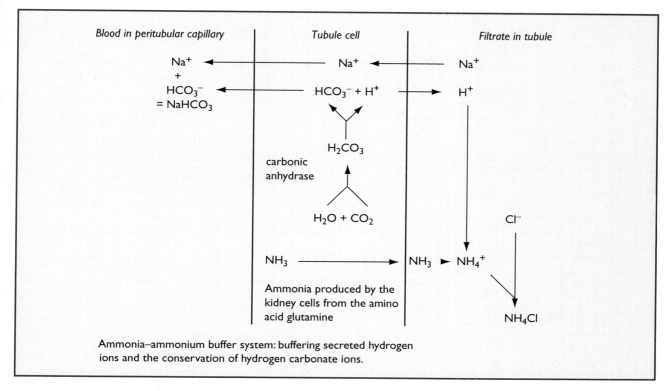

Ammonia–ammonium buffer system: buffering secreted hydrogen ions and the conservation of hydrogen carbonate ions.

Flowchart 15.2

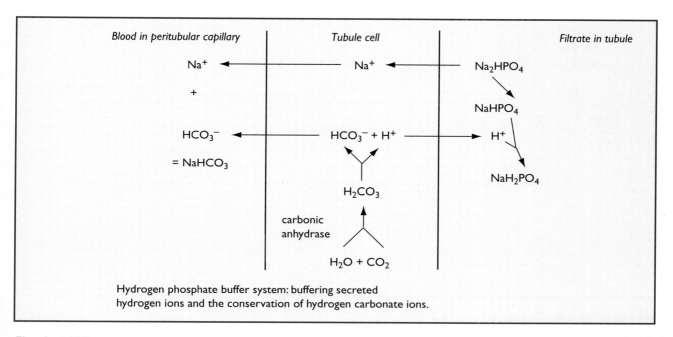

Hydrogen phosphate buffer system: buffering secreted hydrogen ions and the conservation of hydrogen carbonate ions.

Flowchart 15.3

Nursing Practice Application **Observation and testing of urine**

Routine screening of urine for abnormalities is important in:

- Early identification of potential problems; for example, albuminuria (albumin in the urine) during pregnancy may indicate the development of eclampsia (a condition characterized by oedema, albuminuria and high blood pressure, which may progress to fits).
- Diagnosis of disease; for example, the presence or not of bilirubin in the urine is helpful in differentiating between types of jaundice (see Chapter 14).
- Monitoring of existing conditions; for example, the amount of glycosuria (glucose in the urine) is an effective guide to diabetic control where blood glucose monitoring is not possible.

The volume of urine passed will obviously reflect the fluid intake, but abnormally large or small amounts may be associated with disease processes. Polyuria is caused by an inability to form concentrated urine or the presence of large amounts of solutes in the urine. It may be a feature of early renal failure, diabetes insipidus caused by a lack of ADH (see page 352 and Chapter 8) or diabetes mellitus where glycosuria causes an osmotic diuresis (see Chapter 8). Oliguria or anuria indicate a decrease in GFR such as may occur in renal failure or shock. Problems occur when the urinary volume falls below 500 ml/day; this is the minimum amount required to excrete the solutes, e.g. urea.

Before testing a fresh sample of urine it is important to first note the colour, clarity and odour. The colour gives clues about concentration (urine is usually pale when dilute and dark when concentrated) and abnormal contents such as blood (haematuria) give the urine a smoky appearance, or it may be frankly blood-stained. Urine is normally clear with occasional slight turbidity caused by mucus; however, excessive cloudiness may indicate the presence of pus and infection. Fresh urine should not have an offensive odour, but if left to stand the urea undergoes bacterial conversion to ammonia. A 'fishy' odour usually means the urine is infected and in diabetes mellitus the urine may have a sweet odour.

After this important initial examination, the SG can be measured with a urinometer or suitable reagent strip. SG obviously depends on the amount of solutes present and is a guide to other abnormalities; for example, pale (apparently dilute) urine with a high SG may contain glucose or a low SG may indicate an inability to concentrate urine in early stage renal failure, but here a more sensitive test of kidney function would be urinary osmolality (number of solute particles in a kilogram of water) measurement following water deprivation or administration of vasopressin.

Only now are we ready to 'test' the urine with one of the variety of commercially produced reagent strips/tablets. Reagent strips are available to measure or detect all or some of the following: SG, pH, protein, glucose, ketones, blood, nitrites, bilirubin and urobilinogen. For possible significance of abnormal substances in urine see *Figure 15.11*.

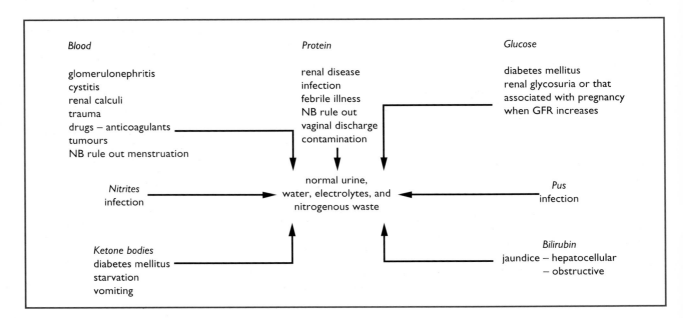

Figure 15.11 Abnormalities in urine.

Special Focus **Renal failure**

The failure of any major organ is always very serious, but support for the failing kidneys is available through dialysis and renal transplant, both of which are now commonly performed and successful procedures.

Renal failure may occur acutely, where renal function is often reversibly impaired, or as a chronic illness, where deterioration with the loss of nephrons progresses irreversibly over months or years.

We will look at some common causes of acute and chronic failure separately, but consider the homeostatic effects of impaired renal function as a whole.

Acute renal failure

Usually the causes are divided into prerenal, renal and postrenal:

Prerenal causes: include reductions in blood volume or cardiac output, e.g. haemorrhage, dehydration and cardiac failure; and haemolysis, e.g. caused by a mismatched blood transfusion, which reduces renal perfusion.

Renal causes: include drugs, toxins and ischaemia, which directly affect renal function by causing acute tubular necrosis, e.g. heavy-metal poisoning; certain types of glomerulonephritis may also cause the kidneys to fail acutely.

Postrenal causes: include obstruction of the urinary tract, e.g. prostatic hypertrophy, bilateral calculi or external pressure, e.g. from advanced tumours of the cervix.

Chronic renal failure

The causes of this gradual reduction in renal function leading to failure include congenital abnormalities of the kidney, e.g. polycystic disease, hypertension, chronic infection, glomerulonephritis and diabetic nephropathy.

Effects on homeostatic balance and management

The effects of failing renal function do not become apparent until GFR has been reduced by 75%. What happens to homeostatic balance when the kidneys fail can be compared with a situation where your household rubbish is not collected and the waste still being produced simply adds to the pile.

When little or no urine is produced the body cannot excrete waste and a toxic state known as uraemia develops. Nitrogenous waste accumulates and the blood urea level (normal 2.5–6.0 mmol/litre) rises.

The electrolyte and acid–base balance is impaired and potassium and hydrogen ions are retained. Excess potassium results in hyperkalaemia, which leads to life-threatening cardiac arrhythmias, and the inability to excrete hydrogen ions produces a metabolic acidosis. Water and sodium are retained which results in oedema and cardiac failure.

Apart from these serious effects, the person concerned, who is, as you can imagine, desperately ill and feels 'rotten', also suffers from:

- Nausea and vomiting – toxins, which include urea, irritate the gastrointestinal tract.
- Hiccups – toxins irritate the phrenic nerve (see Chapter 5).
- Pruritus – the accumulation of toxic waste causes intense skin itching.
- Dyspnoea – due to anaemia caused by lack of erythropoietin associated with renal failure (see Chapter 9); fluid retention will lead to heart failure and pulmonary oedema (see Chapter 10), and acidosis will also contribute to the dyspnoea.
- Confusion, fits and eventual coma – caused by accumulation of toxic waste and possibly severe hypertension, both of which affect brain function (see Chapter 4).

The management of renal failure depends on its cause plus the age and general condition of the individual. Any regimen would include measures to treat the cause if possible and relieve distressing symptoms such as hiccups.

When oliguria/anuria is present the fluid intake is restricted to an amount which reflects urinary and insensible losses and takes account of the water produced during metabolism. Dietary modifications in the form of restricted sodium, potassium and protein are usual. These are combined with a high-energy carbohydrate intake to prevent the use of protein or fat and catabolism of body tissue. Sometimes it is possible

to treat hyperkalaemia by the oral or rectal administration of an ion exchange resin.

Where these measures are inadequate to control the problems it is necessary to commence peritoneal dialysis (see *Figure 15.12*) or haemodialysis. Both forms of dialysis depend upon the basic principles of water movement by osmosis and solute movement by diffusion across a selectively permeable membrane (see Chapter 2) to produce a concentration equilibrium either side of the membrane. The technique of haemofiltration is also used – this involves the ultrafiltration of plasma through a special synthetic membrane to remove unwanted substances.

Peritoneal dialysis utilizes the peritoneum as the selectively permeable membrane and in haemodialysis a synthetic membrane is part of the 'artificial kidney'. Whichever type of dialysis is used, the person's blood is separated from the dialysis fluid only by the selectively permeable membrane; the dialysis fluid contains no nitrogenous waste or potassium, which allows the movement of these substances from the blood to the dialysis fluid.

Hypertonic dialysis fluid can be used to remove excess water and various additions to the fluid can pass in the opposite direction, e.g. to counteract any acidosis. Dialysis may be a temporary measure for a person with acute failure, but in chronic situations some form of intermittent dialysis is required unless a renal transplant is possible.

Peritoneal dialysis may be undertaken as a continuous process [continuous ambulatory peritoneal dialysis(CAPD)]. Here the homeostatic balance is maintained by the use of 3–6 exchanges of dialysis fluid each and every day and provides a more constant internal environment than does haemodialysis.

Unfortunately, not everyone is suitable for transplant or the transplant may fail. This and the shortage of donor kidneys means that many people must depend for long periods upon dialysis, with its attendant physical, psychological and social problems.

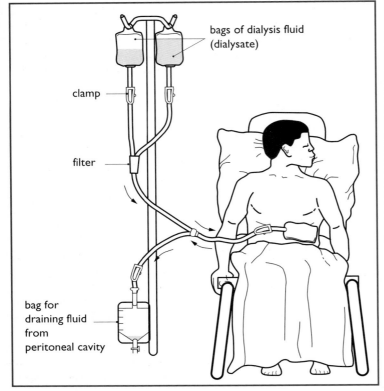

Figure 15.12 Peritoneal dialysis.

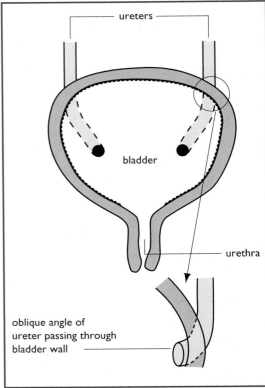

Figure 15.13 Ureters and bladder.

Lower Urinary Tract

Ureters

The two ureters convey urine from the renal pelvis to the bladder (see *Figure 15.1*). They are 25–30 cm in length with a very small diameter of about 3–6 mm and can easily become blocked by calculi (see page 346). The ureters run behind the peritoneum close to the psoas muscle to enter the bladder through its posterior wall. The portion of ureter in the bladder wall runs obliquely (*Figure 15.13*), a useful feature which prevents the reflux of urine by compressing the ureter as the bladder fills and empties.

The ureters have three basic layers: the inner transitional epithelial mucosa (see Chapter 1) continuous with that of the renal pelvis and bladder, two smooth muscle layers and an outer fibrous connective coat.

Urine is moved down the ureters by peristaltic contractions (see Chapter 13). These waves of muscular contraction occur as urine distends the renal pelvis and ureter. A calculus entering the ureter will cause severe colic (see Nursing Practice Application, page 346) as intense muscular contractions attempt to dislodge the calculus and move it into the bladder.

Bladder

The urinary bladder, which lies in the pelvic cavity, acts as temporary storage for urine. It is a collapsible sac which, when empty, is behind the symphysis pubis, but rises into the abdominal cavity on filling. In females the bladder is close to the uterus and vagina; it is close to the prostate gland and rectum in males (see *Figure 1.34*). The bladder has four layers:

- Transitional epithelial mucosa able to withstand the normal variations in urinary pH and composition. This lining forms folds, or rugae, which allow for considerable distension as the bladder fills. We become aware of rising pressure when the bladder contains around 250–300 ml of urine and usually void when it contains 400–500 ml. The bladder can hold more than a litre, but would be very distended, painful and easily palpated (felt) abdominally.
- A submucosa of connective tissue, vessels and nerves.
- A smooth muscle layer formed from the detrusor muscle which thickens at the bladder–urethral junction to form the internal urethral sphincter. During micturition (see page 362) involuntary contraction of the detrusor and opening of the sphincter empties the bladder and allows urine into the urethra. Micturition is further aided by

relaxation of the pelvic floor muscles (levator ani; Chapter 18) on which the bladder sits.

- The outer coat is part peritoneum (superior surface) and part fibrous tissue.

Inside the bladder is a smooth triangular area, formed from the openings of the ureters and bladder neck, known as the trigone (*Figure 15.14*).

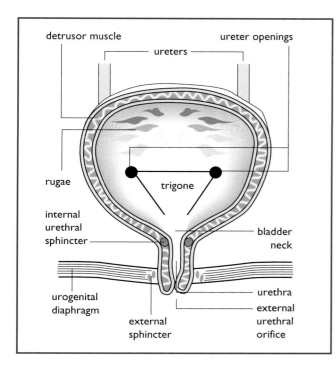

Figure 15.14 Bladder interior.

Urethra

The urethra, which conveys urine from the bladder to the outside, extends from the bladder neck to the external urethral orifice (see *Figure 15.15*). As the urethra leaves the bladder it is lined with transitional epithelium which becomes stratified squamous epithelium. In females this tissue is similar to that lining the vagina and is also influenced by oestrogen hormones. The involuntary internal sphincter (see page 360) keeps the urethra closed except during micturition. A further sphincter, the external urethral sphincter, is formed from skeletal muscle at the level of the pelvic floor. This sphincter is under voluntary control from the age a child achieves bladder control.

The female urethra, which is around 4 cm in length, is attached to the anterior vaginal wall and opens externally just anterior to the vaginal orifice [see *Figure 15.15(a)*]. The short urethra and its proximity to the anus make women particularly susceptible to urinary tract infection. When oestrogen secretion declines during the climacteric (see Chapter 21) it can lead to urethral discomfort (Gould, 1990).

In males the urethra is around 20 cm in length and has dual excretory and reproductive functions (see Chapter 20). It has three parts – the prostatic, where it passes through the prostate gland; the membranous urethra, surrounded by the external urethral sphincter; and the penile urethra, which passes through the penis to open at the external urethral orifice. The ejaculatory and prostatic ducts enter the prostatic urethra and those of the bulbourethral glands empty their secretions lower down in the penile part [see *Figure 15.15(b)*]. The secretions and their role is examined in Chapter 20.

Person-Centred Study **Harry**

Harry has delivered the post for 32 years; he is due to retire next year and plans to spend his extra leisure in the garden and with his racing pigeons. He and his wife Pat feel relieved and rather fortunate that they can now look forward to their retirement. Only 6 months ago Harry was diagnosed as having early bladder cancer and they thought it was the end of all their plans.

Harry had passed some blood in his urine, but as he had no pain did not really think it much to worry about. Pat happened to mention 'the trouble' to their neighbour – a charge nurse at the local

hospital – and he suggested that Harry see his doctor despite having no pain.

Luckily for Harry his painless haematuria was investigated at once and a cystoscopy (endoscopic examination of the bladder) and biopsy confirmed an early bladder papilloma which was destroyed by diathermy through the cystoscope. He will have regular check cystoscopies with further diathermy as required.

Often painless haematuria is the only sign of bladder tumours and it is essential that all such occurrences are investigated. Other treatment modalities include radio-

therapy, cytotoxic drugs and surgery if the tumour is more widespread. The development of photodynamic therapy (photosensitization followed by laser therapy) is seen as a possibility for the treatment of early bladder tumours (Tootla and Easterling, 1989). Certainly early treatment is the key to success, but for this to happen the cancer must be detected. The availability of a test strip which checks for the presence of bladder cancer antigen in urine is another means of detecting transitional cell carcinoma (cancer affecting the transitional cell lining of the bladder) at an early stage.

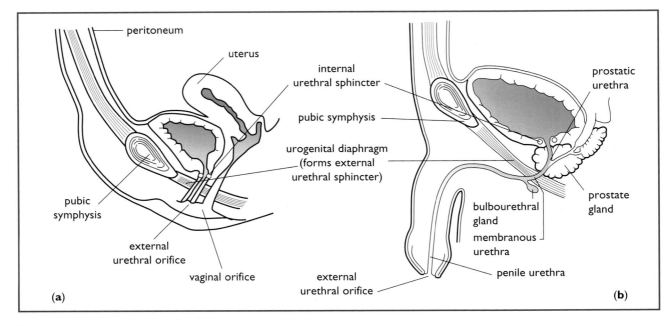

Figure 15.15 Urethra. (**a**) Female; (**b**) male.

Micturition

Micturition is controlled through autonomic and voluntary nerves (*Figure 15.16*). In infants it operates entirely through bladder stretch receptors and a spinal reflex where the bladder empties when full enough, but from the age of 2–3 years nervous system development is sufficient to give awareness of bladder filling and the ability to inhibit the reflex and control the external urethral sphincter.

In adults, as the bladder fills with urine (250–300 ml), stretch receptors in the wall transmit sensory (afferent) impulses in parasympathetic fibres to the sacral region of the spinal cord. Impulses travelling up the cord to higher brain centres make us aware of the need to void urine.

When sufficient urine is present (400–500 ml), parasympathetic motor (efferent) impulses from the spinal cord cause detrusor contraction, bladder neck relaxation with 'funnelling' and internal sphincter relaxation, which allows urine into the urethra. Actual voiding occurs when the somatic motor nerves (pudendal), which normally keep the external sphincter closed, are reflexly inhibited. This relaxes the external sphincter and urogenital diaphragm (pelvic floor), allowing urine to flow out. Complete bladder emptying occurs because a positive feedback mechanism operates while urine is flowing in the urethra. Flow is aided by increased intra-abdominal pressure (Valsalva's manoeuvre) and contraction of the abdominal muscles.

If voiding does not occur bladder contractions cease for a while and the need to void seems to 'wear off' – this is because the reflex becomes refractory. Eventually, bladder stretch receptors start to 'fire' again as more urine enters and distends the bladder, which starts to contract again.

Once we have learnt control, the micturition reflex can be voluntarily inhibited by impulses from higher centres and contraction of the external sphincter. This gives us some choice about where and when voiding occurs, but eventually this option is removed, and when urine volume reaches a critical level the bladder will empty whether convenient or not.

Sympathetic efferents innervating the bladder and ureter may be involved with detrusor relaxation, but this possible minor role is questionable.

The process of micturition is not fully understood and to date much of the current knowledge has been obtained through urodynamic studies. Readers are directed to the Further Reading (Smith, 1984; Abbott, 1992) and References (Gould, 1990) for information regarding urodynamic studies.

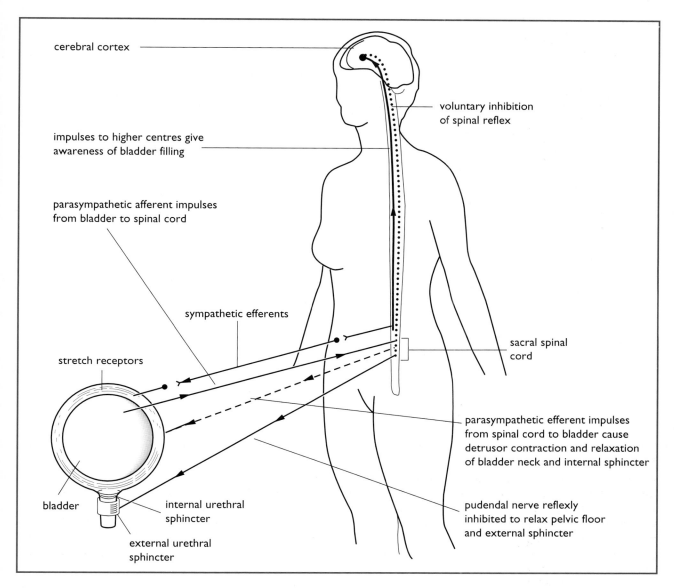

Figure 15.16 Micturition.

Catheterization

We have mentioned the use of urinary catheters in the management of retention (see page 364). Catheterization is a common procedure and 10–12% of people in hospital will have a catheter at some stage. This may be only short term, such as following gynaecological repair surgery, but could be longer term, e.g. management of incontinence where strategies such as pelvic floor exercises or biofeedback have been ineffective. Many of those with long-term catheters are cared for in a variety of health/social care facilities or their own homes. Numerous studies have shown the presence of a catheter to increase greatly the risk of infection (see page 365) and nursing

interventions that prevent contamination are required. Nursing care should include maintaining the integrity of the closed drainage system, adequate cleaning, hand washing for staff, a fluid intake of at least 2.5 litres and appropriate teaching for the patient. In a study of 294 catheterized patients in general hospitals, Crow *et al.* (1988) found that the closed system was broken in 42%, that only 48% had the bag positioned correctly and that cleaning and hand washing by nurses was poor. Roe (1989a) found that the information given to patients/carers by nurses (60 hospital, 46 community) about catheter-care was neither consistent with the literature nor comprehensive. She identified a need for more catheter-care education

Abnormal Function **Problems with micturition**

It is not possible to define 'normal' micturition as there are large variations in healthy individuals. What is important is the recognition of departures from normal or factors which predispose to abnormality for the individual. At this stage it is appropriate to include a brief outline of some problems associated with the elimination of urine, but readers are also directed to the Further Reading and References. Lowthian (1977) states that most micturition problems involve increased frequency and social inconvenience, especially when control is lost.

Frequency

Passing small amounts of urine frequently is often a feature of cystitis (see page 365). This occurs because bladder stretch receptors are stimulated constantly, resulting in detrusor contraction before the bladder is really full. It should not be confused with increased voiding associated with a large fluid intake, e.g. getting up many times to void after an evening drinking beer, which not only increases fluid intake but also inhibits ADH. Frequency also accompanies pregnancy (early and late) due to pressure on the bladder and more seriously with bladder tumours.

Retention

Retention is the inability to pass urine. It is commonly caused by prostatic enlargement in older men (see Chapter 20), but may be associated with other obstructions of the bladder or urethra. Retention with overflow, frequency or incontinence is easily misdiagnosed and it is essential to discover whether the bladder is distended by abdominal examination.

The immediate management of retention involves the introduction of a urinary catheter (see pages 363–364) to drain urine. The catheter is usually introduced through the urethra, but the suprapubic route may be used where the urethra is obstructed.

Incontinence

Inability to control the voiding of urine is extremely common. Norton (1986) states that 2–3 million people in the UK are incontinent of urine, although for many this is very minor and is not seen as a problem. Whatever the exact numbers, they are much greater than those known to the health and social service agencies. The results of a postal survey by Thomas *et al.* (1980) confirm this for all age groups and both genders. The accepted rate for females aged 15–64 was 0.2%, but the study revealed that 8.5% had continence problems. Contrary to popular opinion, incontinence is not confined to the older population but affects all age groups and both genders. Mandelstam (1989) gives examples which include a young man who wets the bed, a new mother, a middle-aged woman and an isolated older person. Research undertaken by Armstrong-Ester and Hawkins (1982), based on the hypothesis that the disturbance of circadian rhythms would manifest as incontinence and nocturnal disturbances, found that many older people had desynchronized renal circadian rhythms in which the cycle was 28 hours, not 24 hours. Their small sample showed that in 15 people, renal and temperature circadian rhythms were affected and in 8 people, the renal was affected alone. Obviously the scale of the problem represents an enormous challenge for practice, and Norton (1986) sees the promotion of continence as the business of every nurse, midwife and health visitor. Further coverage of this important topic can be found in Chapter 20.

Incontinence can be divided into several types, which include:

- Stress incontinence, which is characterized by a leakage of urine when intra-abdominal pressure rises, e.g. coughing, laughing. This type of incontinence, which affects women, is caused by bladder neck displacement and loss of the urethral–vesicular angle caused by weakening of the pelvic floor which follows childbirth, uterine prolapse and the climacteric.
- Detrusor instability with erratic contraction (unstable bladder), leading to urgency and urge incontinence.
- Overflow, where obstruction to the flow of urine, such as an enlarged prostate gland, leads to retention with overflow in the form of stress incontinence or dribbling.
- Neurological incontinence, where conditions such as spinal injury, diabetes or multiple sclerosis (see Chapters 3 and 4) damage the nerves involved in bladder control. The resultant problems depend on where the damage has occurred and include hypotonic/atonic bladder with overflow, reflex emptying of the full bladder and loss of higher centre inhibition with urge incontinence.
- Functional incontinence, where the person has involuntary and completely erratic urine loss without physical problems in bladder or nervous system. Causes include cognitive problems, sensory deficits and immobility.

for nurses, teaching for patients/carers, and for research which considers the effects of teaching on the ability of people to care for their urinary drainage. Another study by Roe (1989b) identified the number of catheterized people being looked after by the community nurses of one district health authority; for the period of the study this was 61 (4%). Roe concludes that this knowledge is important in assessing education needs and costs.

Another problem for people who need long-term catheterization is encrustation and blockage. In a study by Getliffe (1994) 43% of people suffered from recurrent encrustation and blockage. The problem was worse in those catheterized for incontinence and was linked to immobility which reduces access to fluids (particularly in a community setting) and the flow of urine.

Abnormal Function **Problems with micturition *cont.***

During assessment it is essential that the health professional ascertains that the failure to maintain continence is not caused by a simple factor, which is easily rectified, such as an inability to ask for the lavatory because of a speech problem or an older woman too embarrassed to ask a young male care worker; not being able to manage clothing, e.g. people with learning disabilities or after a stroke; and the lack of mobility required to reach facilities in time.

Abnormal function **Urinary tract infection (UTI)**

Complete and regular bladder emptying, high flow rates and the secretion of immunoglobulins and glycosaminoglycans by the bladder mucosa affords some protection against infection, but urinary tract infection is still a common occurrence. UTI represented 30% of hospital-acquired infections in a study by Meers *et al.* (1981). The infection usually enters the urinary tract through the urethra, but it can be blood-borne or spread directly from other structures, e.g. colonic diverticular disease (see Chapter 13).

The vast majority of urinary infections are caused by intestinal bacteria, e.g. *Escherichia coli* and *Streptococcus faecalis*, which spread from the anal/perineal area, but other culprits include *Proteus* spp., *Klebsiella* spp., *Pseudomonas aeruginosa* and *Staphylococcus epidermidis*.

Infection is an unusual event in males with a normal urinary tract, but for reasons we have already discussed UTI is very common in females, and up to 50% will be affected at some stage (Asscher, 1982). The frequency of UTI increases in the population aged over 65 years.

Predisposing factors
The predisposing factors include:
*   Poor perineal hygiene
*   Use of some irritant toiletries.
*   Urethral trauma during intercourse and childbirth.
*   Catheterization, bladder instrumentation, e.g. cystoscopy.
*   Urinary stasis, e.g. urinary obstruction, immobility.
*   Reduced immune function, e.g. immunosuppressed individuals, newborns and older adults.
*   Pregnancy.
*   Diabetes mellitus.
*   Any severe debilitating condition.

Types of infection
*   Asymptomatic or covert bacteriuria (bacteria in the urine) is characterized by at least 10^5 colony-forming organisms/ml in freshly voided urine or a specimen obtained suprapubically (MRC, 1979). With these numbers, and remembering that bladder urine is normally sterile, it is unlikely that the presence of bacteria is caused by contamination. Urine testing, which should form part of every nursing assessment, is important in the detection of asymptomatic UTI (Pitt, 1989).
*   Infection causing inflammation of the bladder (bacterial cystitis) and urethra (urethritis), leading to dysuria, haematuria, offensive cloudy urine which contains leucocytes, increased frequency and urgency, suprapubic pain and possibly pyrexia. The diagnosis is confirmed by culturing a midstream specimen of urine. Usually, treatment with an appropriate antimicrobial drug, e.g. trimethoprim, and a fluid intake of at least 2.5 litres is effective. Analgesia such as paracetamol and a mild alkali, e.g. potassium citrate, to reduce urine acidity will minimize the scalding pain on micturition. In an article by Busuttil Leaver (1996) the use of cranberry juice both as prophylaxis and treatment for some UTI's is discussed, together with its uses in preventing some types of urinary stones and excess mucus in people after urinary diversion surgery.
*   The infection may travel up the ureters to involve the kidneys (pyelonephritis). In addition to the problems of cystitis, the person has loin pain and pyrexia. Pyelonephritis can cause permanent kidney damage which if severe can lead to renal failure (see page 359).

Nursing Practice Application **Anxiety and micturition**

Anxiety and stressful situations can result in changes in normal patterns of micturition. If sufficiently frightened you may not be able to maintain external sphincter control and your bladder will empty as autonomic impulses cause detrusor contraction.

Frequency (voiding small amounts of urine often – perhaps every few minutes) can be a feature of anxiety as well as physical causes. It will come as no surprise that individuals admitted to hospital, waiting for test results or surgery may all have frequency. You will be able to remember specific situations where your own pattern of micturition was disturbed, e.g. examinations, performing in a play/concert and interviews. Frequency may also be experienced by people who have continence problems and fear having an 'accident'.

Sometimes the reverse happens and people cannot pass urine when they want or need to – such as the anxiety associated with producing a specimen of urine for testing or the fear of being disturbed if the lavatory door does not lock. In these cases if voiding does start it may be incomplete, with urine left in the bladder.

Nursing Practice Application **Enuresis and voluntary bladder control**

Enuresis describes the involuntary voiding of urine in a child, after they have attained the age where voluntary bladder control is considered possible. As already stated, most children gain bladder control between the ages of 2 and 3 years. Some children are earlier or later than this, and most children achieve continence during the day before they are dry at night. Nocturnal enuresis may continue for sometime and nappies may be required at night after the fourth birthday. During the early days after daytime continence has been mastered there will continue to be the odd 'accident', especially when the child is involved in a game and simply forgets to ask for the lavatory – they need a timely reminder. A physical illness or emotional upset, e.g. birth of a sibling or not getting their own way, can cause enuresis in a previously continent child. Most authorities do not consider enuresis to require investigation or treatment until the child turns 5 years.

Healthier Living **Preventing UTI**

It may seem to you that UTI is an inevitable consequence of being female, but there are several simple preventive measures that any woman can take for herself:

* Take 2–3 litres of fluid a day, avoiding tea, coffee and alcohol, which are diuretic – this avoids dehydration and keeps the bladder 'flushed out'.
* Pay attention to hygiene, especially after using the toilet – always wipe 'front to back' (avoids bringing bowel organisms towards the urethra).
* Empty bladder every 3–4 hours and before going to bed.
* Make sure the bladder is completely empty after voiding.
* Ensure that hands are washed adequately after passing urine or faeces.
* Empty the bladder before and after sexual intercourse (to 'flush' organisms from the bladder and urethra), and avoid intercourse if symptoms of cystitis are present (to avoid urethral trauma).
* Avoid the use of bubble bath and other preparations which can cause irritation.
* If dysuria/frequency occurs increase intake of water or fruit juice, take a proprietary 'cystitis mixture' (to reduce urine acidity and hence discomfort), start simple measures to give relief, such as analgesia or a warm bath, and arrange to see a GP.

In women who continue to experience attacks of cystitis further investigations may be justified, e.g. an intravenous urogram (radiographic examination of the urinary tract in which the dye injected intravenously is excreted by the kidneys) and cystoscopy.

Summary/Check List

Introduction – early development.

Kidney – gross structure. Blood and nerve supply, Nursing Practice Application – renal calculus. Nephron, juxtaglomerular apparatus. Blood flow.

Functions of the kidney – urine, physical characteristics, composition. Formation of urine. Filtration, GFR and regulation, Nursing Practice Application – renal clearance. Reabsorption. Secretion. Urine concentration and volume, Nursing Practice Application – age and the ability to produce concentrated urine, Nursing Practice Application – diuretics.

Kidney and pH regulation, Nursing Practice Application – observation and testing of urine. Special Focus – renal failure.

Lower urinary tract – ureters. Bladder, Person-centred Study – Harry. Urethra.

Micturition – normal and abnormal. Nursing Practice Application – anxiety and micturition. Nursing Practice Application – enuresis and voluntary bladder control. Urinary tract infection (UTI), Healthier Living - preventing UTI.

Self Test

1 Draw and label the urinary system
2 Put the following in the correct order:
 (a) DCT;
 (b) Bowman's capsule;
 (c) collecting ducts;
 (d) loop of Henle;
 (e) PCT.
3 Which of the following statements are true?
 (a) The kidneys receive around 25% of the cardiac output.
 (b) The afferent arteriole of the glomerulus is larger than the efferent arteriole.
 (c) All nephrons have a vasa recta.
 (d) The nephron has two sets of capillaries.
4 Describe the three processes involved in the formation of urine.
5 Put the following in their correct pairs:
 (a) GFR/min;
 (b) 1200 ml;
 (c) daily urine volume;
 (d) 180 l;
 (e) renal blood flow/min;
 (f) 125 ml;
 (g) filtrate formed daily;
 (h) 1000–1500 ml.
6 Explain briefly how the kidney produces concentrated urine to conserve water.
7 What information can be gained from noting the colour, clarity and odour of a fresh sample of urine?
8 Which of the following statements are true?
 (a) The detrusor muscle is involuntary.
 (b) The ureteric and urethral openings are found in the bladder area known as the trigone.
 (c) The urethra is closed except during micturition.
 (d) Sympathetic nerves control bladder contraction and sphincter relaxation.
9 What type of incontinence is probably present in the following people?
 (a) Farida, who has three small children, is incontinent when she laughs or coughs.
 (b) Maggie finds she has little warning of voiding and cannot get to the lavatory in time.
 (c) Declan, aged 65, who 'dribbles' small amounts of urine without warning.
10 What advice would you give to Sue, aged 23, who asks about preventing UTI?

Answers

1 See page 344.
2 b, e, d, a, c.
3 a, b, d.
4 See pages 349–53.
5 a–f, c–h, e–b and g–d.
6 See page 353.
7 See page 358.
8 a, b, c.
9 (a) Stress;
 (b) detrusor instability (urge incontinence);
 (c) overflow with retention.
10 See page 366.

References

Armstrong-Ester CA, Hawkins LA (1982) Day for night circadian rhythms in the elderly. *Nurs Times* **78**(30):1263–5.

Asscher AW (1982) *Urinary Tract Infection*. London: Update Publications.

Busuttil Leaver R (1996) Cranberry juice. *Prof Nurs* **11**(8): 525–6.

Crow R, Mulhall A, Chapman R (1988) Indwelling catheterization and related nursing practice. *J Adv Nurs* **13**(4): 489–95.

Getliffe KA (1994) The characteristics and management of patients with recurrent blockage of long-term urinary catheters. *J Adv Nurs* **20**(1): 140–9.

Gould D (1990) *Nursing Care of Women*. London: Prentice-Hall.

Heath HBM ed. (1995) *Potter and Perry's Foundations in Nursing Theory and Practice*. London: Mosby.

Lowthian P (1977) Frequent micturition and its significance. *Nurs Times* **73**(46): 1809–13.

Mandelstam D (1989) *Understanding Incontinence: a Guide to the Nature and Management of a Very Common Complaint.* London: Chapman and Hall.

Medical Research Council (MRC) Bacteriuria Committee (1979) Recommended terminology of urinary tract infection. *BMJ* **2**, 717–719.

Meers PD et al. (1981) Report on the National Survey of Infection in Hospitals 1980. *J Hosp Infec* **2**(UTI suppl.): 23–28.

Norton C (1986) *Nursing for Continence*. Beaconsfield: Beaconsfield Publishers.

Pitt M (1989) Fluid intake and urinary tract infection. *Nurs Times* **85**(1): 36–38.

Roe BH (1989a) A study of information given by nurses for catheter care to patients and their carers. *J Adv Nurs* **14**(3): 203–10.

Roe BH (1989b) Long-term catheter care in the community. *Nurs Times* **85**(36): 43–44.

Thomas TM, Plymat KR, Blannin J, Meade TW, (1980) Prevalence of urinary incontinence. *BMJ* **281**:1243–5.

Tootla J, Easterling A (1989) PDT: Destroying malignant cells with laser beams. *Nursing 89 (US)* **19**(11): 48–9.

Further Reading

Abbott D (1992) Objective assessment ensures improved diagnosis. Principles and techniques of urodynamics. *Prof Nurs* **7**(11): 738–42.

Baer CL (1990) Acute renal failure. *Nursing 90 (US)*, **20**(6): 34–9.

Brundage D (1992) *Renal Disorders* London: Mosby.

Kimber E (1997) Peritoneal dialysis. *Prof Nurs* **12**(5): 349–52.

Mandelstam D Ed. (1986) *Incontinence and its Management*, 2nd edn. London: Croom Helm.

Miles P, Everett J et al. (1997) Comparision of blood or urine testing by patients with newly diagnosed non-insulin dependent diabetes: patient survey after randomised crossover trial *BMJ* **315**: 348–349.

Robinson JR (1975) *Fundamentals of Acid–Base Regulation*, 5th edn. Oxford: Blackwell Scientific Publications.

Wheeler V (1990) A new kind of loving? The effect of continence problems on sexuality. *Prof Nurs* **5**(9): 492–6.

Wright E (1988) Catheter care: the risk of infection. *Prof Nurs* **3**(12): 487–490.

Wright E (1988) Minimising the risks of UTI. *Prof Nurs* **4**(2): 63–67.

Wright E (1989) Teaching patients to cope with catheters at home. *Prof Nurs* **4**(4): 191–4.

Useful Addresses

Incontinence Advisory Service
c/o Disabled Living Foundation
380–384 Harrow Road
London W9 2HU

National Kidney Federation
6 Stanley Street
Worksop
Notts
S81 7HX

SPOD (Association to promote the sexual and personal
relationships of people with disabilities)
286 Camden Road
London N7 0BJ

Bone Tissue

Overview

- *Structure and functions of bone tissue.*
- *Ossification (osteogenesis).*
- *Bone homeostasis.*

Learning Outcomes

After studying Chapter 16 you should be able to:

- Discuss the functions of bone.
- Describe lamellar bone tissue – compact and cancellous.
- Classify bones by shape.
- Describe the gross structure of a long bone.
- Describe the microscopic structure and chemical composition of bone.
- Outline the formation of bone.
- Explain how bones grow.
- Describe the different types of fracture.
- Explain how fractures heal.
- Outline normal bone homeostasis and remodelling.
- Discuss some abnormalities of bone homeostasis.

Key Words

Cancellous bone – light, spongy bone.
Compact bone – dense, hard bone.
Diaphysis – the shaft (middle part) of a long bone.
Endosteum – membrane lining the medullary cavity.
Epiphysis – the ends of a long bone. In growing bones the epiphyses and diaphysis are separated by a plate of cartilage.
Medullary cavity – the central cavity of a long bone, containing marrow.
Ossification (osteogenesis) – formation of bone tissue,
either from cartilage and membrane in the fetus or from bone growth after birth.
Osteoblasts – cells involved in bone formation and deposition.
Osteoclasts – cells involved in bone reabsorption and remodelling.
Osteocytes – bone cells derived from osteoblasts.
Osteology – the study of bones.
Periosteum – fibrous connective tissue covering a bone.

Introduction

Try to imagine for a moment what we would be like without bone: no movement would be possible and we would be forever constrained within a mass of flesh. Bone, the hardest body tissue, gives us form, protection, stability and movement. Sometimes mistakenly considered rather dull and static, bones are in fact formed from extremely dynamic tissue that undergoes constant structural changes.

In this chapter we will consider bone tissue and homeostasis prior to looking at muscle tissue in Chapter 17. Chapter 18 brings together the skeleton, joints and major muscles, and considers the integration required for movement and stability.

Functions of bone
Movement and stability
Bones form a supporting body framework and provide attachments for skeletal muscles, ligaments and tendons. They act as a system of levers to allow movement (see Chapter 18).

Protective
The bony framework protects internal structures; for example, the skull encloses the brain and the rib cage protects the thoracic organs.

Storage
Bone is involved in mineral homeostasis. It is a repository for minerals such as calcium, phosphorus and magnesium.

Haemopoietic
Red marrow found in the marrow cavity of some bones produces blood cells (see Chapter 9).

Bone Tissue

Types of bone tissue
Bone is a connective tissue (see Chapter 1) that has been mineralized to produce an extremely hard substance. Mineralization of connective tissue by the addition of mainly calcium salts gives it physical properties that include great tensile (capable of stretching) strength and the ability to withstand considerable compressive forces.

Bone may be the woven type, which is a fragile tissue produced during some stages of rapid ossification (osteogenesis; bone formation), such as in fetal development (see pages 373) or fracture healing (see pages 375, 377). The other type is lamellar bone, the tough tissue which forms healthy adult bones.

The two basic types of lamellar bone tissue are **compact** (cortical) and **cancellous** (trabecular). These differ in structure, function and in location (*Figure 16.1*).

On naked-eye examination, compact bone looks hard and dense; however, it actually consists of many structural units called Haversian systems, or osteons (see page 372 and *Figure 16.4*). Compact bone is found in flat bones, in the shaft (**diaphysis**) of long bones and as the covering of all bones.

Cancellous bone is spongy in appearance; it has fewer Haversian systems and is arranged in a network of trabeculae (tiny, beam-like pieces of bone) that surround marrow-filled cavities. The trabecular arrangement ensures that cancellous bone is well adapted to withstand physical stresses whilst being comparatively light. It is found in the ends (epiphyses; singular **epiphysis**) of long bones, and in short bones, flat bones and irregular bones.

Types of bone
The bones that form the skeleton can be classified by their shape as long, short, flat or irregular (*Figure 16.2*).

Long bones
The long bones form the limbs, e.g. the femur. As already mentioned, they have a diaphysis and two epiphyses. The diaphysis, which is formed from compact bone, encloses the central **medullary cavity**. In young children the medullary cavity is filled with haemopoietic red marrow; this is replaced by yellow fatty marrow in adults. Cancellous bone, containing red marrow, forms the epiphyses and the whole bone is covered with a layer of compact bone. Long bones act as levers which, with muscles, facilitate movement.

Short bones
The short bones are small and light, but very strong. They form, for example, the bones that contribute to the wrist and ankle joints (carpals and tarsals respectively). Short bones are constructed from an inner layer of cancellous bone with a thin outer covering of compact bone.

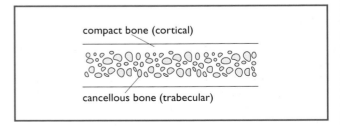

Figure 16.1 Bone tissue – compact and cancellous.

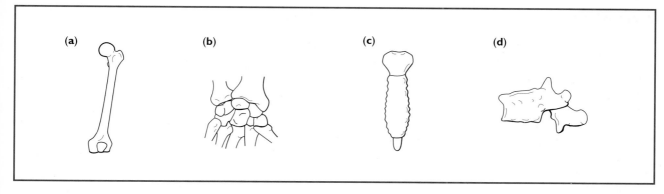

Figure 16.2 Types of bones. (**a**) Long; (**b**) short; (**c**) flat; (**d**) irregular.

Flat bones

Flat bones consist of a sandwich of cancellous bone between two layers of compact bone. Examples of flat bones include sternum, ribs, scapulae and skull. They provide protection, attachment for muscles and, in adults, most contain haemopoietic red marrow.

Irregular bones

Irregular bones are those that cannot be included in the previous groups, e.g. the vertebrae and pelvic bones. They consist of cancellous bone covered with a thin layer of compact bone. In adults the red marrow of irregular bones is an important site of haemopoiesis.

In addition to these groups are the sesamoid bones, which are a type of short bone formed within tendons. They develop close to joints and include the patella found at the front of the knee joint.

Structure of Bone

Gross structure of bone

At this stage it is useful to discuss the gross structural features of bones before looking at their microscopic features and composition in more detail. For our purposes this is best achieved by considering the features of a typical long bone such as the humerus or femur (*Figure 16.3*).

Long bones consist of a diaphysis and two epiphyses. During childhood, the two epiphyses are separated from the diaphysis by epiphyseal plates of cartilage. Growth in bone length occurs at these epiphyseal plates from the growing region of the diaphysis called the metaphysis.

The **periosteum** is a tough, fibrous connective tissue, closely covering the bone except for the articular surfaces of synovial joints (see Chapter 18), which are covered with hyaline cartilage (see Chapter 1). An outer

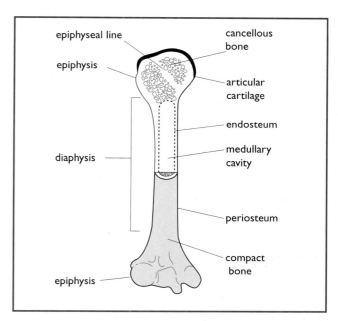

Figure 16.3 A long bone.

fibrous layer of periosteum contains the nutrient arteries and nerves that supply the bone, and under it lies an inner layer of **osteoblasts** concerned with growth in bone girth. The periosteum is attached to the bone by collagen fibres known as Sharpey's fibres. The periosteum also protects the underlying bone and provides attachments for muscles and ligaments.

As already mentioned, there is a central medullary cavity running within the diaphysis. This marrow-filled cavity is lined with a thin membrane, the **endosteum**, which contains both bone-forming osteoblasts and **osteoclasts,** which reabsorb bone.

The various physical features that form the bony landmarks are discussed in Chapter 18.

Microscopic features

The basic structural unit of bone tissue is the Haversian system, or osteon. Compact bone tissue has numerous osteons of regular structure, but in cancellous bone the osteons are far fewer in number.

Compact bone

An osteon comprises a central Haversian canal, which runs along the long axis of the bone surrounded by concentric rings of bone known as lamellae.

The Haversian canals carry the blood vessels, a few lymph vessels and nerve fibres supplying each osteon; these are also carried by smaller channels, called Volkmann's canals, which run at 90° to the Haversian canals.

Between the lamellae are spaces or lacunae that contain mature bone cells (**osteocytes**) and tissue fluid from which the bone cells obtain nutrients and dispose of waste [*Figure 16.4(a)*]. The lacunae connect with each other and the Haversian canal by channels called canaliculi, which are formed by osteoblasts during bone formation. This arrangement of bone tissue gives strength without weight and is sometimes referred to as lamellar bone (see page 370).

Cancellous bone

Cancellous bone is also formed from lamellar bone, but with fewer and larger osteons. In contrast to the regular compact structure, it is formed from a beam-like or trabecular network interspaced with marrow cavities, an arrangement well able to resist stresses placed upon the bone [*Figure 16.4 (b)*].

Composition

Bone contains water, organic molecules, bone cells (osteoblasts, osteocytes and osteoclasts) and inorganic mineral salts. The organic matrix, or osteoid, which consists of collagen and other organic molecules such as proteoglycans (protein plus polysaccharide), is produced by the osteoblasts. It forms around one-third of bone weight and gives bone its incredible tensile strength.

Inorganic salts deposited within the organic matrix during mineralization form the remaining two-thirds of the matrix and confer the extreme hardness characteristic of bone. The inorganic salts are hydroxyapatites, mainly calcium phosphate with some calcium carbonate and calcium hydroxide. Other minerals, present in smaller quantities, include magnesium and fluoride. Mineral crystals align themselves along the collagen fibres to produce bone tissue able to cope with compression forces of over 1400 kg/cm^2 – a massive force directed onto a small area (think about a ballerina's weight directed over a minute area of floor when she is 'on points', compared with when she wears trainers). Operating together, the collagen and minerals provide a material that is immensely strong and stretchy without being brittle, which is very reassuring when considering the forces to which our bones are subjected during most activities.

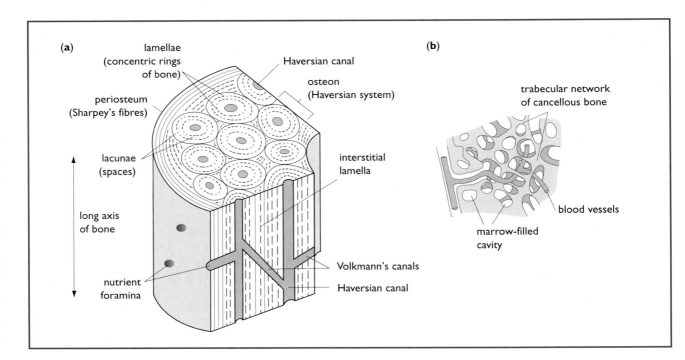

Figure 16.4 Microscopic structure of bone (canaliculi not shown). (**a**) Compact; (**b**) cancellous.

Ossification and Bone Growth

The formation and growth of bone occurs from week 6 of embryonic life as mesenchymal cells (embryonic connective tissue) are converted into cartilage or membranes, and continues after birth until the late teens or early 20s. *Figure 16.5* illustrates the development of bone in a simple long bone.

Ossification

In the fetus, bone develops from the ossification of either hyaline cartilage (endochondral) or fibrous membranes (intramembranous), which act as frameworks or 'patterns' for the developing bone.

Endochondral ossification of cartilage results in the formation of the long and short bones. The process starts as a primary ossification centre in the shaft of the bone 'pattern', and the development of a bone collar around the shaft. Primary ossification commences in the cartilage rods destined to become the long bones between weeks 8 and 12 of fetal development.

Accompanying these structural alterations are changes in blood and nutrient supply, the destruction of chondrocytes (cartilage-forming cells) and the development of osteoblasts, osteoclasts (see remodelling, pages 376–378) and red marrow cells.

Osteoblasts secrete collagen bony matrix (osteoid) into the cartilaginous framework and promote mineralization by the production of the enzyme alkaline phosphatase (see Chapter 14). As bone is produced the osteoblasts ensnared within the lacunae differentiate to form osteocytes, the exact role of which is not yet fully understood. Ossification spreads out towards the epiphyses, which are still mainly cartilaginous at birth, and the medullary cavity is formed as osteoclasts reabsorb bone in the centre of the shaft.

Secondary ossification centres form in the epiphyses during early childhood, resulting in further bone formation until only the epiphyseal growth plates remain as cartilage.

Intramembranous ossification is a less complex process by which bony replacement of fibrous membranes is responsible for flat bones and some irregular bones. A single ossification centre usually occurs in the membrane as mesenchymal cells differentiate into osteoblasts. These cells secrete osteoid matrix, which is soon mineralized to form trabeculae. As before, the osteoblasts are trapped within the lacunae, where they differentiate to osteocytes, and the woven bone is replaced by either compact or cancellous lamellar bone.

The ossification of specific bones occurs at predetermined stages during fetal development – a fact that can be used to assess the gestational age of a fetus. Overall the process of ossification starts and finishes earlier in a female fetus (England, 1983).

Bone growth

Bone growth after birth, which continues throughout childhood and adolescence, is usually complete by the late teens or early 20s (see Chapter 21). Bone growth takes slightly longer in males and certain bones such as the clavicle do not stop growing until as late as 25 years of age.

Even when true growth has ceased there is considerable structural change in adult bones through remodelling (see pages 376–378).

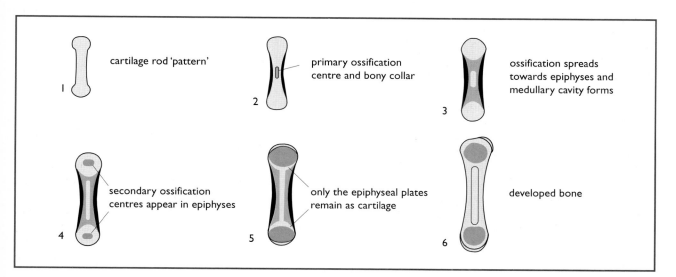

Figure 16.5 Bone development (endochondral).

Nursing Practice Application **Achondroplasia – very short stature**

Once the epiphyseal plates have ossified there can be no more endochondral growth in bone length. If this occurs too early the individual will have short stature because their long bones are abnormally 'short', but the trunk and most of the skull develop normally. This condition is termed achondroplasia and is caused by a faulty gene which codes for disordered cartilage growth and premature ossification of the growing cartilage in long bones, base of skull and pelvis. It is inherited as an autosomal (on one of the 44 autosomes) dominant condition, which is expressed if inherited from one parent, i.e. in the heterozygous state. Not everyone is affected to the same degree, but those in which the abnormal gene is fully expressed will experience considerable difficulties in a world that is generally planned for adults who achieve a height of 150 cm or more.

Imagine for a moment the frustration of trying to cope with furniture and worktops at inappropriate heights, getting clothes that fit, difficulties at work, using public transport and a multitude of situations which disadvantage the person with very short stature.

Growth in length

Growth in bone length continues by endochondral ossification at the epiphyseal plates. The process involves the production of new hyaline cartilage by chondrocytes followed by ossification, as previously described. Growth ceases when the epiphyseal plate is completely replaced by bone and the epiphyses fuse with the diaphysis. A remnant of the original cartilaginous pattern remains as the articular cartilage covering the ends of long bones.

Growth in girth or thickness

Growth in bone girth occurs by appositional growth, where osteoblasts situated in the osteogenic layer of the periosteum produce bone matrix that is then ossified.

Hormones and bone growth

The major hormone that stimulates bone growth at the epiphyseal plate is growth hormone (GH). The importance of GH is illustrated by the problems caused if secretion is disordered prior to epiphyseal plate ossification – gigantism (hypersecretion) and dwarfism (hyposecretion). When hypersecretion occurs after epiphyseal fusion it results in a condition called acromegaly, which is characterized by the growth of the facial bones and bones of the hands and feet (see Chapter 8).

The thyroid hormones (T_3 and T_4) also stimulate bone growth. A deficiency of these hormones in infancy (congenital hypothyroidism) leads to stunted skeletal development and growth (see Chapter 8).

During puberty (see Chapter 21) the sex hormones oestrogen and testosterone influence bone growth and cause the adolescent 'growth spurts'. In girls the secretion of oestrogen leads to the particular female bony changes, e.g. the wide pelvis adapted for child bearing, and in boys testosterone secretion accounts for the masculinization of the skeleton. The sex hormones, however, cause ossification of the epiphyseal plates, which explains why you stop growing in height after the 'growth spurts'.

The many other hormones concerned with bone homeostasis and remodelling, which include parathyroid hormone (PTH), calcitonin, vitamin D and cortisol, are discussed on pages 376, 377 and 378.

Peak bone mass

Peak bone mass (PBM) is usually reached between age 35 and 40 years, but the peak for trabecular bone may occur earlier. Most bone is formed during childhood and adolescence, with less than 10% being added during adulthood. Men achieve a greater PBM than women and Afro-Caribbean individuals have a greater PBM than Asians and Caucasians. Apart from these considerations, PBM is determined by factors that include genetic inheritance and the availability of the correct nutrients (see below). Further coverage of PBM can be found in the Healthier Living box.

Nutritional requirements for ossification and bone growth

Healthy bone formation, both before and after birth, is dependent upon the availability of the correct nutrients in sufficient amounts. Nutrients of particular importance in the formation of bone include protein, calcium and vitamins A, D and C (see Chapter 13). The intake of these, and energy, needs to be increased during periods of bone formation, such as pregnancy (extra calcium may be required in very young mothers), lactation, infancy, childhood and adolescence, and to facilitate the healing of fractures (see page 375).

Healthier Living Peak bone mass (PBM)

It makes good sense to achieve the best possible PBM as insurance against the age-related bone loss and susceptibility to fractures that occur in both men and women. Adequate calcium appears to be important in achieving PBM, especially during childhood, adolescence and early adulthood. In the UK the reference nutrient intake [(RNI) usually enough for 97% of a population] for adolescent females is 800 mg/day and 1000 mg/day for males (DoH, 1991). This intake can be achieved by including bread, milk, cheese and yoghurt in the diet; in addition, some calcium is obtained from drinking water in hard water areas. Rather worryingly, an Australian study (Portsmouth *et al.* 1994) found that 68% of females aged 18 years (sample 113) had calcium intakes less than those recommended (800 mg/day in Australia) and that this was linked to low-energy diets. As discussed earlier, calcium absorption depends on PTH and sufficient vitamin D, and is inhibited by substances which include phytic acid and phosphates (see Chapter 13). Crash diets and some eating disorders may result in low calcium intakes and weight loss, which in the female suppresses the menstrual cycle with its important oestrogenic stimulus for bone growth. Similarly, excessive exercise, which may accompany eating disorders such as anorexia nervosa, can affect the menstrual cycle, causing periods to cease (amenorrhoea).

Another plus for bone growth and PBM, however, is regular weight-bearing exercise in sensible amounts, e.g. walking, which has numerous other benefits, such as cardiovascular and respiratory health. Reaching a respectable PBM can be hindered by sedentary lifestyles, smoking and excessive alcohol intake.

Special Focus Fractures

A fracture or break in a bone is not an uncommon occurrence, despite the incredible strength of bone tissue. Most fractures are caused by trauma resulting from road traffic accidents, sports injuries and falls. Older people, with their weaker osteoporotic (see pages 377–378) bones, are particularly vulnerable to fractures as a result of falls, e.g. fractures of the wrist and neck of femur in older women. Fractures associated with existing bone disorders are said to be pathological. These fractures, which occur spontaneously or after minimal trauma, may be due to conditions such as osteomalacia (see page 377), osteogenesis imperfecta (brittle bone disease) and metastatic malignancy from a primary growth in the breast, prostate or bronchus.

Types of fracture (see *Figure 16.6*)
Fractures can be classified in a variety of ways, including severity, direction of the break and position on the bone, e.g. supracondylar fracture of the elbow (see Chapter 17, Person-centred Study – Dave).

Healing of fractures (see *Figure 16.7*)
The healing of fractures involves haematoma formation and organization (see Chapter 19), callus formation and remodelling.

Haematoma and organization
The initial events of fracture healing are those of the inflammatory process. The bleeding that occurs at the fracture site produces a haematoma and, within 24 hours, organization has commenced within the haematoma. Organization involves the phagocytosis of debris and growth of capillaries and fibroblasts (young cells of fibrous connective tissue) within the haematoma to form granulation tissue. Fibroblasts eventually become the chondroblasts and osteoblasts that produce the materials for the bony repair.

Callus formation
Fibrous connective tissue (callus) appears at the fracture site after about 1 week. The cartilage and osteoid (woven material) produced form a network which is later mineralized and converted to lamellar cancellous bone. The early callus, formed in about 3 weeks, is irregular in structure and relatively fragile. Later, as further ossification occurs, the bony callus becomes stronger and exhibits the usual orderly bone structure of Haversian systems.

Remodelling
Over many months the activity of osteoblasts and osteoclasts return the bone to its original form. The osteoblasts deposit new compact bone as required and osteoclasts restore the medullary cavity and reabsorb excess callus.

NB Readers may wish to compare the process of fracture healing with that of wound healing (Chapter 19).

The time taken for fracture healing to occur obviously depends on the type of fracture and the size of the bone involved; for example, the shaft of the femur will take much longer to heal than the clavicle. Apart from differences between bones, the factors that affect healing include blood supply, age, adequate immobilization of the fracture, apposition of the bone ends, nutritional status, general health and freedom from sepsis (infection).

Healthier Living **Reducing falls and fractures in older adults**

From our discussion about fractures you already know that falls in older adults result in many fractures, especially those of the wrist or femur. Fractures in older adults are associated with increased morbidity and mortality linked to complications of immobility or anaesthesia, e.g. pneumonia complicating a fractured neck of femur. To stress the importance of falls – in England (in 1991), 55% of deaths from accidents in those aged over 65 years were due to falls (DoH, 1993).

It is obviously in everyone's interests to reduce the incidence of accidents involving falls in older adults. The reduction in falls occurring in those aged over 65 years and in deaths from falls in people aged over 75 years is seen as an important local target in the *Key Area Handbook – Accidents* (DoH, 1993). Various initiatives are proposed, which include: monitoring the incidence of falls; home visits and assessment following falls; increasing risk awareness;

increasing safe mobility and exercise; checking visual acuity (see Chapter 7); advising on home safety, e.g. trailing wires; and assessing drug side-effects, such as postural hypotension or sedation, which may predispose to falls (DoH, 1993).

This list contains a few examples of measures that community-based nurses and other health/social care workers can initiate, but you will no doubt think of many more.

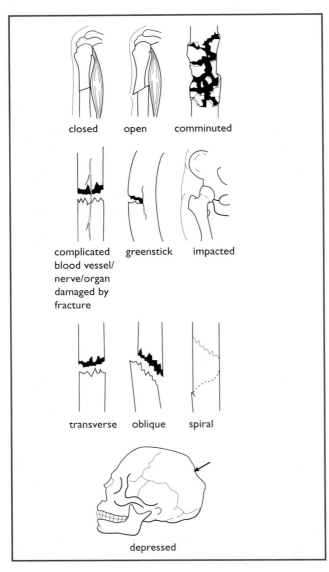

Figure 16.6 Types of fracture.

closed open comminuted

complicated blood vessel/ nerve/organ damaged by fracture greenstick impacted

transverse oblique spiral

depressed

Homeostasis and Bone Remodelling

Earlier we mentioned that bone is subject to constant change, with areas of new bone deposition by osteoblasts and bone reabsorption by enzymes and acids produced by osteoclasts. Deposition and reabsorption occur at both the periosteal and endosteal surfaces. In young adults around 5% of bone tissue is usually involved in the two remodelling processes, but this decreases later in life. The ability to remodel means that bones can respond to mechanical forces in a way that adds bone tissue and consequently strength to an area subjected to particular stresses.

Bone remodelling is controlled by various hormones, especially those whose primary function is calcium/phosphate homeostasis, by vitamin D and by the mechanical forces acting upon the skeleton. These controls maintain the precise balance between osteoblastic and osteoclastic activity, which ensures that the overall bone mass changes very little in healthy adults (remember peak bone mass occurs at age 35–40 years), although a decline in bone mass occurs with normal ageing.

Parathyroid hormone (PTH) secreted by the parathyroid glands, calcitonin secreted by the thyroid gland and vitamin D control calcium/phosphate homeostasis and hence bone remodelling (see Chapter 8). Remember that calcium/phosphate homeostasis is maintained through the action of PTH, calcitonin and vitamin D on bone, kidney and gut.

When blood calcium levels are low, PTH is secreted, which acts to raise calcium levels in several ways. Osteoclasts are stimulated to reabsorb bone matrix, which releases calcium and phosphate into the blood. Meanwhile PTH increases renal reabsorption of calcium and phosphate excretion. The kidneys also produce 1,25-dihydroxycholecalciferol, the active form of vitamin D, which

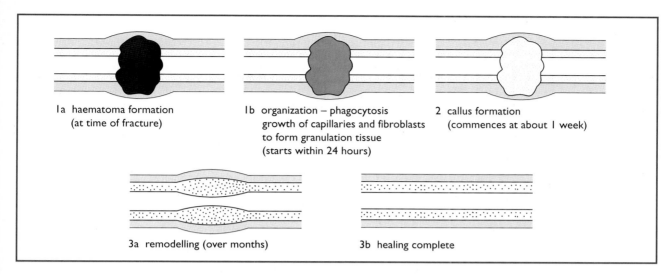

1a haematoma formation
(at time of fracture)

1b organization – phagocytosis
growth of capillaries and fibroblasts
to form granulation tissue
(starts within 24 hours)

2 callus formation
(commences at about 1 week)

3a remodelling (over months)

3b healing complete

Figure 16.7 Healing of fractures.

Abnormal Function **Problems with bone homeostasis**

Rickets and osteomalacia

To associate rickets and its adult equivalent, osteomalacia, exclusively with Victorian inner-city life or developing countries would be incorrect. Unfortunately these disorders both occur within developed economies such as the UK, where they are more common in Asian children and women who may have low levels of vitamin D (DoH, 1991).

Rickets is caused by lack of vitamin D during childhood, which results from a low vitamin D intake or lack of exposure to sunlight. The production of vitamin D from the action of ultraviolet light on sterols present in the skin is discussed in Chapters 13 and 19. Insufficient vitamin D prevents adequate calcium absorption and normal ossification processes cannot proceed. Development is delayed and, if untreated, bony changes occur that lead to permanent deformity, e.g. bow legs.

In adults a lack of vitamin D may also be due to malabsorption (see Chapter 13) or serious kidney or liver disease. Osteomalacia is a softening of the bones caused by a failure to mineralize the osteoid produced. The affected person has bone pain, deformity and an increased risk of fractures, which heal poorly.

Susceptible groups need information about foods rich in vitamin D and available calcium, and in certain situations the advisability of supplementing vitamin D intake, e.g. children living in areas where rickets is endemic. The benefits of exposure, within safe time limits, to ultraviolet light should be explained and where appropriate encouragement given to get out in the sunshine. This will not always be possible, as certain cultures find it unacceptable to uncover the limbs and body.

Osteoporosis

Osteoporosis is the loss of bone mass due to excess reabsorption without the usual balance of bone deposition. The bones, which retain their normal composition, become lighter and weaker. These structural changes lead to bones that deform and fracture more easily. Common sites for fracture are those bones that normally have a high level of trabecular bone, e.g. wrist, vertebrae and neck of femur. Other problems include loss of height and spinal deformity, which can lead to respiratory problems as lung expansion becomes restricted.

Osteoporotic changes are associated with ageing in both sexes, but are especially common in females when oestrogen levels decline during the climacteric. According to Williams and Fletcher (1995), 50% of Caucasian women can expect to sustain an osteoporotic fracture by 80 years of age and the risk for females is three times that for males. Early osteoporotic changes may be seen after a premature menopause and in younger women who have amenorrhoea associated with eating disorders and/or excessive exercise.

Other factors involved in the aetiology include level of calcium intake, which is important in achieving PBM (Francis, 1989) and phosphate intake, immobility, small stature, family history, corticosteroid therapy and Cushing's syndrome.

increases calcium absorption in the gut. In the UK the reference nutrient intake (RNI) for calcium varies with age and gender – for adults aged over 19 years it is 700 mg/day, with an extra 550 mg/day for lactating women (DoH, 1991). However, some authorities, for example, the US government, recommend higher levels.

As blood calcium levels rise, the secretion of PTH is inhibited and calcitonin is secreted. Calcitonin inhibits bone reabsorption and favours the activity of osteoblasts, which produce new bone matrix; as calcium is deposited within the newly formed matrix its level in the blood falls. At the same time renal and intestinal calcium absorption declines. Although the action of PTH and calcitonin do influence the activity of osteoclasts and osteoblasts, it must be emphasized again that their main role is that of calcium homeostasis.

Cortisol from the adrenal cortex increases bone reabsorption, which explains why loss of bone matrix density (osteoporosis) occurs in Cushing's syndrome (see Chapter 8) and is a side-effect of corticosteroid therapy.

Oestrogens and testosterone, so important in bone growth during adolescence, continue to have an influence on bone even after growth has ceased. Oestrogens stimulate osteoblastic activity and their decline during the climacteric is associated with postmenopausal osteoporosis in older women (see page 377, below and Chapter 21).

Mechanical forces and gravity have a profound effect upon the skeleton and bone remodelling – osteoblast activity increases when bone is subjected to prolonged mechanical stress and the bone becomes heavier. These forces, unlike hormones, are primarily concerned with bone dynamics rather than mineral homeostasis. The old adage of 'use it or lose it' is definitely true when applied to bone. Periods of prolonged immobility lead to loss of bone mass, such as that occurring when people become housebound or confined to bed (see Nursing Practice Application – osteoporosis). The decrease in bone mass resulting from immobility and lack of gravity during early space exploration programmes is now prevented by planned physical activity. That bone remodelling and deposition occur in response to mechanical stresses is accepted, but the mechanisms involved are more controversial. One possibility is that electrical activity produced by forces deforming the bone stimulate the cells required for remodelling. The fact that electricity can be used to stimulate bone deposition and speed the healing of fractures does tend to support the idea that electric currents are in some way involved in bone remodelling.

Nursing Practice Application Osteoporosis

The prevention of osteoporosis and its associated problems should start long before old age, through efforts aimed at attaining the best possible PBM and avoiding factors that act against bone deposition (see Healthier Living box). Another weapon in the battle against osteoporosis is the early detection (by measuring bone density) and treatment of low PBM or bone loss (Williams and Fletcher, 1995). In a recent article, Hunt (1996) described a pilot study, involving 76 women (aged 25–88), designed to ascertain the effectiveness of height loss as a means of screening for osteoporosis. The results indicated that height reduction is linked to low bone mass and may predict the occurrence of osteoporotic fractures.

Prolonged immobility at any age can lead to osteoporotic changes. Nurses should encourage exercise and physiotherapy for those who are housebound or confined to bed. It is particularly important that older people continue to undertake weight-bearing exercise, as this appears to slow or prevent age-related bone loss (Chow et al. 1987; Hamdy, 1990).

A diet containing adequate calcium, phosphate, protein and vitamin D should be encouraged, but a study by Stevenson et al. (1988) suggests that dietary calcium supplements in menopausal women have little influence on bone loss. This view is supported by the DoH (1991), who suggest that increasing calcium alone in postmenopausal women will not help because all the components (not just calcium) of bone are lost, and this loss is directly related to the decline in oestrogens. It should be stated, however, that this view is not universally accepted, and some authorities (Riggs and Melton, 1992) advocate an increased calcium intake, of 1000–1500 mg/day, for postmenopausal women. Research in the USA has shown that supplements of calcium and vitamin D, in people over 65 years, reducd bone loss and fracture rates (Dawson-Hughes et al. 1997). For some older women the use of oestrogens in the form of hormone replacement therapy (HRT), with calcium, to prevent bone loss may be appropriate, and here the nursing responsibilities include the planning of an education programme that meets the person's information needs with regard to this type of therapy and its effects.

NB HRT is covered in more depth within the general discussion of changes occurring during the climacteric, in Chapter 21.

Not all women will be able to, or indeed want to, take HRT. Other drugs/substances available to counteract the bone losses include:

- Inhibition of bone reabsorption – calcitonin, biphosphonates, e.g. disodium etidronate
- Stimulation of bone deposition – fluorides, vitamin D with PTH, and anabolic steroids.

Summary/Check List

Introduction – bone functions.
Bone tissue – woven, lamellar, compact, cancellous. Bone types – long, short, flat, irregular, sesamoid.
Bone structure – Gross structure. Microscopic features – composition.
Ossification – endochondral, membranous. Bone growth – length. Nursing practice application – achondroplasia: very short stature, girth, hormonal influences. Peak bone mass.

Nutritional requirements. Healthier living – peak bone mass. Special focus – fractures (types and healing). Healthier living – reducing falls and fractures in older adults.
Bone homeostasis and remodelling – hormones, mechanical forces. Problems with homeostasis – rickets and osteomalacia, osteoporosis. Nursing practice application – osteoporosis.

Self Test

1 Describe the functions of bone.
2 Give one example of each type of bone:
   (a) long;
   (b) short;
   (c) flat;
   (d) irregular;
   (e) sesamoid.
3 Draw a diagram of a typical long bone to illustrate the location of the epiphyses, epiphyseal line, diaphysis, medullary cavity, periosteum and endosteum.
4 Describe the Haversian system/osteon of compact bone.
5 Put the following in their correct pairs:
   (a) osteoclast;
   (b) hydroxyapatite;
   (c) lamellar bone;
   (d) collagen;
   (e) woven bone;
   (f) osteoid;
   (g) osteoblast;
   (h) calcium salts.
6 Which of the following statements are true?
   (a) All fetal bone formation is endochondral ossification.
   (b) Bone growth may continue until the mid-20s.
   (c) Growth hormone (GH) has a major influence on bone growth.
   (d) Increase in bone girth arises from the epiphyseal plate.
7 Describe the control of bone remodelling in a young adult.
8 What information would you give to Tom, aged 65, who asks how he might avoid or delay the bony changes of ageing?

Answers

1 See page 370.
2 (a) Femur, tibia, humerus, radius;
   (b) tarsals, carpals;
   (c) ribs, sternum, skull;
   (d) vertebrae, pelvis;
   (e) patella.
3 See page 371 and *Figure 16.3*.
4 See page 372.
5 a–g, b–h, c–e and d–f.
6 b, c.
7 See pages 376–378.
8 See page 378.

References

Chow R, Harrison JE, Notarius C (1987) Effects of two randomized exercise programmes on bone mass of healthy postmenopausal women. *BMJ* **295**:1441–1444.

Dawson-Hughes B, Harris SS, Krall EA *et al.* (1997) Effect of calcium and vitamin D supplementation on bone density in men and women 65 years of age or older. *New Eng J Med* **337**(10): 670–675.

Department of Health (DoH) (1991) *Dietary Reference Values for Food Energy and Nutrients for the United Kingdom.* Report on Health and Social Subjects, *no. 41* London: HMSO.

Department of Health (DoH) (1993) *The Health of the Nation. Key Area Handbook. Accidents.* London: HMSO.

England MA (1983) *A Colour Atlas of Life Before Birth.* London: Wolfe Medical Publications Ltd.

Francis RM (1989) Calcium's role in preventing and treating osteoporosis. *Geriatr Med* **19**(7): 24–26.

Hamdy RC (1990) Identifying risk factors for osteoporosis. *Geriatr Med* **20**(4): 49–51.

Hunt AH (1996) The relationship between height change and bone mineral density. *Orthopaed Nurs,* **15**(3): 57–66.

Portsmouth K, Henderson K, Graham N *et al.* (1994) Dietary calcium intake in 18-year-old women: comparison with recommended daily intake and dietary energy intake. *J Adv Nurs* **20**(6):1073–1078.

Riggs BL, Melton LJ (1992) The prevention and treatment of osteoporosis. *New Eng J Med* **327**: 620–627.

Stevenson JC, Whitehead MJ, Padwick M *et al.* (1988) Dietary intake of calcium and postmenopausal bone loss. *BMJ* **297**:15–17.

Williams P, Fletcher C (1995) Management and prevention of osteoporosis. *Prof Nurs* **10**(4):233–236.

Further Reading

Aloia JF (1993) *A Colour Atlas of Osteoporosis.* London: Wolfe Medical Publications Ltd.

Munday GR, Martin TJ, Eds (1993) *Physiology and Pharmacology of bone.* Berlin: Springer.

McMurdo MET, Mole PA, Paterson CR (1997) Controlled trial of weight bearing exercise in older women in relation to bone density and falls. *BMJ* **314**:569.

Vaughan JM (1981) *The Physiology of Bone,* 3rd edn. Oxford: Oxford University Press.

Useful Address

National Osteoporosis Society
PO Box 10
Radstock
Bath BA3 3YB

Muscle Tissue

Overview

- *Functions and structure of muscle tissue.*
- *Contraction of skeletal muscle tissue.*
- *Muscle metabolism.*

Learning Outcomes

After studying Chapter 17 you should be able to:

- Discuss the functions of muscle.
- Outline the characteristics of muscle.
- Describe the three types of muscle.
- Compare and contrast skeletal muscle with smooth muscle.
- Describe the gross structure of skeletal muscle.
- Discuss the effects of immobility and disuse on skeletal muscle.
- Describe the microscopic structure of skeletal muscle.
- Outline the events occurring when skeletal muscle contracts.
- Describe the types of muscle contraction and the phases of a twitch contraction.
- Explain how metabolism provides the energy required for muscle contraction.

Key Words

Actin – one of the contractile proteins forming the thin filaments (myofilaments) of the myofibril.

Insertion – the point at which a muscle is attached to the bone that it moves.

Myofibril – longitudinal bundles of contractile protein filaments within the muscle fibre.

Myofilament (filament) – contractile proteins forming the myofibrils; they may be thin (actin, tropomyosin and troponin) or thick (myosin).

Myoglobin – a haem–protein molecule found in skeletal muscle. It acts as a temporary oxygen store for muscle contraction.

Myosin – the contractile protein forming the thick filaments of the myofibril.

Origin – the fixed or immovable point at which a muscle is attached to the bone.

Sarcomere – a segment of myofibril that forms the smallest contractile unit of skeletal muscle.

Tendon – a band of white fibrous connective tissue that attaches muscle to bone.

Tropomyosin – one of the proteins found in the thin filaments of the myofibril.

Troponin – one of the proteins found in the thin filaments of the myofibril.

Introduction

Muscle is formed from excitable cells (cells which produce an action potential by reversibly altering potential difference across their membrane – see Chapter 3) which, in common with nervous tissue, are highly specialized and responsive to stimuli. These specially adapted elongated muscle cells (fibres) produce the contractions required for body movement and the movement occurring within body structures, e.g. peristalsis in the gut. Muscle cells take chemical energy in the form of ATP and convert it to mechanical energy and work.

This chapter is concerned with movement and stability, and we will concentrate on skeletal muscle, which forms over 600 individual muscles and accounts for around 40% of adult body weight. Smooth muscle is discussed in sufficient depth for you to compare it with skeletal muscle, but further coverage of smooth muscle is included in more appropriate chapters (Chapters 12, 13, 15 and 20), as is that of cardiac muscle (see Chapter 10).

Muscle Tissue

Early development

Nearly all muscle tissue develops from myoblasts derived from mesoderm; only iris muscle forms from ectoderm (England, 1983). Muscular activity commences well before birth – the heart is contracting by week 4 and skeletal muscle by around week 7. Fetal movements, however, are not felt by the woman until the middle third (second trimester) of pregnancy, at which time the mother-to-be first becomes aware of 'fluttering' feelings. Skeletal muscles develop mostly from mesodermal cells in the limb buds and from portions of mesoderm, called somites, in the trunk. The actual number of skeletal muscle fibres is complete at birth, but considerable muscular development and improvement in neuromuscular communication and coordination continues during infancy, childhood and adolescence. This is well illustrated by the motor development that occurs as babies and children grow and develop (see Chapter 21).

Functions of muscle tissue

Movement

Movement involving the body requires the contraction of muscle. Skeletal muscles provide the diverse abilities of gross and precise movements that allow us to move within our environment, and to investigate and respond as appropriate. Skeletal muscle contraction is also responsible for: the 'skeletal muscle pump' assisting venous return from the legs (see Chapter 10), eyeball movement (see Chapter 7), certain elements of sphincter control, e.g. external urinary sphincter (see Chapter 15), mastication and facial expression.

The smooth muscle of the alimentary tract moves food and waste (Chapter 13), the bladder empties when its smooth muscle contracts (Chapter 15), smooth muscle controls the diameter of blood vessels (see Chapter 10) and the bronchi (Chapter 12), and uterine smooth muscle contracts during the birth of a baby (Chapter 20).

The vital circulation of blood around the vascular system is totally dependent upon the rhythmic contraction of cardiac muscle, or myocardium (Chapter 10).

Posture and stability

The state of partial contraction (muscle tone) that exists in skeletal muscles helps to maintain stable postures. The ability to stand or sit for considerable periods depends on the activity of proprioceptors (see page 386 and Chapter 3) in muscles, **tendons** and joints. These signal minute changes to the nervous system, which can if necessary modify the partial muscle contraction required to maintain posture.

Heat production and temperature regulation

When you drive a car the engine gets hot whilst producing the mechanical energy required to move the wheels. When muscle is contracting it also produces heat energy in addition to the mechanical energy required for movement. This considerable amount of heat energy is used by the body to maintain temperature homeostasis (see Chapter 19). For instance, on a cold day the contraction of skeletal muscle produces shivering, which acts to increase body temperature.

General characteristics of muscle tissue

All types of muscle tissue possess (to some degree) the following physical properties:
- **Excitability:** muscle fibres react to stimulation (electrical, chemical or mechanical). Skeletal muscle responds to a nerve impulse, which has crossed the chemical synapse to produce an action potential in the muscle (see pages 389–390 and Chapter 3). Muscle tissue is also stimulated by hormones, changes in the local chemical environment and stretching.
- **Contractility and extensibility:** when sufficiently stimulated, muscle contracts (shortens). As muscle relaxes it extends and, in the case of smooth muscle, is capable of considerable stretching. This property allows for distension in hollow organs, e.g. in the stomach after a meal.

- **Elasticity:** this property ensures that muscle length returns to resting proportions following stretching or contraction.

Types of muscle tissue

Skeletal muscle (striated, voluntary) tissue

The skeletal muscles clothe the bony skeleton and facilitate movement. The individual cells or fibres are multinucleate (myoblasts fuse during development; see page 382) and form extended cylinders [*Figure 17.1(a)*]. A microscopic examination reveals banding or striations on the muscle fibre, which produces its striped appearance.

Skeletal muscle is the only muscle tissue that may be controlled consciously – that explains the term 'voluntary muscle'. In many cases, however, this control operates through reflexes that we do not consciously control (Chapter 5).

Skeletal muscle is stimulated by the voluntary motor division (somatic) of the peripheral nervous system (PNS) to produce the rapid, forceful contraction of short duration needed for movement. Although the fibres of skeletal muscle contract in series (one after the other – as the fibres of one motor unit contract others are relaxed), any muscle will eventually tire if required to contract for any period of time without rest, a fact of which you need no reminding after a session of intense muscular activity.

Smooth muscle (unstriated, visceral or involuntary) tissue

Smooth muscle forms part of the structure of the stomach, gut, bronchi, ureter, bladder, uterus and blood vessels. The spindle-shaped smooth muscle fibres, which are uninucleate, form flat sheets of contractile units [*Figure 17.1(b)*].

All smooth muscle is controlled involuntarily and there is no conscious regulation of contraction. Stimulation of smooth muscle occurs through the action of the autonomic nervous system (ANS) and various hormones/regulatory peptides; for example, gastric motility is affected by both vagal activity and local peptides (see Chapter 13).

The contraction of smooth muscle tissue differs from that of skeletal muscle in several respects. Smooth muscle responds more slowly, and the contraction, which is less intense than the contraction of skeletal muscle, is usually more sustained. Contractions of smooth muscle are more widespread, with all the fibres within the sheet able to contract in unison. In addition, some smooth muscle fibres act as 'pacemakers', which are capable of initiating inherent, rhythmic contractions that may be modified by neural or hormonal influences.

Cardiac muscle tissue (see Chapter 10)

Cardiac muscle is found only in the myocardium and, although it forms a distinct muscle type, it has common features with both skeletal and smooth muscle. Cardiac muscle has short branching fibres that may be uni- or binucleate. The fibres, like skeletal muscle fibres, are striated, but contraction is involuntary. The presence of inherent control via a 'pacemaker' produces steady rhythmic contractions which are modified by the ANS and hormones as physiological needs alter. Boundaries between individual fibres, which are not well defined, are formed by intercalated discs [*Figure 17.1(c)*]. This feature allows the wave of contraction to pass easily across the myocardium, which behaves like a syncitium (cell boundaries do not exist or are poorly defined).

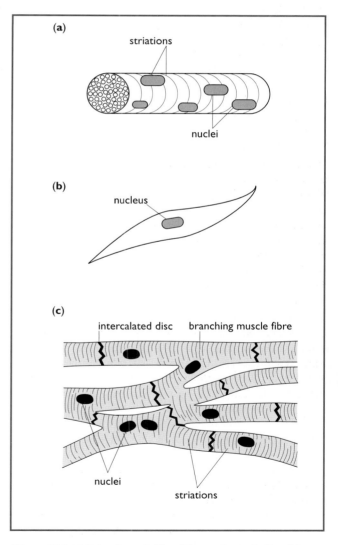

Figure 17.1 (a) Striated muscle fibre; **(b)** smooth muscle fibre; **(c)** cardiac muscle.

Table 17.1 Summary of the characteristics of skeletal, smooth and cardiac muscle tissue

Characteristic	Skeletal muscle	Smooth muscle	Cardiac muscle
Shape of fibre (cell)	Extended cylinders Striated	Spindle-shaped Not striated	Short branched fibres Striated
Nucleus – position and numbers	Multinucleate (peripheral)	Uninucleate (central)	Uninucleate and binucleate (central)
Contraction	Slow ⟶ fast	Very slow	Slow
Spontaneous contraction	No	Yes	Yes
Control	Voluntary	Involuntary	Involuntary
Special features	–	Pacemakers in some Gap junction in some	Pacemakers Intercalated discs between cells
Location and function	Attached to skeleton Body movement	Stomach, gut, bronchi, blood vessels, bladder, ureter and uterus. Moves food and waste through gut. Expels urine from bladder. Alters blood vessel size etc.	Myocardium of the heart. Pumps blood around the circulation

Table 17.1 Summary of the characteristics of skeletal, smooth and cardiac muscle tissue.

Skeletal Muscle Tissue

Gross structure

The 600 or so skeletal muscles are separate organs, which, in addition to muscle fibres arranged in bundles called fasciculi, contain blood vessels, nerves, lymphatics and connective tissue.

Earlier we mentioned that skeletal muscle forms around 40% of the body weight, but there are gender and age differences. In males muscle forms a greater percentage of body weight than in females, and this, with their generally larger body size, accounts for comparatively greater strength on average. Individual muscle fibres are of the same strength in both genders, but androgens are responsible for the increased muscle development in the male.

In normal ageing there is a gradual loss of muscle mass as fibres are replaced with connective tissue. These changes account for the decline in strength and weight loss experienced by older people, especially those over 80 years of age.

At every level a skeletal muscle is enclosed by fibrous connective tissue (remember how much shiny white tissue you remove whilst preparing beef for a stew). The whole muscle is covered by the epimysium; bundles of fibres (fasciculi) are enclosed within the perimysium and a thin layer of endomysium is found around individual fibres. These layers of connective tissue support the muscle as a whole and protect the fragile fibres (*Figure 17.2*).

Muscle attachments to the skeleton may be direct, with the outer connective tissue joining with the periosteum of the bone (see Chapter 16), or indirect by means of tendons. The epimysium merges into the tendons, formed of white fibrous connective tissue and collagen, which attach muscles to bones and other structures. Tendons are either rope-like structures, e.g. those of the biceps brachii in the arm, or flat sheets, known as aponeuroses, which form the attachments of the abdominal muscles.

The tendons, which also transfer the force of muscle contraction to the bone, and their collagen fibres, are well adapted to withstand the stresses involved.

Muscles are generally attached to the skeleton at two or more points: the **origin,** which is usually fixed, and the movable **insertion.** When a muscle contracts, the two points move closer together.

Muscle fibre arrangement

Skeletal muscles can be classified by the arrangement and direction of their fasciculi. The arrangement of the fasciculi will determine a muscle's movement range and power. Two basic patterns exist – the fasciculi may lie either parallel or oblique to the direction of the muscle pull. Generally muscles with long parallel fasciculi tend to have the greatest degree of movement, whereas the obliquely arranged muscles, with more fibres, have increased power. Variations on the two basic patterns include strap, fusiform, unipennate, bipennate, multipennate, circular, spiral and triangular (convergent). Some of these are illustrated in *Figure 17.3*. **NB** Pennate means shaped like a feather.

Muscle blood supply

Skeletal muscles require an abundant supply of oxygenated blood and receive about 1 litre/min, which represents about 20% of the cardiac output at rest.

During strenuous exercise the amount of arterial blood required to supply oxygen to the actively contracting muscles may increase to 15 litres/min or more as precapillary sphincters (see Chapter 10) in the muscles open. The increase in blood flow, which depends on the ability of the heart to maintain supply, is termed exercise or active hyperaemia.

This ability of skeletal muscle to regulate its own blood supply (autoregulation) is based on local chemical conditions, such as pH, potassium, carbon dioxide and oxygen levels, and the release of substances such as lactic acid. This causes the vasodilation and increased blood flow required to supply the metabolically active muscle with oxygen and fuel and to remove waste.

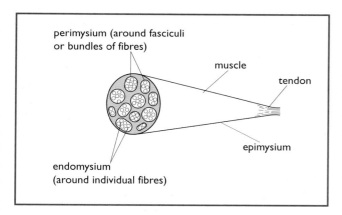

Figure 17.2 A muscle showing connective tissue.

The individual artery that supplies a muscle and its tendon, branches to form an extensive capillary network around individual muscle fibres. Eventually blood drains into the one or more veins required to remove the considerable metabolic waste produced by actively contracting muscle.

If the circulation to or from muscle tissue is impeded the muscle will, in the same way as cardiac muscle, undergo ischaemic changes. The results of ischaemia include necrosis, fibrosis, shortening, formation of deforming contractures (see Person-centred Study – Dave) and muscle atrophy (see Chapter 1).

Muscle nerve supply

Skeletal muscles are innervated by nerves that contain voluntary and autonomic motor fibres and sensory fibres.

Voluntary motor fibres

Muscle fibres are innervated by axons of lower motor neurones. Each axon supplies a group of fibres known as a motor unit (see *Figure 17.4*). The motor units vary in size. Those that cause precise movements contain few fibres, e.g. muscles of the fingers, but where movement is less precise the number of fibres in the motor unit increases, e.g. large muscles of the thigh.

You may wish to refresh your memory with a quick look at Chapter 4, but very briefly, the pyramidal motor pathway is a two-neurone system. An upper motor neurone arising in the motor cortex initiates voluntary muscle contraction on the opposite side of the body. This occurs because the neurone decussates in the medulla prior to continuing down the spinal cord to the appropriate level. Here, in the anterior horn, it synapses with the lower motor neurone that transmits impulses between the spinal cord and neuromuscular junction (see muscle contraction, page 389). Extrapyramidal motor pathways provide innervation for the synergistic muscle contraction necessary for smooth coordinated movement and posture.

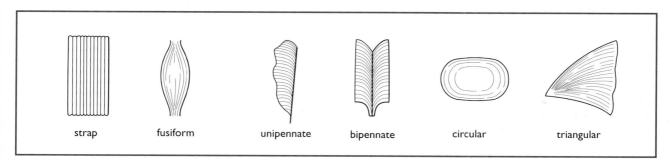

Figure 17.3 Arrangement of muscle fasciculi.

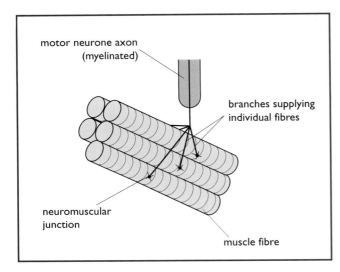

Figure 17.4 Muscle nerve supply – a motor unit.

Microscopic structure of muscle

The extended, cylindrical skeletal muscle fibres have a diameter of 10–100 μm, but there is considerable difference in length, which may range from a few millimetres to several centimetres.

A muscle fibre has a sarcolemma (plasma membrane) surrounding the sarcoplasm (called cytoplasm in other cells) which contains several peripheral nuclei [*Figure 17.5(a)*]. Within the sarcoplasm large quantities of stored glycogen and **myoglobin** (a haem–protein molecule which stores oxygen for muscle contraction) provide for the metabolic needs of contracting muscle.

The sarcoplasm consists mainly of bundles of longitudinal myofibrils [*Figure 17.5(b)*] formed from **filaments** of contractile protein molecules. In each **myofibril** there are thick filaments formed from **myosin** rods, which have the double 'club-like' heads required for binding with **actin** during contraction, and thin filaments comprised of globular G-actin, which form strands of fibrous F-actin, **tropomyosin** and **troponin** (*Figure 17.6*).

The thick and thin filaments are organized alternately in a repeating pattern [*Figure 17.5(c)*]. Because of overlap, this results in a banded appearance, with dark A bands each containing an H zone and an M line, and light I bands each containing a Z line. It is these bands in the myofibrils, which match across the muscle fibre, that give skeletal muscle its characteristic striations.

Each myofibril is divided into several **sarcomeres**, which are the smallest contractile unit of skeletal muscle. The region between two Z lines [*Figure 17.5(c)*] constitutes one sarcomere.

In each muscle fibre/cell there are two sets of tubules – one, formed from tubules of the sarcoplasmic reticulum (SR; a type of endoplasmic reticulum), surrounds the myofibrils in a loose network; and the other, a system of transverse or T tubules lined with sarcolemma, runs from the extracellular space to penetrate deep into the sarcoplasm (see *Figure 17.7*).

Autonomic motor nerves

Autonomic motor nerves are concerned with the regulation of blood flow through the muscle by control of the arteriolar smooth muscle and precapillary sphincters (see Chapters 6 and 10). Apart from neural controls, the metabolites produced within contracting muscle are responsible for the vasodilation and increased blood flow occurring during exercise (see page 385).

Sensory nerves

Sensory nerves relay information from the muscle proprioceptors found in muscle spindles, which are formed from modified non-contractile muscle fibres. This information is required by the CNS for maintaining posture through changes in muscle tone. Sensory fibres also transmit pain impulses such as those you experience the day after unaccustomed exercise.

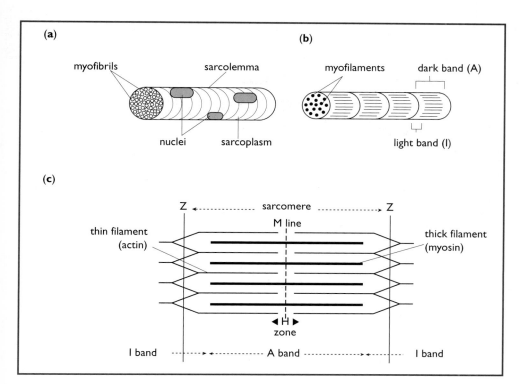

Figure 17.5 (a) Muscle fibre; (b) myofibril; (c) myofilaments.

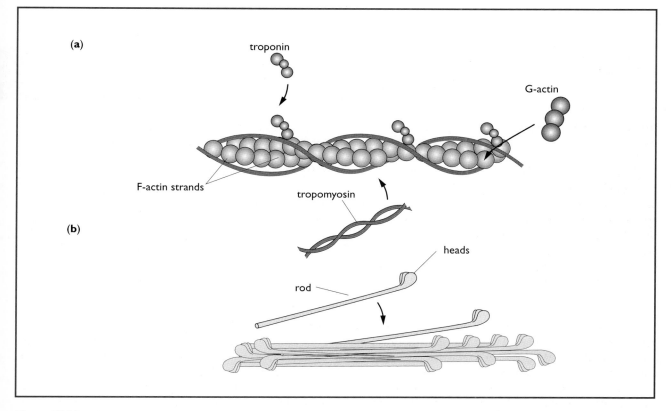

Figure 17.6 Detail structure of myofilaments. (a) Actin; (b) myosin.

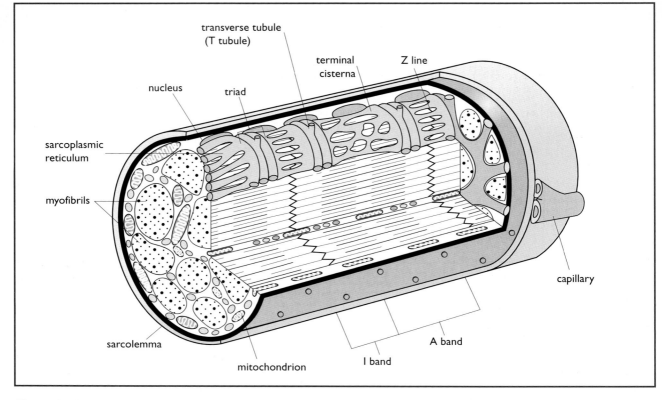

Figure 17.7 Skeletal muscle tubules – transverse tubules and sarcoplasmic reticulum.

Nursing Practice Application **Muscle changes in immobility**

Muscle bulk decreases due to the atrophy resulting from immobility (disuse atrophy), denervation and certain myopathies (disease affecting muscle), e.g. muscular dystrophy (see page 389). Problems of immobility may affect isolated muscles that are under-used when a fractured limb is immobilized (if you get the chance, compare the relative size of the uninjured and injured limb when a cast is removed following fracture healing), or the changes may be more general if someone is extremely immobile or confined to bed. These changes, apart from atrophy, where muscle bulk is replaced with fibrous tissue, also include obvious wasting, muscle weakness, weight loss and a reduction in mobility, which further exacerbates the problem. Older adults, who may be at particular risk, should remain active, which according to Wickham (1989) will maximize their muscle strength, maintain co-ordination and reduce the risk of falls (see Chapter 16).

Nursing interventions should anticipate the known effects of disuse with the introduction of countermeasures, including a full range of passive or active physiotherapy exercises and, where possible, early mobilization.

The risk of other problems of immobility can also be minimized by a regimen of planned exercise/movement, e.g. deep vein thrombosis (see Chapter 9), constipation (see Chapter 13), urinary stasis (see Chapter 15), loss of bone mass (see Chapter 16), joint stiffness (see Chapter 18) and pressure sores (Chapter 19).

Where the SR is in close proximity to the T tubules, it forms distended areas called terminal cisternae. The structural arrangement of a T tubule 'sandwiched' between two terminal cisternae is known as a triad.

The two tubular systems maintain the correct concentration of intracellular calcium and transmit the action potential to the contractile units. The SR is concerned with the amount of intracellular calcium, which it regulates by releasing calcium when required (remember calcium is also needed for synaptic transmission; see Chapter 3). The T tubules function to convey the action potential – when the action potential arrives at the muscle fibre, via the sarcolemma, it 'travels' at high speed through the T tubules to ensure that all the myofibrils in a sarcomere 'get the message' together and are able to produce a co-ordinated contraction.

Muscle Contraction

Shortening of the sarcomeres and hence the myofibrils results in muscle contraction. This can culminate in the whole muscle shortening by as much as 50%. Muscle contraction can be explained by the sliding filament hypothesis (*Figure 17.9*), which proposes that filaments slide against each other to cause shortening – however, the length of individual filaments is unchanged. The molecular structure of the contractile proteins facilitates the movement of the thin filaments (actin, tropomyosin and troponin), over the thick filaments (myosin), towards the centre of the sarcomere. The mobile 'heads' on the myosin filaments form cross-bridges, which attach to and pull the actin filaments (see excitation–contraction coupling, page 390).

Events occurring before, during and after contraction

At this point it might be helpful for you to look again at the transmission of the nerve impulse and synapse in Chapter 3, as skeletal muscle contraction depends on nerve stimulation.

Nerve stimulation and transmission of the action potential

The axons of the motor nerves transmit action potentials to the muscle. Within the muscle the axon forms unmyelinated terminal branches. These conduct the nerve impulse to the neuromuscular junction, or motor end plate [*Figure 17.8(a)*], which forms the communication between the axon terminal and the muscle fibre. This, however, is not journey's end, as the action potential must still cross the synaptic cleft [*Figure 17.8(b)*]. This is facilitated by the influx of calcium ions and the release of the neurotransmitter acetylcholine, from synaptic vesicles, which binds to receptors on the sarcolemma. Following synaptic transmission the acetylcholine is broken down very quickly by the enzyme acetylcholinesterase – this ensures that only one action potential crosses the synapse and prevents continuous muscle contraction.

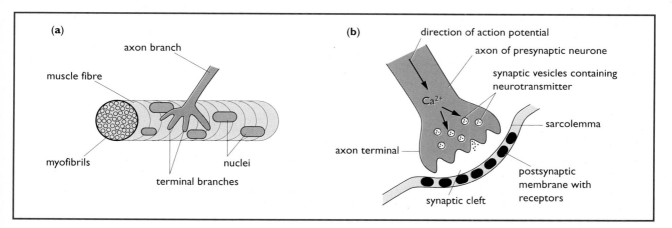

Figure 17.8 (a) Neuromuscular junction; (b) synapse.

Nursing Practice Application **Understanding myasthenia gravis**

Most people with myasthenia gravis have an abnormality of the thymus gland, which fails to control the interactions between its own T lymphocytes and the B lymphocytes responsible for producing autoantibodies, thereby causing loss of acetylcholine receptors (see Chapters 8, 11 and 19). People with myasthenia gravis have muscle weakness, which often causes eyelid drooping (ptosis); double vision (diplopia); problems with speech, coughing and swallowing; and extreme tiredness. The disease process may affect the muscles of respiration, with eventual respiratory failure. The medical management of myasthenia gravis may include drugs that inhibit acetylcholinesterase, so preventing the breakdown of acetylcholine, e.g. pyridostigmine; thymectomy (removal of the thymus); measures that oppose the antibodies (such as corticosteroids and immunosuppressive drugs); and plasmapheresis, where the antibodies are removed from the blood during plasma exchange.

Individuals with myasthenia gravis may need advice to help them structure their daily activities in a way that provides sufficient rest to reduce the tiredness that follows excessive muscle activity and to alleviate the problems of specific muscle weaknesses, e.g. those causing diplopia or the inability to swallow and cough. Another factor for the nurse to consider is that the problems experienced by individuals can be exacerbated by illnesses such as infections, and that, for women, pregnancy can cause a deterioration in condition.

Neuromuscular conduction can be disrupted by a variety of factors, which include:

- Electrolyte imbalances (see Chapter 2) – especially those affecting levels of potassium, which causes muscle weakness or calcium depletion (see tetany, Chapter 8).
- Toxins such as the botulinum toxin produced by the food-poisoning bacterium *Clostridium botulinum*, which blocks acetylcholine release at the synapse (see Chapter 3).
- Myasthenia gravis – an uncommon condition where skeletal muscle contraction does not proceed properly because acetylcholine receptors at the synapse are blocked or destroyed by autoantibodies (see Nursing Practice Application, above).

When a muscle fibre is not contracting its membrane is polarized – the inside of the sarcolemma has a negative resting potential of –90 mV with respect to the outside of the membrane. Depolarization occurs as the membrane (in response to acetylcholine binding) becomes more permeable with the opening of chemically-gated sodium channels to allow sodium ions to move into the muscle fibre (normally the sodium is outside and potassium is inside the fibre). This movement of sodium ions produces an action potential of +30 mV as the inside of the sarcolemma becomes positive, i.e. the membrane potential is reduced, compared with the outside. Now the area of depolarization spreads as more voltage-gated sodium channels open and the action potential is propagated to other areas of the sarcolemma. Lastly, repolarization of the sarcolemma occurs as potassium channels open to allow potassium ions out of the muscle fibre and channels close to stop more sodium ions entering – remember that later the sodium–potassium exchange pump will 'sort out' the normal intra–extracellular balance of ions (see Chapters 1 and 3). The membrane is again in the resting state and the action potential spreads rapidly into the myofibrils via the T tubules (see pages 388–389).

The conduction of the action potential in a muscle fibre obeys the same rules as does a nerve impulse: the all-or-none phenomenon operates, a threshold level of stimulation must first be reached, and absolute and relative refractory periods occur during and after stimulation (see Chapter 3). The actual stimulation to the muscle fibre lasts only a few milliseconds, but the effects in terms of muscle contraction last for several hundred milliseconds.

Excitation–contraction coupling

Myofibril contraction occurs as the action potential rushes into the muscle fibre via the T tubules. When the action potential reaches the triads (see page 388) it causes an enormous release of calcium from the sarcoplasmic reticulum. Calcium ions diffuse through the now permeable membrane of the sarcoplasmic reticulum, resulting in a huge increase in intracellular calcium levels. As calcium binds to the troponin the position of tropomyosin is altered to uncover active sites on the actin filament. In a process requiring ATP, the myosin filament heads form cross-bridges that attach to the actin filaments. The mobile myosin heads attach and move (power stroke), and detach and move (recovery stroke) several times, to slide the actin filament towards the centre of the sarcomere, which causes contraction of the fibre (*Figure 17.9*). It is worth stressing the importance of ATP in the formation, movement and detaching of the cross-bridges – before a cross-bridge can detach, the myosin head must first bind with another molecule of ATP. This is well illustrated by the process of stiffening (rigor mortis) that occurs some hours after death – the muscles contract because the cross-bridges formed, in

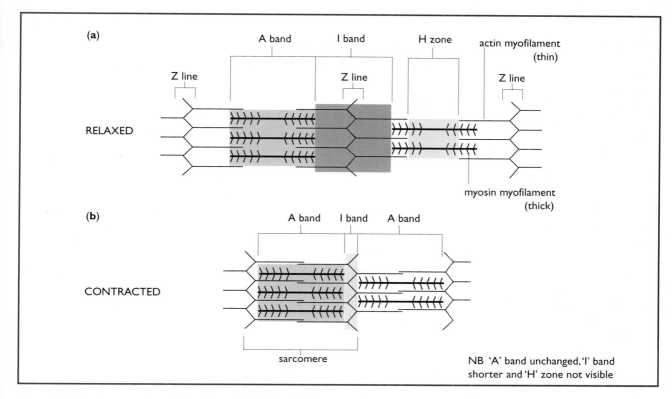

Figure 17.9 Muscle contraction – 'sliding filaments'. (**a**) Relaxed; (**b**) contracted.

response to calcium leaking from the sarcoplasmic reticulum, cannot detach without ATP. (**NB** Rigor later disappears as the myofilaments start to break down as part of general postmortem changes.)

Relaxation

Relaxation occurs when action potentials cease and calcium moves, by active transport, back into the sarcoplasmic reticulum. Troponin loses its calcium ions and, because the tropomyosin moves to block the active binding sites on the actin, no more cross-bridges can form and the filaments return to their resting length.

Types of contraction in a skeletal muscle

Muscles contract to produce the tension which, when transmitted to the skeleton, produces movement or stabilizes the body. The tension or force of contraction must, however, be sufficient to overcome the resistance of the load before the muscle will shorten; for example, your arm muscles must produce enough tension to overcome that exerted by heavy shopping before you can lift a bag.

Twitch contraction occurs in response to an isolated action potential; there is a latent period (period following muscle fibre stimulation before contraction commences) prior to the contraction, which is followed by relaxation (*Figure 17.10*).

In reality the single twitch contraction is unusual; what usually happens is a graded response where summation of contractions occurs. Summation produces smooth, sus-

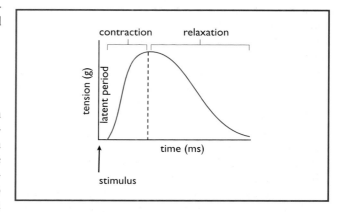

Figure 17.10 Isolated muscle twitch contraction.

tained contraction where tension is increased as required. Wave summation, where increased force is achieved by increasing the frequency of stimulation to a maximum level, which produces a sustained contraction, known as tetanus. (**NB** Remember that tetanus is also the name of a bacterial disease in which bacterial toxins affect motor nerves, causing muscle spasm, rigidity and convulsions.) In multiple motor unit summation or recruitment, extra motor units become involved to increase the force of contraction.

The strength of muscle contraction may show a stepped (treppe) response to stimulation – this is seen in rested muscle fibres when they first start contracting. As the muscle 'warms up', the strength of its response (contraction) to the same degree of stimulation increases to a maximum (see Healthier Living – exercise).

A contraction where the tension is constant is termed isotonic. Here the muscle shortens to produce movement as the load tension is overcome, e.g. walking or lifting your shopping.

The other type of contraction – isometric contraction – is where tension in the muscle increases without muscle shortening. This occurs when you push against a fixed object or hold a posture. The tension is insufficient to overcome that of the load and no movement occurs. Most of our muscle contraction is a combination of isotonic and isometric.

Even when contractions are not occurring skeletal muscles never fully relax – some fibres will be in a state of partial tension known as muscle tone. This muscle tone, which is controlled through stretch receptors and spinal reflexes (see Chapter 5), is vital in sustaining posture and ensures that skeletal muscles are always ready to contract (rather like being 'on call').

Metabolism – Energy for Working Muscles

Active contracting muscle requires ATP to provide the energy to power contraction through the formation and detachment of cross-bridges (see page 390). The ATP is produced in three ways:

- At the start of contraction from a coupled reaction where creatine phosphate, a high-energy molecule stored in muscle, reacts with adenosine diphosphate (ADP) to form ATP:

Creatine phosphate + ADP $\longrightarrow$ ATP + Creatine

The ATP produced in this way will 'tide you over' until other synthetic pathways for ATP have time to get going. The reaction is facilitated by the enzyme creatine kinase. If muscle is damaged the enzyme is released into the blood, where levels can be measured to assist in diagnosis (see Chapter 10).

- From the aerobic use of glucose, glycogen and fatty acids (see Chapter 13) when a continuous supply of oxygen is available from the blood and myoglobin. Most of the ATP is produced during the complex processes involved with the electron transfer chain and oxidative phosphorylation occurring in the mitochondria.
- After prolonged muscle contraction the oxygen supply and utilization is reduced and ATP is produced by the anaerobic metabolism of glucose and pyruvic acid. This process results in an 'oxygen debt' (see Chapters 12 and 13), where increased oxygen consumption may continue for some while, and the formation of lactic acid – the waste product that causes muscle ache felt after exercise. Most of the lactate is converted to carbon dioxide during aerobic processes in other tissues (including slow-twitch muscle; see page 393). Some, however, is recycled, via the Cori cycle (see Chapter 13), where it is converted aerobically to glucose in the liver. This glucose can then be made available for further muscle contraction.

There is a limit to these processes, and when insufficient ATP is forthcoming a condition known as muscle fatigue develops. No amount of will-power can overcome the fatigue as myofibrils cannot contract until ATP is replenished. It does not matter how much you want to complete the last mile of a sponsored run; the muscle fatigue, if it occurs, will dash your hopes. The development of fatigue may include factors such as a fall in pH in the muscle, caused by lactic acid, and local electrolyte imbalance.

Psychological factors also cause fatigue: you may feel that you 'cannot go on', but if there is ATP around you can still be roused to make a further effort – perhaps by the sight of family and friends waiting at the finish line.

An absolute lack of ATP will also cause problems because the cross-bridges are unable to detach – the result is a physiological contracture (contraction is continuous) or cramp (see rigor mortis, pages 390–391).

Fast and slow fibres – contraction speed, duration and degree of fatigue

Earlier we described a general type of skeletal muscle fibre, but in fact individual muscles contain both fast (two types for rapid movement) and slow (sustained movement and posture) muscle fibres, which have very different

Healthier Living **Exercise**

Probably most benefit (increased endurance and strength) is derived from activities that utilize both aerobic and anaerobic muscle metabolism. It is important to think about increasing activity within daily routines, e.g. using stairs rather than the lift – not just thinking of exercise as something we do specially.

Apart from the effects on muscle, regular exercise can produce many beneficial physiological effects. Respiratory and cardiovascular systems function more efficiently; for example, cardiac output increases with improvements in stroke volume (Chapters 12 and 10). Other benefits of exercise include the maintenance of bone (see Chapter 16), joint stiffness prevention (see Chapter 18), avoidance of obesity and prevention of constipation (see Chapter 13). Additionally, there is a sense of well-being associated with improved body image and self-esteem.

It is important, however, to remember some basic rules before increasing activity/exercise:
- You should build up slowly as your fitness increases – with intense unaccustomed exercise there is a real risk of cramp, muscle fatigue, injury and exhaustion.
- There should always be a 'warm-up' period prior to the activity, as muscle functions better when warm (see muscle metabolism, page 392).
- There should be a gradual slowing down at the end of a session.

Some sensible guidelines for activity/exercise are covered in a comprehensive booklet produced by the Health Education Authority (1996) – see Further Reading.

---

characteristics. Imagine for a moment: a cat sits motionless (slow fibres) by a mouse hole until the mouse makes a dash across the room (fast fibres) and then the cat pounces (fast fibres) and you jump (or perhaps think about it) onto a chair (fast fibres). The proportions of fast and slow fibres present will determine your particular athletic ability – whether you are better at darting across a squash court (more fast fibres), or at longer distance running or walking (more slow fibres), or equally proficient in all activities where the fibre mix is more equitable.

Fast-twitch muscle fibres

Many authorities describe two types of fast muscle fibres: one that tires easily – white fast-twitch; and an intermediate fast-twitch type (falling between the extremes of fast and slow fibres) that is more fatigue-resistant.

Fast-twitch fibres are pale because they contain very little myoglobin and their blood supply is not abundant. They are large fibres, have few mitochondria and contain a type of myosin that can use ATP very rapidly – which makes them good at rapid, vigorous contraction for short bursts of intense activity. White fast-twitch fibres are well adapted to produce ATP anaerobically from large (but exhaustible) glycogen reserves. The activity of white fast-twitch fibres, however, is severely limited by early fatigue due to running out of fuel and the build-up of lactic acid.

The intermediate fast-twitch fibres are also concerned with fast contraction, but they have greater fatigue resistance by virtue of their ability to produce ATP by aerobic pathways. They have more mitochondria, a lot of myoglobin and some glycogen.

Slow-twitch muscle fibres

Slow-twitch fibres are red in colour, reflecting their plentiful blood supply and higher myoglobin content. These fibres are small and their myosin uses ATP more slowly than fast-twitch fibres – they contract more slowly and less vigorously, but they can contract for longer before tiring (fatigue resistant). Slow-twitch fibres have many mitochondria, and with their 'in house' supplies of oxygen from myoglobin they are able to produce ATP by aerobic pathways even when the circulation is not providing sufficient oxygen. As you would expect, they have only very small reserves of glycogen.

Exercise and muscle

Both aerobic exercise, e.g. cycling, and anaerobic exercise, e.g. weight training, affect muscle fibres in a variety of ways. Aerobic effects, mainly affecting slow-twitch fibres, are:
- The blood supply improves through capillary proliferation.
- An increase in myoglobin and mitochondria means that ATP is produced more efficiently.
- Fibres develop fatigue resistance and endurance.
- There is a very limited increase in size.

Anaerobic effects, mainly affecting fast-twitch fibres, are:
- Fast-twitch muscle fibres hypertrophy (increase in size; see Chapter 1) and muscle bulk increases.
- Increased glycogen.
- Individual fibres become stronger and more powerful.

NB Compare these effects with what happens with immobility (see page 388).

Nursing Practice Application **Sport and leisure for people with learning disabilities**

Participation in sport and leisure activities can improve many aspects of the health and lives of people with learning disabilities. Activity can improve co-ordination, posture, balance and strength, and help to prevent obesity with its attendant problems. There are also gains for the person in terms of social skills, communications, increased independence and a sense of achievement, e.g. a child who sits upright, for the first time, during a horse-riding session. Individuals may be 'put off' sport and leisure activities by lack of confidence and slower learning skills (McLatchie *et al.* 1995), and nurses and carers can help through encouragement and support.

Abnormal Function **Problems with muscle damage**

Highly specialized skeletal muscle has very little regenerative ability, but relatively minor injuries where nerve and blood supply remain intact will 'heal' with no adverse functional effects. This healing probably occurs by the hypertrophy of existing fibres, not through the production of new fibres. More major damage is repaired by fibrosis, which in some situations leads to impaired function.

Very serious crush injuries (crush syndrome), such as those associated with being trapped under fallen masonry, may be complicated by myoglobin released from the crushed muscles into the circulation (myoglobin 'leaks out' when muscle cells are disrupted). This type of crush injury results in severe shock, with circulatory failure and, possibly, renal failure (see Chapter 15).

Summary/Check List

Introduction. Muscle – functions, general characteristics, types.
Skeletal muscle – gross structure, blood supply and problems. Person-centred study – Dave. Muscle innervation, Nursing Practice Application – muscle changes in immobility. Microscopic structure. Muscular dystrophy.
Muscle contraction – 'sliding filament' hypothesis. Contraction events – neuromuscular transmission. Nursing

Practice Application – understanding myasthenia gravis, excitation–contraction coupling. relaxation. Types of contraction.
Muscle energy – ATP production, oxygen debt, muscle fatigue. Fast and slow fibres. Exercise and muscle. Healthier Living – exercise. Nursing Practice Application – sport and leisure for people with learning disabilities. Muscle damage/crush injuries.

Self Test

1 Complete the following:
Muscle functions include body _ _ _ _ _ _ _ _ , maintaining _ _ _ _ _ _ _ and _ _ _ _ _ _ _ _ _ and _ _ _ _ production.
2 Explain excitability, contractility, extensibility and elasticity.
3 Compare and contrast skeletal and smooth muscle.
4 Which of the following statements are true?
(a) Individual muscle fibres are of the same strength in both males and females.
(b) The endomysium encloses the whole muscle.
(c) Most muscles have at least two attachments, the origin and insertion.

(d) Muscle fasciculi arrangement is either parallel or oblique to the direction of pull.
5 Outline the effects of ischaemia on skeletal muscle.
6 Put the following in decreasing size order:
(a) myofibril;
(b) muscle;
(c) muscle fibre;
(d) myofilament.
7 Outline the 'sliding filament' hypothesis.
8 (a) How does muscle produce the ATP required for contraction?
(b) What happens when insufficient ATP is available?

Answers

1 Movement, posture, stability, heat.
2 See pages 382–383.
3 See page 383 and *Table 17.1*.
4 a, c, d.
5 See page 385.

6 b, c, a, d.
7 See pages 389–391.
8 (a) Creatine phosphate + ADP, aerobic use of fuel molecules, anaerobic use of glucose;
(b) muscle fatigue.

References

England MA (1983) *A Colour Atlas of Life Before Birth*. London: Wolfe Medical Publications Ltd.

McLatchie G, Harries M, King J et al. (1995) *ABC of Sports Medicine*. London: BMJ Publishing Group.
Wickham C (1989) Falls in the elderly. *Nurs Times* **85** (40): 50–51.

Further Reading

Health Education Authority (1996) *Getting Active Feeling Fit*. London: HEA.
Huxley HE (1965) The mechanism of muscular contraction. *Sci Am* **213**(6): 18–27.

Ray WA, Taylor JA, Meador KG et al. (1997) A randomized trial of a consultation service to reduce falls in nursing homes. *JAMA* **278**(7):557-62

Skeleton, Joints and Muscular System

Overview

- *Axial and appendicular skeleton.*
- *Levers.*
- *Joints.*
- *Muscle groups.*

Learning Outcomes

After studying Chapter 18 you should be able to:

- Name the bones forming the axial and appendicular skeleton.
- Name and describe the bones of the skull and face.
- Describe how the skull of an infant differs from that of an adult.
- Describe the location and functions of the paranasal air sinuses.
- Describe the structure of the vertebral column, including the intervertebral discs and ligaments.
- Describe normal spinal curvatures.
- Describe the common features of all vertebrae and the adaptations found in each type that relate to function.
- Outline the causes of prolapsed intervertebral disc and discuss ways in which it may be prevented.
- Describe the sternum and ribs.
- Name and describe the bones of the pectoral girdle, arm and hand.
- Name and describe the bones of the pelvic girdle, leg and foot.
- Discuss the structural differences between the female and male pelvis, relating these to function.
- Describe the foot arches.
- Outline the principles of levers and relate them to body movement.
- Classify joints by structure and function.
- Describe the general features of joints and give examples of fibrous, cartilaginous and synovial joints.
- Name the different types of synovial joint and the movements possible at each.
- Describe some common joint disorders.
- Outline the structure of the shoulder, elbow, wrist, hip, knee and ankle joints; and describe the movements possible at each and the major muscles involved.
- Explain how muscles are named.
- Explain muscle movement relationships and describe the function of prime movers, antagonists and synergists.
- Name and describe the location of some major muscle groups and outline their action.

Key Words

Amphiarthrosis – a slightly movable joint.
Antagonist – a muscle that opposes or limits the action of a prime mover.
Appendicular skeleton – the limbs and limb girdles.

Articulation – a joint formed between two or more bones.
Axial skeleton – the bones that form the longitudinal axis – skull, sternum, ribs and spine (vertebral column).
Diarthrosis – a freely movable or synovial joint.

Key Words cont.

Ligament – fibrous connective tissue that joins bones and stabilizes joints.
Pectoral (shoulder) girdle – the clavicles and scapulae, which join the arms to the axial skeleton.
Pelvic (hip) girdle – the two innominate bones, which join with the sacrum posteriorly and attach the legs to the axial skeleton.
Prime mover – a muscle primarily responsible for a particular movement.

Synarthrosis – an immovable joint.
Synergist – a muscle that assists a prime mover, cancels out unwanted movement or contracts to stabilize joints not involved in a particular movement.
Vertebral column (spine) – consists of 33 vertebrae, of which 24 are unfused (individual bones) and 9 or 10 are fused (joined).

Introduction

This chapter completes our study of movement and stability, with coverage of the skeleton, joints and muscles. It is important to understand the high level of co-ordination existing between bones, joints and muscles, and your knowledge from Chapters 16 and 17 should be integrated with the material in this chapter. Only the early development of joints is covered in this chapter; readers are directed to Chapter 16 for development of bone and to Chapter 17 for that of muscle tissue.

Your understanding will be greatly enhanced if you look at, and feel, the structures in question. Where possible, you should use the 'working model' provided by yourself, or specimen bones and models.

It is not the purpose of this book to give complete detail of every bone and muscle; readers requiring more information are directed to Further Reading (e.g. Williams *et al.* 1995).

Skeleton

The bony skeleton is the framework of the body and consists of some 206 bones (*Figure 18.1*). Its incredibly well designed structure, which acts as levers for movement, supports and protects organs (see Chapter 16), can be divided into two parts:
• The **axial skeleton,** which is the longtitudinal axis of the body and consists of the skull, spine, sternum and ribs and hyoid bone.
• The **appendicular skeleton,** formed from the pectoral (shoulder) girdle, upper limb, pelvic (hip) girdle and lower limb.

Bony landmarks

Before considering specific bones, it might be useful to discuss some bony landmarks. The bones comprising the skeleton have various 'holes, hollows and bumps', none being smooth or completely regular. These landmarks are useful in describing the surface geography of the bone just as we use hills and dales to describe a landscape. Their real purpose, however, is to allow the passage of nerves and blood vessels, provide muscle attachments and form joints (see *Table 18.1*).

Axial Skeleton

The skull

The skull is formed from flat or irregular bones (see Chapter 16) – 8 in the cranium (calvaria) and 14 facial bones (see *Figure 18.2*). The infant cranium is large in relation to the face, and the joints (sutures) are not fully ossified at birth (see pages 402–403).

The cranium

The cranium forms a bony box that surrounds and protects the brain. The upper part forms the vault and a lower part is called the base. The bones that form the cranium – the frontal, two parietal, two temporal, occipital, sphenoid and ethmoid – have a smooth exterior but are grooved and ridged internally to accommodate the brain and vessels. Ridges divide the base of the skull into three fossae – anterior, middle and posterior – each containing a different part of the brain (see *Figure 18.3*). Numerous foramina and other openings in the cranial bones, especially those of the base, allow the passage of nerves and blood vessels.

Frontal bone
The frontal bone forms the forehead, part of the orbit and the ridges (supraorbital margins) above the eyes. The supraorbital margin contains a notch through which

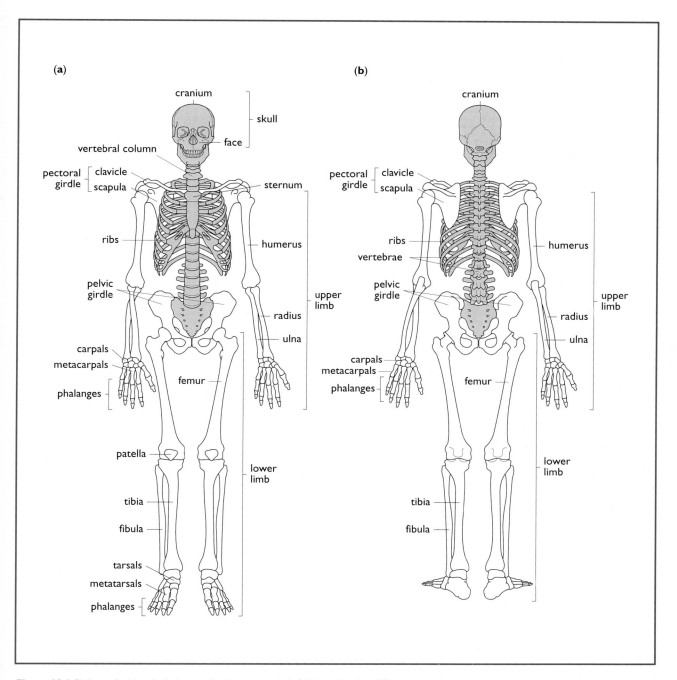

Figure 18.1 Skeleton (axial = shaded, appendicular = unshaded). (**a**) Anterior view; (**b**) posterior view.

vessels and nerves pass. The two halves of the frontal bone are joined by the frontal suture, and the coronal suture unites the frontal and parietal bones. The frontal bone also joins with several other skull bones (see *Figure 18.2*). Two paranasal sinuses are situated in the frontal bone.

Parietal bones

The two parietal bones form the lateral walls and the roof of the skull. They are joined to the frontal bone, to the temporal bone by the squamous suture, to the occipital bone by the lambdoidal suture and to each other by the sagittal suture.

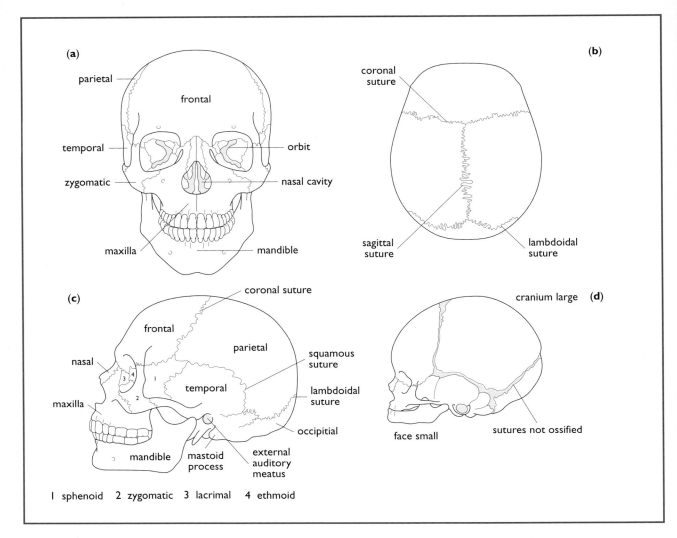

Figure 18.2 Skull and sutures. (**a**) Adult skull – anterior view; (**b**) adult skull – superior view; (**c**) adult skull – lateral view; (**d**) infant skull.

Figure 18.3 Interior of the base of skull.

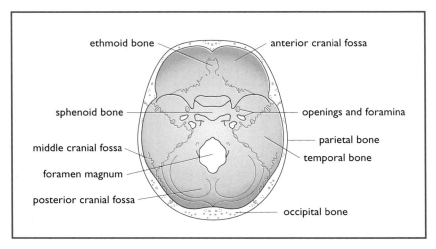

Table 18.1 Common bony landmarks	
Landmark and description	**Examples of particular clinical importance**
Openings and indentations	
Fissure – narrow cleft	Orbital fissure of sphenoid bone
Foramen – an opening	Foramen magnum in occipital bone
Fossa – a shallow cavity	Pituitary fossa in sphenoid bone
Meatus – a passageway	External auditory meatus in temporal bone
Sinus – air-filled cavity within a bone	Maxillary sinuses in the maxillae
Prominences and projections	
a. Providing attachment for ligaments and muscles	
Crest – narrow ridge	Crest of the tibia
Epicondyle – bony eminence upon or above condyle	Medial and lateral epicondyles of the humerus
Process – bony eminence	Mastoid process of temporal bone
Spine – sharper bony eminence	Vertebral spines (spinous processes)
Trochanter – large, irregular prominence	Greater and lesser trochanters of the femur
Tuberosity – rough prominence	Tibial tuberosity
Tubercle – small round prominence	Tubercle at lower end of femur
b. Forming joints	
Condyles – rounded articular surface	Condyles at the upper end of the tibia
Facet – flat articular surface	Facets on thoracic vertebrae for ribs
Head – bony projection on a neck	Head of humerus, which articulates with the scapula
Ramus – thin bony projection	Rami of the lower jaw

Table 18.1 Common bony landmarks.

Temporal bones

The temporal bones form the lower lateral walls and part of the base of the skull (*Figure 18.4*). Each bone is divided into four parts:

- A squamous part that extends upwards to join with the parietal bone. Projecting from the squamous part is the zygomatic process, which joins the zygomatic bone to form the zygomatic arch.
- The tympanic part contains the external auditory meatus. The styloid process projects from its lower border.
- The mastoid process, which is the prominence felt behind the ear, contains tiny air cells which communicate with the middle ear. Infection spreading from the middle ear may cause serious infection of the air cells (mastoiditis), that can spread to infect the brain.
- The petrous portion forms part of the middle cranial fossa of the base of skull and contains the organ of Corti and the semicircular canals of the inner ear (see Chapter 7).

The temporal bones provide attachment for many muscles and articulate with the mandible at the temporomandibular joints.

Occipital bone

The occipital bone forms the back of the cranium and part

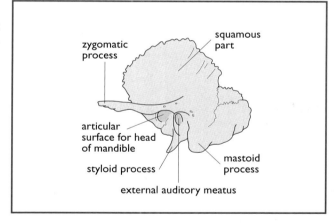

Figure 18.4 Temporal bone (left, viewed from the side).

of the base of the skull (see *Figure 18.5*). It joins with the temporal, parietal and sphenoid bones. It contains an opening, the foramen magnum, through which the spinal cord passes. On each side of this foramen are condyles (*Table 18.1*), which form articulating surfaces for the first cervical vertebra (atlas). The base of the occipital bone forms the posterior cranial fossa, which contains the cerebellum and part of the cerebrum.

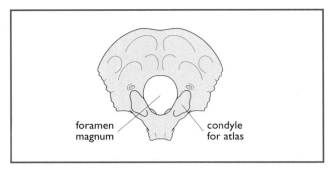

Figure 18.5 Occipital bone (viewed from below).

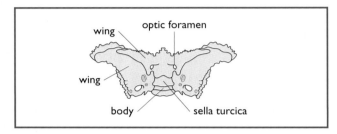

Figure 18.6 Sphenoid bone (superior view).

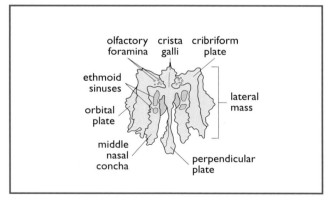

Figure 18.7 Ethmoid bone (anterior view).

Sphenoid bone

The bat-shaped sphenoid bone forms part of the middle cranial fossa of the base of the skull (*Figure 18.6*). A depression in its body, called the sella turcica (pituitary fossa), accommodates the pituitary gland (see Chapter 8). The sphenoid, which joins with all the other cranial bones, contains paired paranasal sinuses. Optic foramina near the sella turcica give passage to the optic nerves and arteries *en route* to the eyes (see Chapter 7).

Ethmoid bone

The complex ethmoid bone, located between the sphenoid and nasal bones, forms part of the orbital and nasal cavities (*Figure 18.7*). The cribriform plate, perforated by numerous foramina for the olfactory nerves, forms the roof of the nose. A close structural relationship exists between the ethmoid and the intracranial structures by which the dura mater (outer meningeal membrane) is secured to its uppermost part, or crista galli (see Nursing Practice Application). A perpendicular plate forms the upper part of the nasal septum. On each side of the perpendicular plate the lateral masses of the ethmoid extend to form the superior and middle nasal conchae, or turbinates, which project into the nasal cavity (see Chapter 12). The lateral masses contain many paranasal sinuses, making the bone spongy and light.

Skull sutures and fontanelles

In adults the serrated joints, or sutures, between the skull bones are fibrous and immovable, which means that any pressure rise within the closed cavity will compress the brain (see Chapter 4). The exceptions are the freely movable joints between the mandible and temporal bones, and the joints between the middle ear ossicles. At birth, however, the sutures are not fully ossified and several membranous spaces known as fontanelles are present (*Figure 18.8*). The anterior fontanelle forms a diamond-shaped opening where the coronal, frontal and sagittal sutures meet; it has usually ossified by 18

Nursing Practice Application **Damage to the ethmoid bone**

Damage to the ethmoid, perhaps during a fight or a road accident, which results in fracture of the cribriform plate can provide an entry route for micro-organisms into the cranial cavity. Assessment of individuals with head and facial injuries should include observation of nasal discharge – drainage of clear fluid may indicate leakage of cerebrospinal fluid from the subarachnoid space (see Chapter 4), but note that the fluid may also be blood stained. Any leakage should be reported as the risk for infection in the form of meningitis is present.

months. The smaller posterior fontanelle, situated where the lambdoidal and sagittal sutures meet, is usually closed within 3 months (see *Figure 18.2*). Abnormally wide sutures and large fontanelles may be observed where the skull has expanded in a baby with hydrocephaly (see Chapter 4).

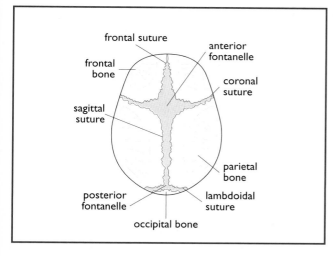

Figure 18.8 Infant skull showing fontanelles.

The facial bones

Except for the mandible, the 14 bones of the face are joined by immovable sutures (*Figure 18.9*). There are six paired bones – nasal, palatine, inferior conchae, zygomatic, lacrimal, maxillae – and a single vomer and mandible. Details of the structure of the orbit and nasal cavity are illustrated in *Figure 18.10*.

Nasal bones

Two small nasal bones join medially to form the bridge of the nose.

Palatine bones

The posterior hard palate (see Chapter 13) is formed from horizontal portions of the two L-shaped palatine bones. The vertical parts extend upwards to form part of the nose and orbit.

Figure 18.9 Bones of the face.

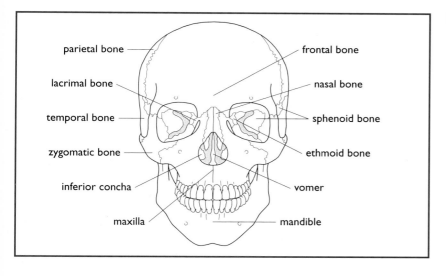

Nursing Practice Application **Moulding of the fetal cranium**

The fetal skull is large in relation to the size of the body, but luckily the joints (sutures) do not fully ossify (page 402) until after birth. This allows for the overlap of the cranial bones, called moulding, as the fetal head passes through the birth canal. Moulding, which depends on fetal presentation – vertex (head first) or breech – and the position of the head as it passes through the pelvis, produces the asymmetrical and sometimes bizarre shape of a newborn's head. New parents can be assured that the moulding will definitely disappear and that a head shape within normal limits will be achieved.

Inferior conchae

Two curved inferior conchae form part of the lateral walls of the nasal cavity. They protrude into the nasal cavity below the middle conchae (ethmoid) and are the largest pair of nasal conchae.

Zygomatic (malar) bones

Paired zygomatic bones form the prominences of the cheeks and part of the orbit. They join with the zygomatic processes of the temporal bone to form the zygomatic arch, and join anteriorly with the maxillae.

Lacrimal bones

Two small lacrimal bones form part of the medial wall of the orbit. The nasolacrimal ducts carrying tears to the nasal cavity pass through foramina in the lacrimal bones (see Chapter 7).

Maxillae

The two maxillae form the upper jaw, anterior hard palate, and part of the orbit and nasal cavity. The maxillae develop in two halves, which normally fuse, in the midline, before birth (see cleft palate, Chapter 13). An alveolar

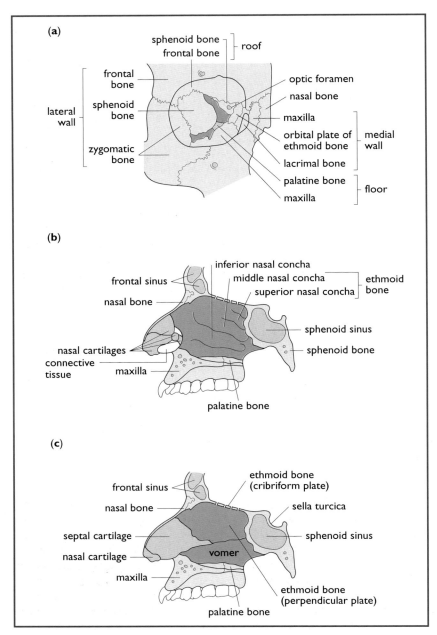

Figure 18.10 (**a**) Orbit; (**b**) nasal cavity (lateral wall); (**c**) nasal septum.

Nursing Practice Application **Mandibular fracture**

Severe jaw injuries, such as those sustained in a road accident, may be stabilized with wires and/or bands. Assessment should include provision for:

- Airway maintenance – while vomiting is a possibility, it is vital that equipment for releasing the wires/bands and for clearing the airway is to hand. Remember that when the mandibular fracture is stabilized the teeth are secured shut. There is high risk for inhalation of vomit if vomiting occurs in a person who cannot open their mouth. Initially, a nasogastric tube may be used, to aspirate gastric contents, and anti-emetic drugs should be prescribed (see Chapter 13); both of these reduce the possibility of vomiting with inhalation.
- Setting up effective communication systems – especially important where the person is unable to speak. The considerable swelling and pain associated with facial injuries and the inability to open the mouth makes speech very difficult. Nurses should be alert to the person's non-verbal communications, administer prescribed pain relief, anticipate the need for clear information and provide resources for writing messages.
- Providing adequate oral hygiene (see Chapter 13) – an essential part of care. The normal cleansing mechanisms are inhibited and the person has actual tissue damage. Keeping the mouth clean, e.g. by gentle irrigation, will minimize discomfort and the risk of complications, such as infection.
- Providing nutritional and fluid requirements in an acceptable and effective way (see Chapter 13). Initially, the person will probably receive intravenous fluid replacement, but if the gut is functioning a quick return to oral or nasoenteric feeding is desirable. Imaginative food presentation, which takes account of what the person likes, needs and can manage to eat, is most likely to be successful. It is worth remembering that this person will require extra calories (they may well have other injuries) to facilitate healing. The nurse, after consultation with the nutrition team, can provide these calories in the form of high-energy fluid supplements, which can be sipped or, if necessary, administered via the nasoenteric route. Attention to oral hygiene after eating or drinking is of particular importance.
- Helping the person and/or family to cope with the altered body image and long-term treatment that will be required.

An individual education programme will be required when the person is discharged with the wires and/or bands still in place.

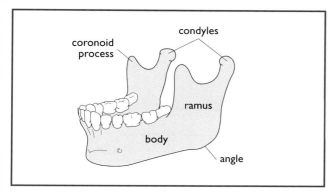

Figure 18.11 Mandible (oblique lateral view).

ridge (margin) contains the upper teeth. A large paranasal sinus or maxillary antrum, running from the orbit to the upper teeth, is present on each side.

Vomer

A single slight vomer forms the lower part of the bony nasal septum.

Mandible

The mandible, or lower jaw, forms the chin and contains the lower teeth in an alveolar ridge or margin (*Figure 18.11*). It has a curved horizontal body, and on each side a ramus extends upwards from the body from a point known as the angle of the jaw. The ramus terminates in two processes: the coronoid process, which provides attachment for a muscle (temporalis) concerned with mastication; and the mandibular condyle, which articulates with the temporal bone at the temporomandibular joint. This joint allows you to open and close your mouth, and to retract and protract your jaw and move it slightly from side to side.

Paranasal sinuses

The paranasal sinuses are mucous membrane-lined cavities or air sinuses that communicate with the nose and are located within the frontal, maxillary, ethmoid and sphenoid bones (see *Figure 18.12*). These air-filled cavities lighten the skull and give resonance to the voice, but their close proximity to the nose renders them easy prey to infection (see Chapter 12).

Spine

The spine, or **vertebral column,** (see *Figure 18.13*) supports the head, allows us to adopt the upright position by providing axial support, protects the all-important spinal cord (see Chapter 4) and acts as a 'shock absorber', e.g. when you jump down the last few stairs. It also provides attachment for muscles and other parts of the skeleton. The importance of the spine is well illustrated by expressions such as 'spineless', which implies weakness, and by describing a person of strong character and courage as having 'backbone'.

The spine, which measures some 60–70 cm in length in an adult, consists of 24 individual vertebrae (7 cervical, 12 thoracic, 5 lumbar) and 9 or 10 bones (5 sacral, 4–5 coccygeal), which fuse during childhood.

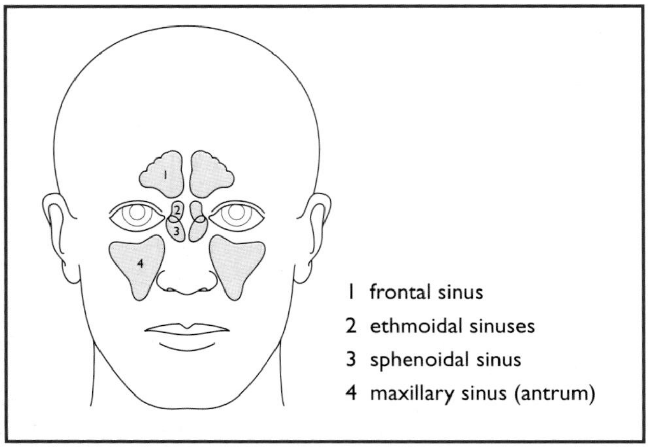

Figure 18.12 Paranasal sinuses.

1 frontal sinus
2 ethmoidal sinuses
3 sphenoidal sinus
4 maxillary sinus (antrum)

The bony arrangement, with its supporting muscles and ligaments, gives the spine great strength, and the number of joints present confers considerable collective flexibility.

Spinal curves

At birth the spine describes a C-shaped curve, created by two primary curves where the thoracic and sacral regions are convex posteriorly (fetal position). The two secondary curves, which are convex anteriorly; occur in the cervical region when the infant lifts its head and the second in the lumbar region when the infant sits up and then stands. All four curves together give the normal adult spinal curvature (*Figure 18.14*).

General features of vertebrae

Vertebrae all have certain features in common (*Figure 18.15*). There is an anterior part called the body and a vertebral (neural) arch, which together surround the vertebral foramen. The foramina of the unfused vertebrae

---

Abnormal Function **Abnormal spinal curves**

Various abnormal curvatures exist; these may be congenital, due to disease or result from age changes. A lateral curvature known as scoliosis may occur in the thoracic region. An exaggerated lumbar curve that gives rise to lordosis may be due to disease, e.g. rickets (see Chapter 16), or to an alteration in the centre of gravity such as occurs in late pregnancy. Kyphosis is an abnormally pronounced thoracic curve, which may result from osteoporotic age changes (see Chapter 16) and intervertebral disc degeneration.

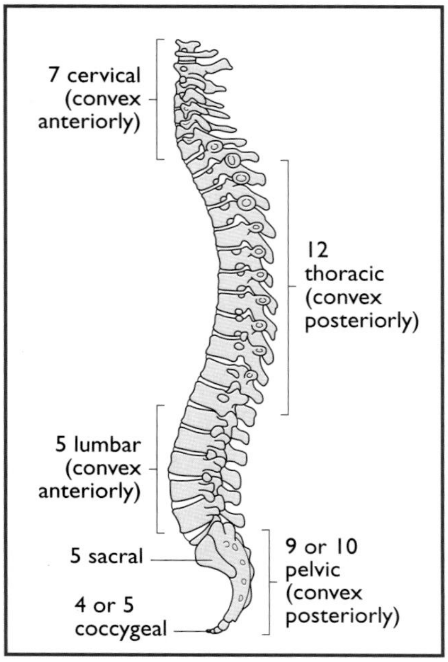

---

7 cervical (convex anteriorly)

12 thoracic (convex posteriorly)

5 lumbar (convex anteriorly)

5 sacral

4 or 5 coccygeal

9 or 10 pelvic (convex posteriorly)

Figure 18.13 Vertebral column, lateral view, showing vertebrae, sacrum and coccyx.

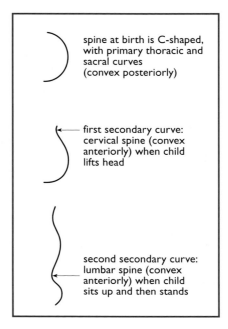

spine at birth is C-shaped, with primary thoracic and sacral curves (convex posteriorly)

first secondary curve: cervical spine (convex anteriorly) when child lifts head

second secondary curve: lumbar spine (convex anteriorly) when child sits up and then stands

Figure 18.14 Curves of the spine.

form the vertebral (neural) canal, in which the spinal cord is situated and protected. The vertebral arch consists of two pedicles, forming the sides, and two laminae posteriorly. Protruding from the arch are three processes and four articular surfaces. There are two lateral transverse processes and a spinous process (spine) that provide attachment for muscles and ligaments. The paired articular surfaces articulate with the vertebra above and below.

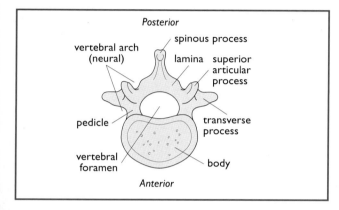

Figure 18.15 Vertebra, showing general features.

Individual vertebrae
Cervical (seven vertebrae)
The first two vertebrae, the atlas and axis, are atypical and will be described separately. Generally the cervical vertebrae have a body that is wider side-to-side than front-to-back, and all except the seventh have a bifid spinous process [*Figure 18.16(a)*]. The spinous process of C7 (the seventh vertebra) can be felt as the prominence at the base of the neck.

The transverse processes of the cervical vertebrae contain foramina for the vertebral arteries that supply the brain, and the vertebral foramen is enlarged to accommodate the spinal cord.

The atlas (C1), a ring of bone without body or spinous process, supports the skull [*Figure 18.16(b)*]. It articulates with the occipital condyles to allow you to nod your head. It might be easier to remember the position of the atlas if you think of Atlas who, according to mythology, supported the universe.

Below the atlas is the axis (C2), which has a large process called the odontoid process (dens) protruding superiorly from its body [*Figure 18.16(c)*].

The odontoid process, which represents the body of the atlas, fits into the vertebral foramen of the atlas. The atlas rotates around the odontoid process, which acts as a pivot for the movement of shaking the head [*Figure 18.16(d)*].

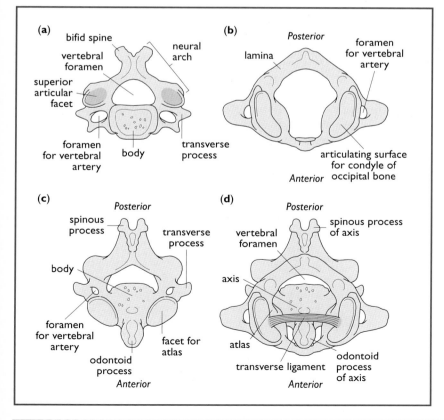

Figure 18.16 (**a**) Cervical vertebra; (**b**) atlas; (**c**) axis; (**d**) atlas and axis. All viewed from above.

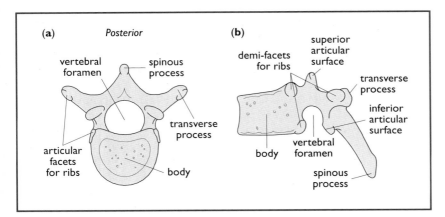

Figure 18.17 Thoracic vertebra viewed from (**a**) above and (**b**) the side.

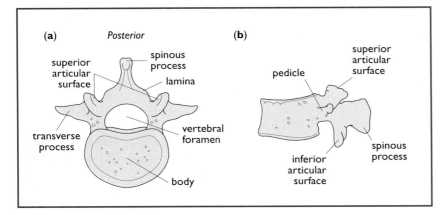

Figure 18.18 Lumbar vertebra viewed from (**a**) above and (**b**) the side.

Thoracic (12 vertebrae)

The thoracic vertebrae, all larger than the cervical vertebrae, show an increase in size from T1 to T12. The heart-shaped body has facets on both sides that articulate with the ribs (heads) (*Figure 18.17*). Facets on the transverse processes also articulate with the rib tubercles. The spinous process is long and projects downwards.

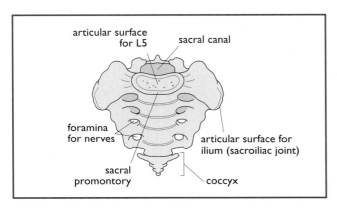

Figure 18.19 Sacrum and coccyx (anterior surface).

Lumbar (five vertebrae)

The strong lumbar vertebrae, with kidney-shaped bodies, are the largest of the vertebrae, a fact that reflects their weight-bearing role. The transverse processes are long and thin. The spinous process, which provides attachment for back muscles, is short, wide and hatchet-shaped (*Figure 18.18*).

The positioning of the articular surfaces prevents rotation and increases stability in this region, which, however, remains notoriously prone to 'back problems' (see page 410).

Sacrum

The wedge-shaped sacrum consists of five fused bones in the adult (*Figure 18.19*). The base, which is uppermost, articulates with the fifth lumbar vertebra. The anterior edge of the base forms the sacral promontory, which bulges forwards into the pelvic cavity. The sacrum, which forms the posterior part of the pelvis, also articulates with the innominate bones at the sacroiliac joints. The anterior surface of the sacrum is concave, with foramina for the passage of nerves and vessels. Running within the sacrum is the sacral canal, which is a continuation of the vertebral canal. The sacral apex articulates with the coccyx below.

Coccyx

Four or five fused vestigial tail bones form the triangular coccyx in adults (*Figure 18.19*). It articulates with the sacrum above. We only really become aware of its existence when it is damaged. Injuries to the coccyx commonly follow a heavy fall, e.g. slipping on a step, and result in pain and problems with sitting. Recovery may take many months and the unfortunate person is forced to rely heavily upon analgesics and several cushions. Those people who continue to experience pain may obtain relief from local injections of anaesthetic and corticosteroids, or from surgery.

Spinal ligaments

The vertebral column is connected and stabilized by various **ligaments** (fibrous connective tissue that joins bones and stabilizes joints), which include [*Figure 18.20(a)*]:

- Anterior and posterior longitudinal ligaments, that run in front of and behind the vertebral bodies for the entire length of the column.
- A transverse ligament [see *Figure 18.16(d)*] that secures the position of the odontoid process.
- Several ligaments that connect adjacent vertebrae, e.g. supraspinous ligament, ligamenta flava and interspinous ligaments.

The muscles of the trunk are also involved in supporting the vertebral column.

Intervertebral foramina and discs

Intervertebral foramina formed by the pedicles of adjacent vertebrae allow the passage of spinal nerves (see Chapter 5) and blood and lymph vessels. They are present on both sides of the vertebral column along its entire length.

The cartilaginous joints (see page 419) between the vertebrae, except C1 and C2, are formed from an intervertebral disc of fibrocartilage (annulus fibrosus) surrounding a semi-solid core (nucleus pulposus). The discs, which contribute to spinal flexibility and act as shock absorbers, are held in place by the posterior longitudinal ligament. There is very little movement between individual vertebral joints, but collective flexibility produces considerable movement. This flexibility allows bending forwards (flexion), bending backwards (extension), bending from side to side (lateral flexion) and rotation. Back pain and prolapsed intervertebral disc (slipped disc) are occupational hazards for nurses and other carers (see Nursing Practice Application).

Thoracic (thorax) cage

The structures forming the thorax, or chest, are the sternum, costal cartilages, 12 pairs of ribs and the thoracic vertebrae (see *Figure 18.22*) (see also page 408). The thoracic cage protects the organs and great vessels of the chest, provides attachment for back and chest muscles, and supports the pectoral girdle. The intercostal muscles are situated between the ribs (see Chapter 12).

The sternum

The sternum (breastbone) is the flat dagger-shaped bone situated in the midline of the anterior part of the chest (see *Figure 18.21*). It is around 16 cm in length and consists of an upper part, the manubrium, connected to its body by a cartilaginous joint that normally remains unossified. Projecting downwards from the body is the xiphisternum (xiphoid cartilage). This provides attachment for some abdominal muscles and the diaphragm. The xiphisternum usually becomes ossified later in life.

The manubrium articulates with the clavicles at its clavicular notches and with the first two pairs of ribs. The body articulates with the costal cartilages of ribs 3–7.

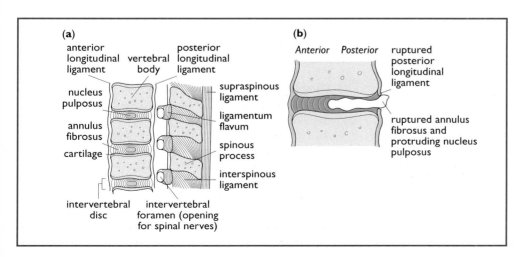

Figure 18.20 (a) Section through the vertebral column showing intervertebral joints, discs and ligaments; **(b)** prolapsed intervertebral disc.

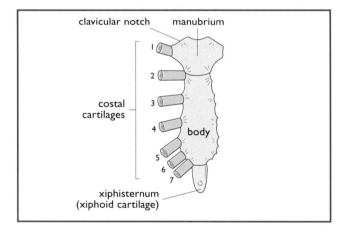

Figure 18.21 Sternum (anterior view).

Ribs generally have a curved shaft, tubercle, neck and head. The inferior border is grooved for the passage of blood vessels and nerves. The head of the rib has two facets that articulate with facets on adjacent vertebral bodies, while the tubercle articulates with the transverse process of the lower vertebral body.

The first, eleventh and twelfth pairs are atypical ribs: the first pair is short and broad and all three pairs (1, 11 and 12) only articulate with one vertebra.

Anteriorly the ribs join with the costal cartilages (hyaline cartilage), which allow the flexibility required for chest movements during respiration. The chest movements that change thoracic volumes (see Chapter 12) are facilitated by the external and internal intercostal muscles (see page 429).

Appendicular Skeleton

Pectoral girdle and arm

The pectoral girdle, which joins the arm to the axial skeleton, consists of a clavicle (collar bone) and scapula (shoulder blade) (see *Figure 18.1*). The upper limb is formed from a humerus, radius, ulna, carpals (8), metacarpals (5) and phalanges (14).

Clavicle

The two clavicles are long bones with a double curvature (*Figure 18.23*). They articulate medially with the sternum

The ribs

The lateral walls of the thorax are formed from 12 pairs of ribs. They are curved bones attached posteriorly to the thoracic vertebrae (see page 408).

The ribs can be divided into seven pairs of true ribs, which articulate with the sternum via costal cartilages, and five pairs of false ribs. The false rib pairs 8–10 are attached indirectly to the sternum by their costal cartilage joining to the costal cartilage above, but pairs 11 and 12, which have no sternal attachment, are known as floating ribs.

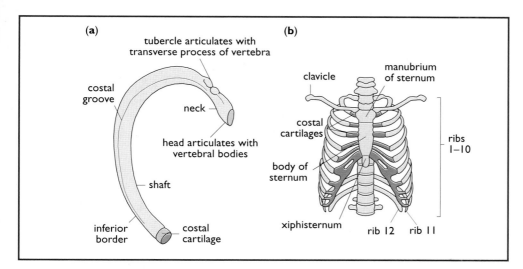

Figure 18.22 (a) A rib; **(b)** thoracic cage.

and laterally with the scapulae at the acromioclavicular joints. The clavicles act as an anterior brace (support) for the shoulder, and provide muscle attachments. Clavicular fractures are common in contact sports such as rugby football and following a fall on the outstretched arm.

Scapula

The scapulae are two large, flat, triangular bones situated on the posterior thoracic wall. A layer of muscle separates the scapulae and ribs (*Figure 18.24*). Each scapula has two surfaces, three borders and three angles. The posterior surface is marked by a prominent ridge, or spine, which extends to the acromion process. The scapula articulates with the clavicle at the acromioclavicular joint. A shallow fossa known as the glenoid cavity, situated at the lateral angle, accommodates the head of the humerus to form the shoulder joint. The coracoid process provides attachment for the biceps brachii muscle responsible for elbow flexion (bending).

Humerus

The humerus is the long bone forming the upper arm (see *Figure 18.25*). It articulates with the scapula at the shoulder joint and the radius and ulna at the elbow joint.

The head of the humerus fits into the glenoid cavity to give a good range of movements at the shoulder. Below the head is the anatomical neck, with two projections called the greater and lesser tubercles (tuberosities by some authorities), which are separated by a groove that accommodates the biceps tendon. The region where the extremity becomes the shaft is called the surgical neck, which is a frequent site for fractures. The shaft, which is triangular in section, has a tuberosity that provides attachment for the deltoid muscle and a groove for the radial nerve. At its distal end the humerus is broad and flattened. It has

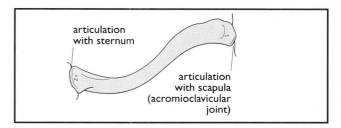

Figure 18.23 Clavicle (left – upper surface).

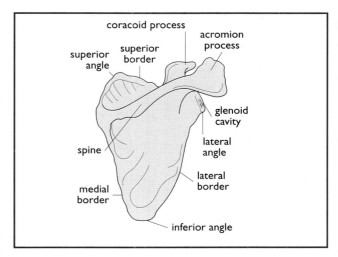

Figure 18.24 Scapula (right – posterior surface).

a lateral and medial epicondyle and two articulating condyles – the capitulum for the radius and the trochlea for the ulna. Above the articulating surfaces are fossae (which receive the processes of the ulna and radius when

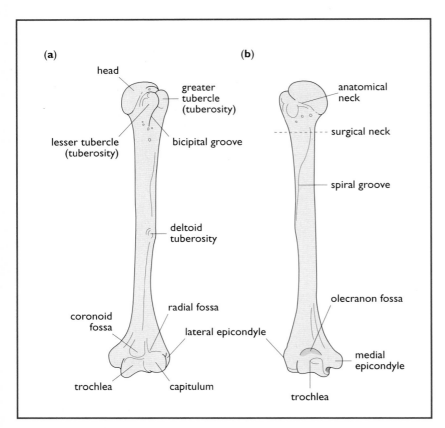

(a)

head
greater tubercle (tuberosity)
lesser tubercle (tuberosity)
bicipital groove
deltoid tuberosity
coronoid fossa
radial fossa
lateral epicondyle
trochlea
capitulum

(b)

anatomical neck
surgical neck
spiral groove
olecranon fossa
medial epicondyle
trochlea

Figure 18.25 Humerus (left) – **(a)** anterior and **(b)** posterior views.

the elbow flexes or extends) – the coronoid and olecranon fossae for the ulna and the radial fossa for the radius. The ulnar nerve, situated behind the medial epicondyle, accounts for the excruciating pain felt when you knock your elbow ('funny bone').

Radius and ulna

The two long bones of the forearm are the radius (lateral side) and ulna (medial side) (*Figure 18.26*). With the arm in the anatomical position (see *Figure 1.35*) they lie parallel to each other, with the radius lateral to the ulna. The two bones articulate with the humerus at the elbow, with the carpals at the wrist and with each other at the proximal and distal radioulnar joints. They are also joined along their complete length by the interosseous membrane.

The ulna is the longer of the two bones. It stabilizes the forearm and contributes to the elbow joint with the coronoid and olecranon processes. The olecranon prevents elbow hyperextension by 'fixing' the arm when the elbow is straight. The shaft of the ulna gives attachment to many muscles of the forearm and, at its lower extremity or head, a styloid process provides attachment for some wrist muscles.

The radius is less important at the elbow than the ulna but is more significant at the wrist joint, where it 'carries

the hand'. The small radial head articulates with the capitulum of the humerus at the elbow. Below the head the radial tuberosity provides attachment for the biceps brachii muscle. The shaft, which provides attachment for many muscles, is narrow and rounded but widens at its lower end. The lower extremity has a lateral styloid process and a concave surface that articulates with the carpal bones.

Wrist and hand

The eight carpals (the carpus), which form the wrist joint, are short bones connected to each other by ligaments (*Figure 18.27*). They are arranged roughly in two rows – a proximal row (lateral to medial) of scaphoid, lunate, triquetral and pisiform, and a distal row (lateral to medial) of trapezium, trapezoid, capitate and hamate. The scaphoid and lunate articulate with the radius at the wrist, and with some distal carpals.

Five 'little' long bones, the metacarpals (metacarpus) (numbered from the thumb inwards), form the palm of the hand. Their proximal ends articulate with the carpals (carpo-metacarpal joints) and the distal ends (heads) articulate with the proximal phalanges.

The digits are formed from 14 'little' long bones called phalanges – two in the thumb and three in each finger.

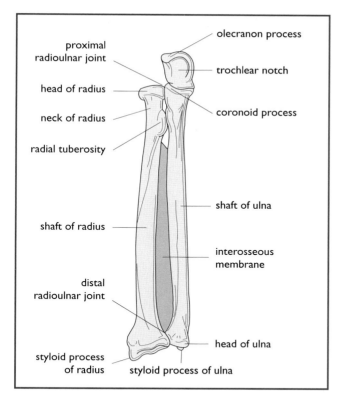

Figure 18.26 Radius and ulna (right – anterior view).

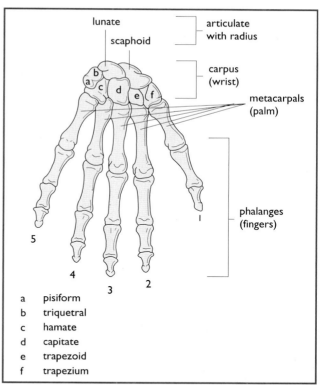

Figure 18.27 Bones of the wrist and hand (left – anterior aspect).

a   pisiform
b   triquetral
c   hamate
d   capitate
e   trapezoid
f   trapezium

Articulation occurs between the proximal phalanges and the metacarpals and the phalanges articulate with each other.

Pelvic girdle and leg

The pelvic girdle, which joins the leg to the axial skeleton, consists of two innominate bones and the sacrum (see page 408 and *Figure 18.1*). The lower limb consists of a femur, tibia, fibula, patella, tarsals (7), metatarsals (5) and phalanges (14).

Innominate (hip) bones

The innominate bone is formed from the fusion of the ilium, ischium and pubis. These unite at the deep depression (acetabulum) that accommodates the femoral head to form the hip joint. The innominate bones articulate with the sacrum to form the sacroiliac joints, and with each other at the symphysis pubis, a slightly movable joint between the pubic bones (see *Figure 18.28*).

The ilium is the large upper bone and has a crest bounded by anterior and posterior superior iliac spines; it is at the anterior spines that you measure your hips. Many large muscles of the back, buttock and abdomen are attached to the ilium.

The ischium forms the strong posterior and inferior parts of the innominate bone. It has an ischial spine and, at its lowest point, an ischial tuberosity, which supports your weight when sitting.

The pubis, which forms the anterior part of the innominate, has a body and two rami. The two pubic bones unite in the midline at the symphysis pubis to form the pubic arch.

The ischium and pubis together surround the obturator foramen, which, although being nearly filled with membrane, allows the passage of vessels and nerves from pelvis to thigh.

Pelvis

The pelvis, as already mentioned, consists of two innominate bones and the sacrum, which form the bony and cartilaginous ring surrounding the lower part of the trunk (see *Figure 18.29*). Apart from the functions already stated, the pelvis protects the organs of the pelvic cavity, e.g. bladder, and in the case of the female provides space for a developing fetus and its exit into the world at the end of pregnancy (see Chapter 20).

The pelvis is divided into two by the pelvic brim, formed from the iliopectineal line and the sacral promontory; the part above is the false pelvis and that below, the true pelvis.

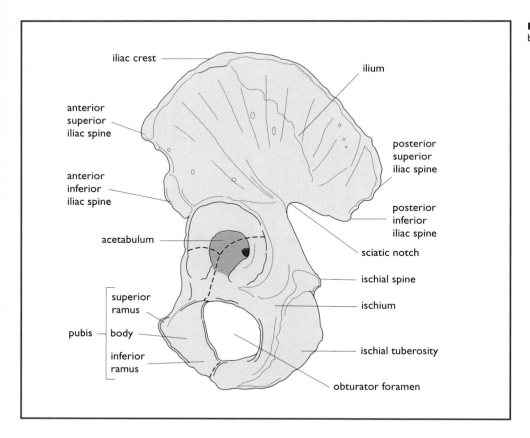

Figure 18.28 Innominate
bone (left – external surface).

iliac crest

ilium

anterior
superior
iliac spine

posterior
superior
iliac spine

anterior
inferior
iliac spine

posterior
inferior
iliac spine

acetabulum

sciatic notch

ischial spine

ischium

superior
ramus

pubis — body

ischial tuberosity

inferior
ramus

obturator foramen

Structural differences between the female and male pelvis

The majority of babies are born by the vaginal route, a process for which the female pelvis is generally well adapted:

- The female pelvis is lighter than the male and the true pelvis is wider and shallower.
- Females have a wider pelvic arch than males and their acetabula are further apart.
- The female sacrum is broad and short, and its promontory encroaches less into the pelvic cavity.
- The pelvic brim in females is oval, whereas in males it is heart-shaped [*Figure 18.29 (a), (b)*].
- In the female the ischial spines are more widely spaced, the ischial tuberosities are more lateral and the coccyx is straighter than in the male – all of which increase the size of the pelvic outlet.

Occasionally the fetal head cannot fit into, and pass through and/or out of the pelvis. This may be caused by a large head and or a small or deformed pelvis, and the mismatch is termed cephalo-pelvic disproportion. If this situation exists it is necessary to deliver the infant by caesarean section, which with early diagnosis can be performed as an elective (planned) operation. Babies born by elective caesarean section do not have moulding of the cranial bones because they have not been subjected to the deforming forces associated with a journey through the pelvis.

Femur

The femur is the long bone forming the thigh, and is the strongest and most substantial bone of the body. It articulates with the innominate bone at the hip joint and the tibia at the knee joint [*Figure 18.30(a)*].

The large femoral head fits into the acetabulum to give a stable joint that still retains a good range of movements. A small pit on the head provides attachment for the ligamentum teres, which holds the femur in the acetabulum. Below the head is the femoral neck, that is a frequent site for the 'hip' fractures that occur so commonly in older women as a result of falls and osteoporotic bone changes (see Chapter 16).

The greater and lesser trochanters mark the boundary between the head and the shaft. The shaft is cylindrical and provides attachment for powerful thigh muscles. At its lower extremity the femur forms medial and lateral condyles, which articulate with the patella and tibial condyles. On the posterior aspect, above the condyles, is the popliteal surface for vessels and nerves.

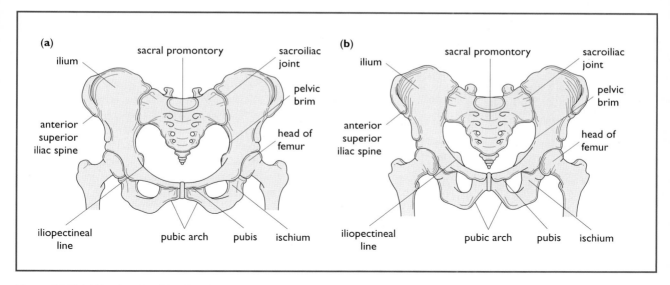

Figure 18.29 (a) Female pelvis; **(b)** male pelvis.

The patella (kneecap) [*Figure 18.30(b)*] is a sesamoid bone, which forms within the patellar tendon of the quadriceps femoris muscle. It is positioned (see *Figure 18.1*) over the femoral condyles and lies anterior to the knee joint, which it protects.

Tibia and fibula

The two long bones of the lower leg are the tibia and fibula (see *Figure 18.31*). The tibia forms the shin bone and is positioned medial to the fibula. The two bones articulate with each other at the superior and inferior tibiofibular joints; the tibia articulates with the femur and both tibia and fibula articulate with the talus at the ankle. The tibia and fibula are also joined by an interosseous membrane.

The tibia is the more important bone. At its upper extremity lateral and medial condyles present flat articulating surfaces for the femur. The semilunar cartilages of the knee joint are situated on the tibial condyles.

The tibial shaft is triangular, with a very prominent crest that can be felt just under the skin. Poorly protected, this area is easily damaged, e.g. by walking into furniture. At its lower extremity the tibia has an articulating surface for the talus and a projection, the medial malleolus (felt as the lump on the inner aspect of the ankle).

The fibula is the lateral non-weight-bearing bone. At its upper extremity the head articulates with the tibia and the shaft provides muscle attachment. The lower extremity projects to form the lateral malleolus, which articulates with the talus.

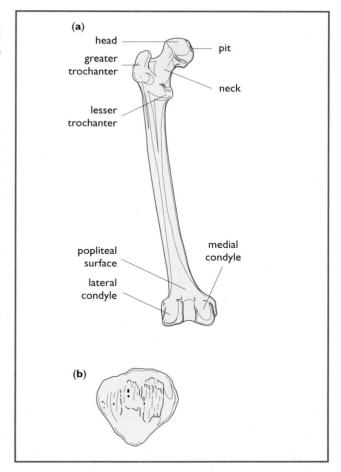

Figure 18.30 (a) Femur (left – posterior view); **(b)** patella (anterior view).

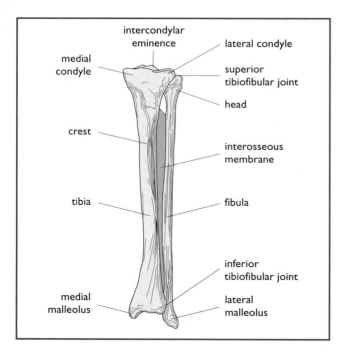

Figure 18.31 Tibia and fibula (left – anterior view).

Ankle and foot

The seven short tarsals (the tarsus), which form the ankle and heel and support the body weight are the talus, which forms part of the ankle joint; the calcaneus or heel bone, which provides attachment for the massive Achilles tendon [see *Figure 18.50(b)*] of the calf muscle; and the navicular, cuboid and three cuneiforms [*Figure 18.32(a)*].

Five metatarsals (metatarsus) (numbered from medial to lateral aspects), which are 'little' long bones, form the dorsum, or instep, of the foot. The proximal extremities articulate with the tarsals, and the distal extremities with the proximal phalanges.

The 14 phalanges that form the toes are much shorter than the fingers, but are arranged in the same way. There are three in each toe apart from the great toe, which has two.

Arches of the foot

Look at a wet footprint and you can see that the foot is not flat on the ground but arched [*Figure 18.32(b)*]. The three arches of the foot produce a bridge-like structure capable of supporting weight while remaining flexible

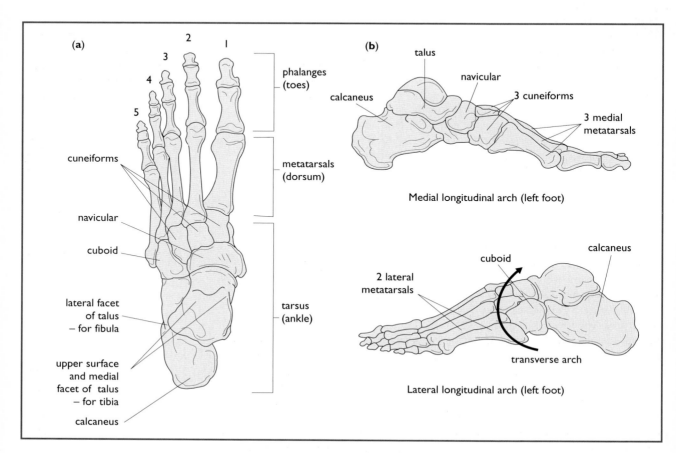

Figure 18.32 (a) Bones of the ankle and foot (left – dorsal aspect); **(b)** arches of the foot.

enough to give 'spring' on walking. The arches are joined by strong ligaments and supported by muscles.

The medial longitudinal arch is the highest and is formed from the calcaneus, navicular, cuneiforms and three inner metatarsals. A less pronounced lateral longitudinal arch is formed by the calcaneus, cuboid and two outer metatarsals. A transverse arch is present and runs across the foot in a line marked by the tarsometatarsal joints [see *Figure 18.32(b)*].

The problem of 'flat feet' is due either to congenital absence of the foot arches or later loss of the arches. Loss may be caused by the prolonged standing associated with certain occupations or damage caused by running on hard surfaces without proper footwear.

Levers and Movement

Bones, joints and muscles operating together produce movement through a system of levers (leverage). A brief look at the principles of levers is appropriate before the consideration of body movement.

A lever is a rigid structure, with a fixed point or fulcrum (plural, fulcra), which moves if force is applied to it. This force (effort) is used to shift a load (resistance). The distance between the effort and the fulcrum is termed the effort arm, and that between the load and the fulcrum, the load or resistance arm.

In the body the bones are the levers and the joints are the fulcra. The effort is supplied by the muscles at their insertions on bones, and load consists of the bone, the relevant part of the body and whatever you are lifting or carrying.

Levers may be classified as first, second or third class, according to the positions of the load, effort and fulcrum relative to each other (see *Figure 18.33*). A first-class lever has the fulcrum between the load and effort, e.g. a seesaw. This type of lever may require an effort less than the load, which makes it very efficient, but in the body, e.g. elbow extension, the effort required is greater than the load. Second-class levers, e.g. wheelbarrows, have the load located between the effort and the fulcrum; these are generally efficient levers and a body example

would be standing on tip toes. Third-class levers, e.g. fire tongs, have the effort located between the fulcrum and the load; they are not efficient and always require an effort greater than the load. The levers operating in the body are generally of this type, e.g. elbow flexion and adduction of the thigh.

Different lever types in the body reflect their particular role in providing for the diverse functions of the musculo-skeletal system (muscles, bones, joints and connective tissue): rapid movement, stability, moving large loads, strength and a wide range of movements.

The equation below shows the equilibrium situation with the lever balanced:

Effort x EA = Load x RA
(effort arm length)   (resistance arm length)

e.g. 5 kg x 10 cm = 25 kg x 2 cm
(50 = 50)

Levers either operate at a mechanical advantage, where little effort is required to move the load, or at a mechanical disadvantage, where much greater effort is needed. Mechanical efficiency is dependent upon the distances EA and RA, and when these are altered the effort and load relationship changes:

1. If EA is increased then effort required will be less:
2.5 kg x 20 cm = 25 kg x 2 cm
(50 = 50)
e.g. using a crowbar to shift a rock too heavy to move by hand.

2. If EA is decreased then effort required will be more:
10 kg x 5 cm = 25 kg x 2 cm
(50 = 50)

In the body, where EA and fulcrum are fixed, it is the RA that changes to maintain the equilibrium. When the RA is lengthened a greater effort is required than if the RA is shortened – try lifting a heavy textbook at arm's length and then close to your body. With this in mind, it becomes clear that carrying heavy objects close to the body requires less effort than holding the same weight away from the body.

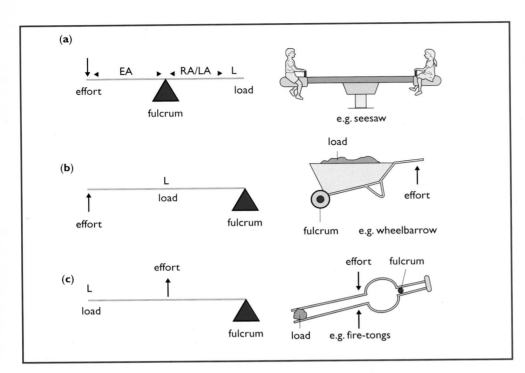

Figure 18.33 Levers. (**a**) First class; (**b**) second class; (**c**) third class. EA = effort arm; LA/RA = load or resistance arm.

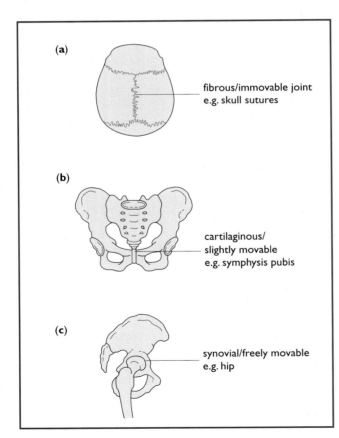

Figure 18.34 (**a**) Fibrous – skull sutures; (**b**) cartilaginous – symphysis pubis; (**c**) synovial – hip.

Joints

A joint, or **articulation** (point at which two or more bones meet), can be classified by its structure and the degree of movement it allows.

Types of joint

Joints may be fibrous (immovable), cartilaginous (slightly movable) or synovial (freely movable). The three main types are all described here, but synovial joints and movement are discussed in more detail (*Figure 18.34*).

Early development of joints

In common with bones (see Chapter 16), the joints develop from mesodermal tissue. At week 6 there are no joints – these start to form at week 8. Fibrous joints are formed as mesoderm becomes dense fibrous tissue. The cartilaginous joints develop as mesoderm differentiates to form fibrocartilage. The complex synovial joints and their components develop as mesoderm forms capsules around the bone ends. Later the articular surfaces are covered with smooth hyaline cartilage, the synovial membranes develop and by the fourth month fluid-filled spaces in the mesoderm have increased to form the joint cavity. Movement at the joint is now possible, and because skeletal muscles are contracting strongly the first fetal movements are felt by the woman (see Chapter 17).

Fibrous joints (synarthroses) — immovable joints

The bones in a fibrous joint are united by fibrous tissue. Examples include sutures, e.g. skull bones (page 402), where the joint is fixed and allows no movement; gomphoses, e.g. the teeth in their sockets, where a tiny amount of movement occurs; and syndesmoses, where a membrane connecting the bones allows some 'give', e.g. the inferior tibiofibular joint.

Cartilaginous joints (amphiarthroses) — slightly movable joints

In cartilaginous joints the bones are joined by cartilage and slight movement is possible. There are two types:

- Synchondroses, formed from the epiphyseal plates present in long bones during growth. These become ossified in adults, after which movement is no longer possible.
- Symphyses, where a fibrocartilage pad separates the hyaline cartilage articular surfaces, which provides strength and some movement. Examples of symphyses include the intervertebral joints (page 409), the manubrium and body of the sternum (page 409) and the symphysis pubis (page 413).

Synovial joints (diarthroses) — freely movable joints

Synovial joints form the freely movable joints of the skeleton, which allow a variety of movements, e.g. hip, elbow. The articulating bones are separated by a membrane-lined joint cavity.

Synovial Joints

General characteristics

All synovial joints have the following common characteristics (*Figure 18.35*):

- **Joint capsule:** a capsule of fibrous tissue encloses the joint cavity, which may be further reinforced by intracapsular and extracapsular ligaments. The capsule is well supplied with blood vessels, motor nerves and specialized sensory nerves, or proprioceptors, which convey data regarding position to the brain.
- **Articular cartilage:** the articular surfaces of the bones are covered with smooth hyaline cartilage.
- **Synovial membrane and fluid:** the joint cavity, except for areas covered with hyaline cartilage, is lined with synovial membrane. The membrane secretes a small amount of viscous, slippery synovial fluid, which occupies the spaces in the joint cavity. The synovial fluid contains protein, fat and polysaccharides such as hyaluronic acid, which confer the characteristic viscosity. Synovial fluid, which thins on

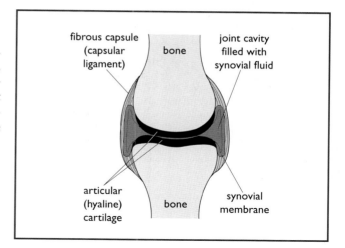

Figure 18.35 A synovial joint.

warming during joint movement, lubricates joint activity and reduces friction and erosion in much the same way as the oil in a car engine. The fluid has a role in joint nourishment, and contains phagocytic cells that remove unwanted material from the joint.

Associated with some joints, e.g. the knee, are small sacs, or bursae, which are lined with synovial membrane. They act to prevent friction between structures such as bone and tendon. Bursitis (inflammation of a bursa) is an extremely painful condition caused by excessive or prolonged use of joints, e.g. tennis elbow or housemaid's knee. Rest, anti-inflammatory drugs and analgesics usually relieve the condition, but in some cases local corticosteroid injections are required.

The muscles and tendons that cross a joint are involved with its movement and in contributing to its stability.

The special features present in individual joints are included in the coverage of specific joints (pages 422–425).

Movements occurring at synovial joints (see *Figure 18.36*)

- Flexion – bending. Reducing the angle of a joint and bringing the bones closer, e.g. bending the elbow.
- Extension – straightening. The opposite to flexion, e.g. straightening the elbow.
- Abduction – movement away from the midline, e.g. moving the straight arm away from the body.
- Adduction – movement towards the midline, e.g. moving the arm back to the body.
- Circumduction – a movement that combines flexion, extension, abduction and adduction, by which the limb traces a cone in the air, e.g. circular movement of the straight arm from the shoulder.

Nursing Practice Application **Joint stiffness and immobility**

Your knowledge of the range of movements (ROM) occurring at individual joints can be put to good use during mobility/immobility assessments and in the prevention of one of the problems of immobility – joint stiffness.

Joints suffer from lack of use just as do bones and muscles (Chapters 16 and 17). Disuse causes joint stiffness, which can seriously affect mobility and stability. Activity should be encouraged, but where this is not possible the nurse works with the physiotherapist and occupational therapist to prevent or minimize joint stiffness. This can be achieved by careful positioning to keep joints slightly flexed and supported, use of aids such as splints, encouraging active movements or by moving the person's joints through a full range of passive movements.

Abnormal Function **Problems with joints – common injuries**

Injuries occur when the joint structures are stretched, stressed or torn; they range from sprains to the major disruption of dislocation, which may be associated with a fracture.

Sprains

Joint sprain occurs when the supporting ligaments are stretched or torn. A common example is the sprain that results when the ankle is twisted.

Dislocation

The damage caused by dislocation is more severe than that caused by a sprain, with joint disruption and displacement of articular surfaces. Dislocations, e.g. of shoulder and finger joints, are commonly sustained during contact sports or can result from a fall. A partial dislocation is termed a subluxation.

NB See also congenital dislocation of the hips (page 425).

Joint injuries can reduce stability, with risk of repeated injury, and an already damaged joint is more likely to develop degenerative changes of osteoarthritis (see Special Focus – Joint conditions, page 428).

- Rotation – turning of a bone as it moves around its axis, e.g. the movement between the atlas and axis when you turn your head.
- Inversion – turning the sole of the foot medially (inwards).
- Eversion – the movement opposite to inversion, where the sole is turned laterally (outwards).
- Pronation – e.g. movement of the radius across the ulna, which turns the palm downwards.
- Supination – e.g. the radius and ulna lie parallel to each other and the palm is turned upwards.
- Elevation – movement upwards, e.g. the scapulae when the shoulders are lifted.
- Depression – downward movement – the reverse of elevation.
- Protraction – forward movement, e.g. thrusting out the mandible.
- Retraction – the backward movement opposite to protraction, e.g. returning the jaw to its normal position.

Movement at a specific joint is limited by the shape of the bones, by the ligaments and by soft tissue such as muscle. The normal range of movement is also modified by increasing age and pathological processes.

Varieties of synovial joints and movements possible

The variety of joint types allows for movement in one plane (monoaxial or uniaxial), two planes (biaxial) or through all planes (multiaxial). The actual movements (see above) can be described as being angular, e.g. flexion/extension; gliding, e.g. slight movement at the wrist as the carpals move against each other; circular, e.g. rotation of the head; or special, such as inversion/eversion.

Ball and socket joint

A ball and socket joint has a rounded extremity that articulates within a cavity in another bone, e.g. hip and shoulder joints. This type of arrangement allows extensive movement – flexion, extension, adduction, abduction, circumduction and rotation.

Hinge joint

A hinge joint has a bony projection that articulates with a concave surface on another bone to give movement in one plane, e.g. elbow, knee, ankle and interphalangeal joints. The only movements possible are flexion and extension.

Pivot joint

A pivot joint allows rotation only; for example, the ring of the atlas rotates around the odontoid peg of the axis or the proximal radioulnar joint, which allows supination and pronation.

Saddle joint

A saddle joint consists of two bones with both convex and concave surfaces that fit together. The only example is the joint at the base of the thumb (carpometacarpal). Movement in two planes is possible: extension, flexion,

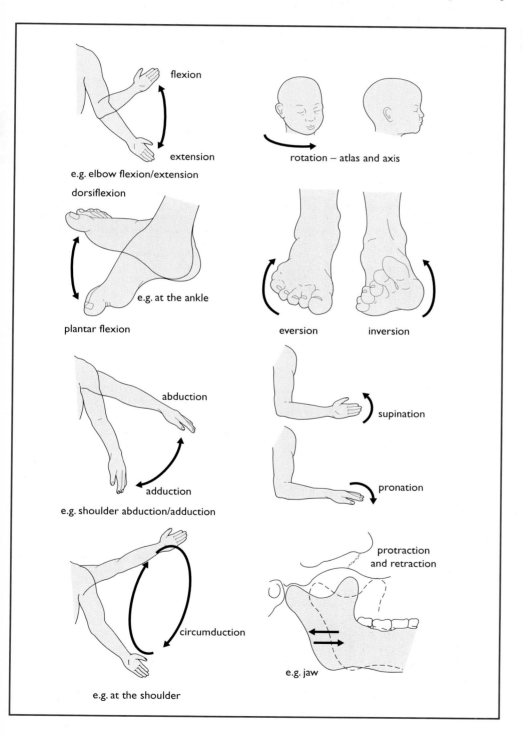

Figure 18.36 Some movements at synovial joints.

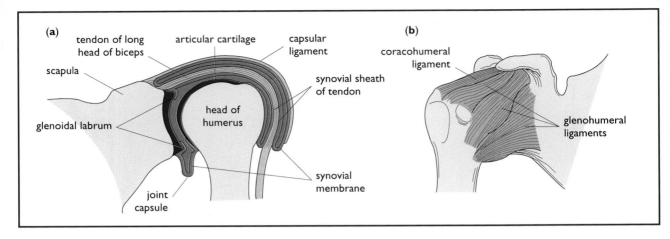

Figure 18.37 (a) Shoulder joint; **(b)** ligaments reinforcing the shoulder (anterior view simplified).

adduction, abduction and circumduction. The thumb can also be opposed to the fingers.

Condyloid (ellipsoid) joint

Condyloid joints are similar to hinge joints, but movement in two planes is possible. Examples include the wrist and metacarpophalangeal joints, where extension, flexion, adduction, abduction and circumduction are possible.

Gliding (plane) joint

A gliding joint comprises two flat surfaces that glide on each other in all directions, e.g. intercarpal, intertarsal and sternoclavicular joints. Movement is generally very limited because of the ligaments present.

Specific synovial joints – structure, movements and muscles

A description of some joints is given here, along with their range of movements and some of the muscles involved with those movements. The major muscle groups are mentioned again later in this chapter.

Shoulder joint (humeroscapular) – ball and socket

The shoulder joint consists of the head of the humerus articulating within the glenoid cavity of the scapula. The glenoid cavity, which is relatively shallow, is deepened by a rim of cartilage known as the glenoidal labrum [*Figure 18.37(a)*]. Extensive movement at the shoulder (*Table 18.2*) is possible because the cavity is shallow and because of the looseness of the ligaments around the joint. However, the price of increased mobility is reduced stability and dislocation (see page 420). The major ligaments reinforcing the shoulder are the coracohumeral ligament,

Table 18.2 Movements and muscles at the shoulder (see also *Figure 18.45*)	
Movement	**Muscles involved**
Extension	Latissimus dorsi, teres major, deltoid (posterior fibres)
Flexion	Pectoralis major, deltoid (anterior fibres), coracobrachialis
Adduction	Pectoralis major, latissimus dorsi, teres major, coracobrachialis
Abduction	Deltoid, supraspinatus
Rotation – medial	Pectoralis major, teres major, deltoid (anterior fibres), latissimus dorsi, subscapularis
– lateral	Deltoid (posterior fibres), infraspinatus, teres minor
Circumduction	Shoulder muscles acting in sequence

NB Four muscles form the 'rotator cuff' that helps to stabilize the shoulder – teres minor, infraspinatus, supraspinatus and subscapularis.

Table 18.2 Movements and muscles at the shoulder (see also *Figure 18.45*).

running from the coracoid process to the humerus, the three glenohumeral ligaments [*Figure 18.37(b)*] and a transverse humeral ligament (not shown in figure). Some shoulder muscles also help to stabilize the joint.

Elbow joint – hinge

The elbow joint is formed by the trochlear surface of the humerus and the ulnar notch, and the capitulum of the humerus and the radius [*Figure 18.38(a)*]. The relatively loose joint cavity of the elbow is attached to the ulna, both coronoid and olecranon fossae and the annular ligament, which is vital to the proximal radioulnar joint. Medial and lateral collateral ligaments stabilize the elbow, as do the muscles which cross the joint [*Figure 18.38(b)* and *Table 18.3*].

Radioulnar joints

The proximal radioulnar joint (*Figure 18.39*) is formed by the radial head rotating in a notch on the ulna. Joint stabilization is achieved by the annular ligament, which surrounds the radial head [*Figure 18.38(b)*].

The lower end of the radius rotates on the head of the ulna to form the distal radioulnar joint.

These joints produce the movements – pronation and supination of the hand – needed when using a screwdriver or turning a door knob (*Table 18.4*).

Wrist joint – condyloid

The wrist, or radiocarpal, joint is formed by the distal radius and a disc of cartilage below the ulna, which articulate with the scaphoid, lunate and triquetral carpal bones [see *Figure 18.40(a)*]. Lateral and medial collateral ligaments and tough transverse ligaments (from the radius to the lunate) stabilize the joint [see *Figure 18.40(b)* and *Table 18.5*].

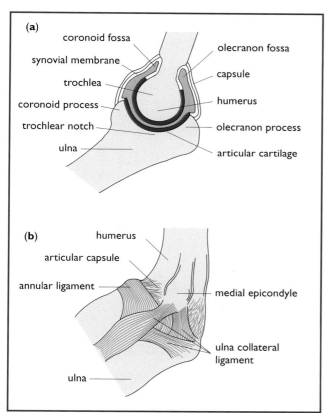

Figure 18.38 (**a**) Elbow joint; (**b**) ligaments reinforcing the elbow.

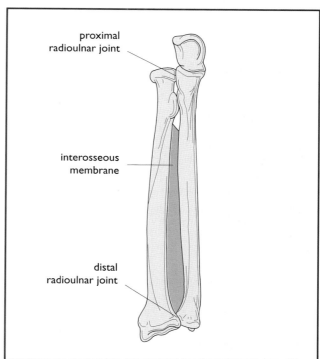

Figure 18.39 Radioulnar joints (right – anterior view).

Table 18.3 Movements and muscles at the elbow (see also *Figure 18.45*)	
Movement	**Muscles involved**
Extension	Triceps brachii, anconeus
Flexion	Biceps brachii, brachialis, brachioradialis (when arm is partially flexed and pronated)

Table 18.3 Movements and muscles at the elbow (see also *Figure 18.45*).

Table 18.4 Movements and muscles at the radioulnar joints (see also *Figure 18.45*)	
Movement	**Muscles involved**
Pronation	Pronator teres, pronator quadratus
Supination	Supinator, biceps brachii

Table 18.4 Movements and muscles at the radioulnar joints (see also *Figure 18.45*).

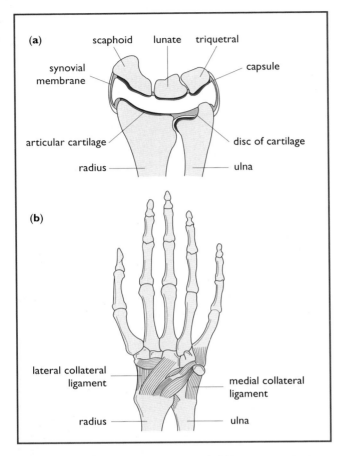

Figure 18.40 (a) Wrist joint (diagrammatic); **(b)** ligaments reinforcing the wrist (anterior view).

Hand and finger joints

The joints between the carpals are of the gliding type, as are the carpometacarpal joints, except for the joint at the base of the thumb, which is a saddle joint.

The metacarpophalangeal joints are of the condyloid type, allowing extension, flexion, adduction and abduction. The interphalangeal joints are of the hinge type, allowing flexion and extension. The thumb can be opposed to the fingers – this provides our ability to grasp objects.

The powerful and fine movements of the hand and digits are produced by various forearm muscles (extensors and flexors) and many small intrinsic hand muscles, e.g. thenar, lumbricals. The extensor and flexor tendons run to the hand within synovial sheaths and are secured by strong ligaments – the extensor and flexor retinacula.

Hip joint – ball and socket

The hip joint is formed by the femoral head and the acetabulum of the innominate bone. A rim of cartilage called the acetabular labrum deepens the acetabulum [*Figure 18.41(a)*]. The hip, which is less mobile than the shoulder, is very much more stable (*Table 18.6*). This stability is provided by the ligamentum teres and a strong capsular ligament, which are reinforced by the iliofemoral, pubofemoral [*Figure 18.41(b)*] and ischiofemoral ligaments (not shown in figure). Some of the strongest muscles in the body also contribute to hip stability.

Table 18.5 Movements and muscles at the wrist (see also *Figure 18.45*)	
Movement	**Muscles involved**
Extension	Extensor carpi radialis (longus, brevis), extensor carpi ulnaris, extensor digitorum
Flexion	Flexor carpi radialis, flexor carpi ulnaris, flexor digitorum
Adduction	Flexor and extensor carpi ulnaris
Abduction	Flexor and extensor carpi radialis, abductor pollicis longus
Circumduction	Wrist muscles acting in sequence

NB Usual movements at the wrist are extension/abduction and flexion/adduction.

Table 18.5 Movements and muscles at the wrist (see also *Figure 18.45*).

Table 18.6 Movements and muscles at the hip (see also *Figure 18.50*)	
Movement	**Muscles involved**
Extension	Gluteus maximus, hamstrings, adductor magnus
Flexion	Iliopsoas (iliacus and psoas), rectus femoris, sartorius, adductors (longus, brevis), pectineus
Adduction	Adductors (magnus, longus, brevis), pectineus, gracilis
Abduction	Gluteus medius and minimus, piriformis
Rotation – medial – lateral	Gluteus medius and minimus Gluteal muscles (lateral rotators), sartorius, adductors, pectineus, piriformis and others
Circumduction	Hip muscles acting in sequence

NB Hamstrings comprise three muscles – biceps femoris, semitendinosus and semimembranosus.

Table 18.6 Movements and muscles at the hip (see also *Figure 18.50*).

Knee joint – hinge

The knee is a modified hinge joint formed by the femoral condyles, tibial condyles and the patella, which glides over the patellar surface of the femur [see *Figure 18.42(a)*]. The knee is stabilized by two intracapsular cruciate ligaments (see *Table 18.7*). The tibial articular surfaces are deepened by the semilunar cartilages (menisci), which also stabilize the knee by preventing lateral movement and act as shock absorbers [see *Figure 18.42(b)*]. The joint is further strengthened by a capsular ligament, various extracapsular ligaments and muscles and tendons.

The knee joint has the largest synovial membrane in the body. This membrane lines the joint cavity, extends upwards beneath the patellar tendon to form the suprapatellar bursa and lines other bursae associated with the joint (see page 419).

Ankle joint – hinge

The ankle joint is formed by the tibia and its medial malleolus and the lateral malleolus of the fibula, which both articulate with the talus [see *Figure 18.43(a)*]. The joint is strengthened by ligaments that include a strong medial ligament (deltoid) [see *Figure 18.43(b)* and *Table 18.8*].

Foot and toe joints

The joints between the tarsals are of the gliding type, as are the tarsometatarsal joints. In addition to the gliding movements, there is some slight adduction and abduction possible between the talus and calcaneus. Movement between the talus and navicular, and calcaneus and cuboid respectively, facilitates eversion and inversion of the foot.

The metatarsophalangeal joints are of the condyloid type, allowing flexion, extension, adduction and abduction. Interphalangeal joints are of the hinge type, allowing only extension and flexion.

The movements of the foot and digits are produced by various leg muscles (extensors and flexors) and many intrinsic foot muscles, e.g. interossei, lumbricals. The intrinsic muscles and the very long tendons of the leg muscles are also important in supporting the foot arches (see pages 416–417). The long extensor and flexor tendons that run to the foot are enclosed within synovial sheaths and are secured by strong ligaments, the retinacula.

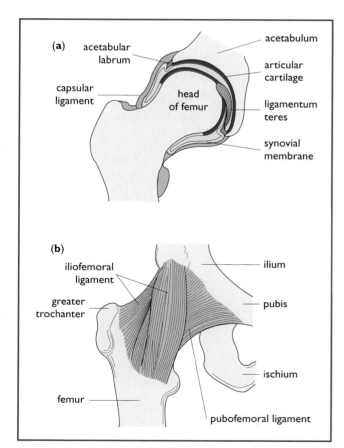

Figure 18.41 (a) Hip joint; (b) ligaments reinforcing the hip (anterior view).

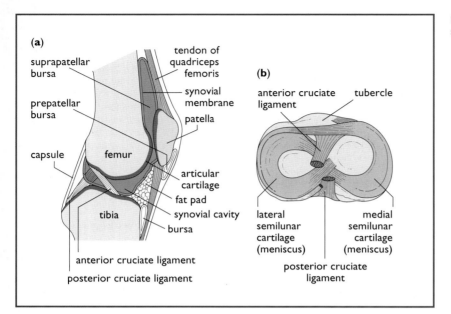

Figure 18.42 (a) Knee midsagittal section; **(b)** semilunar cartilages.

Table 18.7 Movements and muscles at the knee (see also *Figure 18.50*)	
Movement	Muscles involved
Extension	Quadriceps femoris (rectus femoris and three vasti)
Flexion	Hamstrings, gastrocnemius, sartorius, gracilis, plantaris
Medial rotation (slight)	Popliteus (also flexes)

Table 18.7 Movements and muscles at the knee (see also *Figure 18.50*).

Table 18.8 Movements and muscles at the ankle (see also *Figure 18.50*)	
Movement	Muscles involved
Extension (plantarflexion)	Gastrocnemius, tibialis posterior, soleus, long flexors of the toes, peroneus (longus and brevis), plantaris
Flexion (dorsiflexion)	Tibialis anterior, long extensors of the toes, peroneus tertius
Inversion	Tibialis anterior, tibialis posterior, toe flexors
Eversion	Peroneus (tertius, longus and brevis)

Table 18.8 Movements and muscles at the ankle (see also *Figure 18.50*).

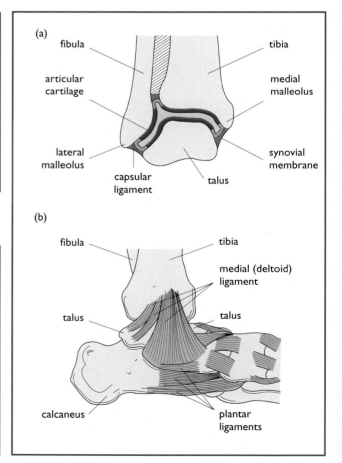

Figure 18.43 (a) Ankle; **(b)** ligaments reinforcing the ankle (medial view).

Person-centred Study **Brian**

Knee injuries involving the medial meniscus or anterior cruciate ligament commonly occur when the knee is twisted in sports such as soccer or squash.

Brian, who plays soccer with a local team, has had pain and increasing problems with his knee, which has 'locked up' completely on a couple of occasions.

Brian's GP referred him to an orthopaedic consultant, who diagnosed damage to the medial meniscus. It was possible to rectify the damage via an arthroscope (instrument for viewing the inside of the joint cavity), which meant that Brian was able to go home the same day without the need for more extensive surgical

treatment (meniscectomy – removal of the meniscus). Following this procedure Brian's knee will function as before, apart for some possible loss of stability (remember the menisci help to stabilize the knee joint by preventing lateral movement).

Special Focus **Joint conditions – arthritis and gout**

Arthritis is not a single condition – it comes in many forms, affects all age groups and may vary in severity from a mild ache to severe joint pathology with pain, disruption, deformity and disability. The word arthritis, which means joint inflammation, tends to be an over-simplification because the aetiology may be immunological, infective, inflammatory or degenerative.

Classifications of arthritis are complex, with dozens of different types existing, but for our purposes a brief consideration of rheumatoid arthritis, osteoarthritis (osteoarthrosis) and gout will give you an outline of the common joint-damaging conditions.

Rheumatoid arthritis

Rheumatoid arthritis (RA) is a generalized chronic inflammatory condition of connective tissue, mostly affecting joints. RA occurs worldwide and affects all ages and ethnic groups. It is characterized by polyarthritis (of fingers, hand, wrist, hip, knee or ankle) and systemic effects, which include fatigue, high temperature and weight loss. Other serious extra-articular manifestations of RA include pericarditis (see Chapter 10) and normocytic anaemia (see Chapter 9).

The aetiology of RA is autoimmune (see Chapter 19) but, as yet, the exact initiating mechanisms are unclear. The abnormal immunological situation with T lymphocyte activity and cytokine release, e.g. of interleukin 1, autoantibodies and immune complexes, will in genetically susceptible people cause synovitis (inflammation of the synovial membrane) with membrane proliferation, eventual loss of articular cartilage and joint destruction. These joint changes cause pain, swelling, severe deformity and progressive loss of mobility with increasing dependence and disability.

Management includes:

- General rest.
- Rest for joints with splints to reduce deformity.
- Measures to deal with systemic effects, e.g. treatment of anaemia.
- Local warmth, e.g. wax baths, gloves and socks, warm baths, or cold applications.
- Physiotherapy and mobility aids.
- Occupational therapy and aids to maintain independence, e.g. large handles on cutlery.
- Change of occupation, environmental adaptations and appropriate housing changes.
- Drugs: analgesics, e.g. aspirin (also used for its anti-inflammatory effects), and other NSAIDs, e.g. ibuprofen; systemic corticosteroids, e.g. prednisolone – prescribed for its anti-inflammatory effects (**NB** aspirin, ibuprofen and prednisolone may cause peptic ulceration and bleeding – see Chapter 13); intra-articular corticosteroids; chloroquine (antimalarial drug); sulphasalazine; gold salts; penicillamine; cytotoxic drugs such as methotrexate and cyclophosphamide; immunosuppressives, e.g. azathioprine and cyclosporin A, which modify immunological responses. Newer techniques such as using monoclonal antibodies (see Chapter 19) to deliver immunlogically active substances to specific areas are being developed and evaluated.
- Radiotherapy – medical synovectomy (destruction of the synovial membrane without surgery) using radioactive colloids in older adults.
- Joint surgery, e.g. synovectomy, arthrodesis.
- Joint replacement surgery (replacement arthroplasty), introduced over 30 years ago, has revolutionized the management of arthritis. Commonly used to replace hip and knee joints, arthroplasty is a highly effective and efficient means of improving quality of life over long periods; for example, a standard hip replacement should function maintenance-free for 10–15 years (Green, 1989). The 'limited life' of the original-type (metal – head of femur; plastic – acetabulum) replacement joint meant that there was some reluctance to replace joints in younger individuals. Advances in material science, with the development of flexible carbon fibre joints that last much longer, means that a younger age group can be offered joint replacement in the knowledge that the need for a second operation is greatly reduced. Other, less extensive, techniques being developed include covering the femoral head with metal and placing a metal cup in the acetabulum, which is attached using hydroxyapatite (see Chapter 16). This metal-on-metal joint replacement apparently increases its life by reducing the 'wear and tear' associated with the original metal–plastic joint and the hydroxyapatite fixes the new component more naturally.

Special Focus **Joint conditions – arthritis and gout** *cont.*

Osteoarthritis (osteoarthrosis)

Osteoarthritis (OA) is characterized by the destruction of the articular cartilage, which usually affects the large weight-bearing joints, e.g. knee and hip, and the intervertebral and phalangeal joints. It occurs commonly in older people (60+) as joints 'wear out', but can be secondary to existing joint problems, e.g. congenital dislocation of the hips (see page 425) or trauma. OA occurs more frequently in Caucasians and genetic factors appear to increase the predisposition to some forms of this joint disease.

The loss of articular cartilage, development of bony spurs (osteophytes) and thickening of the synovial membrane results in pain, crepitus, swelling, stiffness and loss of function with reduced mobility. Obesity increases the prevalence of OA affecting the large weight-bearing joints such as the knees.

Management includes:

- Minimizing damage, e.g. weight reduction, as obesity contributes to damage, or reducing activities to rest the joint.
- Analgesia, anti-inflammatory drugs, intra-articular corticosteroids.
- Physiotherapy to increase muscle strength and mobility.
- Hydrotherapy – can relieve muscle spasm and pain.
- Mobility aids.
- Arthroplasty (see RA) and other joint surgery, e.g. osteotomy to relieve pain and correct early deformity.

Gout (gouty arthritis)

Gout describes a group of diseases characterized by an abnormality of metabolism that leads to excess uric acid (hyperuricaemia) in the blood. Uric acid is a normal waste product of purine-containing nucleic acid metabolism (see Chapter 1), which is mainly eliminated in the urine (see Chapter 15).

Problems occur, however, if production or ingestion of purines increases or the elimination of uric acid, via the urine, is inadequate (a genetic predisposition exists in many individuals). The excess uric acid, in the form of crystals, is deposited in joints, most commonly the first metatarsophalangeal (remember the stereotypical portrayal of gout with the overweight 18th century male with heavily bandaged foot on a stool and a glass of port to hand), where it causes swelling and severe pain.

During an acute episode NSAIDs (for pain relief and anti-inflammatory action) are used plus colchicine, which stops leucocyte movement into the joint. Allopurinol (reduces uric acid production) plus colchicine are used to control gout after an acute episode or to prevent its occurrence where increased purine turnover is anticipated, e.g. in some types of chronic leukaemia (see Chapter 9). Drugs that increase urinary excretion of uric acid, e.g. probenecid (sulphonamide derivative), may be used in situations where excretion of uric acid is a problem, such as with Down syndrome, alcohol misuse and renal failure. Advice regarding resting the joint, weight reduction, limiting intake of high purine foods, e.g. offal, and restricting alcohol intake, which inhibits uric acid elimination, is also useful.

Muscular System

It is appropriate here to give a brief outline of the muscular system – a process that includes naming muscles, movement relationships and the major muscle groups. Some muscles associated with joints have already been discussed in terms of their action at a specific joint and you should refer to the appropriate tables.

Naming muscles

The naming of skeletal muscles, which may at first appear rather complex, is often based on characteristics that include size, position, function, shape, number of origins, direction of fibres, origin and insertion and a combination of these:

- Size – e.g. gluteus maximus (largest) and minimus (smallest).
- Position – e.g. intercostal (between the ribs).
- Function – e.g. pronator teres (pronates).
- Shape – e.g. deltoid (triangular).
- Number of origins – e.g. triceps brachii has three.
- Direction of fibres – e.g. rectus (straight) femoris.
- Origin and insertion – e.g. brachioradialis originates in the brachium (arm) with its insertion on the radius.
- Combination – e.g. extensor digitorum longus (function, location and size).

Movement relationships

The great variety of movements initiated by skeletal muscles are interdependent and co-ordinated just like the steps of a dance. Imagine for a moment the chaos that would ensue if muscles or dancers operated in isolation. It is the co-ordination between muscles that allows the smooth and often very precise movements needed for us to function effectively.

Muscles around a joint most often function in pairs: if a muscle initiates a certain movement there must be another muscle that has the opposing effect. Muscles that have the main responsibility for an action are known as **prime movers** (agonists), e.g. the biceps brachii flexes the elbow. The muscles that limit and counter their action are **antagonists**, e.g. the triceps brachii extends the elbow. The same muscles reverse

Nursing Practice Application **Tardive dyskinesia – a disorder of movement**

Individuals, especially older adults, treated with phenothiazine drugs (neuroleptics used widely in the management of mental health problems such as psychotic disorders), e.g. fluphenazine, can develop tardive dyskinesia. The affected person experiences involuntary movements, often involving the muscles of the head and neck, but they can involve other muscle groups in the trunk or limbs. The involuntary movements result in facial grimaces and tongue and chewing movements, which may distress the person and their family and friends, and in mobility problems if the limbs and trunk are affected. Tardive dyskinesia may take months or years to appear and is unfortunately difficult to treat, but it might help if the offending phenothiazine is replaced with a drug that causes fewer motor problems.

roles when necessary – the prime mover for one movement can be the antagonist for another.

Many movements also require the action of muscle groups that act together as **synergists**: they contract together to assist the prime mover, stabilize a joint and cancel out unwanted movements produced by prime movers where the muscles cross more than one joint. Some synergists, when they prevent a movement by stabilizing a joint, are called fixators.

Major muscle groups

It is unnecessary for you to attempt to memorize the details of every muscle, but the ability to apply the principles of movement and posture to your practice is of paramount importance. The following overview is not intended to provide a complete coverage of skeletal muscles and readers requiring more detail are referred to Further Reading (Williams *et al.*, 1995). It is worth noting that attempts to classify muscles into rigid groups can cause difficulties; for example, the latissimus dorsi is a back muscle that acts at the shoulder.

Muscles of the head and neck

The paired and unpaired muscles of the head and neck (see *Figure 18.44*) are concerned with movement, support, facial expression, e.g. smiling (zygomaticus), speaking, chewing and swallowing.

Damage to the sternocleidomastoid muscle of the neck, which may occur during birth, can result in congenital torticollis (wry neck), where the infant's head is tilted and rotated to one side. After birth, torticollis can occur acutely as a result of the pain and muscle spasm associated with neck injuries. Individuals with certain neurological problems may develop muscle dystonia (abnormal muscle tone), which causes a painful spasmodic torticollis and other abnormal postures.

Muscles of the shoulder and arm

The muscles of the shoulder and arm (see *Figures 18.45* and *18.46*) are concerned with the movements of the shoulder, elbow, wrist, hand and fingers (see also *Tables 18.2–18.5*).

Muscles of the trunk

The superficial and deep muscles of the trunk (see *Figures 18.46–18.49*) are collectively concerned with movement of the trunk, maintaining erect posture, support, respiration and increasing intra-abdominal pressure to assist defaecation, micturition and parturition.

Back

The large back muscles found either side of the spinal column include the trapezius, latissimus dorsi, erector spinae group, or sacrospinalis (see *Figure 18.46*), which consists of three columns, and the quadratus lumborum and psoas, which also form part of the posterior abdominal wall [see *Figure 18.48(b)*]. These powerful muscles support, maintain posture and allow movement at the trunk.

Thoracic wall

The thoracic wall has a superficial layer, which includes muscles involved with movements of the upper limb, e.g. pectoralis major [see *Figure 18.45(a)*] and minor, those that move the scapula, such as the serratus anterior and rhomboids [see *Figure 18.46*], and those confined to the chest wall, e.g. serratus posterior (see *Figure 18.46*). A middle layer consists of the external intercostal muscles [see *Figure 18.47(a)*], which lift the rib cage to enlarge the thorax during inspiration, and the internal intercostals, which are only used during forced expiration (remember that expiration is normally passive) to reduce thoracic capacity (see Chapter 12). During forced inspiration other muscles are used, e.g. scalenes and sternocleidomastoids, and the back and abdominal muscles assist with forced expiration. The innermost layer of muscle consists of subcostal muscles and the transversus thoracis; these may act with the internal intercostals to depress the ribs.

Logically the diaphragm [see *Figure 18.47(b)*], which divides the thoracic and abdominal cavities, is included here as it is concerned with respiration. During inspiration it contracts and flattens to enlarge the thorax, and during expiration it relaxes to decrease thoracic size. The diaphragm also increases intra-abdominal pressure to facilitate venous return (see Chapter 10), defaecation (see Chapter 13), micturition (see Chapter 15) and parturition (see Chapter 20).

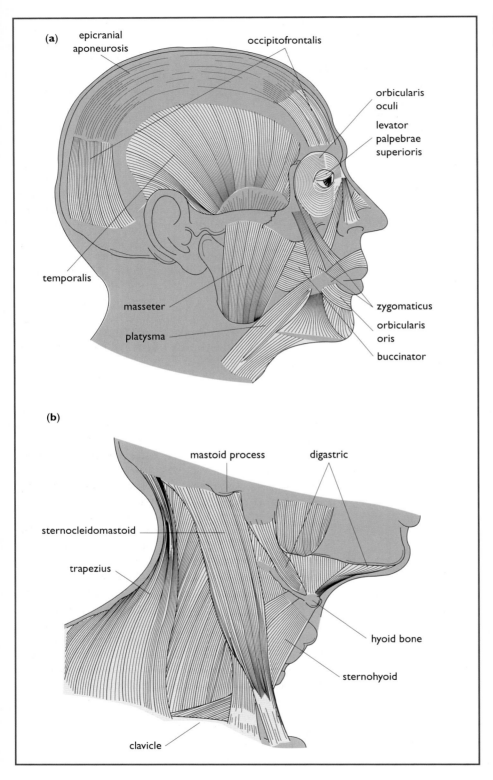

Figure 18.44 Main muscles of **(a)** Head and face; **(b)** neck (platysma not shown).

Abdominal wall

Three layers of muscle form the anterolateral walls of the abdomen [see *Figure 18.48(a)*]. They allow trunk movement, support viscera, compress the abdomen during evacuation and the lifting of objects, and assist with expiration. Working with the diaphragm, they increase abdominal pressure during the Valsalva manoeuvre (see Chapters 12 and 13). The different directions of the fibres of the three layers produce a very strong muscular wall.

The layers, from the outside, are the external oblique, internal oblique and transversus abdominus. The aponeuroses of these three muscles merge with the strap-like rectus abdominus, the medial muscle running from sternum to pubis. The linea alba, a tendinous cord formed from the aponeuroses of the abdominal muscles, divides the rectus abdominus in the midline.

The inguinal canal, which carries the round ligament in females and the spermatic cord in males (Chapter 20), is an intermuscular canal running obliquely through the abdominal muscles at the level of the inguinal ligament formed from the aponeurosis of the external oblique muscle.

The inguinal canal is a 'weak spot' where herniation occurs (inguinal hernia); other sites of herniation include the femoral canal (femoral hernia), the area around the umbilicus (umbilical hernia), the oesophageal opening in the diaphragm (see hiatus hernia, Chapter 13) and the site of an incision (incisional hernia).

Another problem associated with the abdominal wall can occur during embryonic development should the abdominal wall fail to enclose the intestines. This results in the congenital abnormality exomphalos in which the intestines protrude through the defective abdominal wall (see Chapter 13).

The posterior abdominal wall is formed by the quadratus lumborum, psoas and iliacus muscles with their fascia [see *Figure 18.48(b)*].

Pelvic floor and perineum

The muscles and ligaments (strung between the bones of the pelvis much like a cane seat on a wooden chair) that support the pelvic organs consist of the pelvic floor and, inferiorly, the perineum, which includes the urogenital diaphragm. Two main muscles, the levator ani and coccygeus, form a funnel-shaped structure consisting of identical halves that join in the midline [see *Figure 18.49(a)*] to form the pelvic floor or diaphragm. Below the pelvic floor is the wedge-shaped perineum that anteriorly forms the triangular urogenital diaphragm and posteriorly the anal sphincter. The structures contributing to the perineum include the transverse perineus muscles and the urinary and anal sphincters, and over the urogenital diaphragm an overlay of superficial muscles [see *Figure 18.49(b)*]. The pelvic floor is perforated by the urethra and anus, and by the vagina in the female. The role of the pelvic floor is to control voiding and defaecation, maintain continence (see Chapters 13 and 15), keep the pelvic structures in position, and maintain erection of the penis and clitoris during the sexual response (see Chapter 20).

Problems that occur when the pelvic floor malfunctions include urinary incontinence (see Healthier Living box and Chapter 15) and genital prolapse, which is discussed in Chapters 20 and 21.

Muscles of the hip and leg

The muscles of the hip and leg (see *Figure 18.50*) are concerned with the movements of the hip, knee, ankle, foot and toes (*Tables 18.6–18.8*), and maintaining stable postures.

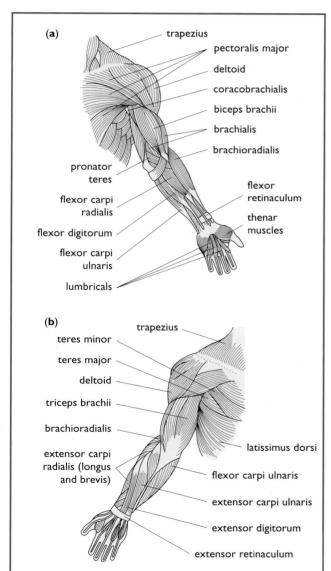

(a)
trapezius
pectoralis major
deltoid
coracobrachialis
biceps brachii
brachialis
brachioradialis
pronator teres
flexor carpi radialis
flexor digitorum
flexor carpi ulnaris
lumbricals
flexor retinaculum
thenar muscles

(b)
trapezius
teres minor
teres major
deltoid
triceps brachii
brachioradialis
extensor carpi radialis (longus and brevis)
latissimus dorsi
flexor carpi ulnaris
extensor carpi ulnaris
extensor digitorum
extensor retinaculum

Figure 18.45 Main muscles of the shoulder and arm. **(a)** Anterior view; **(b)** posterior view. NB Some muscles not shown.

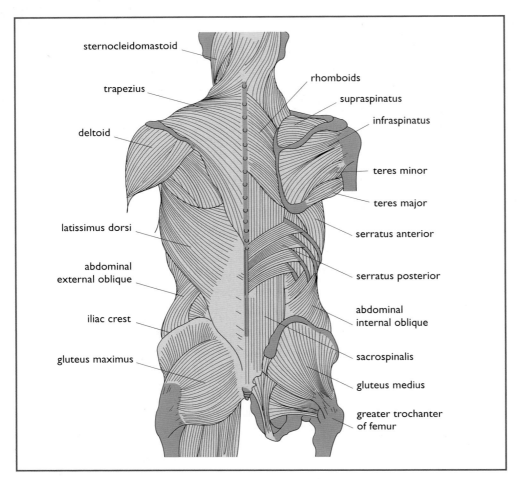

Figure 18.46 Main muscles of the back (superficial muscles removed on the right).

- sternocleidomastoid
- trapezius
- deltoid
- latissimus dorsi
- abdominal external oblique
- iliac crest
- gluteus maximus
- rhomboids
- supraspinatus
- infraspinatus
- teres minor
- teres major
- serratus anterior
- serratus posterior
- abdominal internal oblique
- sacrospinalis
- gluteus medius
- greater trochanter of femur

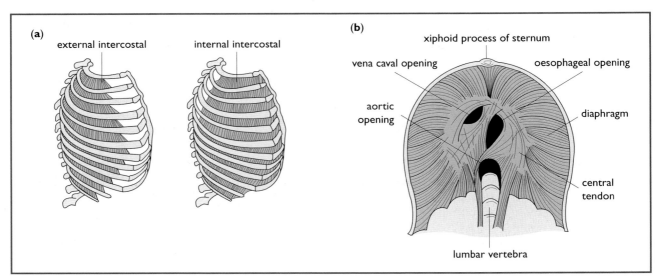

(a)
- external intercostal
- internal intercostal

(b)
- xiphoid process of sternum
- vena caval opening
- oesophageal opening
- aortic opening
- diaphragm
- central tendon
- lumbar vertebra

Figure 18.47 (**a**) Deep muscles of the thorax; (**b**) diaphragm (inferior view).

Healthier Living **Pelvic floor maintenance and continence**

Urinary continence relies heavily upon the proper functioning of the pelvic floor and perineum. Keeping these muscles in 'good shape', with care and exercise, is an important part of more general health maintenance and exercise programmes. Damage to the pelvic floor muscles during parturition and their functional decline during the climacteric make women particularly high risk for urinary incontinence (see Chapter 15) – aspects of labour and the replacement of female hormones (HRT) during the climacteric are discussed in Chapters 20 and 21.

The first objective is to raise awareness about the pelvic floor muscles and their function – Candy (1994) states that women have little awareness in this regard. Pelvic floor health should be a priority throughout life, not just after giving birth or reaching the climacteric. Women, once they know where the muscles are sited, can learn various exercises (such as stopping the flow of urine whilst voiding) that enhance pelvic floor efficacy. Steps can also be taken to avoid raised intra-abdominal/pelvic pressure by lifting objects correctly and treating a chronic cough, which can weaken the pelvic floor.

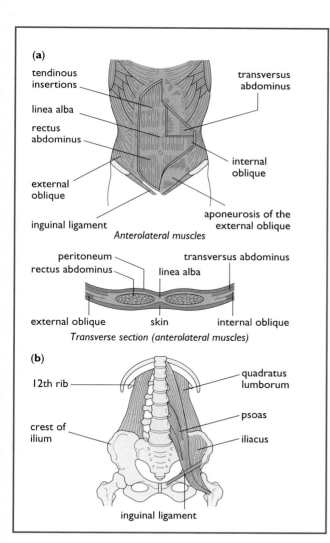

Figure 18.48 Abdominal wall. (**a**) Anterolateral; (**b**) posterior.

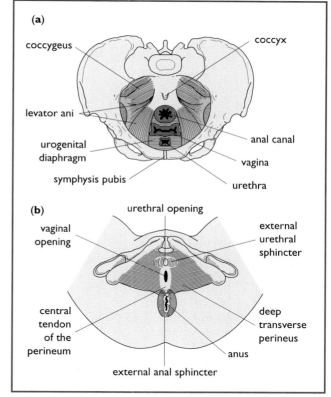

Figure 18.49 Pelvic floor (female). (**a**) Main muscles (superior view); (**b**) urogenital diaphragm (inferior view).

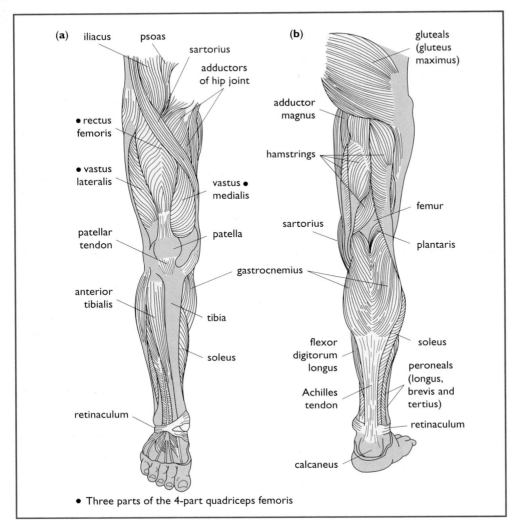

(a) iliacus psoas sartorius adductors of hip joint
• rectus femoris
• vastus lateralis
vastus • medialis
patellar tendon patella
anterior tibialis tibia
soleus
retinaculum

(b) gluteals (gluteus maximus)
adductor magnus
hamstrings
femur
sartorius
plantaris
gastrocnemius
flexor digitorum longus
soleus
peroneals (longus, brevis and tertius)
Achilles tendon
retinaculum
calcaneus

• Three parts of the 4-part quadriceps femoris

Figure 18.50 Main muscles of the hip and leg. (**a**) Anterior; (**b**) posterior. **NB** Some muscles not shown.

Summary/Check List

Introduction
Skeleton – bony landmarks.
Axial skeleton – skull, cranium, Nursing Practice Application – damage to the ethmoid bone, sutures, fontanelles, Nursing Practice Application – moulding of the fetal cranium. Facial bones, Nursing Practice Application – mandibular fracture, paranasal sinuses. Spine: curves, vertebrae, spinal ligaments, intervertebral foramina and discs, spinal movements. Nursing Practice Application – back problems. Thoracic cage, sternum, ribs.
Appendicular skeleton – pectoral girdle and arm, clavicle, scapula, humerus, radius, ulna, wrist and hand. Pelvic girdle and leg, innominate bones, pelvis (female/male), femur, patella, tibia, fibula, ankle and foot, arches.

Levers and movement
Joints – types: fibrous, cartilaginous, synovial.
Synovial joints – characteristics, movements, varieties. Nursing Practice Application – joint stiffness/immobility. Injuries to joints. Specific synovial joints, movements and muscles, shoulder, elbow, radioulnar, wrist, hands/fingers, hip. Nursing Practice Application – CDH, knee joint. Person-centred Study – Brian. Ankle, foot/toes. Special Focus – joint conditions.
Muscular system – naming muscles. Movement relationships. Major muscle groups. Nursing Practice Application – tardive dyskinesia. Healthier Living – pelvic floor maintenance and continence.

Self Test

1 Name the bones of the axial and appendicular skeletons.
2 Put the following in their correct pairs:
   (a) occipital bone;
   (b) odontoid process;
   (c) axis;
   (d) nucleus pulposus;
   (e) ribs;
   (f) foramen magnum;
   (g) annulus fibrosus;
   (h) costal cartilage.
3 How does the female pelvis differ from the male?
4 Explain how carrying loads close to the body is more efficient.
5 Give an example of:
   (a) fibrous,
   (b) cartilaginous and
   (c) synovial joints.
6 Draw a diagram of a synovial joint showing general characteristics.
7 You are asked to teach Maud a full range of arm exercises. What movements would you teach for the shoulder?
8 Outline the function of the following: bursae, semilunar cartilages, foot arches, glenoidal labrum, ligamentum teres.
9 What can the name tell you about a muscle?
10 Complete the following:
   (a) The _ _ _ _ _ _ _ _ _ separates the thoracic and abdominal cavities.
   (b) The levator ani is a muscle of the _ _ _ _ _ _ _ _ _ _ _/_ _ _ _ _ _ _ _ _ _ .
   (c) The Achilles tendon is the insertion of the _ _ _ _ _ _ _ _ _ _ _ _ muscle into the _ _ _ _ _ _ _ _ _ .

Answers

1 See page 398.
2 a–f, b–c, d–g and e–h.
3 See page 414.
4 See page 417.
5 (a) skull sutures, teeth, tibiofibular;
   (b) symphysis pubis, epiphyseal plate, sternum;
   (c) hip, shoulder.
6 See page 419.
7 Extension, flexion, adduction, abduction, medial and lateral rotation and circumduction.
8 See pages 419, 425, 416, 422, 424.
9 Shape, position, size, function, number of origins, site of origin and insertion, and fibre direction.
10 (a) diaphragm;
   (b) pelvic floor/diaphragm;
   (c) gastrocnemius, calcaneus.

References

Candy M (1994) Raising awareness of a hidden problem. Pelvic floor promotion. *Prof Nurs* 9(4): 278–284.

Green A (1989) What's happening to hips? *Nurs Times,* 85 (46): 32–33.

Griffiths BL (1988) Have you ever had a pain in your back? *Prof Nurs* 3(4): 125–130.

Hignett S (1996) Work-related back pain in nurses. *J Adv Nurs* 23(6):1238–1246.

Seymour J (1996) Patient handling safe practice. *Nurs Times* 92 (32): 46–48.

Further Reading

Disabled Living Foundation (1994) *Patient Handling Equipment Advice and Information.* London: Disabled Living Foundation.

Klippel JH, Dieppe PA *et al.* (1994) *Rheumatology.* London: Mosby.

Health and Safety Commission (1992) *Guidance on Manual Handling of Loads in the Health Service.* London: Health and Safety Commission.

National Back Pain Association/RCN (1997) *The Guide to the Handling of Patients,* 4th edn. London: NBPA/RCN.

Royal College of Nursing (1996) *Code of Practice for Patient Handling.* London: RCN.

Royal College of Nursing (1996) *Introducing a Safer Handling Policy.* London: RCN.

Royal College of Nursing (1996) *Manual Handling Assessment in Hospital and the Community.* London: RCN.

Williams PL, Warwick R, Dyson M *et al.* (1995) *Gray's Anatomy,* 38th edn. Edinburgh: Churchill Livingstone.

Useful Addresses

Arthritis and Rheumatism Council (ARC)
Copeman House
St Mary's Court
St Mary's Gate
Chesterfield
Derbyshire S41 7TD

Royal Association for Disability and Rehabilitation (RADAR)
Unit 12, City Forum
250 City Road
London EC1V 8AF

Body Defences and The Skin

Overview

- *Non-specific defences (innate): skin and membrane barriers, cells, chemicals and inflammation.*
- *Specific defences (adaptive): humoral and cell-mediated immunity.*

Learning Outcomes

After studying Chapter 19 you should be able to:

- Describe the structure of the skin and its appendages.
- Discuss normal skin pigmentation and changes that may be abnormal.
- Describe the functions of the skin and relate these to structure.
- Explain how the skin contributes to temperature homeostasis.
- Use physiological knowledge to explain the rationale for the nursing practices involved in monitoring body temperature, and to explain failures of temperature homeostasis.
- Outline the protective role of other innate barriers.
- Describe phagocytosis and the role of non-specific cellular defences.
- List important inflammatory and antimicrobial chemicals.
- Describe the events of the inflammatory response and discuss its defensive role.
- Describe the events of wound healing and use this knowledge in wound care practices.
- Discuss factors that predispose to pressure sores, and measures used in their prevention.
- Outline the characteristics of a specific (adaptive) defence.
- Describe humoral immunity.
- Outline the classes of antibodies and their functions.
- Explain active and passive immunity.
- Outline the immunization programme available to children in the UK.
- Describe cell-mediated immunity.
- Outline the role of cell-mediated immunity in cancer surveillance.
- Discuss the relevance of cell-mediated immunity in organ transplantation.
- Describe abnormal immune responses: hypersensitivity reactions, autoimmunity and immunodeficiency.
- Discuss the aetiology and effects of acquired immune deficiency syndrome (AIDS).
- Discuss aspects of health promotion aimed at reducing the spread of AIDS.

Key Words

Antibody – a protein produced by plasma cells that binds to a specific antigen.

Antigen – a molecule or part of a molecule that is identified as foreign by body defences and which therefore stimulates the immune response, e.g. a virus. It binds specifically to T cell receptors or antibodies.

Autoimmune response – abnormal immune response where the body defences fail to recognize self-antigens. It results in tissue damage.

Cell-mediated immunity – part of the specific adaptive immune response involving the action of T lymphocytes, which destroy abnormal/foreign cells and release regulatory chemicals.

Key Words *cont.*

Commensals – micro-organisms that live in close association with a host. They benefit from the relationship and generally cause no harm.

Complement – a collection of serum proteins involved in both inflammation and the immune response.

Cytokines – a generic term describing cellular signalling chemicals such as the interferons involved in body defences.

Dermis (true skin) – the layer below the epidermis.

Epidermis – the superficial layer of the skin.

Humoral response – part of the immune response involving the production of antibodies by plasma cells.

Hypothermia – abnormally low body temperature where core temperature is below 35°C.

Immune response – specific adaptive defences provided by B and T lymphocytes.

Immunity – resistance to disease.

Immunoglobulin (Ig) (see antibody) – proteins present in blood and other body fluids.

Inflammatory response – non-specific innate tissue response to injury characterized by redness, heat, swelling, pain and loss of function. The local tissue changes are caused by chemicals, cells, vascular events and fluid exudation.

Integument – the skin and its appendages.

Lysis – breakdown/disruption of cells, e.g. by micro-organisms.

Lysozyme – bactericidal enzyme present in many body fluids, e.g. tears.

Melanin – dark pigment found in varying degrees within the skin, hair and other sites, e.g. the iris.

Normal flora – the micro-organisms that normally live on or in the body, e.g. *Escherichia coli* in the gut.

Pathogen – a disease-producing micro-organism.

Phagocyte – a cell able to engulf micro-organisms and other debris by phagocytosis.

Pyrexia (fever, febrile) – elevated body temperature, usually between 37.2 and 41°C. Temperature elevated above 41°C is termed 'hyperpyrexia'.

Introduction

Body defences, which are vital to our survival, consist of two main functional components. The first line of defence is provided by the non-specific innate defences of intact skin and mucous membranes which prevent the entry of **pathogens** (disease-producing micro-organisms) into the tissues. If pathogens do breach the barriers various second line **phagocytes** and inflammation come to the rescue.

Our defence strategies are completed by the **immune response** (specific adaptive defences provided by B and T lymphocytes), e.g. **antibody** (protein produced by plasma cells that binds to a specific **antigen**) production. The components of the immune response deal with pathogens that slip past the innate barriers and also recognize and destroy abnormal or foreign cells, e.g. malignant cells.

Non-specific and specific defence systems work closely in their protective role; for example, phagocytosis (the process by which phagocytes engulf micro-organisms and other debris) is enhanced by the presence of **immunoglobulin IgG** (see antibody).

Defence, which is part of most body systems/structures, cannot be attributed to a particular organ or system. For a wider understanding of surveillance and defence, it will be necessary for you to make frequent reference to other relevant chapters (Chapters 9 and 11).

Throughout this book emphasis has been placed upon the degree of integration required to maintain homeostasis – there is a necessary interdependence between all body systems. The innate defences and immune response, which protect most body systems, have important links with both endocrine and nervous control systems (see Section 3).

Examples of these links include:

- Stress hormones – corticosteroids – are known to suppress both inflammation and immune responses (see wound healing, pages 450–451, and Chapters 6 and 8).
- Thymic hormones process T lymphocytes (see Chapter 8 and pages 456–457).
- Some neurotransmitter chemicals may have a role in modulating the immune response, as may our emotional state.

Non-specific Innate Components – Skin and Membrane Barriers

Skin

The skin (*Figure 19.1*), so often taken for granted, covers and protects the body, and is continuous with the mucous membranes lining body cavities and orifices opening at the surface. Your skin or **integument** (skin and appendages) weighs around 4 kg, covers an area of some 1.4 m² and normally varies in thickness between 0.5 mm on the eyelid to 3–4 mm on the soles of the feet. The skin can become much thicker in certain situations, e.g. going barefoot causes 'hard skin' to form.

Functions of the skin include: control of water loss, protection, sensation, storage, temperature regulation, excretion and vitamin D synthesis. The skin is divided into two layers, the **epidermis** (the superficial layer of the skin) and **dermis** (true skin – the layer below the epidermis), which are secured to the underlying structures by the subcutaneous tissue (hypodermis) and adipose tissue.

Early development

The integument arises from surface ectoderm (epidermis and appendages) and mesoderm (dermis) during development. As early as week 7 primitive epidermis is forming and surface cells are shed (desquamation) – it is these cells that are later collected during amniocentesis for testing for fetal abnormality (see Chapter 21). Over the next few weeks the skin appendages, e.g. sweat glands, and the dermis develop, and by the fourth month the components of the adult skin are in place. Fetal skin is extremely thin and adipose tissue is not deposited until around week 28 – neonates born very early are thin and wrinkled (no adipose deposits), and because the blood vessels are visible through the skin they look very red. The skin is protected

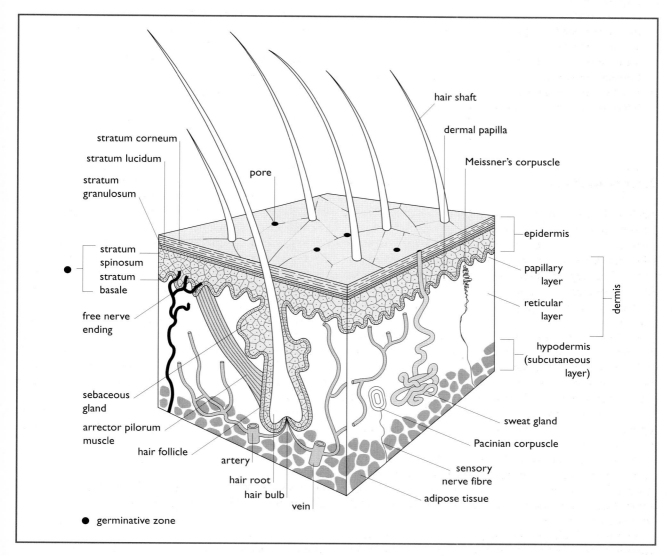

Figure 19.1 The skin.

from the 'watery' intrauterine environment by a white fatty substance called vernix caseosa, which consists of sebum (see page 441), hair and cells. Vernix has mostly disappeared by birth and is usually found only in the skin creases of mature neonates. Another adaptation to fetal life is the presence of fine hair, or lanugo, which develops from the fourth month to cover the body by week 20. Lanugo is lost before and just after birth, and is eventually replaced by vellus and terminal hair (see page 442).

Structure of the skin

Epidermis

The epidermis is formed from several layers of stratified epithelium (see Chapter 1), which have no blood vessels or nerves (*Figure 19.2*). Cells present in the skin are mostly keratinocytes, which produce keratin (tough fibrous protein found in epidermis, hair and nails); modified macrophages called Langerhans' cells (dendritic cells), concerned with immune defences; and melanocytes, which produce **melanin** (dark pigment found in varying degrees within the skin, hair and other sites, e.g. the iris) on exposure to ultraviolet light (see page 442).

The epidermis has an outer horny zone consisting of three layers – stratum corneum (horny cells), stratum lucidum (clear cells) and stratum granulosum (granular cells) – which overlay the germinative zone. The germinative zone has two layers: stratum spinosum (prickle cells) and stratum basale, (basal cells), which contains the melanocytes responsible for melanin and skin pigmentation.

The epidermis undergoes renewal as the stratum corneum is continually shed (desquamation or exfoliation) to be replaced by new cells formed in the stratum basale which move upwards through the layers over a period of 5–7 weeks. This renewal is under the influence of a protein epidermal growth factor. Epidermal cohesion is maintained during the renewal processes by the desmosomes (see Chapter 1), which bind the keratinocytes together and help to prevent structural damage. Various changes occurring as the cells migrate upwards are nuclear disintegration, keratinization (addition of keratin) and flattening. As a result the stratum corneum comprises dead cells containing keratin.

The renewal process, which is most rapid during childhood, stabilizes during adult life to decline as ageing occurs – a point that has relevance when you consider the time required for wounds to heal at different ages.

Next time you undress or make your bed take note of the dust, which is in fact your exfoliated epidermal cells. The dust is only a nuisance at home, but in a surgical area it can present a potential infection risk (if cleaning is inadequate) as micro-organisms that are shed with the epidermis could be transferred to wounds when the dust is disturbed.

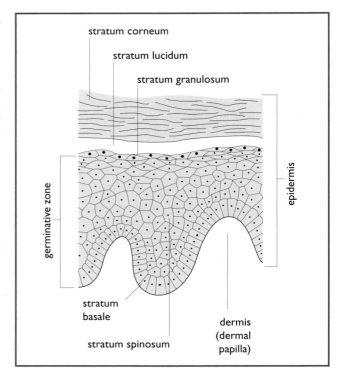

Figure 19.2 Layers of the epidermis.

The epidermis is attached to the dermis by an undulating line consisting of dermal papillae. On the palms (and soles) the papillae are more prominent, and are reproduced on the epidermis as epidermal ridges with the whorls and ridges of your 'fingerprints'. The interlocking layers of epidermis and dermis may be disrupted when subjected to the excessive shearing forces that predispose to pressure sores (page 452) and heel blisters.

Dermis

The dermis is connective tissue containing collagen, elastin and reticular fibres, cells such as fibroblasts and macrophages, blood and lymph vessels, and nerve endings. The dermis is divided into the papillary (containing the dermal papillae – see above) and reticular layers (see *Figure 19.1*). The arrangement of fibres gives rise to a pattern of cleavage lines, which were first described by Langer in 1861. These cleavage lines are of particular interest to surgeons because wounds following the lines heal with less scarring than do those that cross cleavage lines.

The wrinkles of normal ageing are caused by loss of dermal fibres, a process much accelerated by exposure to wind and sunlight. If the skin is stretched, e.g. during pregnancy or severe obesity, the rupture of elastin fibres leads to the formation of 'stretch marks', or striae.

The physical effects of Down syndrome (individuals have an extra chromosome – see Chapter 21) are numerous and varied, e.g. congenital heart defects. Infants with Down syndrome have an abnormality of the dermal/epidermal ridges, evidenced by a single transverse palmar crease (normally there are two creases).

Structures derived from the skin – the appendages

Structures derived from the skin include: sweat glands, ceruminous glands, sebaceous glands, hair follicles and nails.

Sweat glands

Sweat glands are widely distributed over the body and are of two types: eccrine and apocrine. Eccrine sweat glands are the most abundant. They are concentrated on the palms, soles of the feet, and forehead. These coiled glands produce watery sweat, which leaves via a duct to empty onto the surface through pores (see *Figure 19.1*). The major role of eccrine sweat glands is temperature homeostasis, wherein the evaporation of sweat from the body causes heat loss. This principle applies when tepid sponging is used to reduce elevated body temperature and increase comfort.

Sweat, which contains electrolytes (sodium and chloride), nitrogenous waste, and other waste, such as drugs and food residues, also has a minor excretory role. Sympathetic nerve stimulation and adrenaline (see Chapters 6 and 8) cause sweat production in response to changes in skin temperature and emotional states such as nervousness and fear. Insensible water loss also occurs by diffusion, and this plus sweat may total 800–1000 ml/day under normal conditions in a temperate climate. This amount is obviously very variable and depends on factors such as environmental temperature and activity level. In situations where sweating is excessive, e.g. heavy work in hot conditions, where 10 litres/day may be lost, there is risk of dehydration and electrolyte imbalance (see Chapter 2).

Apocrine glands are found in the axillae, areola, groin and external genitalia. They produce a thicker fluid which, when subjected to bacterial action, has a distinctive musky odour. It is possible that apocrine secretions contain chemicals known as pheromones, which influence human sexual behaviour as they do in other species. This view is supported by the fact that apocrine activity does not commence until puberty and is influenced by sex hormones and the catecholamines produced during stressful situations.

Ceruminous glands are modified sweat glands present in the external auditory meatus. They produce cerumen (wax), which traps particles and prevents them entering the ear (see Chapter 7).

NB The milk-producing mammary glands (see Chapter 20) are modified sweat glands.

Sebaceous glands

Sebaceous glands are abundant on the face, neck and back. They secrete a fatty substance, containing cholesterol and other lipids, known as sebum. The glands may discharge their sebum into hair follicles or directly onto the skin surface (see *Figure 19.1*). Sebum is important in keeping hair and skin supple and resistant to cracking, in waterproofing and in providing a bactericidal/fungicidal barrier.

Sebaceous gland activity increases at puberty and is especially stimulated by the action of androgens. Bacterial action on the sebum, with associated blockage of the follicles, inflammation and bacterial infection, explains the development of 'spots' (acne) that cause so much distress during adolescence.

The activity of sebaceous glands is low at the extremes of age, which renders the skin more prone to damage and reinforces the view that babies and older adults need particularly gentle skin care.

Hair and follicles

Hair helps to protect the skin, the eyebrows/lashes protect the eyes and nasal hair traps large particles. Hair also assists minimally in temperature regulation and is used in the expression of self-image (a new hairstyle can do wonders for your self-esteem).

The hair follicles are formed from epidermal tissue that grows down into the dermis or subcutaneous layer (see *Figure 19.1*). Blood vessels and nerves supplying the follicle enter at its base via a papilla. Hair, which consists of keratinized cells, has a bulb or growing region at the base of the follicle, a root within the follicle and a shaft above the surface of the epidermis. Associated with the hair follicle is the involuntary arrector pilorum (plural, pili) muscle (see *Figure 19.1*), innervated by sympathetic fibres, which erects the hair to give you 'goose flesh' or 'pimples' when cold or frightened. Animals such as cats can make their fur 'stand on end', making themselves appear larger and more ferocious. This mechanism is also important in heat conservation in such animals, as a layer of warm air is trapped next to the skin. Humans can in no way match this, but you can still feel the neck hairs become erect while watching a very scary film.

Nursing Practice Application **Hair condition**

Assessments of physical condition should include the hair in the examination. Considerable information can be obtained – not only about the hair, but also about the person's general health and ability to self-care. General appearance, cleanliness and grooming may give clues about mental health – a depressed person may lack the motivation or energy to bother about grooming. Head lice are very common in children from all backgrounds and, although the lice are hard to spot, the nurse should look for eggs sticking to the hair shaft (in adults lice may also infest pubic and body hair). Assessing hair thickness is important as the causes of abnormal hair loss or thinning include scalp disease, autoimmune conditions (see pages 461–462), cytotoxic drugs (see Chapter 9), hypothyroidism (Chapter 8) and protein deficiency (Chapter 13). Other problems that might be noted include abnormal hair distribution, e.g. terminal facial hair in women, which may indicate excess testosterone, or the presence of fine lanugo hair on the body/limbs of a person with the eating disorder anorexia nervosa.

Hair types and growth

There are three types of hair:

- Lanugo (see page 440).
- Vellus hair, the soft, 'fluffy' fair hair that forms the body hair of children and women. It also appears on the scalp when head hair thins.
- Terminal hair, the coarse pigmented hair of the scalp and eyebrows.

During puberty, under testosterone influence, terminal hair replaces the axillary and pubic vellus hair of both genders, and male body and facial hair. The amount of terminal body hair varies between individuals – some men may have very little, while some women have increased terminal hair growth on the arms and legs.

Hair grows in cycles – a period of growth is followed by a resting phase before the old hair is shed and new hair develops. Hair follicles remain active for various periods and those on the head may be active for years. Natural loss of head hair or male pattern baldness, which has an inherited basis, only affects males and is linked with testosterone secretion, which stimulates hair growth on the face but not on the head. Additionally, the hair thins with normal ageing in both sexes as more and more follicles become inactive.

Hair colour (from pale blonde to deepest black) is genetically determined and depends on the amount of melanin present. When the amount of melanin declines, a process that is also genetically controlled, the hair turns grey or white.

Nails

The nails are keratinized sheets that protect the distal ends of the digits (*Figure 19.3*). Nails increase manual dexterity and allow us to deal with annoying itches. They are derived from epidermal tissue and are similar to the hooves and claws of other species. Each nail grows on a nail bed from a matrix of germinative cells. It has a root, body and free edge. At its proximal edge the nail is thickened to form the white lunula, which is covered by eponychium (cuticle). In health the nail appears pink because of the presence of numerous capillaries in the dermis.

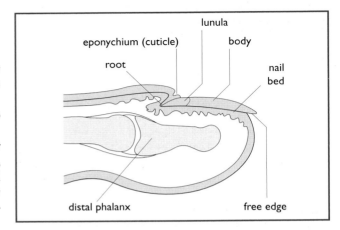

Figure 19.3 Section through distal phalanx and nail.

Skin pigmentation

Skin pigmentation (colour) is due to the presence of haemoglobin, melanin and carotene. The pink colour of Caucasian skin is caused by haemoglobin. Melanin is a brown–black pigment responsible for: racial differences in skin colour (increased melanin = darker skin); pigmented areas such as the nipple/areola; freckles; moles; and the changes occurring when light skin tans. The presence of melanin gives the skin some protection from ultraviolet light (UV) (see page 447). Melanin is derived from the amino acid tyrosine (see phenylketonuria, Chapter 13) and is produced by the epidermal melanocytes when they are stimulated by UV light and hormones (see Chapter 8). Rarely, yellow–orange coloration can be produced by the deposition of carotene in the skin and may be associated with high dietary intakes of carotene-rich foods.

Functions of the skin

Normally functioning skin plays a vital part in maintaining homeostasis and provides physical, chemical and biological protection.

Nursing Practice Application Skin colour and condition

During a nursing assessment important clues about general health can be gained from skin colour and condition. Some examples include:

- Pallor – cold conditions, shock, anaemia.
- Redness (erythema) – hot conditions, emotions (e.g. nervousness), pyrexia, allergy, inflammation, early stage pressure sore, polycythaemia (Chapter 9), 'hot flushes' of the climacteric (Chapter 21) and after exercise.
- Bruising/haematoma/petechiae (escape of blood into the tissue) – bleeding disorder (Chapter 9) or abuse.

- Cyanosis (Chapter 12) – blue discoloration of the skin caused by poor oxygenation of the haemoglobin. Occurs in chronic respiratory conditions and heart failure. Cyanosis, which may be peripheral or central, is easily observable in Caucasians, but is much more difficult to detect in Asian or Afro-Caribbean individuals, in whom a careful examination of the nail beds and mucous membranes is required.
- Yellow – jaundice (Chapter 14), fading bruises (due to haemoglobin breakdown), suntan.
- Normal pigmentation changes –

increased pigmentation, e.g. of the face during pregnancy, dark 'age spots' on the hands of older adults.
- Abnormal pigmentation – the bronze discoloration seen in Addison's disease (Chapter 8) caused by increased secretion of ACTH, which is very similar chemically to MSH. Patchy areas of depigmentation known as vitiligo.
- Rashes/local swellings or lesions/dryness/oedema – may indicate a variety of abnormal states, e.g. dry skin in dehydration; scars of different ages may indicate self-harm.

Waterproofing

The skin forms an effective waterproof layer that prevents excess water loss or entry – which is just as well when you soak in the bath. The outer layers and sebum work as well as any waxed jacket. If this barrier is breached, as with severe burns, the consequent fluid (serum) loss results in hypovolaemic shock (Chapter 10). Indeed, fluid replacement, based on the percentage of body area involved (calculated using charts for age and size, e.g. Lund and Browder's), is a priority in the management of burns.

Temperature regulation

The skin is a major contributor to temperature homeostasis. Humans are homeothermic ('warm-blooded') and adults are able to maintain a constant core temperature (organs in the cranial, thoracic and abdominal cavities) within the range 36–37.6°C by balancing heat gained with heat lost (*Table 19.1*). In contrast, the temperature of the outside shell of the body varies, with site and environmental conditions, from the feet at 20°C to the forehead at 35°C. The control mechanism, or thermostat, set at 37°C, is situated within the hypothalamic heat-regulating centres (see Chapter 4).

Infants have a wider range for body temperature, but their heat-regulatory ability is poorly developed – shivering and sweating is limited. They have a special adipose tissue, called brown fat, situated in the neck, back and chest, which gives up its heat energy with ease – an adaptation that helps to offset their inability to produce heat.

A constant core temperature is critical for the proper functioning of the enzymes that facilitate the reactions required for physiological processes (see Chapter 1). A rise in temperature of 1°C will cause the metabolic rate to increase by some 7%, a fact that explains why **pyrexial**

Table 19.1 Heat gain and loss

Heat gain	Heat loss
Metabolism of fuel molecules	Through the skin by:
Muscular activity/shivering	evaporation
Environmental temperatures	conduction
Hormones increasing metabolism, e.g. thyroxine	convection
	radiation
Female sex hormones	Via the lungs
Body fat	Urine and faeces
Hot food/fluids (minimal)	

Table 19.1 Heat gain and loss.

(having an elevated body temperature – usually between 37.2 and 41°C) people need extra calories.

Body temperature shows a diurnal variation of 0.5–1.0°C. It is lowest during the night (1–4/5 a.m.) then gradually increases until late morning, remains static during the day and reaches a peak late afternoon/early evening (5/6 p.m.), after which it starts to fall. This pattern is reversed in people who do shift work involving long periods of night work, but not during short spans of night duty.

Earlier we mentioned core temperature – the centres of the head, chest and abdomen are much warmer than the shell or skin surface. When recording body temperature it is important to remember that tympanic membrane recordings correspond closely to core temperature, followed by the oral (only with a sensor placed in the sublingual area, close to the lingual artery with the mouth closed) and rectal sites (usually reliable, but the presence of faeces will affect accuracy); the sites least representative of core temperature are the axillae and groin.

Temperature control

The cells of the heat-regulating centre receive impulses from skin thermoreceptors and monitor the temperature of the blood passing through the hypothalamus.

When core temperature rises above the 'set point' of 37°C the hypothalamus inhibits heat production (see below) and initiates sweat gland activity (sympathetic stimulation) and peripheral vasodilation (sympathetic inhibition) (*Figure 19.4*). Sweating causes heat loss as moisture evaporates from the skin surface whilst environmental humidity is low, which is why we find humid conditions so much more uncomfortable than dry heat. Vasodilation of the arterioles in the dermis, which diverts blood to the skin capillaries and accounts for the red colour of hot skin, causes heat to be lost. This loss occurs by:

- Radiation to the surrounding air.
- Conduction to objects such as a chair.
- Convection as warm air currents move away from the skin to be replaced by cooler air.

Most heat is lost from the body by radiation, conduction and convection, and all can be utilized to reduce pyrexia, e.g. by fanning, reducing clothing, taking a cool bath, changing bed linen. Where possible we also take steps to 'cool off' when feeling too hot by removing a jumper or moving out of the sun.

Conversely, when the core temperature drops below 37°C or environmental temperatures fall, the heat-regulating centre initiates heat conservation/production mechanisms via the sympathetic pathways. Sympathetic stimulation causes vasoconstriction and the skin becomes pale and cold as blood is diverted from the surface to prevent heat loss.

A short-term increase in catecholamine release, e.g. of noradrenaline, speeds up the metabolic rate and more heat is produced (see Chapter 8). Catecholamines also increase sympathetic vasoconstriction. Shivering (intense muscular contraction), which produces large amounts of heat, will occur if the temperature fails to rise. A small amount of warm air trapped by body hair may also contribute. Longer term, when summer turns to winter and environmental temperatures fall, the thyroid gland is stimulated to release more thyroxine, which increases the metabolic rate, thereby allowing us to adapt to the environmental change (see Chapters 8 and 13). In adults the subcutaneous adipose layer serves as insulation, which we enhance by wearing several layers of clothes in cold weather.

Certain adaptive features operate in very cold weather: cold-induced vasodilation prevents hypoxic changes if skin blood flow is shut down for too long. In response to local hypoxia (see Chapter 12) the vessels dilate to restore blood flow, which accounts for the red hands and nose on a cold morning. Another feature is an arrangement by which venous blood regains heat before returning to the body core. The veins (venae comitantes) run close to the main arteries of the limbs, and use them as a countercurrent heat exchanger in much the same way that a cold water supply is warmed by running close to hot water pipes. This prevents cold blood reducing core temperature.

Blood flow through the skin, which is central to temperature control, is regulated by arteriovenous shunts and precapillary sphincters (see Chapter 10) that divert blood to or from the skin capillaries as needs change.

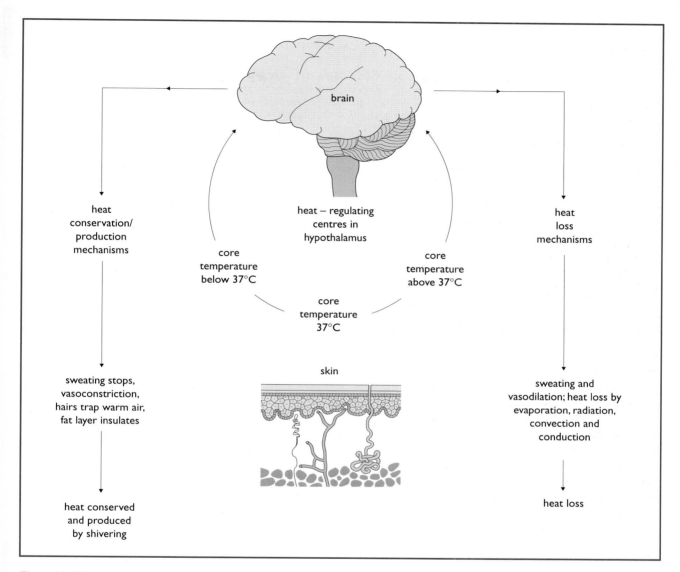

Figure 19.4 Temperature regulation and the skin.

Sensation

The skin is a major part of the environmental sampling kit vital to survival. It contains different sensory receptors that are able to distinguish various stimuli, from the touch of a feather to extremes of temperature. Receptors which respond to temperature, touch, pressure and pain relay the sensory data to the CNS for integration and, where appropriate, for the initiation of motor activity (see Chapter 3).

Skin receptors include: free dendritic nerve endings (pain, touch and temperature), Meissner's corpuscles (light pressure), Pacinian corpuscles (deep pressure), Krause's bulb (pressure) and the Ruffini organ (stretch and pressure). There is, however, some overlap of receptor function. Receptors

in the skin protect by alerting us to potentially harmful external factors, e.g. moving your hand rapidly (by reflex) when you touch a hot cooker ring. They also allow you the pleasurable sensations such as the feel of fresh bed linen.

Protection

Many skin functions protect – prevention of water loss, temperature homeostasis and the recognition of harmful stimuli have already been discussed. Intact skin also protects by providing physical, chemical and biological barriers to harmful agents.

The epidermis is a physical barrier against microorganisms. It is able to withstand some chemicals, e.g. mild acids; melanin blocks some UV light; and alpha ion-

Abnormal Function **Problems with temperature homeostasis**

Fever

In this situation the hypothalamic set point is reset to a higher temperature by the presence of exogenous pyrogens (chemicals producing fever) released by micro-organisms or by the action of endogenous pyrogens (**cytokines**) released from blood cells and injured tissue. Physical problems within the heat-regulating centre, e.g. severe head injury (see Chapter 4), have similar effects on the thermostat. The hypothalamus continues to initiate heat-conserving/producing mechanisms, which explains the vasoconstriction, feeling cold, shivering and rigors, as your core temperature rises to the new setting.

Once treatment with antibiotics or antipyretics, or natural defence mechanisms, have dealt with the cause of the fever, the thermostat is reset to normal and the whole system goes into reverse to initiate heat loss. There is vasodilation, profuse sweating and the person feels very hot.

Increased body temperature is one of the defence mechanisms of the body – it inhibits bacterial reproduction and the acceleration in metabolic rate can aid healing. An excessive or prolonged fever, however, will have profound negative effects upon physiological processes. The excessively increased metabolic rate causes an increase in pulse and respiration, and with

it the demand for energy and protein. With hyperpyrexia (body temperature above 41°C) there is a serious loss of enzyme efficiency, and brain damage (see below).

Heat stroke

Much more serious is the uncontrolled situation that occurs if body temperature reaches 41–42°C. The hypothalamus ceases to function properly and heat loss mechanisms fail to operate. The skin is hot and dry, and sweating and vasodilation do not occur. The rise in core temperature increases metabolic rate, which in turn produces more heat (a maladaptive positive feedback mechanism). If this dangerous state is not reversed the person will suffer convulsions and brain damage or death, when the body proteins become denatured at around 43°C. Heat stroke may result from unaccustomed or prolonged exposure to high environmental temperatures. It is likely to follow strenuous exercise in very hot conditions.

Hypothermia

At the opposite end of the scale is accidental hypothermia, which affects newborns, older adults (see Person-centred Study – Mavis) and those whose occupation or life-style may expose them to harsh environmental conditions, e.g. people 'living rough' or those who go ill-prepared for climbing expeditions.

Small babies are at risk because they lose heat through the head, become

uncovered, do not shiver and because their heat regulation system is underdeveloped. Older adults have reduced subcutaneous adipose tissue and poor homeostatic control (see Chapter 2), and may simply not feel cold or shiver as their temperature falls.

When body core temperature falls below 34°C the normal heat conservation mechanisms, such as shivering, fail to work. All body systems are sluggish, and the person becomes drowsy and eventually unconscious. Unresolved hypothermia leads to cardiac arrhythmias (see Chapter 10) and death when the temperature falls to around 20°C.

Various factors that increase the risk of accidental hypothermia include:
- The socio-economic situation of older adults, who may have poor housing, reduced income for heating or food, and less motivation.
- Physiological causes, e.g. falls, hypothyroidism, alcohol misuse, sedation, confusion and reduced mobility in the older population.
- Mental health problems and learning disabilities that may prevent awareness of the effects of cold (Heath 1995).

NB Hypothermia is sometimes used during cardiac surgery to reduce metabolism and hence the cellular oxygen requirements.

Person-centred Study **Mavis**

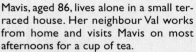

Mavis, aged 86, lives alone in a small terraced house. Her neighbour Val works from home and visits Mavis on most afternoons for a cup of tea.

When Val got no answer at the door she used the key that Mavis had given her for just such an eventuality. Val feared the worst, and when she saw Mavis slumped on the sofa in her nightie she thought that

she had died. On closer examination Val found that Mavis was drowsy and felt cold.

While Val waited for the ambulance she put Mavis into the recovery position (Chapter 12), covered her with two blankets and lit the gas fire. The paramedics wrapped Mavis in an aluminium foil 'space blanket' prior to the journey to hospital. The rationale here is to prevent further

heat loss by radiating the heat back to the body. Mavis was admitted to hospital for gradual rewarming (temperature 30°C) and rehydration. On recovering Mavis revealed that she had fallen on her way to bed and had just managed to get on the sofa, but had felt too shaken to light the fire or summon help before falling asleep in the unheated room.

izing radiation does not penetrate the skin. The fat layer provides varying amounts of 'padding', which gives some protection against trauma. It is worth mentioning that some lipid-soluble substances can enter the skin – a feature used increasingly in drug delivery systems such as

patches for transcutaneous administration.

The skin, which is usually acid (secretions are acidic), keeps out micro-organisms by forming a chemical barrier or 'acid mantle', and both sebum and sweat are bactericidal.

Biologically the skin protects against infection through its own **normal flora** (micro-organisms normally living on or in the body) or via **commensal** (micro-organisms living in close association with a host; they benefit from the relationship and generally cause no harm) organisms resident on the surface or within the deeper layers. These commensals, which are well adapted to their environment, tend to 'crowd out' other, more harmful organisms, which find it difficult to become established. The normal flora changes after admission to hospital, where the skin may be colonized by a different set of organisms, which increase the risk for infection. Although we have talked in terms of 'normal' flora it should be remembered that these organisms may operate as pathogens if they find their way into a different site, e.g. a wound. Langerhans' cells and dermal macrophages, which are part of the biological barrier, 'deal with' pathogens that do get through.

Synthesis of vitamin D

Vitamin D (see Chapters 8, 13, 15 and 16) is produced by the action of UV light on the sterol 7-dehydrocholesterol, which is present in the skin. Although some exposure to sunlight is beneficial, it is important to stress the dangers inherent in excessive 'sun-bathing', which include: 'sunburn', sun stroke, dehydration, premature ageing and, most serious of all, malignant skin changes. The incidence of skin cancers, including malignant melanoma, is increasing (for all skin types, but especially in Caucasians) in areas that enjoy good weather, e.g. Australia and the southern USA, and because the annual holiday is often spent sun-bathing in a hot country.

Excretion

Compared with the lungs and kidneys, the skin excretes only small amounts of waste. Water, sodium, chloride, urea and a minute amount of carbon dioxide leave via the skin.

Storage

The skin acts as a store for water, which can augment blood volume as required. Subcutaneous adipose tissue forms a substantial part of fat reserves. These reserves can be utilized as a source of energy when the body is otherwise depleted. The amount and type of fat stored depends on factors that include:

- Gender: females have a greater percentage of adipose tissue.
- Inheritance: the tendency to inherit a lean or plump build.
- Age: infants have brown fat cells (see page 443), which yield their heat energy more easily than other fat cells, and some individuals may retain brown fat into adult life. Older people have less subcutaneous fat, in some body areas, to act as insulation.

Other innate barriers

Most of these are covered in the relevant chapters, but during our discussion of non-specific defences a summary of the innate protective barriers will be helpful.

Gastrointestinal tract (see Chapter 13)

- Saliva contains **lysozyme** (a bactericidal enzyme present in many body fluids) and immunoglobulin IgA.
- Gastric HCl (pH 1.5–3.0) kills most micro-organisms, but cannot deal with large numbers of food poisoning micro-organisms.
- Gastric mucus protects the stomach lining from acid attack.
- Reflex vomiting occurs, e.g. after ingesting 'bad' food.
- Normal flora of the gastrointestinal tract helps to prevent colonization by pathogens. Fungal infection, e.g. by *Candida albicans* ('thrush'), can be a problem following antibiotic therapy, which may kill off the normal flora.
- Lymphoid tissue and immunoglobulins are present in the intestinal wall.

Nursing Practice Application **Skin hygiene**

Before starting we should perhaps reflect upon what Armstrong-Esther (1981) had to say about the subject of daily bed baths: 'the patient is not in contact with the water long enough to suffer effects other than mild exposure, hypothermia and discomfort'. Put this way, the daily bed bath does seem to fail in terms of providing hygiene and comfort without harm. The concept of skin as a physical, chemical and biological barrier to bacteria has important implications for practice. It is imperative that nursing interventions aimed at assisting with personal cleansing do not in fact compromise the integrity of this barrier. Moisture should not be allowed to accumulate in areas such as the axillae, the groin and where skin surfaces meet, as this encourages the growth of pathogens. Another aspect to consider is the frequent and often ritualistic use of alkaline soap and water, which alters the pH of the skin and has a drying effect that can lead to cracking. This is particularly serious in older adults, who already have a thinner, drier skin with reduced sebaceous gland activity. Pembroke (1983) suggests that problems in this age-group can be aided by reducing the use of soap and water and by using emollients instead.

Genitourinary tract (see Chapters 15 and 20)

- Frequent/complete voiding flushes bacteria from the urethra/bladder.
- The length of the male urethra.
- Normal flora of the vagina produces an acid environment (pH 4.5) which, during the reproductive years, keeps most pathogens out.
- The vagina has a 'tough' lining of stratified squamous epithelium.
- Regular shedding of the endometrium during menstruation may militate against chronic uterine infections.

Eyes (see Chapter 7)

- The presence of eye lashes.
- The occurence of the blinking reflex.
- Tears contain lysozyme.

Respiratory tract (see Chapter 12)

- The shape of the upper respiratory tract, hairs, cilia, and mucus prevent the entry of debris and many pathogens.
- Nasal secretions contain lysozyme.
- The sneeze reflex prevents the entry of unwanted material.
- Mechanisms which protect the larynx during swallowing.
- Cilia and mucus in trachea and bronchi trap microorganisms and move them out.
- The cough reflex expels unwanted material from the lungs.
- Phagocytic cells and lymphoid tissue are present in the bronchial walls.

Non-specific Components – Cells and Chemicals

Many cellular and chemical processes operate as part of the non-specific body defences. The major components are: phagocytes, natural killer (NK) cells, antimicrobial chemicals, e.g. lysozyme, **complement** (a collection of proteins involved in both non-specific and specific defences), interferons and the **defensive inflammatory response.**

Phagocytes and phagocytosis

The process of phagocytosis, in which phagocytic cells engulf and destroy foreign particles or dead cells, is a vital part of non-specific defences (see *Figure 9.10*). Phagocytes are found in most tissues and include some types of leucocyte, e.g. neutrophils, eosinophils and monocytes (Chapter 9), and the very important macrophages. Some phagocytic cells are fixed, e.g. Kupffer cells of the liver (Chapter 14), whilst others, such as free macrophages, are mobile and can congregate in areas of inflammation.

Phagocytosis is aided by immunoglobulins and complement (see below), which both coat the invading particle for destruction with opsonins. This process, called opsonization, makes it easier for the phagocyte to bind to the particle. Once the bacterium is inside the phagocyte it is killed by chemicals, such as activated oxygen species and nitric oxide, and then destroyed by lysosomal enzymes. Phagocytes can also kill other cells without engulfing them.

After dealing with the foreign particle, neutrophils are themselves destroyed and form part of the pus resulting from the encounter. The macrophages are not destroyed and can perform their role many times. Phagocytosis occurs as part of the inflammatory and healing processes – see healing of fractures (Chapter 16) and wound healing (pages 450–451) – and performs a vital role in both parts of the immune response (page 438).

Natural killer cells

Non-phagocytic NK cells belong to a group of large granular lymphocytes (LGLs) found in the blood and tissues, and they form part of the non-specific defences. These leucocytes can recognize and destroy, by chemical **lysis** (cell disruption/breakdown), a malignant or virus-infected cell. In the case of viral infection, the NK cells are attracted by the release of chemicals called interferons (see below). They also have a regulatory role in the production of blood cells in the bone marrow.

Antimicrobial chemicals

Lysozyme

Lysozyme is an enzyme found in many body fluids (see page 448) and in the lysosomes (see Chapter 1) of phagocytes. Its role is to destroy bacteria by cell wall disruption.

Acute phase proteins

These are a group of serum proteins, e.g. C-reactive protein, which are made in the liver. Their role is not well understood, but their release increases when inflammation occurs.

Interferons

Virus-infected cells produce antiviral proteins called interferons (IFNs). These IFNs help to prevent the destruction of surrounding cells by viruses, and stimulate macrophages and NK cells, which also destroy malignant cells. This has led to considerable interest in their development as antiviral agents, e.g. in hepatitis and acquired immune deficiency syndrome (AIDS), and as a treatment for malignancy, but as yet the results have been variable. Interferons are produced by many leucocytes, fibroblasts and T lymphocytes, acting as cytokines (a generic term describing cellular signalling chemicals) to modulate the immune response (see pages 458–459).

Complement

Complement is a complex of about 20 plasma proteins that are concerned with both non-specific and specific defences. Complement is activated in one of two ways: by an alternative pathway in non-specific defences and by the classical pathway in specific defences. Complement acts through cascades, where the first protein activates the second and so on. The activated complement is concerned with enhancing phagocytosis (see earlier text), bacterial lysis and the inflammatory response; and inflammatory chemical release, vasodilation and chemotaxis (see below).

Inflammatory response (inflammation)

Inflammation is the response of tissues to physical or chemical injury. The tissue injury may be due to micro-organisms, trauma, extremes of temperature (burns, scalds and frostbite), UV light, extremes of pH or ionizing radiation.

The important non-specific inflammatory response operates locally to limit tissue damage, remove the cause, and 'clear away' dead cells and other debris so that healing may occur. The tissue changes of inflammation are caused by chemicals, cells, vascular events and fluid exudation, which interact to produce an effective defence mechanism.

Acute inflammation is characterized by: redness (erythema) and heat as hyperaemia (excess blood in an area) occurs; swelling due to fluid exudation; pain caused by inflammatory chemicals and pressure on nerve endings; and loss of function, especially if a joint is involved. The degree of loss of function is directly related to the amount of swelling and pain present, as well as the injury site. If widespread or systemic inflammation occurs, these signs and symptoms are accompanied by leucocytosis (see Chapter 9) and the release of pyrogens with an elevation in body temperature, which under controlled conditions has beneficial effects (see page 446).

Events of the inflammatory response

- Immediate, but short-lived vasoconstriction.
- Next comes the release of inflammatory chemicals or mediators, e.g. histamine, prostaglandins and kinins, by damaged tissue, mast cells and basophils; the release of lymphokines (cytokines released specifically by lymphocytes); and complement activation. This leads to vasodilation and local hyperaemia as blood flow to the area increases.
- The release of inflammatory chemicals also increases capillary permeability, with exudation of fluid and proteins (fibrin and antibodies), which leak from the blood to the tissues. The exudate brings extra supplies of oxygen, fuel and leucocytes, helps to dilute any microbial toxins and commences the 'walling off' process with fibrin, which limits the damage – much like closing a fire door.
- More leucocytes are released from the bone marrow in response to chemicals released by damaged tissue. The extra leucocytes – neutrophils initially, monocytes (which become macrophages) later – and lymphocytes where pathogens are involved migrate to the inflamed area, attracted by inflammatory chemicals and chemicals released by micro-organisms, in a process called positive chemotaxis (see Chapter 9). Meanwhile the movement of plasma proteins results in slower blood flow, which allows the leucocytes to marginate (move to the sides of the capillaries).
- The leucocytes, having marginated, will stick to the capillary endothelium by virtue of vital adhesion molecules on both leucocyte and endothelial surfaces. They are now poised to move through the capillary wall to the damage zone by a process called diapedesis (see Chapter 9), which is initiated as chemotaxis continues. Individuals who lack a leucocyte adhesion molecule cannot fight bacterial infections because their leucocytes do not adhere or move into the tissues.
- Once the neutrophils, and later the macrophages, reach the damage zone they start to remove micro-organisms and damaged tissue by phagocytosis. Where inflammation is chronic the macrophage is the predominant cell. The phagocytic cells engulf the particles, which are then dealt with by chemicals and lysosomal lytic

enzymes (see page 448). Pus, if formed, is a mixture of dead leucocytes, tissue debris, micro-organisms and exudate. Phagocytosis is enhanced by the presence of immunoglobulins and complement.

- The last stage of the inflammatory response is for the macrophages to clear the debris from the battle zone so that the processes of healing can proceed (see wound healing, below).

NB Before healing can occur it may be necessary for a collection of pus (abscess) to be drained surgically.

Wound healing

Wound healing and inflammation are closely related processes. Healing, which aims to restore tissue integrity and normal function, may take place by rapid primary/first intention (*Figure 19.5*) or the more protracted secondary intention.

Clearly, the desired method is primary intention healing, which occurs in clean surgical incisions where the wound edges are in apposition. Where there is tissue loss, however, such as pressure sores, leg ulcers or a gaping wound, the healing occurs slowly by secondary intention as the cavity heals from the bottom.

Stages of wound healing

The stages of healing are: traumatic inflammation (acute), destructive phase (days), proliferative phase (days) and maturation, which can take months (Westaby, 1985). The inflammatory (see earlier text), destructive and early proliferative phases do, in fact, occur concurrently.

The major events of healing by first intention are:
- Blood clot fills the wound and the inflammatory response is initiated.
- Neutrophils and macrophages commence clearing clot and cellular debris by phagocytosis.
- Macrophages stimulate the development of fibroblasts, which synthesize the collagen needed to form the scaffolding or framework required for healing.
- New capillaries appear and, with collagen, form the glistening pink granulation tissue, which eventually fills the gap.
- Epidermal cells regenerate from the wound edges and grow across the granulation tissue in a process termed epithelialization. NB at this stage the wound is still very fragile and requires gentle handling.
- When epithelialization is complete the 'scab' is dislodged to expose the new pink scar tissue, which gradually fades to white. The wound repair continues to be strengthened by further synthesis and remodelling of collagen and usually reaches maximum strength by about 12 weeks, but can take longer.

Healing by secondary intention or granulation is basically the same but requires some modification:
- Infection must first be overcome by the inflammatory and immune responses.
- Necrotic tissue must be removed by the macrophages.
- Foreign bodies, e.g. splinters, must be removed by natural mechanisms. When this proves ineffective it may be necessary to intervene surgically.
- The process of filling the cavity with granulation tissue, which takes much longer, commences on the cavity floor.
- Epithelialization takes longer.
- The resultant fibrous scar will be larger because wound edges were not originally in apposition.

Factors that delay healing

Factors known to influence wound healing include:
- Normal ageing – this slows all phases of healing.
- Infection.
- Poor apposition of wound edges and tissue loss.
- Presence of foreign bodies and necrosis.
- Repeated wound trauma, e.g. coughing and inappropriate dressing techniques.
- Stress (physiological and psychological) and other reasons for high corticosteroid levels, e.g. Cushing's disease and 'steroid' therapy (see Chapter 8), which suppress inflammation and collagen synthesis.
- Poor blood and oxygen supply, e.g. anaemia (see Chapter 9), cardiovascular disease and shock (see Chapter 10).
- Diabetes mellitus (see Chapter 8), which impairs microcirculation.
- Nutritional status – protein and energy depletion, lack of vitamin C and zinc, which are all needed for healing. In obesity, adipose tissue has a poor blood supply (see Chapter 9).
- Widespread malignancy and immune problems, and their treatment, e.g. radiotherapy, cytotoxic drugs and immunosuppression.

For many of these factors competent nursing practice can prevent or minimize the negative effects. Wound care practices should also take account of those factors that fall within the responsibilities of the medical officer, such as diabetes control. Holistic care, which includes high standards of aseptic technique, choice of appropriate dressings (see Nursing Practice Application), use of research-based wound care protocols, consideration of nutritional status (see Chapter 13) and minimizing stress with information and support, can contribute considerably to wound healing.

A considerable body of reseach-based knowledge is available regarding all aspects of wound healing, pressure sores and leg ulcers, and readers are urged to make full use of this in their practice. Gould (1986) used the

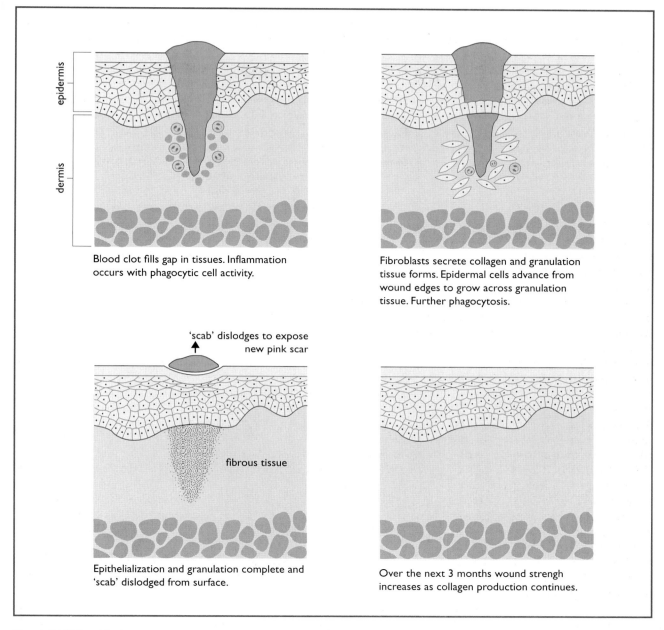

Blood clot fills gap in tissues. Inflammation occurs with phagocytic cell activity.

Fibroblasts secrete collagen and granulation tissue forms. Epidermal cells advance from wound edges to grow across granulation tissue. Further phagocytosis.

'scab' dislodges to expose new pink scar

fibrous tissue

Epithelialization and granulation complete and 'scab' dislodged from surface.

Over the next 3 months wound strengh increases as collagen production continues.

Figure 19.5 Wound healing – primary intention.

prevention and treatment of pressure sores as an example of where nurses fail to implement research findings. She explored the reasons (proposed by Hunt, 1981) why nurses do not apply research findings: they do not know about them, do not understand them, do not believe them, do not know how to apply them or are not allowed to use them.

The Further Reading includes a few examples of the wide selection of articles and books available, and reference is made to others within the text.

Specific Adaptive Components – the Immune Response

Specific adaptive defences of the immune system form our last line of defence against foreign particles such as pathogens that slip past the non-specific defences, as well as transplanted cells and abnormal cells arising in the body.

The components of the specific defences (see *Figure 19.6*) that produce the immune response are two lymphocyte populations – B lymphocytes (**humoral immunity** – part of the

Special Focus **Pressure sores**

Pressure sores cause suffering and use scarce resources – their development means that the person requires expensive nursing time, dressings and drugs, and where the sore is extensive surgical debridement and skin grafting may be necessary. Pressure sores increase morbidity and may contribute to death, e.g. from infection.

A complete coverage of pressure sores is not appropriate here, but a brief discussion is included.

Aetiology

Pressure sores develop when part of the body is subjected to unrelieved pressure sufficient to collapse the capillaries and disrupt the microcirculation. This happens when the skin and underlying tissues are squeezed between bone and a hard surface, e.g. of a trolley. Unrelieved pressure leads to tissue hypoxia, ischaemia and necrosis, with inflammation and ulcer formation.

Shearing forces also disrupt the microcirculation when they cause the skin layers to move against one another. Shearing occurs when a person slips down the bed or is dragged instead of moved properly. This type of tissue injury damages the deeper layers and results in a very extensive pressure sore.

Friction caused by continual rubbing of the skin leads to blisters, abrasions and superficial pressure sores. This type of tissue injury is exacerbated by the presence of moisture such as sweat or urine.

Assessment of risk

Initial risk assessment should be completed as soon as possible, and again at regular intervals or whenever circumstances change. Financial considerations make this essential as prevention costs money and nursing interventions should be targeted at those people at risk. Prevention is obviously better in every respect and is a great deal cheaper than the management of newly created sores.

Risk scales are in common use (e.g. Norton *et al.* 1962; Waterlow, 1985, 1991), but all have limitations, including a lack of community-based research or proper investigation as to their reliability and validity (Edwards, 1994). Spenceley (1988) thought that although risk calculators were valuable there was nothing to replace good nursing observations. This view is also supported by Edwards (1994), who states that scales were never meant to replace clinical judgement.

Factors that predispose to pressure sore formation

- Age over 65–70 years.
- Immobility, e.g. due to pain.
- Incontinence (see Chapters 13 and 15).
- Systemic infections, diabetes mellitus, malignancy and circulatory disorders, e.g. shock.
- Altered consciousness, e.g. by sedation.
- Sensory loss, e.g. after spinal injury (see Chapter 4).
- Dehydration (see Chapter 2) and or malnutrition, e.g. PEM (see Chapter 13), and lack of vitamin C, iron and zinc.
- Damage sustained from; wrinkled sheets or clothes, nurses' rings, watches etc.; plasters and splints.
- Oedema (see Chapter 10).

NB For many 'high risk' people there may be several factors operating together, e.g. being unconscious, immobile and incontinent following a stroke (see Chapter 4).

Assessment of skin and existing pressure sores

Assessment of pressure sore severity is vital for nursing management – without a standardized severity scale it is difficult to apply research findings or choose the most appropriate treatment. One such assessment tool is the four-stage Stirling Pressure Sore Severity Scale, which grades pressure sores from 1.1 – erythema (not blanchable) with local heat to 4.2 – sinus leading to tendon, bone or capsule; a stage 0 is available to record skin condition where no pressure sore exists (Reid and Morison, 1994).

Factors important in prevention

- Relief of pressure, e.g. special mattresses/beds and position change.
- Frequent assessment of high-risk areas.
- Avoiding skin trauma and shearing, e.g. by correct handling techniques (see Chapter 18).
- Assessing nutritional status (see Goodinson, 1987a–d, referred to in Chapter 13) and providing adequate hydration and nutrition.
- Planning care that minimizes the effects of incontinence, insomnia and confusion.
- Skin care and hygiene (see page 447).

Before leaving this topic we should perhaps reflect upon the statement: 'prevalence and incidence of pressure sores do not appear to be diminishing' (Land, 1995).

Nursing Practice Application **Wound healing and dressings**

Earlier we discussed the importance of holistic practice, where all requisites for wound healing are ensured, e.g. adequate nutrition and infection prevention. Another nursing responsibility is the provision of the correct microenvironment for healing, by the choice of appropriate dressings. The characteristics of an 'ideal' dressing, which provides such a microenvironment, have been identified (Turner, 1985):

- Provides thermal insulation – heat loss at the wound site impairs healing.
- Is non-adherent, causing no trauma on removal.
- Removes excess exudate and toxic substances – excess moisture impedes healing.
- Maintains high humidity – drying delays epithelialization.
- Allows gaseous exchange (possibly).
- Impermeable to micro-organisms.
- Leaves no contaminants in the wound.

NB Any dressing must also be comfortable and acceptable to the patient, and available and affordable.

Nursing Practice Application **Assessment of leg ulcers**

Most people with leg ulcers are managed at home and they form a large part of the workload of community-based nurses. Leg ulcers cost the health services millions each year, and accurate assessment is imperative for improving treatment, prognosis and reducing costs (financial and human).

Dale and Gibson (1993) suggest that assessment should include: the whole person; past history; examination of the leg and ulcer; noting other signs/symptoms; monitoring foot pulses (see Chapter 10); and Doppler ultrasound scanning to check blood supply by calculating ankle/brachial pressure index (API). In a literature review Shipperley (1997) stresses the importance of holistic assessment.

Although the aetiology of most leg ulcers is venous, about 20% of people will also have the risk of arterial disease and assessment must be research-based if the dangerous use of compression (in arterial disease) is to be avoided (Moffatt and O'Hare, 1995), they go on to say that the use of Doppler ultrasound is a vital additional assessment technique.

---

immune response involving the production of antibodies by plasma cells) and T lymphocytes (**cell-mediated immunity** – part of the immune response involving the action of specific lymphocytes that destroy abnormal foreign cells and release regulatory chemicals), antibodies and various chemicals. The ubiquitous macrophages, although part of the innate non-specific defences, are also concerned with the activities of B and T lymphocytes.

Co-operation between the specific defences confers **immunity** (resistance to disease) against a wide range of antigens (a molecule or part of a molecule that is recognized as foreign by the body defences and which therefore stimulates the immune response) by the recognition and subsequent neutralization or destruction of the foreign substance or particle. Some substances are incomplete antigens (or haptens), e.g. the drug penicillin; they only achieve antigenicity if they combine with serum proteins to cause allergies, which are certainly not protective. The correct functioning of the immune system, where the T and B lymphocytes have become immunocompetent, provides the body with considerable protection. There are, however, numerous examples of what happens when the immune system 'gets it wrong': **autoimmune** (abnormal immune response where body defences fail to recognize 'self', results in damage) disease, allergies, tumours and immunodeficiency, e.g. AIDS.

The early development of components of the immune response is linked closely to that of the thymus (Chapter 8), lymphoid tissue (Chapter 11) and haemopoietic tissue (Chapter 9). During fetal life the T and B lymphocytes start to develop immunocompetence and immune tolerance as the lymphocytes 'learn' to differentiate self from non-self antigens. The thymus eliminates those lymphocytes that do not react correctly to glycoprotein self antigens – the major histocompatibility molecules (MHCs) on body cell surfaces (genetically determined by the MHC gene cluster on chromosome 6). MHCs are also called human leucocyte antigen (HLA) because they were first described on leucocytes. It is worth noting that the concept of self and non-self is not absolute – some lymphocytes remain capable of attacking normal cells under certain conditions, thereby causing autoimmune disease. Although the immune system is not fully developed at birth, neonates derive some passive protection from maternal antibodies, received via the placenta or in colostrum (see Chapter 20) and breast milk.

At the other extreme the immune system in older adults tends to degenerate, which may help to explain why malignant and autoimmune diseases occur more frequently as we age.

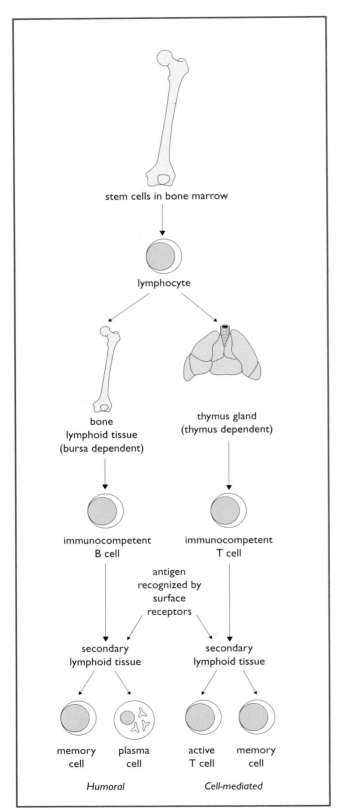

stem cells in bone marrow

lymphocyte

bone
lymphoid tissue
(bursa dependent)

thymus gland
(thymus dependent)

immunocompetent
B cell

immunocompetent
T cell

antigen
recognized by
surface
receptors

secondary
lymphoid tissue

secondary
lymphoid tissue

memory
cell

plasma
cell

active
T cell

memory
cell

Humoral

Cell-mediated

Figure 19.6 Development of B and T lymphocytes.

Characteristics of a specific defence

A specific defence has antigen specificity – the defence is mobilized by a specific antigen, e.g. a bacterium, but it is possible for antibodies to act against similar antigens (see page 455). 'Memory' cells remember how to destroy a particular antigen so that when it is confronted on subsequent occasions the defence response is more vigorous. Specific defences operate throughout the body and in this respect are quite different to the rather parochial inflammatory response.

Although they are quite different, it is important to remember just how much the non-specific and specific defences co-operate to enhance each other's activity; for example, phagocytosis is enhanced by the presence of antibodies, and macrophages present antigens to the T lymphocytes.

Humoral immunity

Humoral immunity is conferred by the presence of antibodies within the body fluids. Some lymphocytes, derived from the bone marrow stem cells, become B cells (bursa dependent), which eventually produce antibodies (*Figure 19.6*). The B cells are so called because in birds they are processed by gut lymphoid tissue known as the bursa of Fabricius; in humans the equivalent processing probably occurs in the lymphoid tissue of the bone (see Chapters 9 and 11). When the immunocompetent B cells in the blood or lymphoid tissue, e.g. lymph nodes and spleen, are exposed to an antigen that their surface receptors recognize, they undergo further changes within the secondary lymphoid tissue. This involves clonal selection, whereby huge numbers of identical B cells (a clone), which recognize the same antigen, are formed. Two distinct cell types emerge from the clone: plasma cells and memory cells (*Figure 19.7*). The transient plasma cells secrete the antibody that disarms the antigen, and the clone of memory cells, which 'remember' how to produce that particular antibody, circulate in the blood until required.

The memory cells, which may persist for many years, retain the ability to produce the specific antibody if they are again challenged by the antigen. This explains the increased vigour of response to second and subsequent antigen exposures, and forms the basis of immunization (see pages 456–457).

Antibodies (immunoglobulins)

Antibodies are proteins secreted by the activated B cells in response to a specific antigen (also usually a protein), e.g. bacteria, bacterial toxin and virus particles, but remember that smaller molecules can act as haptens (see page 453). When the antigen is a bacterial toxin the antibody that neutralizes its effects is termed an antitoxin. Antibodies that circulate in the gamma globulin part of the plasma proteins (see Chapter 9) are also known as immunoglobulins (Ig), of which there are five classes: IgG, IgM, IgA, IgD and IgE. These perform diverse defensive roles in a variety of body sites (*Table 19.2*).

Antibodies are Y-shaped proteins formed from four polypeptide chains (two heavy (H) chains and two light (L) chains). They have a variable region, with binding sites for specific antigens, and a constant region, with sites for complement and macrophage binding.

Antibodies function in different ways to inactivate antigens, but all involve the formation of an antibody–antigen complex (immune complex) where the specific (or very similar) antibody and antigen interact together (*Figure 19.7*). A helpful analogy is that of a jigsaw puzzle, in which each piece is specifically shaped to fit a space; a very similar piece may also physically fit, but a differently shaped piece will never fit the space in the puzzle.

Once the complex has been formed the antigen is inactivated by neutralization of toxins, precipitation and agglutination, or by complement fixation where complement fixes to the antigen. Later the antigens are destroyed by the immune-complex-driven processes, especially complement fixation, enhanced inflammation, phagocytosis and cell lysis by T lymphocytes, which follow on to 'clear up'. It is worth noting that some of the reactions, such as

Table 19.2 Antibody/immunoglobulin classes	
Ig Class	**Site and function**
IgG (gamma, γ)	Commonest antibody found in plasma, also in other body fluids. Passes across the placenta to confer passive immunity on the fetus. Binds to antigens, enhances phagocytosis and fixes complement.
IgM (mu, μ)	Largest antibody, found only in the plasma. First Ig released in response to a new antigen. Concerned with agglutination and fixes complement. Does not cross the placenta.
IgA (alpha, α)	Present in the plasma, respiratory, and gastrointestinal tracts, and other secretions, e.g. milk and tears. Acts to protect the mucosal surfaces.
IgD (delta, δ)	Large Ig present only in the plasma. Role not entirely clear but involved with B cell activity.
IgE (epsilon, ε)	Small amounts present in the plasma and bound to basophils and tissue mast cells (see Chapter 9). Involved with histamine release from these cells in allergic reactions such as asthma.

Table 19.2 Antibody/immunoglobulin classes.

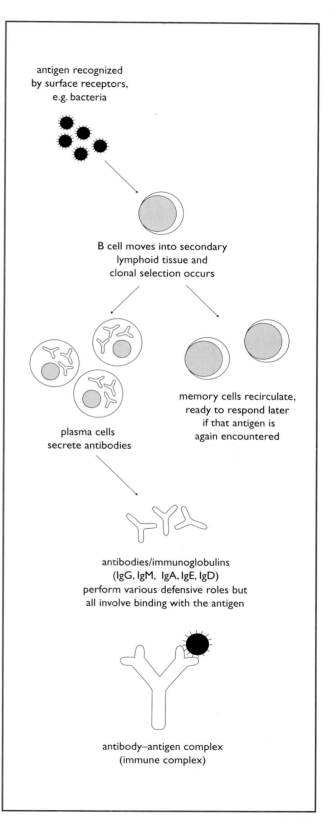

Figure 19.7 Summary of humoral immunity.

agglutination, may adversely affect the body, e.g. agglutination of donor red cells by IgM during a mismatched blood transfusion (see Chapter 9).

Many of these immunoglobulin reactions are used in diagnostic tests, and include blood grouping, and testing for certain infections and pregnancy. A recent development is the use of identical monoclonal antibodies, which are specific to a single antigen, for research and diagnosis of diverse conditions, including some early cancers, but most interesting of all is their use in transplant immunosuppression and cancer treatment. For example, monoclonal antibodies can be joined to cytotoxic drugs which, when introduced into the body, 'target' the specific antigen (cancer cells) and facilitate their destruction by the cytotoxic drug. This area of work is still developing, but the possibilities for effective cancer treatment without side-effects are very promising; this is especially so where the monoclonal antibody can also be made to stimulate body defences.

Immunity and immunization

As we have already mentioned, the presence of antibodies confers humoral immunity against many microbial diseases. During the first exposure to an antigen there is a lag phase of 2–3 weeks before antibody production (primary response) reaches a protective level. If we survive this first exposure the B lymphocyte memory cells can produce the antibody much more quickly (secondary response), with a very much reduced lag phase, if that antigen is again encountered. This exposure to the antigen, i.e. having the disease, is a form of active immunity in which the immune system is naturally stimulated to produce antibodies.

Active immunity, which is generally of long duration, can also be produced artificially by injecting vaccines. The vaccines contain inactivated or attenuated (weakened/changed strain) organisms or toxins that retain sufficient antigenicity to stimulate antibody production without the pathogenicity which would cause the disease. Many vaccines provide protection by active immunity, including those against tetanus, diphtheria, pertussis (whooping cough), poliomyelitis, mumps, morbilli (measles) and rubella (German measles).

The type of vaccine and its level of antigenicity determine the number of doses required: vaccines containing inactivated organisms, such as pertussis, are administered on three occasions, whereas those vaccines with live attenuated organisms need fewer doses, e.g. measles.

The other type of immunity is passive immunity, which results from the transfer of antibodies from one person or animal to another. This type of immunity is short-lived because the antibodies 'on loan' are eventually destroyed and, without antigenic stimulation, the immune system does not 'learn' to produce that particular antibody.

Passive immunity occurs naturally as maternal immunoglobulins are transferred to the fetus through the placenta (IgG) or to the infant via colostrum and breast milk (IgA, which protects against gastrointestinal infections). If you are wondering how proteins can survive the digestive processes – IgA is resistant and some authorities suggest that the immaturity of the infant's digestive tract allows the whole antibody to be absorbed by endocytosis and released into the blood by exocytosis.

Artificial passive immunity can be provided by injecting various immunoglobulins obtained from immune humans or, rarely, antisera (serum, obtained from animals, containing antibodies to a specific antigen) from animals (see note below). There are several situations where the provision of temporary but immediate immunity is appropriate: for non-immunized individuals during an epidemic; for protection during short trips abroad; following contact with the organism; or where an individual is immunosuppressed. The injection of gamma globulin, specific immunoglobulins and antitoxins give protection against diseases, which include hepatitis A and B, rabies, tetanus and botulism.

NB Antiserum, which causes allergic reactions, has been replaced with immunoglobulins.

The prevention of rhesus (Rh) blood group incompatibility and haemolytic disease of the newborn is another area that utilizes passive immunity. Anti-D immunoglobulin (containing anti-D antibodies to Rh-positive blood) administered to Rh-negative women within 72 hours of delivery, miscarriage or termination stops natural antibody production by destroying any fetal Rh-positive red cells that have entered the maternal circulation. Without this injection of anti-D, the woman would produce her own anti-D and, next time she is pregnant with a Rh-Positive fetus, the memory cells would produce anti-D antibodies which would cross the placenta and harm the fetus (see Chapter 9).

NB There is no danger to future pregnancies because the injected anti-D is short-lived.

Cell-mediated immunity

Cell-mediated immunity is facilitated by the activation of T lymphocytes (see *Figures 19.6, 19.8*). Some lymphocytes derived from the bone marrow stem cells become the T lymphocytes, which eventually form the effector and regulatory T cells. The T lymphocyte population is processed by the thymus gland in the mediastinum (see Chapters 8 and 9) and is said to be thymus-dependent. The thymus does most of the T lymphocyte processing before birth and during early childhood, which explains the gradual reduction in thymus size throughout adult life. Remember that the thymus is the site where T lymphocytes develop immunocompetence and immune tolerance. Immunocompetent T cells, circulating between the blood

Nursing Practice Application Immunization information

Nurses and midwives will often need to answer basic questions and give information regarding immunization programmes during their work. Varied questions for example, from new parents, people worried about contact with infectious diseases or someone planning a trip abroad may be encountered.

A basic immunization programme is outlined in *Table 19.3*, but sources of detailed information include: health visitors, child health and school health clinics, health centres/family doctors, and health promotion units. Where travel is involved, occupational health departments in companies where employees are required to travel, and DoH leaflets obtained direct or from travel agents and the appropriate embassy, can help.

Special groups such as health care workers, the immunocompromised and people travelling abroad require an individualized programme, e.g. health care workers should have hepatitis B protection.

NB Many authorities, including the World Health Organization, recommend that hepatitis B immunization is offered routinely during childhood.

Table 19.3 Basic immunization programme: from birth to leaving school.

Table 19.3 Basic immunization programme: birth to leaving school

Immunization	Timing	Remarks
Diphtheria Tetanus Pertussis (whooping cough)	2, 3 and 4 months (3 doses of each)	Injection (DPT), but pertussis can be excluded if parents wish or if there are contraindications
Poliomyelitis		Oral
Haemophilus influenzae type b (Hib)		Injection
Measles Mumps Rubella	12–15 months	Injection (MMR)
Preschool booster		
Diphtheria Tetanus	3–5 years	Injection (DT)
Poliomyelitis		Oral
Measles Mumps Rubella		Injection (MMR)
BCG (Bacillus of Calmette-Guerin) tuberculosis protection	10–13 years	For tuberculin-negative children (skin test)
Boosters: Diphtheria Tetanus	14–19 years	Injection (DT)
Poliomyelitis		Oral

NB Babies can be given BCG after birth – no skin test needed.
Hepatitis B vaccine given to babies born to hepatitis B positive mothers.

and lymphoid tissues, will react to antigen fragments that their specific surface receptors (T cell receptors, or TCRs) recognize. They only function, however, if an antigen-presenting cell (APC) first processes the antigen before presenting it to the T cell 'on a plate'. APCs, which include macrophages, B lymphocytes and special dendritic cells found in lymphoid tissue and elsewhere, e.g. Langerhans' cells in the skin, use their MHC proteins (class I for endogenous antigen, e.g. cancers, and class II for exogenous antigen, e.g. bacteria) to carry the processed antigen

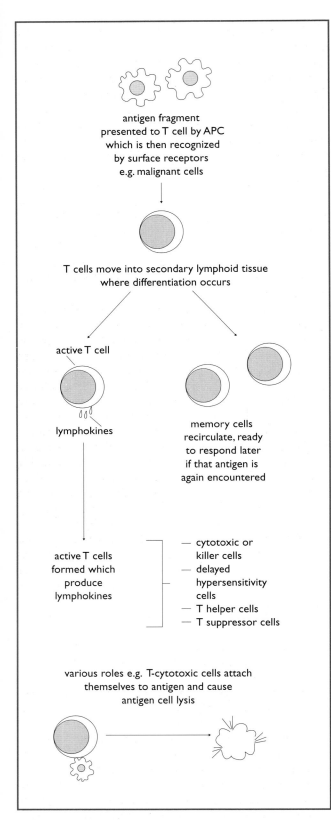

antigen fragment
presented to T cell by APC
which is then recognized
by surface receptors
e.g. malignant cells

T cells move into secondary lymphoid tissue
where differentiation occurs

active T cell

lymphokines

memory cells
recirculate, ready
to respond later
if that antigen is
again encountered

active T cells
formed which
produce
lymphokines

— cytotoxic or
  killer cells
— delayed
  hypersensitivity
  cells
— T helper cells
— T suppressor cells

various roles e.g. T-cytotoxic cells attach
themselves to antigen and cause
antigen cell lysis

Figure 19.8 Summary of cell-mediated immunity.

fragment. Once in the lymphoid tissue the T cells 'get to work' after using their TCRs to identify the foreign antigen and the APC. T cell differentiation occurs, with multiplication of the most appropriate T cell and memory cell for the task required, before antigen destruction occurs.

Types of T cells, cytokines and their functions

The several types of T cell can be classified functionally as:

Effector cells
- T-cytotoxic or killer cells: these directly destroy cells carrying antigens to which they are sensitive. These T cells provide a mobile immune surveillance as they continually search for malignant cells, transplanted cells and virus-infected cells. The killer cells attach themselves to the specific antigen and destroy it by chemical lysis. Here the entire T cell acts much like an antibody by 'locking on' to the cell carrying the antigen fragment. The memory cells continue to circulate between the blood and lymphatics until called upon to 'remember' that particular antigen, should it again threaten the body.
- Delayed hypersensitivity T cells: these are involved in the response of macrophages and other T cells in chronic inflammation and cell-mediated delayed hypersensitivities (see page 461).

Regulatory cells
- T-helper cells: these are vitally important to the immune response. They are alerted by macrophage APCs and start to stimulate the proliferation of killer cells, B lymphocytes and other immune cells by producing lymphokines, e.g. interleukins.
- T-suppressor cells: as their name suggests, these stop or slow T and B lymphocyte activity, by releasing lymphokines, once immune responses have dealt with the antigen. In this way they act to limit the immune response to an appropriate level and are thought to have a role in preventing autoimmunity.

A more recent classification based on the presence or not of two surface molecules (CD4/CD8) is often used in clinical situations:
- T-helper cells and delayed hypersensitivity cells are CD4 or T4 cells.
- T-suppressor and T-cytotoxic cells are CD8 or T8 cells. Loss of balance between T-suppressor/CD8 and T-helper/CD4 cells may result in abnormally intense immune responses or an immunodeficiency such as that caused when T-helper cells are destroyed by HIV infection (see Special Focus, page 463). Overactivity of T suppressor cells is linked to this and other types of immunodeficiency (see page 462).

Cytokines

T-cell-mediated immunity protects the body against virus-infected cells, some bacteria, malignant cells and transplanted foreign cells. The destruction of these antigens may be by direct attack and lysis, or by the release of cytokines. Before we look at cytokines in more detail it is worth mentioning that the nomenclature is used in several different ways, but for our purposes cytokines describe all the signalling molecules, and lymphokines are cytokines released by lymphocytes. Cytokines/lymphokines are chemical mediators that bind to surface receptors to produce effects that augment the immune response by stimulating macrophages, other lymphocyte (T, B, NK) proliferation and activity, and they also stimulate the inflammatory response. Individual cells generally produce several different types of cytokine, each of which may perform many tasks.

The lymphokines produced by activated T cells are a group of non-specific chemicals which include:

- Gamma interferon (IFN): affects B, T and NK cell activity, and stimulates macrophages to become killers. **NB** interferons are also made by virus-infected cells (see page 449).
- Interleukins (IL): signal between leucocytes to cause NK cell activity, B and T cell proliferation, and antibody secretion.
- Transforming growth factor (TGF): acts to suppress the immune response.
- Macrophage migration inhibitory factor (MIF): stops the movement of macrophages to keep them where they are needed.
- Lymphotoxin (LT): kills cells marked down for destruction.

In addition, the macrophages also produce cytokines (sometimes called monokines), which enhance the immune and inflammatory responses, e.g. interleukins and tumour necrosis factor (TNF) involved in chemotaxis, phagocytosis and fever production.

Our list of cytokines is far from complete – new ones are being discovered all the time. As knowledge increases, their suppression or use as routine therapeutic agents for modulating immune responses becomes a real possibility. To date examples include the treatment of multiple sclerosis and enhancing the action of monoclonal antibodies in treating bowel cancer.

Organ transplants and rejection

Organ transplant is now a common life-saving measure for people with end-stage kidney, heart, lung or liver disease. The degree of success in most, however, depends upon finding a 'good match' between recipient and donor and, where necessary, T cell suppression to prevent graft rejection. Liver transplants do not require a particularly good match because the liver is less immunogenic, but immunosuppression is still

needed. As you already know, body cells have genetically determined surface antigens – ABO blood groups on erythrocytes (see Chapter 9), and on all other cells, e.g. leucocytes, the MHC molecules coded by the MHC gene cluster (remember they are called HLA on leucocytes). The closer the match between MHC antigens the greater is the chance of a successful transplant. First-time kidney transplants from cadaveric donors have a good success rate, with 80% functioning for at least a year (*Lancet*, 1990). Heart–lung transplants now enjoy similar degrees of success.

The very best 'match' possible is an autograft, where tissue is transplanted from one site to another in the same person, e.g. via a skin graft. Here the MHC antigens are identical and, in the absence of other problems, e.g. infection, the graft is likely to be successful. This will also be the case where an isograft between identical twins is used, as again the genetic make-up and hence the MHC antigens are identical.

Most of us, however, do not have an identical twin, and the best MHC match between non-identical individuals, called an allograft (homograft), offers the best chance. Allografts are usually cadaver donations (see brain death criteria, Chapters 4 and 21) and, more rarely, the donation by a living person of a kidney to a close relative (genetically similar) suffering from end-stage renal failure (Chapter 15). Although the number of living donors varies across the UK, they do provide a vital source of much-needed kidneys. To reduce the risk of allograft rejection, a close MHC match, determined by tissue typing, is highly desirable, and obviously there must be ABO compatibility. Even when tissue typing reveals a close match between donor and recipient MHC antigens it will be necessary to suppress the immune response, especially the activity of T cells and macrophages, which would recognize and destroy the 'foreign' cells of the graft. Organ transplants may also fail because antibody-mediated reactions cause thrombus production and other vascular problems in the donated organ.

Various measures are taken to prevent rejection:
- Drugs
  Azathioprine (cytotoxic immunosuppressant).
  Corticosteroids, which suppress the immune and inflammatory responses.
  Antilymphocyte serum (immunoglobulin from horses).
  Cyclosporin, which primarily prevents rejection by T-cell-mediated immunity. It is also used to prevent graft-versus-host disease that follows a bone marrow transplant where the donor T cells become sensitized to the host, the cells of whom they regard as 'foreign'.
  Newer approaches include the use of monoclonal antibodies to carry the immunosuppressant to the specific area required, e.g. the site of a transplanted kidney.
- Radiation may be used to produce immunosuppression.

An important side-effect of immunosuppression is bone marrow depression, with a reduction in the leucocytes that would normally defend against infection. This is overcome by giving 'just enough' immunosuppressive therapy to prevent rejection; administration of antimicrobial drugs; and very careful monitoring for signs of infection.

The last type of graft, a xenograft (heterograft) between different species, is fraught with immunological problems. Recently, however, there have been rapid advances in the research concerning the use of transgenic (contain human genetic material) pigs as a source of organs for transplant. There are considerable problems to overcome in this type of transplant and Bach (1996) identifies the problems as being vascular, immunological and potential disease transmission; however, clinical trials are planned at the time of writing. Apart from the physical problems there are ethical, emotional and cultural issues to consider – individuals may not condone this use of animals and some people may find pig organs unacceptable on moral/religious grounds.

MHC (HLA) antigens and disease

The inheritance of certain MHC (HLA) antigens appears to make that individual more susceptible to diseases as diverse as insulin-dependent diabetes, autoimmune Addison's disease and Graves' disease (see Chapter 8), some types of rheumatoid arthritis (see Chapter 18), multiple sclerosis (see Chapter 3) and myasthenia gravis (see Chapter 17). Some of these conditions have an autoimmune or allergic basis, but considerable work remains to be done in this field.

Abnormal Immune Responses

We have given considerable thought to the protective role of the immune response, but sometimes the reaction to an antigen can cause harm. The same highly versatile immune system that carries out cancer surveillance and produces immunoglobulins is also responsible for the 'over the top' anaphylactic response to bee stings and the production of autoantibodies that destroy your own erythrocytes.

At the other extreme there may be an immunodeficient state, where a much-needed immune response does not occur, leaving the individual exposed and vulnerable to antigen attack.

A brief mention of some abnormal responses is appropriate here, but readers requiring more details should consult Further Reading, e.g. Staines *et al.* (1993).

Hypersensitivity (allergy)

A hypersensitivity reaction to a particular allergen (antigen that produces an allergic reaction) may be classified by its timing and whether it involves antibodies or is cell-mediated.

Immediate (within minutes or hours of exposure)

Antibody-mediated type I reaction (anaphylaxis)

An antibody-mediated type I reaction occurs when IgE binds to an allergen such as dust or pollen. This causes mast cells and basophils to release chemicals, which include histamine, prostaglandins and leukotrienes (see also inflammatory response, pages 449–450). The chemicals produce vasodilation, vessel permeability and smooth muscle contraction, which may be local or systemic. An anaphylactic reaction causes oedema and other problems specific to the site – skin redness, diarrhoea, excess mucus with nasal discharge and bronchoconstriction. Anaphylactic reactions, in common with normal immune responses, are more intense following a second exposure to the allergen. Some families, where the individuals are described as atopic, show a definite propensity to anaphylactic reactions such as eczema, hay fever and asthma.

Abnormalities caused by an anaphylactic reaction include drug, food (see Healthier Living) and bee sting sensitivities, eczema, hay fever and allergic asthma. Treatment involves reducing the allergen load, providing antihistamine drugs and desensitization to some allergens – here increasing doses of the allergen are injected over a period of time to stimulate IgG, which binds to the allergen and blocks IgE (desensitization should be effected where resuscitation facilities are available, since severe anaphylaxis can occur).

Rarely, a very severe systemic reaction known as anaphylactic shock occurs. This is caused by widespread chemical release following the second exposure of the susceptible individual to the allergen. Often the allergen enters the circulation by injection, such as via an insect sting or drug administration, e.g. of penicillin. It is characterized by bronchospasm, laryngeal oedema, hypovolaemia and shock. The immediate life-saving management includes giving adrenaline by injection, provision of an airway, e.g. by tracheostomy (see Chapter 12), and administering antihistamines, e.g. chlorpheniramine.

Antibody-mediated type II reaction (cytotoxic)

An antibody-mediated type II reaction involves IgG or IgM, the activation of complement, lysis and subsequent phagocytosis of the body cell antigen. An example of a cytotoxic allergic reaction is a mismatched (ABO) blood transfusion causing donor red cells to become agglutinated (see Chapter 9). A similar reaction occurs in rhesus incompatibility, as Rh-positive fetal red cells are destroyed by maternal anti-D immunoglobulin (see page 456).

Antibody-mediated type III reaction (immune complex)

An antibody-mediated type III reaction involves antibodies and the activation of complement. Prolonged exposure to the antigen produces huge numbers of immune complexes, which lodge within the tissues or vessel walls; the effects vary according to the severity and the site involved.

There are various forms of immune complex hypersensitivity, which include localized reactions, such as farmer's lung (extrinsic allergic alveolitis), caused by inhaling antigens from mouldy hay. Immune complexes may cause a more local Arthus reaction, with swelling, inflammation and necrosis at the point of antigen entry by injection. In this case the antigen may be found within a drug, e.g. insulin.

A more widespread immune complex hypersensitivity, called serum sickness, may follow injection of a foreign antigen such as bacteria, e.g. streptococcal infections, viruses and antibiotic drugs. Serum sickness used to occur more frequently when horse antibodies were used for production of passive immunity. The immune complexes are lodged in various sites, such as the heart (myocarditis or endocarditis), kidneys (glomerulonephritis) and joints (arthritis). In addition, there may be local swelling, enlarged lymph nodes and urticarial rashes (nettle rash or hives).

Immune complex hypersensitivity may be linked to some autoimmune diseases in which the antibodies contributing to the immune complexes are autoantibodies that act against body cells.

Delayed (24–48 hours after exposure)

Cell-mediated type IV reaction

Cell-mediated type IV hypersensitivity, which involves T cell and macrophage activity and lymphokine release, occurs 24–48 hours after exposure to the antigen. There is chronic inflammation and a tissue reaction that may persist for weeks. Examples of commonly implicated antigens are the bacteria responsible for tuberculosis and syphilis, intracellular malarial parasites, metals (such as nickel), cosmetics and plants, e.g. poison ivy. Delayed hypersensitivity affecting the skin is called allergic contact dermatitis. The inflammatory effects of delayed hypersensitivity, which are due to lymphokines, may be treated with corticosteroids as antihistamines are ineffective.

An example of type IV hypersensitivity is the local reaction seen after skin testing (Heaf or Mantoux tests) with tuberculin antigens to determine the need for BCG immunization.

Mixed antibody/cell-mediated type V reaction

Mixed reactions involving antibodies, T lymphocytes and phagocytes are implicated in responses to some viruses and in a type of autoimmune hyperthyroidism (Graves' disease; see Chapter 8), where autoantibodies stimulate hormone production.

Autoimmune disorders

A large number of autoimmune conditions exist, ranging from organ-specific conditions such as autoimmune haemolytic anaemia to more generalized conditions such as rheumatoid arthritis (see Chapter 18) and systemic lupus erythematosus, which may involve the kidneys, connective tissue, skin and CNS. Autoimmune conditions, which have a genetic link (see page 460), result from changes in the normal immune tolerance that we have to our own cell antigens. The changes may occur spontaneously or be due to some extrinsic factor such as drugs or micro-organisms.

Various mechanisms by which autoimmunity develops have been proposed and include:

• Exposure of body proteins not previously in contact with the immune system, e.g. spermatozoa, which are not produced until long after immunocompetence has been completed. The development of autoantibodies to spermatozoa, which may occur after inflammation of the testes, is a cause of male infertility. The proteins of the lens of the eye are also normally isolated from the immune system and if the two should meet, e.g. after an eye injury, the resultant autoantibodies can damage the eye.

- An extrinsic agent, e.g. a micro-organism or drug, may alter the 'self' antigens in such a way that the immune system regards them as foreign – they are altered by their combination with antibodies formed against bacterial infection, e.g. with certain streptococci. This explains the carditis and glomerulonephritis (see Chapter 15) caused by immune complex deposition following a streptococcal sore throat.
- There may be a failure of lymphocyte processing that fails to remove T and B cells that do not respond appropriately to self antigens.

The actual damage of autoimmunity is caused by autoantibodies, immune complexes or T cells sensitized against body cells, or a combined antibody/cell-mediated reaction. By now you will have realized, even after our brief discussion, that many links exist between normal immune responses, hypersensitivities and autoimmune reactions.

Immunodeficiency

The large number of immunodeficient states reflects the complexity of a body defence system that involves so many innate and adaptive components. Classification is difficult and readers should consult Further Reading for detailed descriptions.

For our purposes it is sufficient to outline the major immunodeficiencies that may be present at birth (congenital) or acquired after birth:

Congenital defects (genetic)
- Lack of complement.
- Agammaglobulinaemia, where the individual is unable to produce immunoglobulins or has a deficiency of B cells.
- T cell deficiency and thymic defects.
- Absence of both B and T cells – severe combined immunodeficiency (SCID).
- Abnormal or decreased phagocytes.

Acquired defects
- Phagocyte deficiency resulting from bone marrow depression caused by malignant disease or drugs.
- Inadequate complement when general protein synthesis is reduced.
- Hypogammaglobulinaemia (reduced immunoglobulins) due to protein deficiency or loss, e.g. PEM, kidney disease.
- Deficiency of lymphocytes caused by radiation; immunosuppressive or cytotoxic therapy; Hodgkin's disease (see Chapter 11); corticosteroids; infections, e.g. AIDS (see page 463).
- Abnormal immunoglobulins produced at the expense of the normal range, e.g. multiple myeloma.

Whatever the cause of the immunodeficiency, the major problem is infection due to an increased vulnerability to pathogens and opportunistic organisms that normally cause little harm. The management of immunodeficient states depends on individual circumstances but may include provision of a clean or even sterile environment, immunoglobulins and antimicrobial drugs, bone marrow transplant, meticulous hygiene, careful monitoring for signs of infection and, where possible, measures to reduce the feelings of isolation and loneliness.

Developments in immunology and clinical applications

Many exciting developments can be expected as immunological research and clinical application continue to expand. Specific areas include: immunization, use and suppression of cytokines, AIDS control, xenograft organ transplant/control of rejection, contraception, treatment of some types of infertility, cancer diagnosis and treatment, autoimmune mechanisms and MHC/HLA disease susceptibility.

Special Focus **Human immunodeficiency virus (HIV)/acquired immune deficiency syndrome (AIDS)**

AIDS is one of the most serious and potentially catastrophic health problems to emerge during the 20th century. The first case was diagnosed in 1981 on the west coast of the USA, but the disease is known to have existed in Africa for much longer. Infection with HIV, a retrovirus, causes an initial B and T cell response, but later depresses T cell immunity by reducing T-helper cell (CD4) and macrophage numbers. In addition, there is an increase in T-suppressor cells (CD8). (The CD4:CD8 ratio is measured to assess the course of established disease.)

Antibodies for HIV first appear in the blood (seropositive) 3 months or more after initial infection, but they do not confer immunity – which means that the person is capable of passing on the virus although they may well be asymptomatic. This idea has caused some confusion for both the public and health professionals. Searle (1987) found that 38% of senior doctors, dentists and nurses at sister level did not know what a positive HIV serotest meant.

Not surprisingly the virus-induced havoc among the immune cells leaves the individual open to attack by micro-organisms (pathogens and opportunists), for example, causing fungal infections, meningitis (*Cryptococcus neoformans*), tuberculosis, bowel disease (*Cryptosporidium* spp.) and fungal pneumonia (*Pneumocystis carinii*), which usually occurs only after immunosuppression. Another problem linked to the breakdown in immune processes is the development of the otherwise rare Kaposi's tumour, which affects blood vessels in the skin and viscera.

There is a great deal yet to learn about HIV infection. HIV has a very variable incubation period, which may even be more than 10 years. The virus is present in the blood, semen and vaginal secretions, and to a limited extent in other body fluids such as saliva and tears.

AIDS, which is characterized by weight loss, lymphadenopathy, diarrhoea, night sweats and repeated infection, may be preceded by an AIDS-related complex (ARC), which is similar to but less severe than fully developed AIDS. Throughout the 1980s AIDS infection was most commonly associated with 'high-risk' activities, such as sharing needles or syringes and some types of sexual behaviour, e.g.

anal intercourse. Some individuals, however, were also infected by contaminated blood or blood products, e.g. those suffering from haemophilia (see Chapter 9), or via the placenta, where the virus passes from mother to fetus. Rarely, infection has occurred following 'needlestick' accidents in health workers. The risk of HIV infection from 'needlestick' injury, where the patient is HIV positive, has been estimated to be 0.25% (McKeown, 1992). Pratt (1994) describes the risk to health professionals as depending upon factors that include: the prevalence of HIV in the population (higher in large cities), professional experience, type of exposure (skin or mucous membrane) and amount of blood/fluid involved.

There are differences in infection transmission worldwide, e.g. vertical spread from mother to fetus is less likely to occur in Europe, and there are marked regional variations within the UK. Current patterns of infection in the UK appear to indicate that more children are now infected with HIV and that people are being exposed to the virus through sexual contacts whilst travelling abroad (Far East and sub-Saharan Africa).

The considerable prejudice and ignorance concerning AIDS is unfortunate, because many people still think that the infection has 'nothing to do with them'. In a survey of nurse education, McHaffie (1994) found that intolerance and prejudice was common and recommended that HIV/AIDS education take place within the broader issues of sexuality, infection control and death.

Another commonly held, but erroneous, view is that you can 'catch' AIDS from normal social contact, such as shaking hands. This is certainly untrue, as AIDS is spread by sharing needles or syringes, 'high-risk' sex (including vaginal intercourse with an infected person), or exposure to infected body fluids, blood or blood products, and sometimes via the placenta or breast milk.

There is as yet no cure for AIDS, which at present is almost always fatal, but there are drugs that may prolong and improve the quality of life, e.g. antimicrobial drugs (for opportunistic infections); zidovudine (AZT), didanosine (ddI); zalcitabine (ddC), alpha interferon

(for Kaposi tumour); and recently the protease inhibitors such as ritonavir, which attack the virus at a different point in its life cycle. Interestingly the drug thalidomide, which caused fetal limb malformation in the late 1950s to early 1960s, may alleviate the effects of *Cryptosporidium*, but because of its toxicity it is vigorously controlled and supplied on a named patient basis.

Until effective treatment or immunization is available the most important aspects of AIDS management and containment are health staff education at all levels (Searle, 1987) and health education programmes to inform all groups about high-risk activities. Other initiatives, such as heat-treated blood products, screening blood donors and needle exchange schemes for drug users, are all helpful, but the major task is to convince people that they are at risk and help them to take responsibility for and modify their behaviour. The most important message is that 'all sexually active individuals have the potential to be infected and to infect others' (Kuykendall, 1992).

Various studies have considered the risks of HIV infection in people who inject drugs. In 1989 Hart *et al.* studied the risk behaviours of drug users in London; most were sexually active, with one-third having experienced 2–20 sexual partners, and most had shared injection equipment. Skidmore *et al.* (1990) found that many of the drug users studied in Edinburgh had modified their intake of drugs, but the changing patterns of HIV spread suggests that heterosexual transmission will be a future problem.

Health education aimed at reducing the spread of AIDS includes:

- Practice 'safer sex', e.g. use condoms; limit sexual partners; and consider alternatives to 'high-risk' activities.
- Injecting drug users should not share needles/syringes, and used equipment should be disposed of safely.
- It is safest not to share razors, toothbrushes and other equipment that may be contaminated with blood, e.g. earpiercing equipment.

NB There is no risk of being infected with AIDS when donating blood for transfusion; only sterile, single-use equipment is used.

Summary/Check List

Introduction.
Non-specific components – skin and membrane barriers: skin structure. Nursing Practice Application – Down's syndrome and the palmar creases. Skin appendages. Nursing Practice Application – hair condition. Skin pigmentation. Nursing Practice Application – skin colour/condition. Skin functions: waterproofing, temperature regulation. Nursing Practice Application – recording temperature. Problems with temperature homeostasis – fever, heat stroke, hypothermia. Person-centred Study – Mavis. Sensation, protection, Nursing Practice Application – skin hygiene. Synthesis of vitamin D – exposure to UV light, Healthier Living – safe sun, skin excretion, storage. Other innate membrane barriers.

Non-specific components – cells and chemicals: phagocytes, phagocytosis, natural killer cells, acute phase proteins, interferons, complement, inflammatory response, wound healing. Nursing Practice Application – wound healing and dressings. Special Focus – pressure sores. Nursing Practice Application – assessment of leg ulcers.
Specific components – the immune response. Humoral immunity – B lymphocytes. Antibodies/immunoglobulins. Immunity, immunization. Nursing Practice Application – Immunization information. Cell-mediated immunity – T lymphocytes. Organ transplants and rejection. MHC and disease.
Abnormal immune responses – hypersensitivities (allergies). Healthier Living – peanut allergy. Autoimmunity. Immunodeficiency. Special Focus – HIV and AIDS.

Self Test

1 Put the following in their correct pairs:
   (a) sebum
   (b) eccrine gland
   (c) ceruminous gland
   (d) sebaceous gland
   (e) germinative layer
   (f) wax
   (g) sweat
   (h) epidermis.
2 Describe the heat loss mechanisms of the skin that maintain body temperature homeostasis on a hot day.
3 Describe how the following protect: lysozyme, normal flora, mucus.
4 Describe the events of inflammation and link these to its signs and symptoms.
5 Which of the following statements are true?
   (a) Phagocytes, NK cells and complement are part of the non-specific defences.
   (b) Clean surgical incisions usually heal by primary intention.
   (c) Wound repair reaches maximum strength at about 14 days.
   (d) Circulatory disorders predispose to pressure sores.
6 What is meant by antigen specificity and 'memory' in relation to specific defences?
7 Complete the following statements:
   (a) humoral immunity is conferred by the presence of _ _ _ _ _ _ _ _ _ .

   (b) B cells are said to be _ _ _ _ _ dependent.
   (c) antibodies are also known as _ _ _ _ _ _ _ _ _ _ _ _ _ _ _ _ .
   (d) antibodies destroy antigens in different ways, but all involve the formation of _ _ _ _ _ _ _ _ /_ _ _ _ _ _ _ /_ _ _ _ _ _ _ _ _ .
8 Explain active and passive immunity, and give examples of how each may be achieved.
9 Complete the following statements:
   (a) Activation of T cells confers _ _ _ _ /_ _ _ _ _ _ _ _ immunity.
   (b) T cells are _ _ _ _ _ _ dependent.
   (c) T-helper cells are also known as _ _ _ cells.
   (d) Chemicals such as interleukins and TNF are known collectively as _ _ _ _ _ _ _ _ _.
10 What information would you give in the following situations:
   (a) Stefan, a health care assistant, asks how HIV causes immunodeficiency.
   (b) You and the health visitor are asked about the risks of having a child who is HIV positive in school.
   (c) Your friend says that he will not donate blood because of the AIDS risk.
   (d) Paul, who injects drugs and has never had an AIDS blood test, asks if he and his girlfriend should use condoms.

Answers

1 a–d, b–g, c–f and e–h.
2 See pages 444–445.
3 See pages 447–448.
4 See pages 449–450.
5 a, b, d.
6 See page 454.
7 (a) Antibodies;
  (b) bursa;
  (c) immunoglobulins;
  (d) antibody–antigen complexes.
8 See page 456.
9 (a) Cell-mediated;
  (b) thymus;
  (c) CD4;
  (d) cytokines.
10 See page 463.

References

Armstrong-Esther CA (1981) Skin introduction. *Nursing (1st Series)*, 1115.

Bach FH (1996) Transplanting porcine hearts to humans. *BMJ* **312**: 651–652.

Closs J (1987) Oral temperature measurement. *Nurs Times* **83**(1): 36–39.

Dale J, Gibson B (1993) Leg ulcer management. *Prof Nurs* **8** (5):(suppl.) 5–7.

DoH (1992) *The Health of the Nation*. Summary. London: HMSO.

Edwards M (1994) The rationale for the use of risk calculators in pressure sore prevention, and the evidence of the reliability and validity of published scales. *J Adv Nurs* **20** (2): 288–296.

Gould D (1986) Pressure sore prevention and treatment: an example of nurses' failure to implement research findings. *J Adv Nurs* **11**: 389–394.

Hart GJ, Sonnex C, Petherick A *et al.* (1989) Risk behaviours for HIV infection among injecting drug users attending a drug dependency clinic. *BMJ* **298**: 1081–1083.

Heath HBM, ed (1995) *Potter and Perry's Foundations in Nursing Theory and Practice*. London: Mosby.

Hunt J (1981) Indicators for nursing practice: the use of research findings. *J Adv Nurs* **6**(3): 189–194.

Kuykendall J (1992) Families and HIV – rebels at risk. *Nurs Times* **88**(5): 26–28.

Lancet (1990) Organ donors in the United Kingdom – getting the numbers right. (Editorial). *Lancet* **335**: 80–82.

Land L (1995) A review of pressure damage prevention strategies. *J Adv Nurs* **22**(2): 329–337.

McHaffie HE (1994) HIV and AIDS: a survey of nurse education in the United Kingdom. *J Adv Nurs* **20**(3): 552–559.

McKeown M (1992) Sharpening awareness. *Nurs Times* **88** (14):66–68.

Moffatt C, O'Hare L (1995) Ankle pulses are not sufficient to detect impaired arterial circulation in patients with leg ulcers. *J Wound Care* **4**(3):134–138.

Nichols GA and Kucha DH (1972) Taking adult temperatures: oral measurements. *Am J Nurs* **72**: 1091–1092.

Norton D, McLaren R, Exton-Smith A (1962) *An Investigation of Geriatric Nursing Problems in Hospital*. Edinburgh: Churchill Livingstone.

Pembroke AC (1983) Preventing skin problems. *Geriatr Med* **13** (11): 797–781.

Pratt R (1994) Safe practice. *Nurs Times* **90** (21): 64–68.

Reid J, Morison M (1994) Towards a consensus: classification of pressure sores. *J Wound Care* **3**(3): 157–160.

Searle ES (1987) Knowledge, attitudes and behaviour of health professionals in relation to AIDS. *Lancet* **i**: 26–28.

Shipperly T (1997) The importantance of assessing patients with leg ulceration. *Br J Nurs* **6**(2): 71–80.

Sims-Williams AJ (1976) Temperature taking with glass thermometers: a review. *J Adv Nurs* **1**(6): 481–493.

Skidmore CA, Robertson JR, Robertson AA, Elton RA (1990) After the epidemic: a follow up study of HIV seroprevalance and changing patterns of drug use. *BMJ* **300**: 219–223.

Spenceley P (1988) Norton v Waterlow. *Nurs Times* **84** (32): 52–53.

Turner TD (1985) Which dressing and why? In: Westaby S, ed, *Wound Care*. London: Heinemann Medical.

Waterlow J (1985) A risk assessment card. *Nurs Times* **81**(48): 49–55.

Waterlow J (1991) A policy that protects: the Waterlow pressure sore prevention/treatment policy. *Prof Nurs* **6**(5): 258–264.

Westaby S, ed (1985) *Wound Care*. London: Heinemann Medical

Further Reading

Crow R (1988) The challenge of pressure sores. *Nurs Times* **84** (38):68–78 (literature review).

Dealey C (1994) *The Care of Wounds*. Oxford: Blackwell Scientific Publications.

DoH (1997) *Animal tissue in humans: a summary of the main conclusions and recommendations*. London: DoH.

HEA/DoH (1996) *A Guide to Childhood Immunizations*. London: Health Education Authority.

Morison MJ (1997) *A Colour Guide to the Nursing Management of Wounds*. 2nd edn London: Mosby.

Pratt RJ (1995) *HIV and AIDS: A Strategy for Nursing Care*, 4th edn. London: Edward Arnold.

Royal College of Nursing (1994) *Universal Precautions against Hepatitis B and AIDS*. London: RCN.

Staines NA, Brostoff J, James K (1993) *Introducing Immunology*, 2nd edn. London: Mosby.

Thompson J (1989) Fact sheet – the cold that kills. *Nurs Times* **85** (46): (Community Outlook) 21–25.

Weir DM, Stewart J (1993) *Immunology*, 7th edn. Edinburgh: Churchill Livingstone.

Useful Addresses

Terrence Higgins Trust
52–54 Grays Inn Rd
London
(Tel: 0171 242 1010)

National AIDS Helpline
(Tel: 0800 567 123)

Reproduction

Overview

- *Structure and function of the male and female reproductive systems.*
- *Conception, pregnancy, parturition and lactation.*

Learning Outcomes

After studying Chapter 20 you should be able to:

- Outline sexual differentiation of the reproductive structures.
- Describe the male reproductive system, ducts and accessory glands.
- Describe meiosis and spermatogenesis.
- Discuss the hormonal control of male reproductive function.
- Describe the structures of the female reproductive system.
- Outline the structure of the mammary glands.
- Describe oogenesis and the ovarian cycle.
- Describe hormonal control of the ovarian cycle.
- Describe the menstrual (uterine) cycle.
- Discuss the sexual response in both male and female.
- Describe some sexually transmitted diseases and discuss their effects on the reproductive system.
- Discuss methods of contraception.
- Describe fertilization and the determination of genetic sex.
- Outline the events of pre-embryonic development, implantation and formation of the placenta.
- Describe important maternal changes occurring during pregnancy and discuss the major hormones involved with pregnancy.
- Outline the initiation of labour and describe its three stages.
- Describe the process and control of lactation.

Key Words

Diploid (2n) – a cell that has a full set of paired chromosomes (46 arranged in 23 pairs; in humans $n = 23$, therefore $2n = 46$); seen in all cells except the gametes. There are 44 autosomes and 2 sex chromosomes.

Embryo – the early developmental stage from the third week until the end of the eighth week of gestation.

Fertilization – union of the spermatozoon (male) and oocyte (female) nuclei to form the diploid (2n) zygote.

Fetus – the developmental stage from the ninth week of gestation until birth.

Gametes – the haploid (n) reproductive cells, oocytes and spermatozoa.

Gametogenesis – the process by which gametes are formed in the ovary (oocytes) or testis (spermatozoa).

Genitalia – the generative/reproductive structures (internal and external).

Gonad – the primary reproductive structure: ovary (female) and testis (male).

Gonadotrophins – pituitary hormones that control gonad functioning, e.g. follicle stimulating hormone, luteinizing hormone.

Key Words cont.

....

Haploid (*n*) – a cell which has a set of unpaired chromosomes (23 only), seen only in the gametes following meiosis. There are 22 autosomes and 1 sex chromosome.

Meiosis – a complex reduction division by which a diploid reproductive cell produces four haploid cells.

Menstrual (uterine) cycle – the uterine changes occurring as the lining of the uterus responds to the secretion of ovarian hormones. It corresponds to the ovarian cycle.

Oocyte – an immature ovum, the female gamete prior to penetration by a spermatozoon.

Oogenesis – the formation of oocytes (female gamete) by the ovaries.

Ovarian cycle – the events occurring as an ovarian follicle matures and female sex hormones are released under the

influence of gonadotrophins.

Ovulation – the release of the secondary oocyte from the surface of the ovary.

Ovum – the female gamete after penetration by a spermatozoon.

Sex hormones – the steroid hormones that control reproductive function: oestrogens and progesterones (female) and the androgen testosterone (male).

Spermatogenesis – the formation of spermatozoa (male gametes) by the testes.

Spermatozoon – a mature, male gamete.

Zygote – the fertilized ovum following fusion of the female and male nuclei.

Introduction

Each chapter so far has dealt with functions that are vital to homeostasis. In this chapter, however, we discuss reproduction, which, while being essential to species continuity, has nothing to do with individual survival. The reproductive organs are not functional until puberty and in the female cease to function during mid-life. The chapter looks at male and female reproductive function and includes conception, early development, pregnancy from the maternal viewpoint and birth, and some associated problems. It is important to remember that reproductive functioning is much more than the workings of a physiological system: the complexity of human sexual behaviour goes far beyond the basic need to reproduce. The business of expressing sexuality, which includes reproduction, is subject to considerable environmental and sociocultural influence as well as physiological controls. Another feature is that, for the most part, sexual behaviour is not intended by the participants to lead to reproduction. In this humans differ from other species.

Chapter 21, which completes Section eight, includes basic genetics, embryonic/fetal development and changes occurring at birth. It outlines major developmental events from birth through the lifespan to ageing and death.

Early development

Genetic sex (see pages 498–499) is determined by the sex chromosomes – the chromosomes X and Y. One sex chromosome is inherited from each parent and individuals have one pair – XX in females and XY in males (see *Figure 20.23*).

This, however, is only part of the story because gender is derived from a dual system of embryonic ducts which can be influenced to become either male or female. Early in development there are close links between the urinary tract (see Chapter 15), the external **genitalia** and the internal reproductive structures that develop from the ducts (*Figure 20.1*). The early **embryo**, although genetically sexed, is said to be 'sexually indifferent' – both male and female duct systems are in place with gonadal mesoderm (adjacent to the primitive kidney – mesonephros) which can become testes (male **gonads**) or ovaries (female gonads).

Similarly, the external genitalia develop from identical structures present in both males and females:

- Genital tubercle (penis or clitoris).
- Urethral groove as the opening of the urogenital sinus (bladder and urethra); in females the urethral groove will form the vestibule (see *Figure 20.14*).
- Labioscrotal swellings (fused as scrotum or unfused as labia majora).
- Urogenital folds (fused as part of penis or unfused the labia minora).

The male genitourinary (reproductive/urinary) tract starts to develop around week 7 from the primitive embryonic Wolffian (mesonephric) ducts when they are stimulated by testosterone, secreted by the fetal testes. Although the male Y chromosome causes the development of testes from the gonadal ridges of mesoderm, it is testosterone that ensures the proper formation of a male tract and external genitalia. By weeks 7–8 the male (XY) embryo has formed male structures and the 'female' ducts are disappearing. Meanwhile, around week 8, the male external genitalia (penis and scrotum) start rapid development under the influence of testosterone. Various problems can occur during this stage, e.g. hypospadias, where the urethra opens on the ventral surface of the penis – this occurs when the urogenital folds fail to fuse over the urethral groove.

Female development starts slightly later, around week 8. As before, the sex chromosomes determine the type of gonad formed – the genetically female embryo (XX) forms ovaries from the gonadal ridges because the male Y chromosome is absent. The female genital tract develops from the same embryonic ducts as does the male tract (*Figure 20.1*), but now the Mullerian (paramesonephric) ducts develop and the Wolffian ducts degenerate. It is mainly the lack of testosterone that leads to the formation of female genitalia, but there may be some oestrogenic effect from the fetal ovaries. The external genitalia in the female form from the same structures as for the male (see page 468).

It is interesting to note that without testosterone all **fetuses,** genetic males included, will develop a female duct system and external genitalia.

Male Reproductive System

The function of the male reproductive system is the production of male **gametes** (**haploid** (*n*) reproductive cells) and the transfer of these spermatozoa to the female during sexual intercourse. Research during the latter part of the 20th century has led to developments that allow for **fertilization** without sexual intercourse, e.g. *in vitro* fertilization (IVF).

Structure of the male reproductive system

The male reproductive system (see *Figure 20.2*) consists of: testes (two) in the scrotum, epididymis (two), vas deferens (two), ejaculatory ducts (two), seminal vesicles (two), prostate gland, bulbo-urethral glands (two) and the urethra as it passes through the penis.

NB The scrotum and penis are known as the external genitalia.

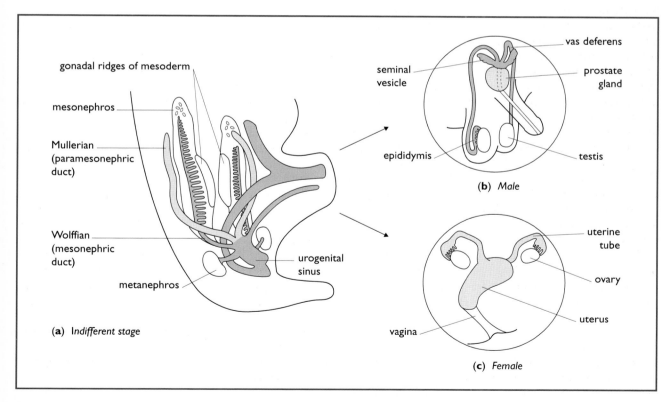

Figure 20.1 Sexual differentiation of the internal reproductive structures.

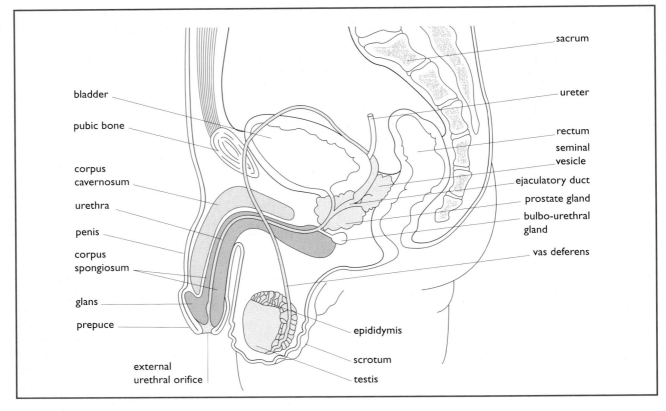

Figure 20.2 Male reproductive structures (midsagittal section).

Testes

The male gonads (primary reproductive structures), or testes, produce spermatozoa and act as endocrine organs (see Chapter 8) by secreting the male hormone testosterone, which is discussed further on pages 477–478. Each testis is around 4.5 cm in length and 2.5 cm in diameter (*Figure 20.3*). During fetal development the testes, which start off high in the abdomen, descend with their spermatic cord through the right and left inguinal canals (see Chapter 18) and are present in the scrotum by the eighth month of development. Occasionally the testes fail to descend. If both testes fail to descend and this is not corrected, it could lead to sterility because the testes need to be 2–3°C cooler than body temperature. Testes that remain in the abdomen are more likely to become malignant – another reason for surgical correction.

Normally the oval testes, suspended by their spermatic cords within the scrotum, are outside the body cavity. The scrotum is a bag of pigmented skin and fascia (fibrous connective tissue) that hangs between the thighs anterior to the rectum. It may appear to be somewhat risky having the structures that confer maleness in such a vulnerable position, but this adaptation keeps the testes at the slightly lower temperature required for the production of healthy spermatozoa. To maintain a constant temperature the position of the scrotum can be changed by muscle contraction. This occurs in response to temperature changes; for example, heat causes the scrotum to hang loosely away from the body, but it moves closer to the body when cold.

Each testis, which occupies a separate compartment (formed from fascia) within the scrotum, has two coverings – a double serous layer, the tunica vaginalis, and the inner fibrous tunica albuginea, which forms the septa dividing the testis into 200–300 wedge-shaped lobules. Individual lobules contain the convoluted seminiferous tubules, the site of **spermatogenesis** (formation of spermatozoa), and Leydig (interstitial) cells, which secrete androgen hormones. The seminiferous tubules from the lobules form tubuli recti which converge at the rete testis. From here the spermatozoa enter the efferent ductules and the duct system of the epididymis (see below).

The spermatic cord, which passes through the inguinal canal, encloses blood vessels, lymphatics and autonomic nerves of both divisions travelling to and from the testes and the vas deferens (ductus deferens), which carries the spermatozoa. Arterial blood supply to the testes is via the

Nursing Practice Application **Testicular tumours – screening and early detection**

Testicular tumours are rare and represent between 1 and 2% of male malignancies. Although only a small number occur each year, it is worth remembering that in the UK this is the commonest cancer affecting young men of age 20–34 years, it is becoming more common and early diagnosis increases the chance of successful treatment.

A study by Thornhill *et al.* (1986), involving 500 men aged 21–65, revealed that 32% did not know about testicular tumours, 92% did not know about self-examination and 90% wanted more information. Regular monthly self-examination of the testes, after a bath or shower, can be helpful in detecting changes, and nurses can encourage adolescents and men to undertake this simple screening test. Alterations such as a lump, general enlargement or a testis that 'feels' different, although these changes may not be due to malignancy, should be reported to their family doctor as soon as possible.

Some men may find screening, for conditions that directly affect sexuality, distressing or embarrassing; however, nurses can be sensitive to individual needs when giving information about testicular tumours and self-examination. The leaflets published by the Health Education Authority (HEA, 1993) and other visual aids can be used to overcome difficulties. Testicular self-examination and awareness initiatives are described by Paolozzi (1994).

testicular arteries, which branch directly from the aorta (see Chapter 10), and venous blood leaves in the pampiniform plexus of veins. Occasionally the spermatic cord becomes twisted (testicular torsion), which results in damage to the testis if treatment is delayed.

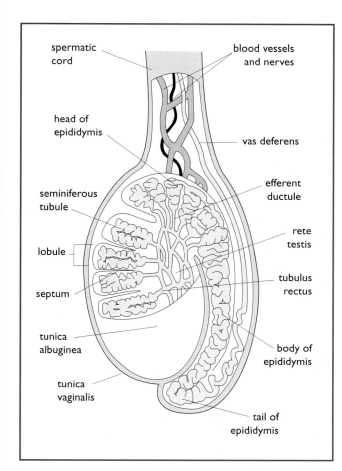

Figure 20.3 Testis.

Duct system

The convoluted epididymis, a tube some 6 m in length, is coiled on the posterior part of each testis (*Figure 20.3*). Immature non-motile spermatozoa leaving the testis move into the epididymis, where they become fully mature and motile during the 3 weeks or so they take to travel its length.

The epididymis is continuous with the vas deferens, which travels in the spermatic cord to enter the pelvic cavity. The vas deferens runs anterior to the pubic bone, over the ureter and behind the bladder, where it dilates to form the ampulla. The vas deferens contains a muscle layer capable of the rapid contraction that conveys mature spermatozoa into the urethra during ejaculation.

Male sterilization or vasectomy involves removal of a small portion of each vas deferens, which ensures that they are no longer continuous. It should be considered to be permanent, however, reversal is possible in some cases. Vasectomy, which is usually performed under local anaesthetic as an out-patient, should have no effect other than sterility. It is important that couples understand that sterility is not immediate, as spermatozoa already in the duct system may remain viable for some weeks. An alternative method of contraception is required for about 2–3 months until all spermatozoa have been ejaculated. The actual time depends upon the frequency of ejaculation, and usually samples of ejaculate are examined to confirm the absence of spermatozoa before contraception is abandoned.

A duct from a seminal vesicle (an accessory gland; there are two of these) opens into the ampulla of each vas deferens, which is then known as the ejaculatory duct. The two ejaculatory ducts merge with the urethra as it passes through the prostate gland.

The male urethra, which is some 20 cm in length, transports both urine (see Chapter 15) and semen. It is divided into three parts: prostatic, membranous and penile urethra, which opens at the external urethral orifice and forms around 75% of urethral length (see penis, page 472).

The accessory glands

Seminal vesicles

The seminal vesicles are tubular glands with muscular walls (see *Figure 20.2*). They are lined with secretory epithelium that produces a viscous alkaline fluid. This secretion, which contains fructose, amino acids, ascorbic acid, clotting enzymes and prostaglandins, forms about 60% of the volume of semen (fluid produced at ejaculation).

Prostate gland

The first part of the male urethra is surrounded by the prostate gland (*Figure 20.4*). This walnut-sized structure consists of several glands, fibrous tissue and smooth muscle,

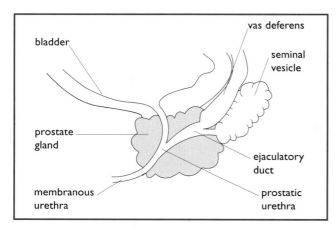

Figure 20.4 Prostate gland.

all enclosed within a capsule. Prostatic secretion, which accounts for around 30% of the total volume, is added to semen during ejaculation. Prostatic secretion is a thin milky fluid (pH 6.5), containing chemicals such as spermine (alkali) and enzymes (fibrinolysins, acid phosphatase), which assist spermatozoa activity/motility and modify vaginal acidity.

Bulbo-urethral glands (Cowper's glands)

The two tiny bulbo-urethral glands are located inferior to the prostate (see *Figures 20.2* and *20.5*). These glands secrete a small amount of lubricating mucus into the penile urethra before ejaculation.

Penis

The penis, through which the spongy (penile) urethra runs, is the male organ of copulation. The penis has a root embedded in the perineum (see Chapter 18) and a body/shaft that terminates at the expanded glans penis (*Figure 20.5*). The glans is normally covered with a loose double fold of skin known as the prepuce (foreskin).

The penis consists of three columns of erectile tissue containing vascular spaces, connective tissue and involuntary muscle. There are two lateral columns, the corpora cavernosa and the ventral corpus spongiosum, surrounding the urethra. Normally the penis is flaccid but during sexual excitement the vascular spaces fill with blood, causing erection as the penis becoming enlarged and rigid (see page 494). The penis is well supplied with arteries, veins and autonomic parasympathetic nerves, which run in its dorsal aspect.

Special Focus **Prostatic problems**

Enlargement of the prostate gland is extremely common from mid-life onwards. This enlargement, which may be caused by benign hypertrophy (see Chapter 1) or malignant changes, will obstruct the urethra and affect micturition – the man may complain of hesitancy, dribbling, poor stream, nocturia and retention with overflow incontinence (see Chapter 15).

Prostatic problems usually affect men aged over 60, but can occur earlier. Other manifestations are urinary tract infection and renal damage due to urinary stasis or acute retention.

The management of benign hypertrophy involves relief of retention, if present, by catheterization prior to surgery. In many instances the prostatic enlargement is removed by transurethral resection

(TURP). The ability to achieve erection should not be affected following transurethral resection, but ejaculation may be altered (less volume, retrograde ejaculation into the bladder). It is important to note that medical treatment with anti-androgens may be offered and other means of reducing prostate size, for example, laser treatment are increasing in use.

Prostatic malignancy (second commonest cause of cancer death after lung cancer), which may spread locally in the pelvis or to nearby bone, e.g. vertebrae, is increasingly common with age. The tumours are hormone-dependent and the management involves surgery, radiotherapy and modification of androgen levels for metastatic tumour – anti-androgen drugs to block androgen receptors, gonadotrophin ana-

logues to prevent gonadotrophin release, oestrogens and removal of the testes (orchidectomy). These treatments, which may cause feminization, e.g. breast development, sterility, impotence and reduced libido, can result in considerable distress for men and their families. Very careful explanation and support is required by individuals needing these treatments. Unfortunately prostatic tumours are not always amenable to treatment, but early detection is possible with education aimed at early reporting of symptoms and with screening, which includes rectal examination and blood tests for the presence of the tumour marker prostate-specific antigen (some disagreement exists as to its suitability in screening, but it is used to monitor existing disease).

Functioning of the male reproductive structures

In order to understand spermatogenesis and **oogenesis** (**oocyte** formation) it is necessary for us to first consider the process of meiosis. Readers will also find it helpful to revise the events of DNA replication and mitosis (Chapter 1) so that the two processes may be compared.

Meiosis

Meiosis is the term given to the complex nuclear divisions by which a **diploid** (**2n**) (cell with a full set of paired chromosomes – 46 arranged in 23 pairs) cell forms four haploid (*n*) (cell with a set of unpaired chromosomes – 23 in total) gametes. This process ensures that the resultant gametes have only half the normal chromosome number (23) and that random genetic variation occurs. When the male and female gametes fuse at fertilization the diploid chromosome number of 46 is again restored.

NB Meiosis, which is divided into stages, is preceded by interphase and replication of DNA, which doubles the amount of chromatin in the nucleus.

Stages of meiosis I (see *Figure 20.6*)
Prophase I

In meiosis this stage takes longer than in mitosis. During prophase I the chromosomes coil, condense and become visible. In a process unique to meiosis there is pairing or synapsis of homologous (similar) chromosomes to form a bivalent, consisting of two chromosomes. The paired chromosomes coil around each other. Towards the end of prophase I the chromosome pairs undergo incomplete separation and each chromosome can be seen to have two chromatids; each unit now consists of four strands and is quadrivalent (two bivalents). At this stage several 'cross-over' points, or chiasmata, can be seen between the chromatids. These chiasmata are the means by which genetic material is exchanged between the chromosomes of a homologous pair to produce gametes of infinite genetic variability. Separation of the two bivalents continues and the nucleolus and nuclear membrane disappear, ready for the next stage.

NB The process of oogenesis, which commences in fetal life, is arrested during prophase I and does not resume until puberty (see pages 487–488).

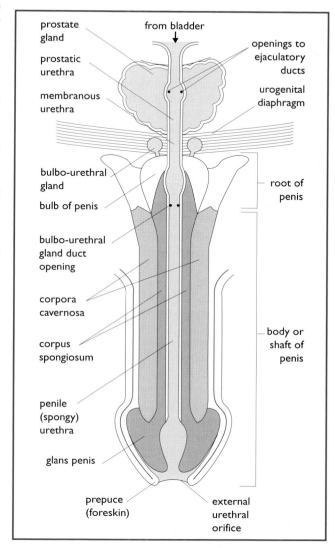

Figure 20.5 Penis.

Nursing Practice Application **Phimosis and paraphimosis**

Sometimes an abnormally tight prepuce cannot be drawn back over the glans penis – a condition known as phimosis. This is treated by circumcision (excision of the prepuce) to prevent hygiene problems where secretions collecting under the prepuce cause inflammation of the glans penis (balanitis).

The opposite problem of paraphimosis occurs when the retracted prepuce cannot be drawn back over the glans penis, which swells. Paraphimosis may occur when the prepuce is not drawn over the glans after catheterization or where a tight prepuce has been forcibly retracted.

Metaphase I

This stage sees the appearance of the spindle apparatus, consisting of contractile proteins. The bivalents position themselves on the spindle equator in such a way as to ensure that each new cell receives only one chromosome from a homologous pair.

Anaphase I

One chromosome, consisting of two chromatids, from each homologous pair migrates to opposite poles of the cell. Here there is no separation of the chromatid strands at the centromere as there is during mitosis. Each pole of the cell will contain the haploid (*n*) number of 23 chromosomes.

Telophase I

During this stage nuclear membranes form around each haploid set of chromosomes.

Cytokinesis, which follows telophase, forms two haploid 'daughter' cells.

To summarize: the events of meiosis I produces two haploid (*n*) cells that are genetically quite unlike the original cell.

It is important to note that there follows a second interphase, but in this instance no DNA replication occurs prior to the start of meiosis II.

Stages of meiosis II (*Figure 20.6*)

Meiosis II, which commences with two haploid cells, follows the same four stages as mitosis. During prophase II the events already described occur but with only 23 chromosomes, not homologous pairs. During metaphase II the chromosomes, each of which consists of two chromatid strands, arrange themselves on the spindle equator. This time, however, the chromatid strands separate at the centromere, as they do in mitosis, and during anaphase II the daughter chromatid strands from each chromosome migrate to opposite poles of the cell. The events of telophase II and cytokinesis result in each of the two haploid 'daughter' cells becoming two haploid cells. In this way four haploid gametes with a mix of genetic material are formed.

To summarize:

```
                        Meiosis I
One diploid cell (2n) ─────────────▶  Two haploid cells
                                          (n) + (n)


                            Meiosis II
Two haploid cells (n) + (n) ─────────────▶  Four haploid gametes
                                              (n) + (n) + (n) + (n)
```

Spermatogenesis

Spermatogenesis, which occurs within the seminiferous tubules of the testes, is a continuous process, starting at puberty (see Chapter 21). Surrounding the seminiferous tubules are the Leydig cells. These produce the androgen hormone testosterone so important in the stimulation of spermatogenesis (see pages 477–478). Situated in the seminiferous tubules of an adult testis are two cell types: germ cells and Sertoli cells. The germ cells are all at different stages of development and will eventually become spermatozoa; the supporting Sertoli cells help to nourish the germ cells, secrete controlling hormones and, with their tight junctions, provide the blood–testis barrier that prevents the immune system 'getting a look at' the spermatozoa antigens formed long after immunocompetence was achieved (see autoimmunity, Chapter 19).

Diploid stem cells known as spermatogonia produce germ cells by continuous mitosis (see *Figure 20.7*). Prior to puberty this mitotic division results in the production of identical spermatogonia, but following puberty some cells formed will differentiate into primary spermatocytes. The first meiotic division involves the primary spermatocytes, which divide to form two haploid secondary spermatocytes. The secondary spermatocytes then undergo the second meiotic division, resulting in four haploid cells known as spermatids.

Each spermatid still needs considerable modification before it becomes a highly specialized motile **spermatozoon** with a head, midpiece and tail (see *Figure 20.8*). These modifications, which occur in the seminiferous tubules and the duct system, include changes to the nucleus, loss of excess cytoplasm and the formation of a tail. The genetic material (DNA) of the spermatid nucleus is condensed to form the head of the spermatozoon, which is topped by an acrosome formed from the Golgi region (see Chapter 1). Lytic enzymes present in the acrosome allow the spermatozoa to pass through the cervical mucus and ultimately to penetrate the oocyte.

The midpiece contains many mitochondria (see Chapter 1), arranged in a spiral, which produce the ATP required to power the movements of the tail. The tail, which has a typical flagellum configuration of two central microtubules surrounded by a further nine pairs (2 + 9), is formed from one of the centrioles present in the spermatid (see Chapter 1).

The process of spermatogenesis takes about 70–75 days, but further maturation occurs within the epididymis, where the spermatozoa become motile and fully fertile. Many millions of spermatozoa are produced each day and those not ejaculated are dealt with by phagocytosis and absorbed.

Meiosis I

interphase
DNA replicated

chromatin diploid cell (2*n*)

Prophase I

 synapsis of homologous chromosomes to form bivalent

 chromosomes coil around each other

 each chromosome can be seen to have 2 chromatids, each unit now has 4 strands (quadrivalent), 'cross-over' occurs

Metaphase I

 spindle forms bivalents form so that each new cell receives only one chromosome from the homologous pair

Anaphase I

 a chromosome (2 chromatids) migrates to each pole

Telophase I and cytokinesis

  2 haploid cells (*n*)

Meiosis II

short interphase
no DNA replication

Prophase II

 usual events of prophase occur

Metaphase II

 chromosomes (2 chromatid strands) arrange themselves on the spindle

Anaphase II

 chromatid strands separate at centromere and each migrates to opposite poles

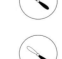

Telophase II and cytokinesis

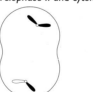

4 haploid gametes (*n*)

Figure 20.6 Stages of meiosis (events are shown in a hypothetical cell with only one pair of chromosomes).

Semen

Semen is the viscous white fluid consisting of motile spermatozoa and the secretions of the accessory glands. The fluid part of semen provides a vehicle for the spermatozoa and contains nutrients and chemicals necessary for spermatozoa survival.

Semen is slightly alkaline (pH 7.2–7.6), which helps to counteract the vaginal acidity – an important property as spermatozoa need an alkaline environment for motility.

Nutrients such as fructose are supplied by the secretions from the seminal vesicles. The presence of hormones and prostaglandins in semen facilitates the movement of spermatozoa through the female reproductive tract and enzymes enhance their ability to penetrate the cervical mucus. Semen contains clotting enzymes that cause initial coagulation after ejaculation, thus ensuring that a mass of semen is delivered to the top of the vagina. Later, other enzymes (fibrinolysins) cause this mass to liquefy and pass through the cervix.

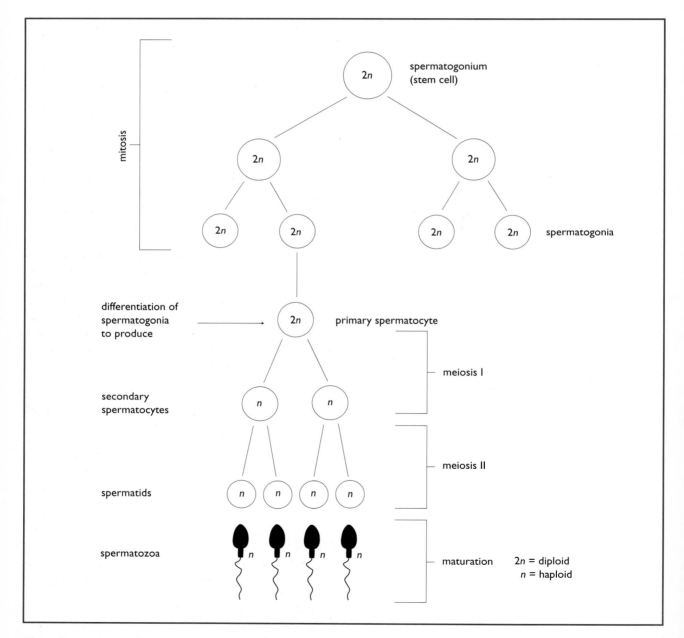

Figure 20.7 Spermatogenesis.

The volume of semen produced at each ejaculation is normally 2–6 ml and contains 50–150 million spermatozoa/ml; this volume and number of spermatozoa decreases as the frequency of ejaculation increases. During investigations for subfertility (see Further Reading, e.g. Winston, 1986) the numbers (sperm count), motility, coagulability and morphology (shape) of the spermatozoa are determined, as are the pH, chemical content and volume of the semen.

Hormones and control of male reproductive function

Spermatogenesis and the release of testicular androgens are controlled by hormones produced by the hypothala-mus, anterior pituitary and the testes (see Chapter 8 and *Figure 20.9*).

From puberty onwards, a gonadotrophin-releasing hormone (GnRH) released by the hypothalamus stimulates the anterior pituitary to produce two **gonadotrophins** (hormones controlling gonad function): follicle stimulating hormone (FSH) and luteinizing hormone (LH), the latter also being known as interstitial cell stimulating hormone (ICSH) in the male.

FSH acts upon the Sertoli cells in the seminiferous tubules to stimulate spermatogenesis, a process which also requires some LH. The major role of LH, however, is to stimulate the Leydig cells surrounding the seminiferous tubules to produce testosterone, an androgen steroid hormone, which in turn stimulates spermatogenesis. Testosterone circulates in the blood and shows effects elsewhere in the body, which we will consider separately. Paradoxically, LH also stimulates the testes to produce small amounts of oestrogens (female steroid hormone), which may have some regulatory role.

In common with many hormones, the gonadotrophins are subject to negative feedback/inhibition. High levels of testosterone act to inhibit the release of the hypothalamic and/or pituitary hormones. Also involved in the inhibition of FSH and LH release is the protein hormone, inhibin, which is produced by the Sertoli cells in response to a rising spermatozoa count.

Following puberty the adult males hormonal patterns and level of spermatogenesis remain fairly constant, although a general decline occurs with ageing. These hormonal patterns are not, as in the adult female, cyclical. Hormonal control of male reproductive function is dependent upon the relationships between hypothalamic releasing hormone, FSH and LH from the anterior pituitary, and testicular testosterone and inhibin.

Testosterone

Testosterone is the major androgen hormone, it has a steroid (see Chapter 1) structure and is derived from cholesterol. Most testosterone originates from the testes, but small amounts are produced by the adrenal glands in both sexes. Apart from its effects upon spermatogenesis, testosterone exerts widespread anabolic (see Chapters 13, 16 and 21) effects by stimulating protein synthesis in both reproductive and somatic tissue. Testosterone circulates in the blood to reach its many target cells, where it influences libido (sex drive) in both sexes, and is responsible for the development of the male secondary sexual characteristics at puberty (see Chapter 21) and the continued correct functioning of the accessory reproductive structures. A drastic fall in testosterone production, e.g. as a result of bilateral orchidectomy, causes spermatogenesis to decline and atrophy of the reproductive structures, resulting in impotence and loss of fertility.

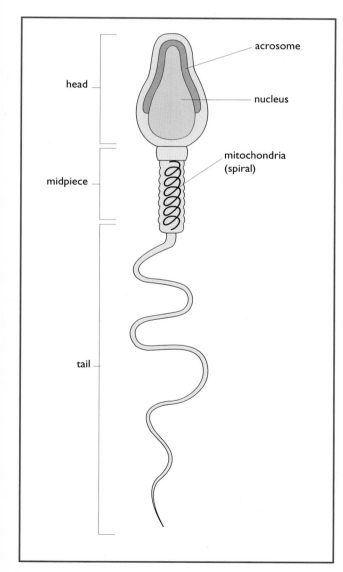

Figure 20.8 A mature spermatozoon.

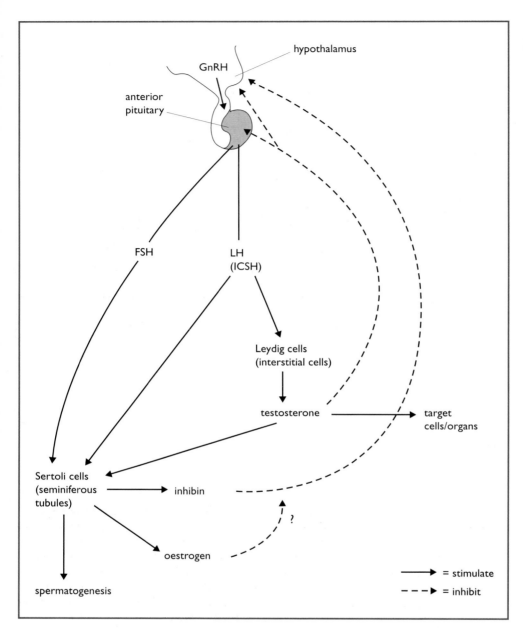

Figure 20.9 Hormone control of male reproductive function.

Female Reproductive System

The female reproductive system has an intricate role which consists of producing the female gametes (oocytes), providing the site for fertilization and providing an environment suitable for the nurture of a developing embryo (from fertilization to the end of the eighth week of gestation) and fetus (from the ninth week of gestation until birth) should conception occur. It is more complex than that of the male and is completely separate from the urinary tract.

Structure of the female reproductive system

The female reproductive system (*Figure 20.10*) can be divided into two parts. The internal genitalia consists of the ovaries (two) in the pelvis, uterine/fallopian tubes (two), uterus and vagina; the external genitalia consists of the structures comprising the vulva. The mammary glands (breasts) are usually included in a discussion of reproductive structures because of lactation.

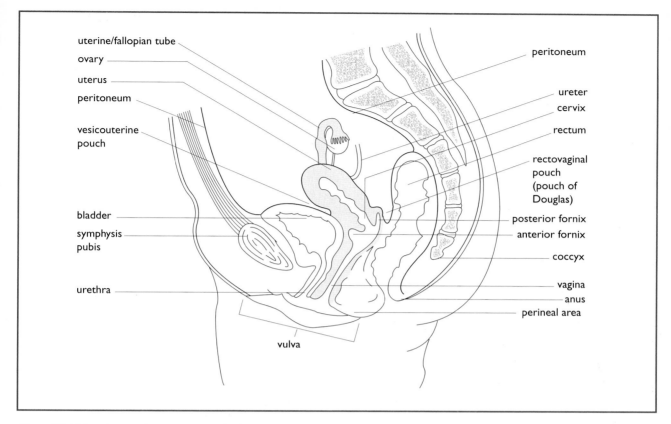

Figure 20.10 Female reproductive structures (midsagittal section).

Ovaries

The female gonads, or ovaries, produce the cells destined to become ova, and act as endocrine organs (see Chapter 8) by secreting female hormones – oestrogens and progesterone – and small amounts of male androgens. During fetal life the ovaries, in common with the testes, develop high in the abdomen, but unlike the testes the ovaries descend only to the pelvic cavity, where they remain.

The almond-shaped ovaries lie in shallow fossae on the lateral pelvic walls. One ovary is situated on either side of the uterus, to which they are attached by ovarian ligaments. The ovaries are attached by the mesovarium to the posterior part of the broad ligament, the fold of peritoneum (see Chapter 13) which encloses and supports the internal genitalia. Blood vessels and autonomic nerves of both divisions run in the mesovarium to enter the ovary at its hilum. The arterial supply is via the ovarian arteries, which branch directly from the aorta and from a branch of the uterine artery. A plexus of veins drains venous blood from the ovaries. The ovary is covered by a thin layer of germinal epithelium, which is so named

because it was once thought, quite erroneously, to be the site of oocyte development. Under this layer is the fibrous tunica albuginea, which encloses an outer cortex of connective tissue stroma and follicles containing the oocytes and an inner medulla containing blood vessels (see *Figure 20.11*). Scarring on the outer surface, which is due to repeated follicle rupture at **ovulation**, increases with the age of the woman. The adult ovary varies in size during the **ovarian cycle** (see pages 488–489) and contains follicles at different stages of maturation (see *Figure 20.11*) – primary, maturing, and mature Graafian follicles – and a structure known as the corpus luteum that develops following follicle rupture (see page 489).

Uterine/fallopian tubes

The paired uterine tubes (fallopian tubes) extend laterally from the uterus to open into the peritoneal cavity; they are about 10 cm long, with a diameter of about 1 cm; however, the tube varies considerably in diameter along its length.

Person-centred Study **Lucy**

Lucy, aged 49, had been worrying about cancer since the death of a close friend, from ovarian cancer, the previous month. Ovarian tumours, which kill around 4500 women each year in the UK, are more commonly diagnosed as investigations improve, and represent an important malignancy of the female reproductive structures.

Unfortunately few women are even aware of the possibility of ovarian cancer, probably because it has received little publicity compared with tumours of the cervix (see pages 483–484) and breast (see page 486). Many ovarian tumours are diagnosed too late for an effective cure with surgery and cytotoxic drugs because their growth deep in the pelvis gives rise to few symptoms in the early stages.

Lucy decided to see her family doctor and was able to discuss her fears about cancer. Her doctor suggested that she have a pelvic examination – which proved to be normal – and told Lucy that had there been any doubt she would have referred her for further tests that usually include ultrasound scan and a computed tomography scan, if indicated. What she did suggest, however, was that Lucy make an appointment for Well-woman Screening with the practice nurse (continued on page 487).

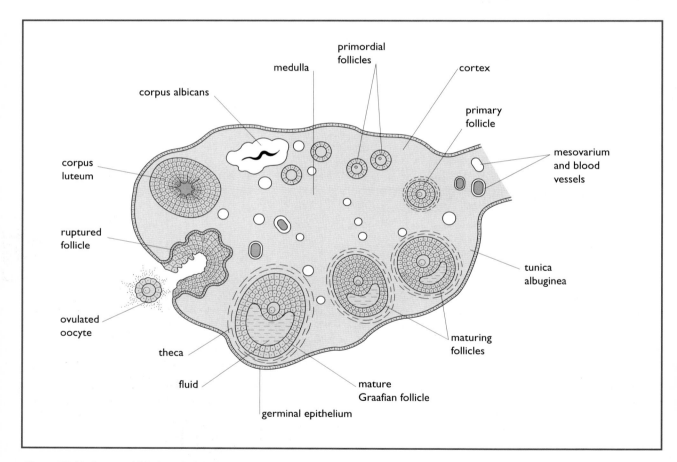

Figure 20.11 Ovary and follicles at all stages.

It is important to note that this arrangement of the uterine tubes opening into the peritoneal cavity means that infection from other parts of the reproductive tract can spread to the pelvic cavity and cause pelvic inflammatory disease (PID; see below and page 495).

Each tube is divided into a funnel-like infundibulum ending in the fimbriae (finger-like projections), which help to waft the oocyte from the ovary into the tube, which consists of a dilated ampulla where fertilization usually occurs, an isthmus and an interstitial part within the uterine wall, which is very narrow (1 mm) (*Figure 20.12*).

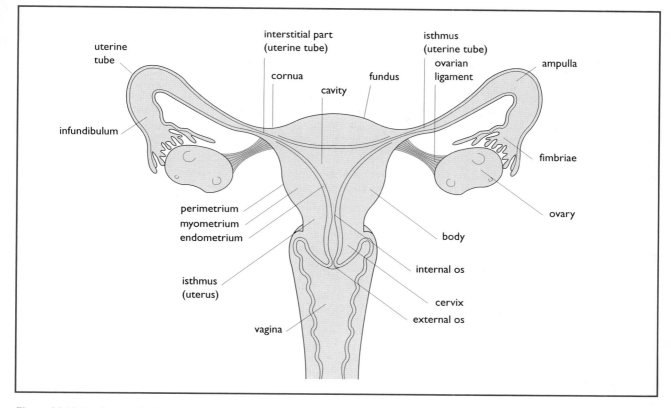

Figure 20.12 Female reproductive structures (anterior view).

Abnormal Function **Tubal problems – ectopic pregnancy**

Any extrauterine pregnancy is termed ectopic. Most commonly this occurs within the uterine tube, but rarely implantation may be in the pelvis or ovary. As you can imagine, a structure as delicate as the uterine tube is easily occluded by congenital defects, pelvic surgery, PID (see page 495) or a blood clot from a previous ectopic pregnancy. A partial or unilateral blockage may lead to ectopic implantation, whereby the early embryo, finding its route to the uterus barred, starts to develop within the uterine tube.

This abnormal event may have several outcomes, but all result in the loss of the pregnancy. Most dramatically, the growing embryo may rupture the uterine tube, resulting in pain, severe haemorrhage, hypovolaemia and shock (see Chapter 10). The management of tubal rupture includes blood transfusion followed by surgical removal of the affected tube (salpingecto-my) as life-saving measures. Where the clinical presentation is subacute or atypical the diagnosis is confirmed by ultrasound and laparoscopy (endoscopic examination of the abdominal cavity). Complete bilateral tubal blockage, for whatever reason, will cause subfertility. This type of subfertility may sometimes be overcome by specialized tubal surgery techniques or possibly by IVF (see page 499), which bypasses the blocked tube.

The uterine tubes are covered with and supported by part of the broad ligament known as the mesosalpinx. A middle layer of smooth muscle is responsible for the peristalsis which helps to convey the oocyte towards the uterus. The mucosal lining is highly specialized, with ciliated cells and secreting cells with microvilli. The cilia beat rhythmically to assist the oocyte on its journey to the uterus and the secretions help to keep the oocyte and spermatozoa in a viable condition.

The uterine tubes have an extremely good arterial blood supply via the ovarian and uterine arteries. This vascularity would lead to considerable blood loss if a tube were to rupture.

Uterus

The uterus is an amazing structure; it provides the correct environment for embryo implantation and nurtures the developing fetus, which it expels at the end of pregnancy (hopefully at full term).

A healthy nulliparous (never been pregnant) uterus is pear-shaped and approximately 7.5 cm long, 5 cm wide and 2.5 cm thick, but may be slightly larger following pregnancy. It is a pelvic structure situated between the bladder and rectum. Basically, the thick-walled uterus is a hollow muscular organ, which can be divided into a fundus (top), a corpus (body) and a cervix (neck) (see *Figure 20.12*); the body and cervix are separated by a narrow area (also called the isthmus), which becomes the lower segment in pregnancy. The two uterine tubes insert laterally into the uterus at the cornuae inferior to the fundus, and the cervix protrudes into the vagina.

An abundant arterial supply reaches the uterus via two uterine arteries that branch from the internal iliac arteries. The uterine arteries divide at the level of the cervix, the lower branch supplying the cervix and the vagina, and the upper branch the body, fundus, tubes and ovaries. The branches that run up to the fundus are convoluted to allow for uterine enlargement during pregnancy. We will discuss the further modifications to arterial supply during our consideration of the endometrium. Venous blood leaves the uterus in corresponding veins. The uterus is innervated by both divisions of the autonomic system – parasympathetic fibres from the sacral outflow and sympathetic fibres from the lumbar outflow. Lymphatic vessels drain via aortic and iliac lymph nodes.

A fold of peritoneum called the perimetrium (see *Figure 20.12*) is draped over the uterus to form an adherent outer covering; this is reflected laterally to form the broad ligament. Anteriorly the pelvic peritoneum forms the vesico-uterine pouch between the uterus and bladder and posteriorly the rectovaginal pouch (also called the recto-uterine pouch or pouch of Douglas) between the vagina/uterus and rectum (see *Figure 20.10*). The latter is a common site for the collection of pus or blood resulting from pelvic disease.

Uterine muscle, or myometrium, found in the fundus and body, is formed from a thick layer of interlocking smooth muscle fibres. The myometrium is influenced by both autonomic nerves and hormones when it contracts strongly during labour to expel the fetus. Following delivery of the infant and placenta the interlocking fibres contract as a 'living ligature' and compress the uterine blood vessels to limit blood loss.

The mucosal lining of the body of the uterus, known as the endometrium, consists of highly vascular epithelium containing many tubular glands (*Figure 20.13*). From the menarche (commencement of menstruation) to the menopause (cessation of menstruation) this unique tissue undergoes cyclical changes in response to ovarian hormones (see pages 489–491) and if fertilization occurs the embryo implants into a specially prepared endometrium (see page 498).

The endometrium consists of two layers – the stratum basalis, which is permanent, and the stratum functionalis, which is shed every 28 days or so during menstruation and regenerates under the influence of ovarian hormones.

It is appropriate here to consider the special features of the endometrial blood supply. Branches of the uterine arteries divide within the myometrium to form the arcuate arteries, which send radial branches to the endometrium. These radial arteries form straight arteries that supply the stratum basalis, and the coiled (spiral) arteries that supply the stratum functionalis and that degenerate with each menstrual flow.

The uterine cervix contains mostly fibrous tissue and its mucosa does not show the cyclical changes that affect the endometrium. What does change is the type and quantity of mucus produced by the glands in the cervical columnar epithelium during the **menstrual (uterine) cycle**. Examination of this mucus forms the basis of a 'natural' method of family planning (see page 497). The cervical canal has two openings: the internal os, which communicates with the uterine cavity, and external os, which opens into the vagina (see *Figure 20.12*). The columnar epithelium lining the cervix is replaced by stratified squamous epithelium in the part of the cervix that protrudes into the vagina, affording it some protection from trauma, e.g. during intercourse.

Uterine supports

The position of the uterus is normally anteverted (inclined forward) and anteflexed (bent forward) over the bladder (see *Figure 20.10*). The uterus is supported in this position by the muscles of the pelvic floor (see *Figure 18.49*), ligaments and, to a limited extent, by the pelvic peritoneum (broad ligament). Apart from support, these structures, when healthy, are able to maintain continence, assist with micturition and defaecation, and stretch sufficiently to permit the birth of a baby.

The supporting ligaments are:

- Round ligaments: one from each uterine cornua runs through the inguinal canal to the labia majora (see page 485), offering limited support.
- Transverse cervical ligaments (cardinal): two ligaments running from the cervix to the lateral walls of the pelvis.
- Uterosacral ligament: extends backwards from the cervix to the sacrum. It divides on reaching the rectum but the two parts rejoin at the sacrum.
- Pubocervical ligament: extends from the cervix to the symphysis pubis. It supports the bladder and urethra.

Figure 20.13 Endometrium.

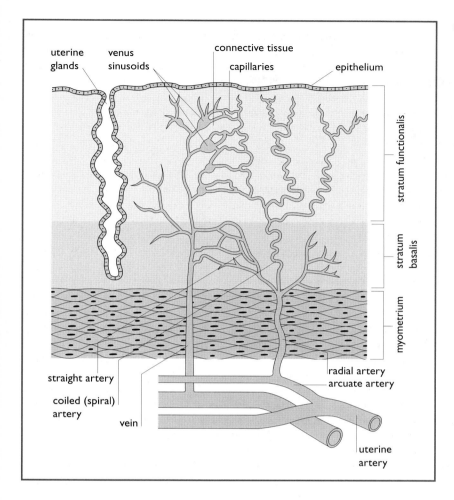

uterine glands
venus sinusoids
connective tissue
capillaries
epithelium
stratum functionalis
stratum basalis
myometrium
straight artery
coiled (spiral) artery
vein
radial artery
arcuate artery
uterine artery

Abnormal Function **Cervical problems – cancer**

Cervical carcinoma kills around 2000 women in the UK each year and many of these deaths could be avoided with regular and effective screening (see Nursing Practice Application, page 484). The disease develops through an early phase known as cervical intraepithelial neoplasia (CIN) where potentially malignant precancerous changes are present in the epithelial cells. CIN and the next stage of early non-invasive malignant change may be detected by 'smear test' and treated successfully by destroying the lesion with lasers and/or removing it surgically by cone biopsy. The cellular changes occurring in the cervix are initiated by viruses,

such as the human papilloma virus (HPV) or herpes simplex virus type 2 (HSV2), which are passed to the woman during sexual intercourse (coitus). A recent study by Lehtinen *et al.* (1996) showed that women with HPV type 16 infection were more likely to develop cervical cancer.

Precancerous and malignant lesions of the cervix are associated with risk factors that include:
• Early first coitus (before stratified epithelium is in place).
• Multiple sexual partners (the disease is least common in women who have never been sexually active).

• Sexual activity with a partner who may have had multiple partners.
• Multiparity.
• Chronic cervical inflammation.
• Sexually transmitted diseases.
• Lower socio-economic groups.
• Smoking.
• Sexual partners not circumcised (cervical cancer is virtually unknown in orthodox Jewish women – the men are circumcised). Cervical cancer is present in some populations where the male is circumcised, but may be due to multiple sexual partners.
• Oral contraceptives (see page 497).

Nursing Practice Application **Screening for cervical disease**

Women are naturally anxious about 'cancer tests' and need adequate information and the opportunity to express their fears. Although screening and diagnostic tests usually cause no pain and are performed without anaesthesia, the need for emotional support should be anticipated. A major problem can be the time waiting for appointments or results, both of which increase anxiety. **Exfoliative cytology:** here cervical cells are obtained via a speculum, using a wooden spatula or brush, and examined microscopically for changes. A cervical smear (Papanicolaou) should cause no pain, but speculum insertion may be painful for women who are anxious or embarrassed and for those who are not sexually active. This potential problem can be overcome by selecting a speculum of the most appropriate size and shape for individual women. False results do occur, but if abnormal cells are found the diagnosis is confirmed by colposcopy.

Colposcopy: this is the examination of the cervix with a colposcope, an instrument that magnifies the cells. Again, this involves speculum insertion; the cells are stained with iodine and any abnormal tissue seen can be biopsied and examined in the histology department.

Opinion differs regarding the frequency of cervical screening and which age groups should be included. Currently the DoH (UK) recommends that women aged 20–64 should have a smear at least once every 5 years, but many experts suggest that tests be repeated more frequently (1–3 years), e.g. annual tests where women or their partners have HPV. Hiscock and Reece (1988) recommended that there should be more pressure for 'high risk' women to attend triennial (at least) screening.

Abnormal Function **Problems with uterovaginal prolapse**

Uterovaginal prolapse, which usually occurs after the menopause, is due to damage incurred by the supporting structures over many years. The damage occurs primarily during childbirth, especially during a difficult or prolonged second stage, but other risk factors include constipation (see Chapter 13), poor handling/moving technique (see Chapter 18) – which has particular significance for both professional and informal carers, poor posture, chronic cough and obesity. The problem occurs during the climacteric (the period of time during which changes in the female reproductive tract result in decline and eventual cessation of reproductive function) because declining oestrogen levels lead to muscle/ligament atrophy with loss of function.

The problems experienced by individual women depend on the type and severity of the prolapse, but the proximity of the bladder and urethra quite often results in frequency or stress incontinence. Some women complain of defaecation difficulties and, where the uterus is prolapsed, they may have discomfort and the feeling that 'something has dropped down'. Management may include: information regarding contributing factors such as constipation, pelvic floor exercises and electrical stimulation, and a supporting pessary (rarely) or surgery, e.g. anterior colporrhaphy (surgical repair of the anterior vaginal wall).

Prevention is, however, much the preferred option, with prophylactic pelvic floor exercises (see Chapter 18), avoidance of risk factors, careful management of labour and suturing of perineal lacerations and episiotomy (incision made in the perineum during the second stage of labour), and possibly oestrogen replacement (see Chapter 21).

Vagina

The vagina is the canal extending from the cervix to the external genitalia (see *Figure 20.10*). Its anterior wall is about 7.5 cm long and lies close to the urethra and bladder, and the posterior wall, which is longer at 9 cm, has contact with the rectum and the rectovaginal pouch. Normally the vaginal walls are in apposition (touching) but, because of rugae (folds), the vagina is capable of the considerable stretching required to facilitate coitus and childbirth.

The vagina runs at an angle of 45°, which is an important point to note prior to inserting instruments or medication. Nurses should also remember to mention this fact when teaching women about medicated pessaries or contraceptive diaphragms. The projection of the cervix into the vagina forms four fornices (deep folds or gutters); the posterior fornix, which receives the semen, is deeper than the lateral, or anterior, fornices. At its distal orifice the vagina is partially occluded by the hymen, a perforated membrane, which is usually ruptured during the first coitus. It may also have been ruptured by tampon use or exercise, and any remnants are completely destroyed by the birth of a woman's first child.

The vagina receives arterial blood from branches of the uterine arteries and from a vaginal artery that may branch direct from the internal iliac artery or from the uterine artery. Venous blood drains via many interconnecting veins

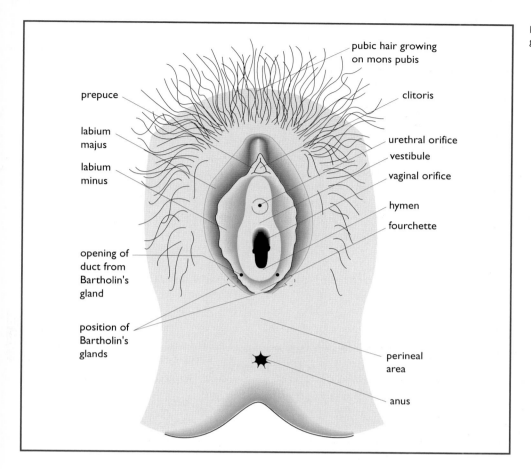

Figure 20.14 External female genitalia.

Labels on figure:

pubic hair growing on mons pubis

prepuce

clitoris

labium majus

urethral orifice

labium minus

vestibule

vaginal orifice

hymen

fourchette

opening of duct from Bartholin's gland

position of Bartholin's glands

perineal area

anus

and venous plexuses which empty into the internal iliac vein. The sensitive lower vagina is innervated by the voluntary pudendal nerve and the upper part by autonomic sympathetic fibres.

Structurally the vagina consists of an outer layer of fibrous tissue, a layer of involuntary muscle, a loose areolar layer and the stratified squamous epithelial lining. The stratified squamous epithelium, which is adapted to withstand the trauma of coitus and childbirth, has no secretory glands. Some fluid may leak through the walls, but the bulk of vaginal moisture originates from the cervical mucus and mucus produced during sexual excitement (see page 494).

During the reproductive years the vagina is acidic (pH 4.5) due to the production of lactic acid by bacteria of the *Lactobacillus* species, which form part of the normal flora (see Chapter 19). The lactic acid produced from bacterial metabolism of glycogen, stored in the mucosal cells, helps protect the vagina from many pathogenic organisms. Vaginal acidity is, however, hostile to spermatozoa, which are normally protected by the alkaline semen and cervical mucus.

Vulva

The vulva consists of the structures known collectively as the external genitalia (*Figure 20.14*); these structures include the mons pubis, labia majora, labia minora, clitoris, structures within the vestibule, hymen (see page 484) and fourchette.

The mons pubis is a pad of fatty tissue situated over the symphysis pubis. It is covered with terminal pubic hair, which first grows during puberty. Moving back from the mons pubis are the fatty labia majora, which merge posteriorly with the perineal skin. The labia majora are skin-covered and contain numerous sebaceous glands; pubic hair grows on the outer part, whereas the inner surface is smooth. Remember the labia majora are homologous with the scrotum – they develop from the same embryonic structures.

Inside the protective outer labia are two smaller folds called the labia minora. Formed from smooth skin, they enclose the area known as the vestibule. Anteriorly the labia minora fuse to form the prepuce, which covers the clitoris; posteriorly they form the fourchette. The clitoris is homologous with the penis; it contains erectile tissue and is abundantly innervated. It is extremely sensitive and is involved in the female sexual response.

Apart from the clitoris, the vestibule contains the openings of the urethra and vagina and the vestibular glands. The ducts of two tiny Skene's glands (lesser vestibular glands) open into the urethral meatus. There are two larger Bartholin's glands (greater vestibular glands) whose ducts open into the vaginal orifice. Bartholin's glands, which are homologous with the male bulbo-urethral glands, produce lubricating mucus, which increases during sexual stimulation to facilitate coitus.

The area between the vagina and rectum consists of soft tissue and skin (sometimes called the clinical perineum) overlying the posterior muscles of the wedge-shaped perineum (see Chapter 18).

Mammary glands

The breasts (mammary glands) are highly specialized sweat glands adapted to produce milk (lactation), when stimulated by the correct hormone environment, follow-ing the birth of a baby. Although breasts are significant in expressing sexuality, their only physiological function is lactation. At puberty in the female (see Chapter 21) the rudimentary breast, which is present in both sexes, responds to oestrogen stimulation by developing and enlarging. The breasts also show cyclical changes during the menstrual cycle, but it is only during pregnancy that the breasts enlarge and become physiologically active in readiness for lactation. When oestrogen levels decline, during the climacteric, there is breast atrophy and later loss of adipose tissue.

Each breast has an area of pigmented skin, the areola, into which the nipple opens. Smooth muscle fibres in the nipple and areola cause nipple erection in response to cold and sexual excitement. The many sebaceous glands (Montgomery's tubules) in the areola help to keep the skin in that area supple and lubricated. The areola darkens during a first pregnancy, when it becomes permanently brown in colour.

Nursing Practice Application **Episiotomy and perineal laceration**

Following episiotomy or perineal lacera-tion a careful repair of the perineum is essential to promote healing (see Chapter 19) and prevent later vaginal prolapse. The perineal area is extremely well innervated and the episiotomy wound or laceration is likely to be painful. This makes sitting uncomfortable and the establishment of breast feeding more difficult. Defaecation will be painful and constipation should be avoided, e.g. by the use of aperients and high fibre intake. Meticulous hygiene reg-imens are required to avoid infection in this damp, warm area, and women are encouraged to wash their hands before and after perineal contact, change pads fre-quently, wash and dry the area after elim-ination and report signs of infection, e.g. increasing pain and discharge.

Pelvic floor exercises, undertaken soon after delivery, improves perineal blood flow, which aids healing, minimizes infec-tion risk and reduces congestion and with it discomfort (Gould, 1990).

Abnormal Function **Breast problems**

Many women have breast pain as part of the menstrual cycle changes (see page 493). Breast lumps are very common, but most prove to be benign breast disease. Although benign disease causes anxiety and sometimes pain, the focus of this discussion will be cancer. In the UK, breast cancer is the most common malignant condition affecting women, where it accounts for 20% of female malignancies and kills around 16 000 women annually. Properly planned and supported screening programmes, which include breast awareness and reporting changes, and mammography (see Person-centred study – Lucy), can detect lesions at an early stage, when cure may be possible and treatment options are acceptable to the women concerned. However, the effectiveness of breast self-examination in prolonging life has not been established by research. Recently genes e.g. BRCA1, responsible for a small minority of breast cancers have been identified. Women with a family history of breast cancer (especially mother, grandmoth-er or sister) may be offered the test to detect a mutant gene, but if they are found to carry the BRCA1 gene there are some difficult decisions to make about possible prophylactic treatment. The management of breast cancer usual-ly involves a combination of:

- Surgery – lumpectomy, where only the lump is excised, or some form of mas-tectomy (breast removal), with its implications for body image, sexuality, self-esteem and relationships.
- Radiotherapy.
- Some tumours are oestrogen-depen-dent and hormone modification, such as removal or destruction of the ovaries in premenopausal women or the administration of tamoxifen (oestrogen antagonist), may be indicat-ed. After the menopause sex steroid production is adrenal, and drugs, such as aminoglutethimide (inhibits conver-sion of androgens to oestrogens) or tamoxifen, are administered.
- Cytotoxic drugs after excision.

Situated anterior to the pectoral muscles (see Chapter 18), each breast consists of 15–20 lobes containing alveolar glands that radiate out from the nipple (*Figure 20.15*). The lobes are supported by fatty and fibrous tissue and separated by suspensory ligaments which also secure the breast to the chest wall. Normal breasts show a large variation in size and shape. Within the breast lobes are the small lobules of alveolar glands whose role is milk secretion. A lactiferous duct draining each lobule dilates to form a lactiferous sinus (ampulla), just below the areola, where milk is stored prior to discharge through the ducts opening on the nipple surface. Further coverage of breast function can be found in the discussion on lactation (page 503).

Functioning of the female reproductive structures – oogenesis

The process of oogenesis occurring within the cortex of the ovary differs from spermatogenesis (page 474) in several ways. Notably the entire stock of female gametes are already present, in an immature state, within the ovaries of a female fetus before birth. The time spent in the immature state may be up to 50 years. Maturation occurs on a cyclical basis, which commences at puberty and continues until the cessation of reproductive function after the climacteric. During maturation there is a second resting stage and an unequal cytoplasmic division.

Readers may care to refresh their memories regarding meiosis (pages 473–475) before our discussion of oogenesis (see *Figure 20.16*). We will, however, first consider the processes occurring in the ovary prior to birth. Early during fetal life primordial germ cells differentiate to become diploid stem cells called oogonia (*2n*). The oogonia multiply by rapid mitotic division to form several hundred thousand primary oocytes (*2n*). Mitosis is followed by a period of growth and the development of primordial follicles, which surround the primary oocytes. At this stage the first meiotic division commences in the primary oocyte, but is arrested at prophase I. The primary oocyte commences a variable-length resting stage before meiosis I is completed, in some 450 cells, some time during the reproductive life of the woman.

At puberty the production of functional oocytes commences with the activation of several primary oocytes during each ovarian cycle. Ovarian follicular changes occurring as part of the ovarian cycle and oogenesis are discussed on pages 488 and 489.

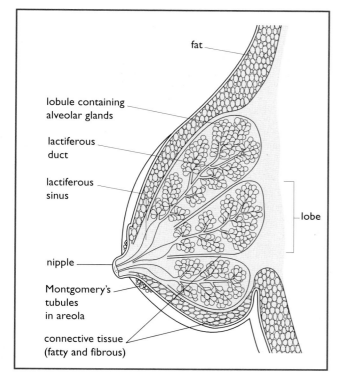

fat

lobule containing alveolar glands

lactiferous duct

lactiferous sinus

lobe

nipple

Montgomery's tubules in areola

connective tissue (fatty and fibrous)

Figure 20.15 Breast.

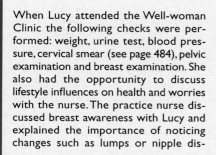

When Lucy attended the Well-woman Clinic the following checks were performed: weight, urine test, blood pressure, cervical smear (see page 484), pelvic examination and breast examination. She also had the opportunity to discuss lifestyle influences on health and worries with the nurse. The practice nurse discussed breast awareness with Lucy and explained the importance of noticing changes such as lumps or nipple discharge, and offered her a leaflet (Cancer Research Campaign, 1991). She also told her about the mammography screening programme, which in the UK is offered by the NHS to women aged 50–64 every 3 years. This service is also available to women with suspicious breast lumps and those over 64 on request. Currently there is debate about whether mammography should be offered at an earlier age (45); in the USA it is recommended more frequently and commences at age 40. One problem of earlier screening is the denseness of younger breasts, which makes cancer detection more difficult. It will be some years before we know if mammography actually reduces breast cancer mortality, but reducing deaths by at least 25% in the population invited for screening by the year 2000 is one of the Health of the Nation targets (DoH, 1992).

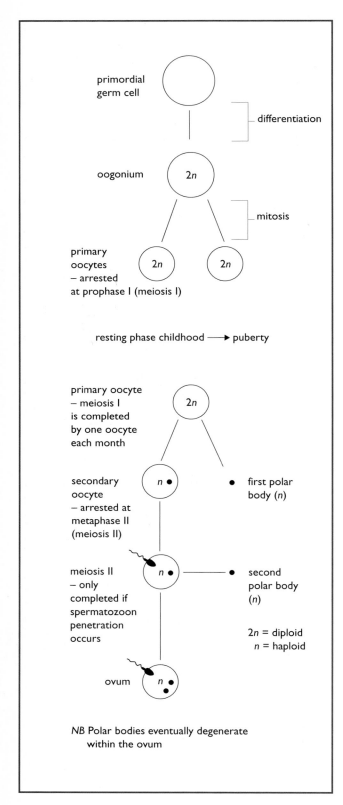

primordial
germ cell

differentiation

oogonium   2n

mitosis

primary
oocytes
– arrested
at prophase I (meiosis I)   2n   2n

resting phase childhood ⟶ puberty

primary oocyte
– meiosis I
is completed
by one oocyte
each month   2n

secondary
oocyte
– arrested at
metaphase II
(meiosis II)   n •   • first polar
body (n)

meiosis II
– only
completed if
spermatozoon
penetration
occurs   n •   • second
polar body
(n)

2n = diploid
n = haploid

ovum   n •

NB Polar bodies eventually degenerate
within the ovum

Figure 20.16 Oogenesis.

The arrested meiosis I is recommenced in several primary oocytes but usually only one is 'chosen' to complete the process. During meiosis I the diploid primary oocyte produces two very dissimilar haploid cells: the secondary oocyte (*n*) and the first polar body (*n*). The secondary oocyte, which still contains the first polar body, is discharged from the surface of the ovary at ovulation.

The first polar body, which has very little cytoplasm to sustain its existence, usually undergoes meiosis II, but eventually all polar bodies degenerate. Meiosis II starts in the secondary oocyte, only to be arrested, this time in metaphase II, and will only be completed if the secondary oocyte is penetrated by a spermatozoon.

If spermatozoon penetration does occur the secondary oocyte completes meiosis II with the production of two haploid cells, a viable **ovum** (*n*) and a second polar body (*n*). The events of fertilization, which take place in the uterine tube, are discussed on pages 496 and 498. Interestingly, the events of oogenesis, which result in four haploid cells, yield only one functional ovum (and thus ensure that the one ovum has enough nutrients to survive prior to implantation), whereas the same meiotic divisions during spermatogenesis produce four functional spermatozoa (large numbers of spermatozoa are lost on their journey to the uterine tube; see page 496).

Ovarian cycle

As already mentioned, the events of oogenesis are accompanied by changes in the ovary that can be divided into two phases: follicular (days 1–14), which includes ovulation, and luteal (days 15–28) (*Figures 20.17* and *20.18*). The ovarian cycle lasts for around 28 days in most women, but may vary (from 21 to 35 days); any changes in cycle length are reflected in the follicular phase, as the luteal phase remains unchanged.

The hormonal influences that control oogenesis and the ovarian cycle are discussed separately, in more detail, on pages 489–491.

During the follicular phase, primordial follicles, enclosing the primary oocytes, develop layers of granulosa cells to become primary follicles. Maturation of the primary follicle into a secondary follicle involves the formation of a zona pellucida around the oocyte and a theca folliculi around the outside of the follicle. Cells of the theca produce oestrogens during maturation. Further development results in the formation of a fluid-filled space around the oocyte, and some granulosa cells develop into a corona radiata, which surrounds the oocyte. The follicle, by this stage, is a mature Graafian follicle ready to release a secondary oocyte at ovulation (remember the ovum is not formed until later).

Ovulation, which usually occurs in alternate ovaries each month, involves rupture of the follicle and discharge of the secondary oocyte into the abdominal cavity. From the abdomen it enters the fimbriated end of a uterine tube. Ovulation is caused by an increase in LH (see page 490), which causes the Graafian follicle to swell, burst and discharge its oocyte. Some women (around 25%) experience 'cramping' pain in the lower abdomen at ovulation; this is known as mittelschmerz, which is German for 'middle pain'.

Usually only one oocyte is released during the ovarian cycle, but the release of two or more oocytes can result in a multiple birth, which is not the norm for humans. In this situation the potential individuals are not identical because they result from the fertilization of different oocytes by different spermatozoa. They are no closer genetically than siblings born at different times.

The follicular phase ends with ovulation and is replaced by the luteal phase. The ruptured follicle 'caves in' and fills with blood clot. Granulosa and theca cells increase to form an endocrine structure called the corpus luteum (yellow body). The corpus luteum secretes progesterone and oestrogen, and is important in preparing for possible fertilization and maintaining pregnancy should it occur. The lifespan of the corpus luteum depends upon the fate of the oocyte released at ovulation. If fertilization does not occur, which is the usual course, the corpus luteum degenerates after about 12–14 days and hormone production stops. The area left after the corpus luteum has degenerated is filled with scar tissue and becomes the corpus albicans (white body). If fertilization does occur the corpus luteum persists and functions to maintain the pregnancy until placental and fetal hormone production are sufficiently developed (see page 500).

Hormones and control of the ovarian cycle

The ovarian cycle and the events of oogenesis are controlled by the gonadotrophins – FSH and LH (see *Figure 20.18*). These two hormones are released cyclically by the anterior pituitary gland in response to hypothalamic GnRH. Although FSH and LH are the same in both sexes, their role in female reproductive functioning is more complex than in the male. FSH and LH levels fluctuate during the ovarian cycle and they control the release of the ovarian hormones oestrogens and progesterone. As you can imagine, this is a finely balanced system that requires precise controls and considerable integration if it is to function correctly.

During puberty the secretion of GnRH causes cyclical release of FSH and LH, which act upon the ovaries to cause the development of adult hormone patterns.

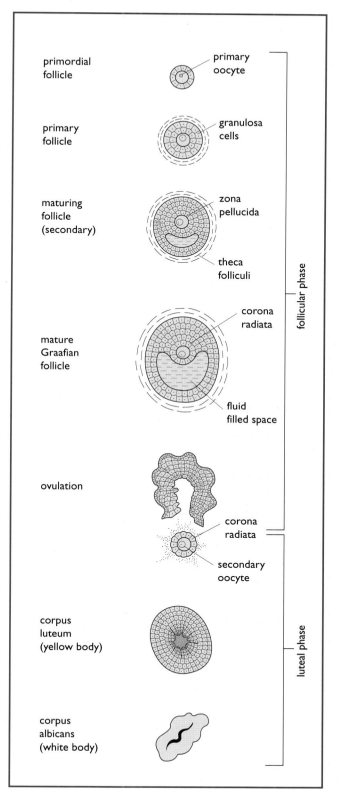

Figure 20.17 Ovarian cycle – follicular development.

Eventually the menarche occurs, but cycles remain largely anovulatory (without ovulation) for the first 2 years until hormonal cycles are stabilized.

In adult women the release of FSH and LH stimulate initial follicular development (see earlier text) and oocyte maturation (see pages 487–488). At this stage the small amount of oestrogen produced by the follicle inhibits pituitary secretion of FSH and LH by negative feedback. In addition the granulosa cells secrete inhibin, which also curtails FSH release (sensible-because follicle development is well underway).

Oestrogen, however, actually increases the effects of FSH and LH locally on the follicle, where development continues and oestrogen levels rise. When oestrogen plasma levels reach a critical point they stop inhibiting the hypothalamus/anterior pituitary and stimulate, by positive feedback, the release of further LH and FSH. Now, at around midcycle, there is a sudden surge of LH, which stimulates ovulation and the formation of the corpus luteum, which LH helps to maintain. FSH released at this time may also be involved with ovulation.

Following ovulation, the corpus luteum secretes progesterone

and oestrogen, which prepare the body for possible pregnancy and together exert negative feedback inhibition on further LH and FSH release. If pregnancy does not occur the decline in LH causes the corpus luteum to degenerate, resulting in reduced levels of oestrogen and progesterone. Now the combined ovarian hormone inhibition is removed and the pituitary can again secrete FSH and LH to start a new ovarian cycle.

It is important to note for events if pregnancy occurs see page 498.

The ovarian cycle is controlled through the integration of hypothalamic releasing hormone, FSH and LH from the pituitary, and ovarian oestrogen, progesterone and inhibin, which exhibit both negative and positive feedback.

Major female steroid hormones
Oestrogens

Oestrogens are steroid hormones derived from cholesterol, and include oestradiol, oestrone and oestriol. Oestrogens are produced by the ovaries, the placenta and, to a limited extent, the adrenal glands. These hormones, which are

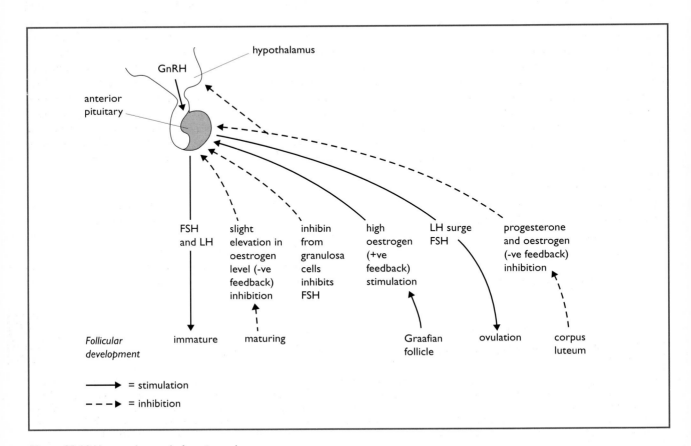

Figure 20.18 Hormonal control of ovarian cycle.

vital for reproductive function, are involved with oogenesis and follicle maturation, development of female secondary sexual characteristics and pubertal growth spurt, and growth and maintenance of reproductive organs.

Oestrogens cause wider metabolic effects, such as a lower serum cholesterol level, which helps to explain why premenopausal women have a lower incidence of coronary heart disease (see Chapter 10) than men of the same age. Another important metabolic influence is the oestrogenic effect upon calcium homeostasis, demonstrated by the increase in the incidence of osteoporosis (see Chapter 16) after the menopause.

Progesterone

Progesterone is another steroid hormone secreted by the ovary and placenta. It is the 'gestation hormone' important in preparing for and maintaining pregnancy. Progesterone increases growth of the endometrium and breasts, causes changes in cervical mucus and inhibits uterine muscle activity.

Menstrual cycle

The menstrual cycle (uterine cycle) involves the changes occurring in the uterus as the endometrium responds to the secretion of ovarian hormones (see *Figure 20.19*). It corresponds to the ovarian cycle and is repeated every 28 days (range 21–35 days) or so, except during pregnancy, from the menarche to the menopause (both the menarche and menopause are discussed in Chapter 21). The menstrual cycle can be subdivided into three phases or stages: proliferative, secretory and menstrual. The whole point of the menstrual cycle is the preparation of the endometrium for possible implantation of the early embryo. Although the menstrual phase comes at the end of the cycle, the first day of bleeding is, by convention, counted as day 1 of the menstrual cycle because it provides an obvious landmark.

Proliferative phase

The proliferative phase corresponds to the follicular phase of the ovarian cycle and starts around day 5 when menstrual bleeding has ceased. After menstruation only the stratum basalis of the endometrium remains. The release of oestrogen causes cell proliferation and regeneration of the stratum functionalis with its blood vessels and glands (see page 482). The proliferative phase ends with the maturation of a Graafian follicle and ovulation at around day 14. At this point the endometrium is approximately 2 mm thick. During the proliferative phase the cervical mucus changes from a thick plug blocking the cervix to profuse amounts of thin slippery mucus that the spermatozoa can penetrate.

Secretory phase

Commencing after ovulation, the secretory phase corresponds with the luteal phase of the ovarian cycle and lasts about 14 days. The oestrogen-primed endometrium is now influenced by progesterone, which causes the glands to enlarge and secrete glycogen, which would nourish the embryo during implantation. The spiral arteries of the endometrium increase in size and become more coiled. Endometrial thickness has by now increased to 5 mm. Cervical mucus becomes thick and again blocks the canal to protect the developing embryo if implantation occurs.

If fertilization does not occur the decline in hormones from the corpus luteum results in spiral artery spasm, initiated by the secretion of endometrial prostaglandins (normally inhibited by progesterone and oestrogen), which causes endometrial degeneration as the endometrium is deprived of nutrients and later autodigestion by lysosomes. This leads, some 24 hours later, to menstruation. The spiral arteries dilate and bleed into the necrotic stratum functionalis, which starts to slough away.

Menstrual phase

It is worth reminding ourselves that the menstrual phase is the last part of the menstrual cycle, in spite of being taken as day 1. The menstrual flow consists of blood, other fluids and endometrial fragments, and lasts on average 3–6 days. Fluid loss at menstruation, which is usually around 75 ml (only 50% is blood), varies considerably and is notoriously

Nursing Practice Application **Learning disability and the menstrual cycle**

The events of the menstrual cycle present additional problems for girls and women who have learning disabilities, and for their carers. Explanations of menstruation need to be geared to an individual's level of understanding, and the practical aspects of providing sanitary protection and hygiene may require modifications to maintain their ability to self-care.

Another difficulty may be behavioural problems associated with fluctuating hormone levels during the cycle. Slevin (1996) reports several studies that have shown an increase in problematic behaviour as progesterone levels decline.

difficult to assess objectively. You might care to consider the amount of blood lost in a year, where in menstruation occurs 13 times with an above average blood loss of 50 ml each time: 13 x 50 = 650 ml lost, which must be replaced – no wonder women need more iron than men during the reproductive years (see Chapter 9). Excessive menstrual loss (menorrhagia) is a common cause of iron deficiency anaemia. Bleeding occurring between menstruations, e.g. after intercourse, should always be investigated to exclude serious pathology, such as endometrial malignancy.

Interestingly, menstrual blood is prevented from clotting within the uterus by the release of fibrinolysins, which ensures that the now useless endometrium is completely expelled through the cervix. At the start of menstruation the uterus contracts, in response to prostaglandins, to expel the blood. These contractions result in the discomfort and pain, experienced by many women, known as dysmenorrhoea.

Body temperature may show variation during the menstrual cycle (*Figure 20.20*). There may be a fall in temperature, which corresponds with the LH surge occurring about 24 hours before ovulation. Progesterone secreted by the corpus luteum then causes a rise in metabolic rate and body temperature of about 0.5°C which persists until menstruation occurs. These changes in

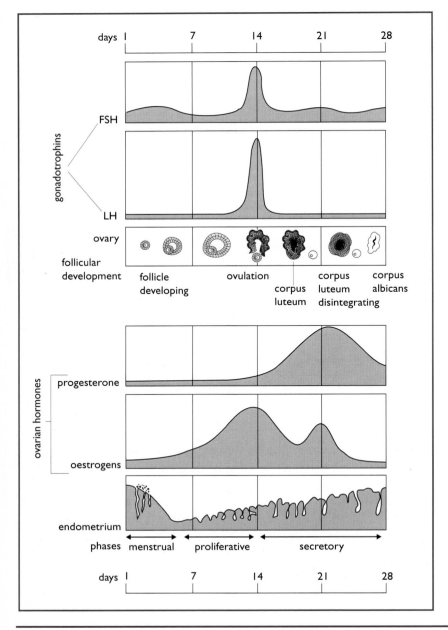

Figure 20.19 Menstrual/uterine cycle (with hormonal and ovarian events).

temperature are a crude guide to the timing of ovulation in some women. The knowledge that ovulation is occurring can be helpful for couples wishing to conceive; they may then time intercourse for the few days when pregnancy is more likely to occur. Conversely, couples who wish to avoid pregnancy can use temperature changes as part of 'natural' family planning, but this has been largely superseded by the use of commercially produced testing kits (see page 497).

Other factors influencing the menstrual cycle have not, as yet, been fully explained. Emotional factors are known to affect menstrual cycle regularity, e.g. grief, leaving home, starting a new course or job and extreme worry. Another interesting observation is the degree of synchrony in menstrual cycle patterns established by women living in close proximity to each other; this is linked to the secretion of pheromones in sweat (see Chapter 19).

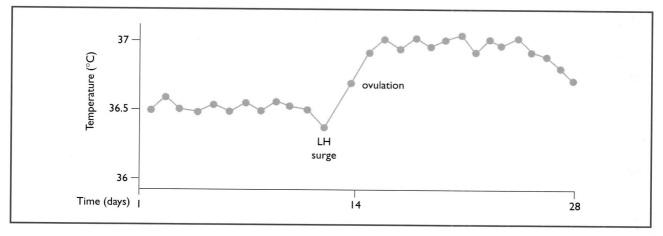

Figure 20.20 Temperature variation during menstrual cycle.

Nursing Practice Application **Premenstrual syndrome (PMS)**

Premenstrual syndrome (PMS) is sometimes called premenstrual tension, or PMT, but either way it describes the physical (mainly due to fluid retention) and emotional effects associated with the 10–12 days before menstruation. Most women experience some changes, but for others the problems cause intense distress, disruption to their lives and relationships, and in severe situations may have serious social implications. Dalton (1980) describes three serious criminal cases where women successfully pleaded diminished responsibility/mitigation due to PMS. The features of PMS include: abdominal swelling; weight gain; breast discomfort and heaviness; ankle oedema; headaches; nausea/vomiting; tiredness; emotional lability, with crying and irritability; insomnia; clumsiness; poor memory; change in bowel habit.

Various studies have shown that women perform less well during the premenstrual and menstrual phases, e.g. in driving, skilled tasks and examinations. It is thought, by some authorities, that during this time women are more likely to commit crimes, have accidents, attempt suicide and require psychiatric treatment.

The aetiology of PMS is not fully understood, but current theories include:
• Reduced progesterone in the secretory phase.
• Elevated prolactin levels.
• A deficiency of pyridoxine (vitamin B$_6$).
• Some, as yet unknown ovarian factor.
With such a diversity of presentation and possible causes, the management of PMS needs to be considered on an individual basis, for what offers relief for one woman will be totally ineffective in another. Treatment regimens may include the administration of natural progesterone or synthetic progestogens. Pyridoxine may relieve PMS by its action on tryptophan (an amino acid), a

precursor of 5-hydroxytryptamine – a neurotransmitter concerned with mood regulation. The use of pyridoxine supplements may also be helpful in reducing high prolactin levels. Diuretics (see Chapter 15) can be prescribed to reduce oedema, as may reducing sodium intake. Essential fatty acids, such as gamma-linoleic acid (GLA) found in the oil of the evening primrose, may relieve some PMS symptoms. NB GLA is needed for the synthesis of prostaglandins.

General measures such as simple analgesia, distraction, exercise and a 'healthy' diet may all help women with PMS. Kirkpatrick et al. (1990) found that self-care measures, especially those related to nutrition and exercise, could be helpful. Women who are informed about and understand what is happening each month can gain considerable benefit from open discussion with their partner or family, or within a self-help group.

Healthier Living **Toxic shock syndrome**

Toxic shock syndrome (TSS) is a potential complication where tampons are used for sanitary protection, but it can affect men and non-menstruating women. It occurs very rarely and is caused by toxins produced by the bacterium *Staphylococcus aureus*. The micro-organism is found at various sites, including the perineal area, in healthy people. Bacteria can be transferred, by the hands, to the tampon, which, when inserted into the vagina, provides an excellent medium for bacterial growth. Toxins entering the blood produce a condition characterized by pyrexia, vomiting and diarrhoea, rash, and possibly life-threatening hypovolaemic shock. Measures aimed at preventing TSS during menstruation include: hand hygiene before and after tampon use; using tampons of the lowest absorbency for the amount of loss; changing tampons every 4 hours; consider using a pad during the night; reporting illness occurring during menstruation; and last, but certainly not least, remembering to remove a tampon at the end of a period. Women who have previously had TSS are advised to use sanitary pads rather than tampons.

Reproductive Physiology

After our separate considerations of the structure and functioning of the male and female reproductive systems, it is highly appropriate to remind ourselves that neither system functions naturally in isolation. Even with the most sophisticated assisted fertility techniques it still requires the presence of an oocyte and a spermatozoon to produce a new life.

This part of the chapter looks at sexual response, conception, pregnancy and parturition. In addition, we will discuss areas relevant to reproductive function, such as sexually transmitted diseases, contraception and subfertility.

Male sexual response

The male sexual response consists of penile erection, which allows the penis entry into the female tract, and the ejaculation of semen within the vagina. Erection takes place as the erectile tissue in the corpora cavernosa and corpus spongiosum fills with blood (see *Figure 20.5*). Arterioles in the erectile tissue are normally constricted and the penis is flaccid, but during sexual excitement the arterioles dilate and the penis enlarges. These vascular changes occur through a spinal reflex and involve an example of parasympathetic-stimulated vasodilation, which is unusual, and nitric oxide release, which also causes vasodilation. Mucous secretion by the bulbo-urethral glands is also stimulated by parasympathetic fibres. As the penis enlarges the venous return is impeded, which results in further rigidity.

Sexual excitement has a variety of triggers, including visual, auditory and olfactory stimuli, emotions, and direct stimulation of the genitalia, for example of mechanoreceptors in the glans penis.

The erection reflex operates through afferent pathways (pudendal nerve) that synapse in the sacral spinal cord, and the efferent parasympathetic outflow from the S2–S4 segments known as the nervi erigentes (see Chapter 6), which initiates vasodilation. There are also descending spinal pathways from the cerebrum, which can either expedite or prevent the erection reflex; for example, thoughts alone can cause erection without any physical stimulation and anxiety or worry can prevent erection.

Impotence is the failure to achieve or maintain an erection. There are many physical and psychological causes, including excess alcohol, anxiety, certain drugs, vascular disease, nerve damage, e.g. during pelvic surgery, spinal injuries (see Chapter 4), diabetes mellitus (see Chapter 8) and multiple sclerosis (see Chapter 3).

Ejaculation of semen also results from a spinal reflex. It is accompanied by an intensely pleasurable sensation known as orgasm and physiological changes that include increased respiration, blood pressure and heart rate. The afferent pathway involved is the same as that for the erection reflex and when afferent impulses reach a critical point, as stimulation continues, the sympathetic efferents to the genitalia, mainly via L1 and L2, are stimulated. These sympathetic effects include: contraction of smooth muscle in the accessory glands and ducts, which discharge their secretions into the urethra; closure of the internal urinary sphincter to prevent retrograde ejaculation of semen into the bladder or the leakage of urine; and vigorous contraction of the skeletal muscles at the base of the penis to expel semen.

Ejaculation is followed by a period of relaxation, known as the latent period, which varies from minutes to hours, during which further erection is impossible.

Female sexual response

The female sexual response is indicated by engorgement and erection of the clitoris and labia minora. This occurs through the same autonomic pathways as in the male. Vaginal lubrication is provided by the vestibular glands, which increase secretion, and the fluid which 'leaks' through the vaginal walls. There is breast enlargement and nipple erection with possible flushing of the skin of the chest and neck. Females may experience orgasm during coitus and, as there is no

Special Focus **Sexually transmitted diseases (STDs)**

In the wake of massive publicity campaigns concerning AIDS (see Chapter 19) you could be forgiven for forgetting the existence of other STDs. These include: syphilis, gonorrhoea, warts, chlamydia, genital herpes, trichomoniasis and candidiasis. It must be stressed, however, that many of these infections may also occur without sexual contact, e.g. chlamydial infection of an infant's eyes during birth.

It is not intended to explore each disease in depth but rather to concentrate on the effects within the reproductive system. Readers should refer to Further Reading for more specific information about individual infections.

Syphilis

Syphilis is caused by the spirochaete (type of bacterium) *Treponema pallidum*. Infection usually occurs during sexual contact, when the organisms enter through the mucosa of the genitalia, anus or mouth. Syphilis may also be transmitted from mother to fetus via the placenta. The disease has well-defined stages: primary, secondary, tertiary and quaternary. In primary syphilis painless lesions called chancres develop, which may affect the genitalia and other sites, including the anus and mouth. Secondary stage manifestations affecting the genitalia include wart-like condylomata lata on the penis or vulva, an associated lymphadenopathy and occasionally a generalized body rash. The tertiary stage is characterized by skin ulcers called gumma, and quaternary syphilis has effects involving the nervous and cardiovascular systems. Very few new cases of syphilis now occur in the UK.

Gonorrhoea

Gonorrhoea is caused by the bacterium *Neisseria gonorrhoeae*, which, being very fragile, does not survive for long outside the body. It infects the genital tract, urinary tract and the mucosa of the throat and anus. Gonorrhoea infection has profound effects within the reproductive system, which can result in subfertility. Men usually have urethritis, with dysuria and discharge. If untreated, this could lead to inflammation of the duct system with stricture formation; however, the vast majority of infections are treatable. Women may have urinary symptoms, but unfortunately they may remain asymptomatic while severe damage occurs. Some women suffer vaginal discharge, abdominal pain and bleeding. The infection can cause PID, which leads to serious ill health and subfertility if the delicate uterine tubes become blocked. Non-sexual spread may occur, e.g. an infant's eyes infected during birth. New cases of gonorrhoea reported to genito-urinary medicine (GUM) clinics are decreasing in line with the Health of the Nation target (DoH, 1992).

Chlamydia

Chlamydia is an increasingly common STD. It is caused by the organism *Chlamydia trachomatis*, which has both bacterial and viral characteristics. In males it causes urethritis and testicular pain but may be asymptomatic. Women infected with chlamydia may have urethritis, vaginal discharge and irregular menstruation. It is the major cause of PID and can lead to serious eye and respiratory infections in infants exposed to the organism during birth.

Warts

Genital warts caused by HPV is one of the commonest reasons for attendance at GUM clinics. The warts occur on the genitalia and in the anal area. They are uncomfortable, but more importantly infection with the HPV predisposes to cervical cancer (see pages 483–484).

Genital herpes

Genital herpes is most commonly caused by HSV2. The infection results in extremely painful blisters on the genitalia and the virus may infect the eyes. Both sexes become carriers as the virus lies dormant within their tissues, but 'flare-ups' or exacerbations of inflammation occur at intervals. An article by Beardsley (1993) outlines ways in which the spread of genital herpes may be reduced. The herpes virus may cause first trimester miscarriage and serious, possibly fatal, infections and malformations in infants born to infected mothers. Also very worrying is the link between genital herpes and the development of cervical malignancy (see page 483).

Trichomoniasis

Trichomoniasis is caused by the protozoon *Trichomonas vaginalis*. Infected women have a foul, frothy yellow vaginal discharge, vulval soreness and irritation. Men and sometimes women may be asymptomatic carriers of the organism.

Candidiasis

Candidiasis (thrush) is caused by many species of fungi including *Candida albicans*. It causes intense pruritus and a thick creamy vaginal discharge. Although it may be sexually transmitted, candidiasis commonly affects women who are debilitated; where hormones have been modified, following antibiotic therapy; and in diabetes mellitus (see Chapter 8). Candidiasis may cause balanitis (see page 473) in the male.

Bacterial vaginosis

The bacterium *Gardnerella vaginalis* infects the vagina and causes a frothy grey/off-white discharge that smells very offensive. Apart from the distress suffered by individual women, the presence of the bacterium is linked to late miscarriage and preterm delivery.

latent or refractory period, some women experience multiple orgasms. Although female orgasm is not essential for fertilization, the rhythmic uterine contractions that occur may assist the passage of semen into the uterus.

As with the male, orgasm is accompanied by an increase in pulse, respiration and blood pressure.

Conception and fertilization

Conception requires that a spermatozoon reaches and penetrates a secondary oocyte that completes meiosis II prior to the fusion of the two nuclei at fertilization (*Figure 20.21*). Time for fertilization is limited as the gametes have a finite life, after which they deteriorate; the oocyte is viable for about 24 hours and spermatozoa for a longer period of up to 48 hours, but some may still be functional up to 72 hours.

After spermatozoa are deposited in the vagina during coitus they must make their way through the uterus and into the uterine tube, but they still need changes (see below) to allow them to penetrate the oocyte. Nature has ensured an abundance of spermatozoa, which is just as well because millions are lost on the way – only a few thousand actually reach

the ampulla of the uterine tube. Spermatozoa are motile, but they do have some help – they secrete prostaglandins that cause contraction of the uterus and tubes.

Before spermatozoa can penetrate an oocyte they must undergo the processes of capacitation and acrosome reaction. You will remember that the spermatozoon carries enzymes that it will use to gain access to the oocyte. These proteolytic and other enzymes must remain intact on the journey but need to be available once the spermatozoa have located the oocyte. Capacitation involves structural changes to the acrosome that make the enzymes available for release. Many spermatozoa must release their enzymes by the acrosome reaction to 'break through' the defences (zona pellucida) around the oocyte, but only one will actually latch onto and penetrate the secondary oocyte. There are vital mechanisms involving oocyte membrane depolarization and an increase in intracellular calcium level that prevent the entry of further spermatozoa (polyspermy).

At last, the secondary oocyte that has been wafted into the ampulla, and the spermatozoon, are together. Once penetration by the spermatozoon head has occurred, the secondary oocyte will complete meiosis II to produce the

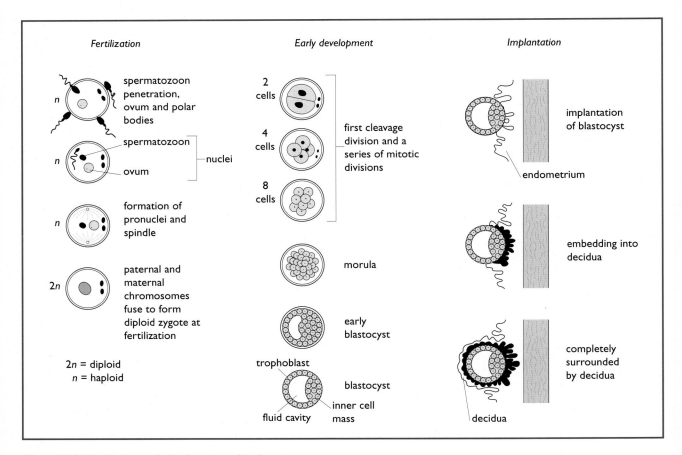

Figure 20.21 Fertilization, early development and implantation.

Special Focus Fertility control and contraception

Over the centuries human beings have devised many ways to control fertility. Some methods, such as wearing a 'magic' charm, were destined to fail, as were more active attempts to prevent the meeting of egg and sperm, e.g. leaping to the vertical position after coitus! The acceptance of fertility control and contraception took a long time – in Great Britain family planning services did not become available until the 1930s and then only for married women. Over the years there have been many developments in methods of contraception, but the only sure way to avoid pregnancy is to abstain from intercourse.

There are numerous methods by which couples may avoid pregnancy; some are highly reliable, such as taking the 'pill', whilst others are nearly as risky as the use of magic charms. Couples should be given sufficient information to allow them to choose the method that best suits them.

Coitus interruptus: this involves the withdrawal of the penis from the vagina before ejaculation occurs. In the absence of research findings, it is probably wise to assume that withdrawal is not reliable because semen may leak from the penis prior to ejaculation.

Natural methods: the fertile period is ascertained by cervical mucus changes (Billing's method), temperature changes (see page 492) or a combination of the two. This requires a high degree of motivation in both partners. Recently a method of ascertaining the timing of ovulation by measuring urine hormone levels has been developed. A test stick is used and then read by a device that indicates whether conception is a risk or not – useful for avoiding pregnancy and for couples hoping to conceive.

Barrier methods:

- Spermicidal chemicals, e.g. nonoxinols, in the form of vaginal foams, gels, pessaries and impregnated film. They are not very effective when used without a vaginal diaphragm, cap or condom.
- Condoms and vaginal diaphragms or caps are reliable when used properly, e.g. use of spermicides with a vaginal diaphragm and applying condoms carefully. Condoms have the additional advantage of reducing the spread of AIDS and other STDs.
- Other barrier methods include use of the female condom (a polyurethane tube that fits inside the vagina). Apart from contraception, the female condom will also reduce the trans-

mission of STDs, but to date it is not widely used.

Intrauterine contraceptive devices (IUCDs): made of polythene with or without copper, they are inserted through the cervix into the uterus. An IUCD or 'coil' probably exerts its contraceptive effect by preventing implantation (see page 498). An IUCD can be used as postcoital contraception if it is inserted within 5 days of unprotected intercourse.

Oral contraception, or 'the pill': this has been, so far, one of the major breakthroughs in fertility control. Either low-dose oestrogen and progesterone combinations, which override the normal hypothalamic–pituitary–ovarian hormonal controls of the ovarian cycle, or a progesterone-only pill can be used. Oral contraceptives act in a variety of ways to prevent pregnancy. The combined oestrogen–progesterone pill produces effects that include: inhibition of FSH-release and failure of follicle maturation; no LH surge or ovulation; possible changes in uterine tube motility (may affect the passage of an oocyte if ovulation does occur); endometrial proliferation inhibited (making implantation unlikely if ovulation occurred); and cervical mucus remains thick and impenetrable to spermatozoa. The progesterone-only pill is less reliable because it does not always inhibit ovulation; its contraceptive effects are achieved mainly by changes to cervical mucus, which remains thick and hostile to the passage of spermatozoa. Progesterone-only pills also affect endometrial proliferation and uterine tube motility. They are taken continuously, at the same time each day (no more than 3 hours late or the effects may be impaired), to provide contraceptive effect.

Taken correctly, the oral contraceptive offers very high reliability and, because the cycles are probably anovulatory, they will be less painful. If all this sounds too good to be true, let us examine the minus points, which include some definite contraindications to use, such as a history of breast cancer, ovarian cancer or thrombo-embolic disorders. There may be side-effects e.g. weight gain, nausea and headache, which are unacceptable to some women. Missed pills, gastrointestinal upsets or drugs such as antibiotics can all reduce the contraceptive effects.

High-dose oestrogen or combined pills can be used as postcoital contraception ('morning after'), but must be commenced within 72 hours of unprotected inter-

course. This type of therapy can be offered, for example, to rape victims or when contraception fails. The anti-progesterone mifepristone (RU486), which is used, with prostaglandins, to terminate pregnancy (as a 'medical' termination) during the first 7 weeks, is also effective if given as a postcoital contraceptive.

Various studies have suggested links between oral contraceptives and the development of breast or cervical malignancy and cardiovascular disease. There may well be a slight increase in the incidence of breast cancer in pill users, but studies have produced conflicting findings. In other studies, women who had taken the combined pill appeared to show an increased incidence of cervical cancer. Most authorities feel that the low oestrogen pills do not increase cardiovascular disease in healthy women, but there have been various 'scares' reported by the media. On the plus side, the combined pill reduces the risk of uterine and ovarian cancer, benign breast disease and PMS.

In the light of rather contradictory evidence it is important to remember that the risks, where they exist, are indeed very small and may well be acceptable to individual women in return for reliable contraception. Also to be noted are the physical risks associated with pregnancy, even in a developed country, plus the emotional and social implications of an unwanted pregnancy.

Hormone-impregnated vaginal rings, progesterone depot injections and subcutaneous progesterone implants are available that provide contraception for from 3 months to 5 years. There are side-effects, and a 'change of mind' means that implants must be removed. Otherwise it is necessary to wait for their contraceptive effects to dissipate before pregnancy is again possible.

A permanent solution for couples wishing to avoid conception is sterilization surgery – vasectomy (see page 471) in the male and tubal ligation in the female. These procedures should be considered to be permanent, although reversal is sometimes possible.

There are several possible developments for future fertility control, which include: inhibition of FSH and LH with continuous GnRH agonists; use of substances such as inhibin to inhibit FSH; and use of anti-progesterones to block the hormones required for successful implantation may be used on a once-a-month basis.

functional ovum and the second polar body. The haploid nuclei of both ovum and spermatozoon enlarge to form the pronuclei. A mitotic spindle forms between the two pronuclei and the maternal and paternal chromosomes combine to form the diploid **zygote** – and the incredible process of fertilization is complete.

Chromosome complement and determination of genetic sex

It is appropriate here to mention chromosomes and the determination of genetic sex (see Chapter 21 for more on chromosomes). Normally the 23 chromosomes – 22 autosomes (a chromosome that is not a sex chromosome) + 1 sex chromosome – from both ovum and spermatozoon, combine to give the zygote 46 chromosomes, or 23 pairs (*Figure 20.22*). Human body (somatic) cells have 22 pairs of autosomes and one pair of sex chromosomes, either XX (female) or XY (male). In females one of the X chromosomes becomes inactivated and appears in the somatic nuclei as a mass known as the Barr body (sex chromatin).

Genetic sex is determined by the spermatozoon, which may carry either the X or Y sex chromosome, whereas the ovum will always carry the X chromosome. An ovum fertilized by an X spermatozoon produces a genetic female, and that fertilized by a Y spermatozoon produces a genetic male (*Figure 20.23*). Remember that inheritance of a sex chromosome only determines genetic sex; it is the presence or not of fetal testosterone that drives genitalia differentiation, and further hormones are required at puberty. Usually more males are born than females, the M:F ratio in the UK currently being around 105:100.

Pre-embryonic development and implantation

The zygote, formed during fertilization, starts to divide by mitosis (cleavage) as it travels through the uterine tube towards the uterus (see *Figure 20.21*). Earlier we mentioned non-identical (dizygotic) twins resulting from the fertilization of two oocytes (see page 489); in contrast, identical (monozygotic) twins result from changes after the fertilization of one oocyte. During early cell division two separate cell masses develop, which are destined to become two individuals who are genetically identical (useful for transplants).

By the time the uterus is reached, 4–5 days after fertilization, a series of cell divisions has resulted in a mass of cells called the morula. The pre-embryo (so called for the first 2 weeks) floats free within the uterine cavity for a further 2 days or so while progressing to the blastocyst stage. The blastocyst consists of a fluid-filled cavity surrounded by an outer layer of trophoblast cells and an inner cell

mass protruding into the cavity. Trophoblast cells will become the placenta and the inner cell mass the embryo and its membrane (amnion). The inner cell mass will form two further cavities, yolk sac and amnion, divided by cells of the embryonic plate/disc (see Chapter 21).

Implantation of the blastocyst into the hormone-prepared endometrium commences about 6 or 7 days after fertilization. The trophoblast layer invades the endometrium, which thickens to become the decidua. After a few days the blastocyst is completely enclosed within the decidua. At this stage the pre-embryo receives nutrients derived from the endometrial cell debris produced by the trophoblastic invasion. The three primary germ layers (ectoderm, mesoderm and endoderm), which will give rise to all body tissues, form as the blastocyst undergoes massive change to become the gastrula. In a process called gastrulation, cell migration prepares the 'plan' for the organism and ensures that cells are in the correct positions when structural development starts.

During these very early days the corpus luteum is maintained by a hormone, human chorionic gonadotrophin (hCG), secreted by the trophoblasts. This is essential to maintain the high levels of progesterone and oestrogen required to prevent menstruation and maintain the pregnancy. The detection of hCG in a woman's blood or urine forms the basis of pregnancy testing. It is possible to obtain a positive test as early as 1–2 weeks after conception, but more reliable results are obtained 6–8 weeks after the last menstrual period (LMP). hCG levels reach their peak about 8–10 weeks after the LMP.

Readers are directed to Chapter 21 for an outline of the embryonic and fetal stages of development and to appropriate chapters for specific organ system formation. We will, however, consider the placenta (although it is both embryonic and maternal), hormones, pregnancy, parturition and lactation.

Placental development and function

The placenta is a temporary structure that forms from the trophoblast layer (embryonic tissue) and the decidua (maternal tissue) (see *Figure 20.24*). Early placental development includes:

- Formation of the chorion, which will become the tough outer membrane surrounding the fetus inside its protective, fluid (liquor amnii)-filled amniotic membrane or 'bag of water'.
- Growth of vascular chorionic villi, from the chorion, into the decidua to form the close contacts with maternal blood vessels required for exchange of substances. Meanwhile the blood vessels are forming in the embryo, which will eventually be linked to the placenta by three blood vessels (one vein and two arteries) that run in the

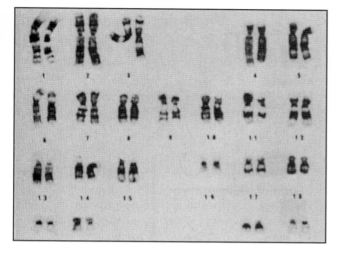

Figure 20.22 Normal chromosomes (male): 22 pairs of autosomes plus one pair of sex chromosomes (XY) = 46 chromosomes. (Baraitser M, Winter R (1990) *A Colour Atlas of Clinical Genetics.* Wolfe Medical Publications, Ltd. Reprinted with permission.)

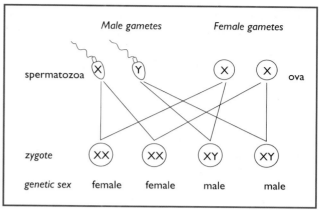

Figure 20.23 Determination of genetic sex.

Abnormal Function **Fertility problems**

Before we continue with our discussion of development it would be helpful to consider some of the obstacles to conception. By now you will be aware of the complexity of reproduction and it will be no surprise to learn that subfertility may be caused by a multitude of factors, including infrequent coitus, impotence (page 494), infrequent or anovulatory cycles, low sperm counts, non-patent uterine tubes following ectopic pregnancy or PID, hostile cervical mucus, and immunological causes where both sexes produce antibodies against spermatozoa (see Chapter 19).

The management of subfertility depends upon the cause, if it can be identified, available resources and the wishes of the couple. Some people will find intimate investigations or treatments unacceptable; for example, postcoital sperm checks near to the time of ovulation require that the couple have intercourse 'to order' and the woman attends the clinic soon after. Couples may have moral objections to treatments using donated semen (artificial insemination-donor AID), and others may feel unable to cope emotionally with seemingly endless visits, treatments and disappointments associated with IVF.

Assisted fertility techniques used to help childless couples are extremely complex and many ideas that challenge established attitudes have been developed, e.g. embryo selection and selective termination. No attempt is made here to consider investigations and only a brief mention of treatments is included. Readers requiring more information are referred to Further Reading.

Management

- Hyperprolactinaemia (increased prolactin in the blood) may be treated with the drug bromocriptine.
- Drugs to stimulate ovulation, e.g. clomiphene 'fertility drug' or gonadotrophins (which may cause multiple ovulation). Treatment for anovulatory cycles is extremely effective, with pregnancy occurring in the vast majority of females.
- Men with low sperm counts may receive gonadotrophins or testosterone.
- Tubal surgery to remove adhesions.
- Artificial insemination using the husband's/partner's semen—may overcome problems with hostile mucus or female anti-sperm antibodies.
- AID, where the male produces few or no spermatozoa or has autoantibod-

ies which inhibit sperm motility.
- Intracytoplasmic sperm injection (ICSI), where a single sperm is injected into an oocyte that is then placed in the uterus, useful for low sperm counts.
- IVF – may be used for low sperm counts, blocked uterine tubes, female anti-sperm antibodies or hostile mucus. In IVF the oocytes collected via a laparoscope are fertilized, using the partner's semen, in the laboratory. Up to three fertilized ova are later introduced into the uterus, with varying degrees of success. Oocytes or spermatozoa may be donated for IVF.
- Gamete intrafallopian transfer (GIFT), a simpler technique used to overcome hostile cervical mucus. Here the oocytes and spermatozoa are mixed together prior to being placed in the uterine tubes. The technique, which is much simpler than IVF, still needs one functional uterine tube.
- Adoption – difficult, with very few small babies available.
- Surrogacy, where another woman agrees to have a baby for an infertile couple – an area for extreme caution with its potentially catastrophic legal, ethical and emotional problems.

umbilical cord. The placenta and vessels start to function within a few weeks and by 10–12 weeks the exchange system between fetus and mother is fully operational. Soon the bag of membranes will completely fill the uterine cavity, with all the chorionic villi concentrated as the placenta.

The placenta forms part of the endocrine unit producing the hormones required to sustain the pregnancy (see page 501). Hormone production by the placenta replaces that of the corpus luteum by 10–12 weeks.

The vessel connection between mother and fetus ensures that oxygen, nutrients and protective antibodies can pass from the maternal blood across the placenta (normally there is no mixing of maternal and fetal blood) into the fetal blood. The low partial pressure of 'second-hand' maternal oxygen in the placenta is overcome by the development of a special fetal haemoglobin (HbF) which has a high oxygen affinity. Fetal waste products, including carbon dioxide, pass in the opposite direction across the placenta into the maternal blood.

Unfortunately agents harmful to the embryo/fetus can also cross the placenta. These include:

- Micro-organisms – viruses, such as rubella, human immunodeficiency virus and cytomegalovirus; bacteria, e.g. causing syphilis (rarely); protozoa, e.g. causing toxoplasmosis. It is important to note that toxoplasmosis, which causes miscarriage and fetal abnormalities such as hydrocephaly, can be detected by a blood test early in pregnancy.
- Drugs, e.g. antibiotics, antithyroid, sedatives and many more. It is important to note all drugs should be avoided around conception (where planned) and during pregnancy, especially in the first trimester (3 months), when organ development occurs – only drugs prescribed by a doctor, who is aware of the pregnancy or its possibility, should be taken.
- Alcohol – may cause fetal alcohol syndrome (FAS).
- Environmental chemicals and chemicals from cigarettes.
- Harmful antibodies such as anti-D (see Chapters 9 and 19).

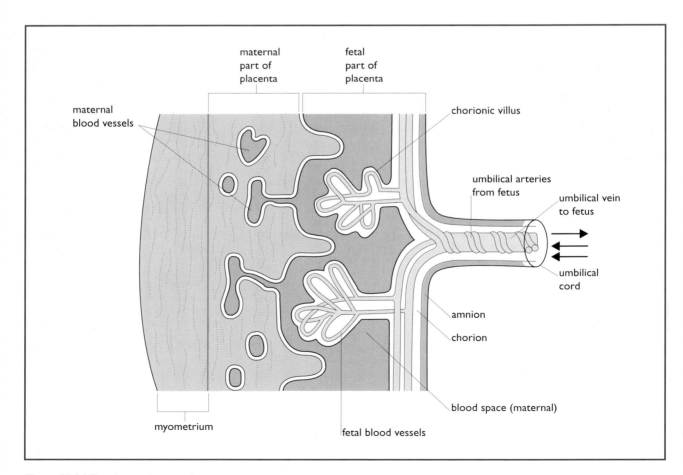

Figure 20.24 The placenta (structure).

Maternal changes during pregnancy

The physical and psychological changes that occur in women during pregnancy may be attributed in part to major structural events, physiological adaptations to the pregnancy or to hormonal effects (see below).

Examples include:

- The uterus grows to fill most of the abdominal cavity and, by term (40 weeks), the fundus has reached the level of the xiphoid process. This enormously enlarged uterus will compress the abdominal structures, causing effects such as 'heartburn', where gastric acid is regurgitated into the oesophagus. Pressure on the bladder causes the frequency and urgency of micturition associated with the last weeks of pregnancy.

- During pregnancy blood volume increases by as much as 40% to cope with the extra demands. The increase necessitates changes in cardiovascular function, including an increased cardiac output.

- Changes in hormone levels have wide-ranging effects on metabolism. The nausea experienced by many women in the first 12 weeks is due to increasing progesterone and oestrogen secretion. Progesterone also reduces peristalsis, which results in constipation. There may be increased skin pigmentation affecting the nose and cheeks (chloasma) and breast areola, and a line from umbilicus to pubis may darken to form the linea nigra. Hormones are also responsible for the mood changes so characteristic of pregnancy; for example, during the later stages women may feel calm and placid.

Although these changes are all part of a normal event, it is important that both woman and fetus are monitored through a programme of antenatal care. This helps to ensure that pregnancy and labour progress normally and that problems are detected early, e.g. glycosuria, hypertension and a fetus who is not growing.

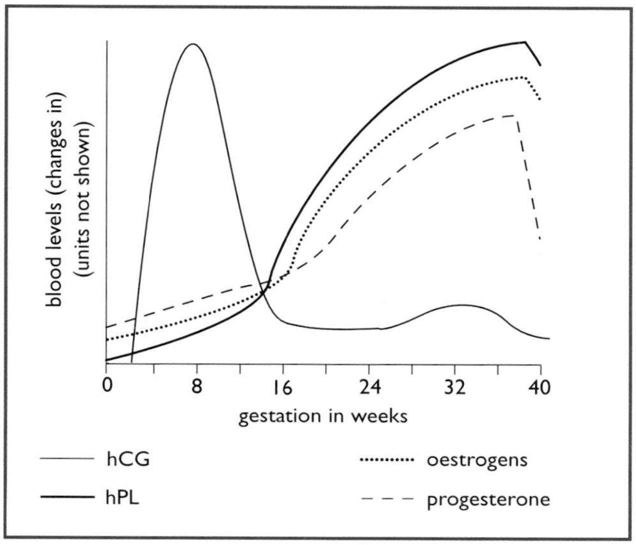

Hormones and pregnancy

Progesterone (Figure 20.25)

Progesterone, produced initially by the corpus luteum and later by the placenta, is essential in sustaining the pregnancy. Its functions include maintenance of the endometrium, inhibition of uterine muscle contraction and helping to prepare the breasts for lactation.

Oestrogens (Figure 20.25)

Oestrogens, which are also produced by the corpus luteum and placenta, are concerned with uterine growth. Development of the breast duct system is stimulated by oestrogens and later in pregnancy oestrogens prepare the myometrium for parturition (see page 502).

Human chorionic gonadotrophin (Figure 20.25)

Human chorionic gondaotrophin (hCG) is initially secreted by the trophoblast cells and later by the chorion. It maintains the corpus luteum and its secretion of progesterone and oestrogens until placental production of these hormones is sufficiently advanced. The level of hCG peaks at around 8–10 weeks, after which it declines suddenly to a low level which persists throughout the pregnancy. The presence of hCG in blood or urine is used to confirm pregnancy (see page 498).

Human placental lactogen (Figure 20.25)

Human placental lactogen (hPL) (or human chorionic somatomammotrophin – hCS), also produced by the placenta, stimulates growth and metabolism of carbohydrates and fat, which liberates glucose for fetal use. It is also involved with breast preparation for lactation.

Oxytocin

Oxytocin, secreted by the posterior pituitary, is concerned with parturition (see page 502) and milk 'let down' during lactation (page 503).

Relaxin

Relaxin, produced by the placenta, prepares the pelvis for labour (see page 502).

Many other hormones are also concerned with the changes occurring during pregnancy, including growth hormone and other anterior pituitary hormones, thyroid hormones, corticosteroids and insulin.

Figure 20.25 Hormone changes during pregnancy.

Parturition

Parturition (giving birth) normally occurs after a gestation period lasting some 280 days (40 weeks) from the first day of the last menstrual period (LMP), or 266 days (38 weeks) from conception (when cycles occur every 26–30 days). Most babies arrive within a fortnight either side of the expected date of delivery (EDD).

'Labour' is the term used to describe the processes required for parturition. The cervix dilates and the uterus contracts to expel the infant plus placenta and membranes, and afterwards prevents excess blood loss.

What actually initiates labour is not completely understood, but several hormones are known to be involved and many authorities consider that an increase in fetal cortisol triggers the hormonal changes that cause labour to start. During the last weeks of pregnancy a change in the oestrogen/progesterone ratio appears to have two effects: the inhibitory effect of progesterone on uterine muscle is reduced and the myometrium becomes very sensitive to the posterior pituitary hormone oxytocin, which is known to stimulate myometrial contraction. Prostaglandin synthesis also increases. Women experience irregular contractions, known as Braxton Hicks contractions, as pregnancy nears completion. The hormone relaxin increases flexibility of the pelvic ligaments, which allows for more 'give' as the fetus passes through the pelvis.

The secretion of placental prostaglandins, e.g. $F_{2\alpha}$, and high levels of oxytocin are known to initiate the contractions of 'true labour'. As labour progresses its momentum increases through a positive feedback loop operating as the fetus moves down to exert pressure on the cervix. Cervical pressure receptors transmit impulses that cause oxytocin release, which in turn increases the rate and intensity of uterine muscle contractions. This pushes the fetus down still further to exert more pressure on the cervix, which gradually dilates.

Both oxytocin and prostaglandins can be used to stimulate labour or terminate pregnancy. The use of antiprostaglandin drugs to inhibit premature labour can be taken as further evidence that prostaglandins are involved in labour.

Labour is divided into three stages (see Family-centred Study):

- First stage, which involves cervical dilatation.
- Second stage, during which the fetus is expelled by powerful contractions.
- Third stage, when the placenta and membranes are expelled.

Puerperium

The puerperium is the 6–8 weeks period following childbirth, during which the reproductive structures involute

---

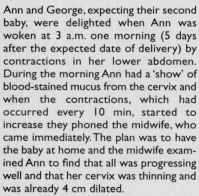

Family-centred Study **Ann, George and Harvey**

Ann and George, expecting their second baby, were delighted when Ann was woken at 3 a.m. one morning (5 days after the expected date of delivery) by contractions in her lower abdomen. During the morning Ann had a 'show' of blood-stained mucus from the cervix and when the contractions, which had occurred every 10 min, started to increase they phoned the midwife, who came immediately. The plan was to have the baby at home and the midwife examined Ann to find that all was progressing well and that her cervix was thinning and was already 4 cm dilated.

Ann started using transcutaneous electrical nerve stimulation (TENS) during contractions (see Chapter 4) and because she was getting good pain relief did not feel that she needed any other analgesia. The midwife, after checking with Ann and George about any last-minute preparations and answering their questions, arranged cover for her other

work, informed the family doctor and arranged for a colleague to join her. Ann, who had formed a good relationship with the community midwives during the pregnancy, felt confident and relaxed.

By 1 p.m. the contractions were coming every 3 min and Ann could feel that they were getting stronger. Although Ann was still coping well with the contractions she now had backache, which was causing some distress. Another examination revealed that the cervix was 8 cm dilated; Ann and George were delighted that the progress was so good. Ann started inhalation analgesia (nitrous oxide + oxygen) while George rubbed her back. At 3.30 p.m. the amniotic membranes ruptured, releasing the fluid, and Ann had a strong urge to 'bear down'. A quick examination revealed that the cervix was fully dilated and that the second stage had started.

The contractions were occurring every 2 min and Ann was pushing with

good effect. By 4.00 p.m. George and the midwives could see the baby's head. This was a great boost to Ann, who was working very hard. At 4.20 p.m. the baby – a boy (Harvey) – was born, who cried (and breathed) at once. The umbilical cord was clamped and cut while Ann and George had a good look at their son, who appeared quite 'perfect'.

Ann was given an injection of ergometrine and oxytocin to contract the uterus and the third stage was completed by 4.40 p.m. The midwife confirmed that Ann's uterus was contracted and that there was no bleeding, and then checked that the placenta and membranes (amnion and chorion) were complete (retained placental tissue could cause infection and haemorrhage). While all the checks and care were being completed George went to fetch their daughter Kay, who had been collected from school by neighbours, so that she could meet her brother.

(return to the non-pregnant state). Structural and physiological changes occur, which include:

- The uterus returns to normal size (it is slightly bigger after childbirth) and position through enzymic autolysis (self-digestion). The progress of this can be assessed by ascertaining the position of the uterine fundus (fundal height). Blood, cell debris and other waste form the vaginal discharge, called the lochia, which may continue for up to 6 weeks. Initially the lochia is red (lochia. rubra), but as less blood is lost from the placental site the discharge becomes pink (l. serosa) and then white (l. alba), and the quantity is much reduced. The process is aided by the release of oxytocin during breast feeding (see below). Menstrual cycles usually return within 8–12 weeks, but may be delayed if lactation is established.
- The pelvic floor, perineum and uterine supports regain tone. This will be accelerated by pelvic floor exercises (see page 484 and Chapter 18). An episiotomy or tear, however, will need time to heal (see page 486 and Chapter 19).
- Breast changes will depend on whether lactation is established and for how long.

Lactation

During pregnancy the secretion of hormones causes breast enlargement and development of the glandular secreting tissue and duct system. Late in pregnancy the breasts are already secreting a fluid called colostrum, which continues during the 2–3 days following parturition.

Colostrum secretion is initiated by the hormones hPL (see page 501) and prolactin from the anterior pituitary (see *Figure 20.26*). Prolactin release, which increases from early pregnancy, may be due to the suppression of prolactin-inhibiting hormone or the presence of a hypothalamic releasing hormone (see Chapter 8). The colostrum, which is replaced by 'true' milk after 3 days, contains more protein, minerals and vitamins but less lactose and fat, than milk. Although prolactin starts off milk secretion, it is the sucking by the infant that ensures continuity of supply. As the infant sucks, it initiates release of prolactin, which in turns stimulates the production of milk for the next feed. Without the stimulation of sucking, prolactin levels fall and lactation is not established.

So far we have only discussed milk secretion; another hormone, oxytocin, is required for milk ejection, or the 'let down' reflex (see *Figure 20.26*). Oxytocin release, which is also stimulated by the infant sucking, causes contraction of myoepithelial cells that surround the glandular tissue and milk is ejected. The release of oxytocin also causes uterine contraction, which helps the uterus to involute (return to the non-pregnant state); this explains the abdominal 'cramps' felt by some women at the start of breast-feeding.

Both colostrum and milk contain immunoglobulins (IgA) that help to prevent gastrointestinal infections in the infant (see Chapter 19). Breast milk contains water, lactose, proteins, fats, minerals and vitamins in a form that the infant can most easily absorb and use.

During full lactation the prolactin levels are usually sufficient to prevent the return of ovarian cycles and menstruation, probably through inhibition of GnRH release by other hormones released in response to the stimulus of suckling. It is, however, unwise to rely upon this as contraception because ovulation can certainly occur during lactation.

Nursing Practice Application Postnatal mental health

Imagine for a moment a couple delighted with their new baby and then, for no apparent reason, the new mother is irritable, crying, tired and cannot manage. A shock for all concerned, but many women experience some mood changes in the days immediately after giving birth – they move from the euphoria felt at the end of labour to feeling 'weepy' and unsure about being able to cope with the demands of this dependent and entirely selfish new human. These are the so-called 'baby blues' that start around the third day and last for a few days. The changes in progesterone and oestrogen levels may be contributing factors. These feelings usually resolve quickly, but women and their families need explanations and support.

Much more severe is the disabling postnatal depression that occurs during the puerperium and which may last for months. Midwives and health visitors need to be alert to the possibility of postnatal depression when women exhibit signs of depression, guilt, fears and anxiety about the infant and a general lack of interest. Support, reassurance and acceptance from professionals and family can do much to help, but antidepressant drugs may be needed.

Very rarely a psychotic illness, known as puerperal psychosis, occurs soon after childbirth. It usually presents as an affective disorder or schizophrenic event. The new mother cannot relate to the infant and in extreme cases may seek to harm herself and the baby. Treatment usually requires admission to a specialist psychiatric unit where, hopefully, mother and baby can be together. Other members of the family will need considerable emotional and practical support.

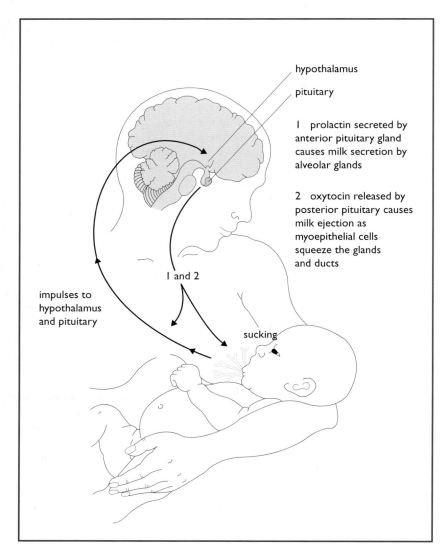

Figure 20.26 Lactation – milk secretion and 'let down'.

hypothalamus

pituitary

1 prolactin secreted by anterior pituitary gland causes milk secretion by alveolar glands

2 oxytocin released by posterior pituitary causes milk ejection as myoepithelial cells squeeze the glands and ducts

I and 2

impulses to hypothalamus and pituitary

sucking

Summary/Check List

Introduction. Early development.
Male reproductive system – structure. Testes. Nursing Practice Application: testicular tumours – screening and early detection. Duct system. Accessory glands. Special Focus – prostatic problems. Penis. Nursing Practice Application – phimosis/paraphimosis. Functioning – meiosis. Spermatogenesis. Semen. Hormonal control, testosterone.
Female reproductive system – structure, ovaries. Person-centred Study – Lucy. Uterine tubes. Uterus, CIN/cervical cancer, Nursing Practice Application – cervical screening. Uterine supports. Vagina. Vulva. Nursing Practice Application – episiotomy/perineal laceration. Mammary glands. Person-centred study – Lucy (continued). Breast cancer. Functioning –

oogenesis. Ovarian cycle and hormonal control. Female steroid hormones. Menstrual cycle. Nursing Practice Application – learning disability and the menstrual cycle. Healthier Living – toxic shock syndrome. Nursing Practice Application – PMS.
Reproductive physiology – sexual response. Special Focus – STD. Special Focus – contraception. Conception/fertilization. Chromosome complement and determination of genetic sex. Subfertility. Pre-embryonic development and implantation. Placental development and function. Maternal changes during pregnancy – hormones and pregnancy. Parturition – labour. Family-centred Study – Ann, George and Harvey. Puerperium, Nursing Practice Application – postnatal mental health. Lactation.

Self Test

1   Which of the following statements are true?
    (a) The testes function best at body temperature.
    (b) The epididymis is continuous with the vas deferens.
    (c) Most of the fluid part of semen is produced by the prostate gland.
    (d) The male urethra conveys both urine and semen.

2   Discuss ways in which spermatogenesis differs from oogenesis.

3   Complete the following:
    (a) Spermatogenesis occurs in the _ _ _ _ _ _ _ _ _ _ _ \ _ _ _ _ _ _ _ .
    (b) A mature spermatozoon has a _ _ _ _ , _ _ _ _ _ _ _ _ and _ _ _ _ .
    (c) Enzymes are carried in the _ _ _ _ _ _ _ _ of the spermatozoon.
    (d) The gonadotrophins _ _ _ and _ _ stimulate spermatogenesis and the release of the male hormone _ _ _ _ _ _ _ _ _ _ _ _ .

4   Which of the following are part of the internal female genitalia and which are external genitalia?
    (a) uterus;
    (b) ovary;
    (c) fourchette;
    (d) fimbriae;
    (e) cornua;
    (f) ovary;
    (g) clitoris;
    (h) external os;
    (i) labia minora;
    (j) Bartholin's glands;
    (k) endometrium;
    (l) mons pubis.

5   Describe the events of oogenesis.

6   Put the following in the correct chronological order:
    (a) primary follicle;
    (b) corpus luteum;
    (c) primordial follicle;
    (d) corpus albicans;
    (e) Graafian follicle;
    (f) maturing/secondary follicle.

7   Describe the phases of the menstrual cycle and the endometrial changes that occur.

8   Which of the following statements are true?
    (a) Fertilization occurs in the ampulla.
    (b) The zygote formed at fertilization is haploid.
    (c) Implantation occurs 6–7 days after fertilization.

9   Put the following in their correct pairs:
    (a) prostaglandins and oxytocin;
    (b) pregnancy testing;
    (c) progesterone;
    (d) initiation of labour;
    (e) hCG;
    (f) longest stage of labour;
    (g) cervical dilatation
    (h) inhibition of uterine contraction.

10 What answers would you give to the following questions asked by Jane, who is breast feeding her first baby aged 2 days?
    (a) Why do I have 'crampy' abdominal pains while breast feeding.
    (b) How does colostrum differ from real milk?
    (c) Why is the baby sucking so important to milk production?
    (d) Is it true that I cannot get pregnant during lactation?

Answers

1   b, d.
2   See pages 487–488.
3   (a) Seminiferous tubules;
    (b) head, midpiece and tail;
    (c) acrosome;
    (d) FSH, LH, testosterone.
4   Internal – a, b, d, e, f, h, k; external – c, g, i, j, l.

5   See pages 487–488.
6   c, a, f, e, b, d.
7   See page 491.
8   a, c.
9   a–d, c–h, e–b and g–f.
10 See page 503.

References

Beardsley J (1993) Education to undermine a taboo. Understanding herpes simplex virus. *Prof Nurse* **8** (5): 322–328.

Cancer Research Campaign (1991) *Be Breast Aware*. Oxford: Cancer Research Campaign.

Dalton K (1980) Cyclical criminal acts in premenstrual syndrome. *Lancet* **ii:** 1070–1071.

DoH (1992) *The Health of the Nation*. Summary. London: HMSO.

Gould D (1990) *Nursing Care of Women*. London: Prentice-Hall.

Health Education Authority (HEA) (1993) *Cancer: How To Reduce Your Risks*. London: HEA.

Hiscock E, Reece G (1988) Cytological screening for cervical cancer and human papillomavirus in general practice. *BMJ* **297**: 724–726.

Kirkpatrick MK, Brewer JA, Stocks B (1990) Efficacy of self-care measures for premenstrual syndrome (PMS). *J Adv Nurs* **15**(3):281–285.

Lehtinen M, Dillner J, Knekt P, Luostarinen, T *et al.* (1996) Serologically diagnosed infection with human papillomavirus type 16 and risk of subsequent development of cervical carcinoma: nested case-control study. *BMJ* **312**: 337–339.

Paolozzi H (1994) Looking after your kit. *Nurs Times* **90** (5): 30–31.

Slevin E (1996) Causation of problematic behaviour in people with learning disabilities I. *Br J Nurs* **5**(9): 546–550.

Thornhill JA, Conroy RM, Kelly DG *et al.* (1986) Public awareness of testicular cancer and the value of self examination. *BMJ* **293**: 480–481.

Further Reading

Adler MW (1990) *ABC of Sexually Transmitted Diseases*, 2nd edn. London: British Medical Journal publications.

Edwards RG, Steptoe PC (1980) *A Matter of Life*. London: Hutchinson.

England MA (1983) *A Colour Atlas of Life Before Birth – Normal Fetal Development*. London: Wolfe Medical Publications Limited.

Ellerby K (1997) Contraception and safer sex. *Practice Nursing* **8**(8): 16–19.

Fullerton D (1997) A review of approaches to teenage pregnancy. *Nurs Times* **93**(13):48–49.

Gould D (1997) Ectopic pregnancy: causes and outcomes. *Nurs Times* **93**(14):53–55.

Lewis S, Bor R (1994) Nurses' knowledge of and attitudes towards sexuality and the relationship of these with nursing practice. *J Adv Nurs* **20**(2): 251–259.

Masters WH, Johnson VE (1966) *Human Sexual Response*. Boston: Little, Brown and Company.

O'Brien PMS (1987) *Premenstrual Syndrome*. Oxford: Blackwell Scientific Publications.

Warnock M (1985) *A Question of Life – The Warnock Report on Human Fertilization and Embryology*. Oxford: Basil Blackwell Limited.

Webb C, Ed (1994) *Living Sexuality (Issues for Nursing and Health)*. Harrow: Scutari Press.

Winston RML (1986) *Infertility: A Sympathetic Approach*. London: Martin Dunitz.

Basic Genetics, Development and Growth – Embryo to Older Adult

Overview

- *Basic genetics.*
- *Development – embryo to older adult.*

Learning Outcomes

After studying Chapter 21 you should be able to:

- Describe normal chromosomes.
- Outline some common chromosomal problems.
- Define gene, allele, genotype and phenotype.
- Outline how genetic variation occurs.
- Describe types of inheritance.
- Outline major events of embryonic and fetal development.
- Discuss how the fetal circulation is adapted for intrauterine life and the changes occurring at birth.
- Describe the characteristics of a mature newborn.
- Outline growth and development during infancy and childhood.
- Describe the events of puberty.
- Outline developmental events of adulthood and mid-life.
- Describe the climacteric.
- Outline current theories of biological ageing.
- Describe the physiological changes of normal ageing.
- Discuss death and dying.

Key Words

Allele (allelomorph) – one of two matched genes that occupy the same site (locus) on homologous chromosomes. They code for inherited characteristics or traits.

Autosome – a non-sex chromosome. In human somatic (body) cells there are 44 autosomes arranged in 22 pairs. The gametes contain 22 autosomes.

Chromosomes – genetic material present in the cell nucleus. They consist of strands of DNA molecules known as genes. Human cells normally contain 46 chromosomes, except gametes which have 23.

Climacteric – the time during which changes in the female result in the decline and eventual cessation of reproductive function.

Development – the process of maturation. An increase in complexity, differentiation and skills.

Embryo – the early developmental stage which commences two weeks after fertilization and lasts until the end of the eighth week of gestation.

Fetus – the developmental stage from the ninth week of gestation until birth.

Gene – the hereditary factors present on for the chromosomes. They consist of DNA and code for a characteristic, or for the precise replication of proteins.

Heterozygous – where the paired alleles (genes) for a particular characteristic or trait are different.

Homozygous – where the paired alleles (genes) for a

Key Words cont.

particular characteristic or trait are the same.
Menarche – the commencement of menstruation. An event occurring during puberty.
Menopause – the cessation of menstruation. An event occurring during the climacteric.
Puberty – the period during which reproductive structures

become functional and the secondary sexual characteristics develop.
Sex chromosomes – the chromosomes (X and Y) that determine genetic sex. One sex chromosome is inherited from each parent. An individual has one pair of sex chromosomes – XX in females and XY in males.

Introduction

At last the end is in sight. Chapter 21 considers how characteristics are inherited and outlines developmental progress from **embryo** to older adult. Although we concentrate on genetic inheritance of characteristics, it is important that you remember the environmental influences on **development** ('nature versus nurture'); for example, malnourished children will not grow properly even with the genes for 'tallness'. The aim is to give an overview of the 'grand plan' that makes us unique and the significant physical events occurring during life. You might like to compare this with Chapter 1, which charts the 'building' of a complete human organism from organic molecules through cells and tissues to the organs and functional systems that maintain homeostasis.

Our story of development starts 2 weeks after fertilization (see Chapter 20) and details of organ system formation can be found in appropriate chapters.

Introduction to Genetics

Genetics is the science of heredity that concerns itself with the study of how traits and characteristics, such as eye colour and blood group, are transmitted from parent to offspring.

Chromosomes

Chromosomes carry the genetic material present in the cell nucleus. They are formed from much-folded chromatin, which consists of double-stranded DNA molecules surrounding proteins called histones. Specific DNA nucleotide sequences on the chromosomes form the individual genes (see page 509). Human cells are diploid ($2n$) and normally contain 46 chromosomes, except the gametes, which are haploid (n) with 23. The 46 chromosomes of somatic cells are arranged in 23 pairs of homologous chromosomes, of which 22 pairs are **autosomes**

Abnormal Function **Problems with chromosomes**

Sometimes the complex meiotic divisions of gametogenesis (see Chapter 20) go wrong and the resultant zygote has a chromosomal error of number or structure, e.g. deletion or translocation of segments. Many errors are incompatible with development and the zygote is lost, but sometimes infants with the wrong number or a chromosomal structural defect are born, e.g. Down syndrome, where infants have 47 chromosomes – because there are

three chromosomes in 'pair 21', this disorder is also called trisomy 21. The only error with 45 chromosomes (monosomy) that is compatible with life is Turner's syndrome, where a female infant has only one X chromosome (XO). Both Down and Turner's syndromes are attributed to non-disjunction, where chromosomes do not separate properly during meiosis (Chapter 20) – one gamete has 24 chromosomes and the other only 22.

Some errors produce abnormalities so severe that the infant is unable to survive, whereas others produce a range of anomalies dependent upon the chromosome affected. The aetiology is not always known, but one theory is the long resting stage of oogenesis; it is possible that agents, e.g. radiation and viruses, affect the oocyte during its wait for maturation.

Nursing Practice Application **Down syndrome**

The incidence of Down syndrome due to non-disjunction increases with maternal age, which supports the 'long resting stage' theory. Down syndrome is the most common autosomal abnormality, with an overall incidence of about 1 in 700 live births. Women over 35 years show an increased risk and by age 45 years the risk is 1 in 50. A much rarer type occurs when chromosome segment translocation occurs between chromosomes 13–15 and 21–22. This results from a genetic carrier state, e.g. a translocation error between chromosomes 14 and 21 occurring at any parental/maternal age.

Down syndrome babies have a typical appearance – low set ears, slanted eyes (with epicanthic folds) and broad hands with a single palmar crease (see Chapter 19). Congenital abnormalities, e.g. heart defects, are more common (see Chapter 10) and they tend to have short adult stature. Some degree of learning disability is usually present, but many people gain employment and live independently. Prenatal testing for Down syndrome is discussed on page 513.

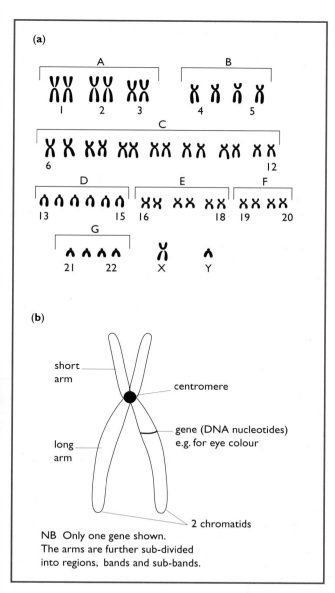

(a)

(b)

short arm

centromere

gene (DNA nucleotides) e.g. for eye colour

long arm

2 chromatids

NB Only one gene shown. The arms are further sub-divided into regions, bands and sub-bands.

Figure 21.1 Chromosomes. (**a**) Karyotype – normal chromosome structure and numbers (male); (**b**) chromosome (2 chromatids) detail.

(non-sex chromosomes) and one pair constitute the **sex chromosomes**. One half of a homologous pair is inherited from the oocyte (maternal) and the other from the spermatozoon (paternal), which you will remember only have 23 chromosomes each.

A diagrammatic representation (karyotype, *Figure 21.1*) of a set of chromosomes arranges the homologous autosome pairs in groups A–G plus the sex chromosomes, XX (female) or XY (male).

Genetic material is only visible as chromosomes just before cell division by mitosis (see Chapter 1) or meiosis (see Chapter 20); at other times it exists as a network of chromatin threads.

Genes

Genes are the hereditary factors present on the chromosomes (*Figure 21.1*). Consisting of DNA nucleotides, they code for a characteristic, or for the precise replication of proteins (see Chapter 1). With the complexity of the human organism in mind it is easy to see why thousands of genes are packed into each chromosome.

The matched pair, of genes (one from each parent) sited at the same locus (site) on homologous chromosomes are called **alleles** (**allelomorphs**). Both alleles code for an inherited trait, either the same or in its alternative form. Allele interaction determines which form is expressed physically. If the alleles are the same the individual is described as being **homozygous** for the trait controlled by that **gene**, but if the alleles are different they are said to be **heterozygous**.

The gene collection of an individual is termed the genotype; however, not every gene will express itself in a physical trait. The physical traits, e.g. hair colour, which result from your unique collection of genes is called your phenotype. Remember that genotype and hence phenotype will be the same in identical twins – which is why people cannot tell them apart.

Genetic variation

Being unique depends upon an ability to create gametes of infinite genetic variability. This is achieved by processes occurring during meiosis I – the formation of 'crossover' points (chiasmata) between chromatids (2 strands of the chromosome) allows the exchange of genetic material between homologous chromosomes (see chapter 20). The subsequent segregation and independent assortment of the paternal and maternal chromosomes that end up in the haploid cells results in the 'never to be repeated' gametes with their unique genetic mix at the end of meiosis II. Maintaining genetic variability is a good reason for not marrying your first cousin as any children would have an increased risk for genetic disease – with grandparents and too many genes in common.

Inheritance patterns

The inheritance of a particular trait depends on: the frequency with which the alleles occur in a population; whether the person is homozygous or heterozygous for the trait; and whether the allele is dominant, depicted by an uppercase letter, or recessive, with the corresponding lowercase letter (see below).

Dominant and recessive genes

Dominant genes are expressed in both the homozygous and heterozygous condition (dominance over the recessive gene – only one is needed), but recessive genes are only expressed in the homozygous state (two needed). We can illustrate this with the inheritance of a dominant trait such as freckles. The dominant allele is (F) and recessive allele is (f). A person will have freckles if they inherit FF (homozygous) or Ff (heterozygous), but will need to be ff (homozygous) to escape freckles (*Figure 21.2*).

Diseases caused by dominant genes include Huntington's disease (see Chapter 4) and achondroplasia (see Chapter 16). Individuals who are heterozygous (being homozygous results in fetal death) for the faulty gene will have the disease, and if they have children there is a 1-in-2 chance of transmitting the disease.

There are, however, traits where dominant genes are not always fully expressed (incomplete dominance). Examples of these are the haemoglobinopathies (see Chapter 9). There is a 'halfway' state where individuals who are heterozygous for the faulty gene have a milder form of the disease.

Recessive genes are responsible for physical characteristics, e.g. having the correct number of digits. They also cause diseases that include phenylketonuria (see Chapter 13) and cystic fibrosis (see Chapter 12). The important point with recessive diseases is that healthy people may be carriers of the gene and if they meet up with another healthy carrier their children have a one in four chance of having the disease (see earlier – first cousin or other consanguineous unions and *Figure 21.2*).

Table 21.1 gives further examples of dominant and recessive traits.

Single, multiple allele and polygene inheritance

Sometimes inheritance is simple, involving a single gene pair, e.g. freckles, but it may involve multiple alleles at the same locus, e.g. ABO blood groups. Inheritance can also be very complex, with the interaction of many genes (polygene), e.g. eye colour and height (remember height also has environmental determinants).

Sex-linked inheritance

The inheritance patterns discussed so far have involved autosomal genes. There are many non-sexual traits and recessive conditions coded by sex chromosome genes that are said to be sex-linked.

Interestingly, the male Y chromosome has fewer genes than the female X chromosome – unlike the autosomes they are not homologous. Apart from the vital gene (sex-determining region Y – SRY) that produces the factor causing development of embryonic testes, the only trait known to be coded by Y chromosome genes is hairy ear lobes, transmitted from father to son (Holandric inheritance).

The X chromosome is more significant and carries genes that code for colour vision and blood clotting factors. If a male inherits a faulty recessive gene via the X chromosome from his mother (healthy carrier) he will have the sex-linked condition – with only one X chromosome he has no allele pair to counter the recessive gene, which is expressed in the heterozygous state.

Sex-linked conditions include fragile X syndrome (learning disability), red–green colour blindness (see Chapter 7), haemophilia (see Chapter 9) and Duchenne-type muscular dystrophy (see Chapter 17).

Theoretically, females pass the recessive gene to 50% of their sons, and 50% of their daughters will be carriers. Females only have sex-linked conditions if a female carrier has a daughter with an affected male.

Other forms of inheritance

Genetic material is also present in cell organelles – it is not exclusive to the nucleus. Mitochondria have circular chromosomes (coding for metabolic activity) that can also be responsible for the inheritance of conditions via the oocyte (only the oocyte contributes cytoplasm to the zygote), e.g. optic nerve atrophy.

Sometimes chromosomes altered structurally during gametogenesis may affect the way a particular allele is expressed, but what is interesting is that the outcome

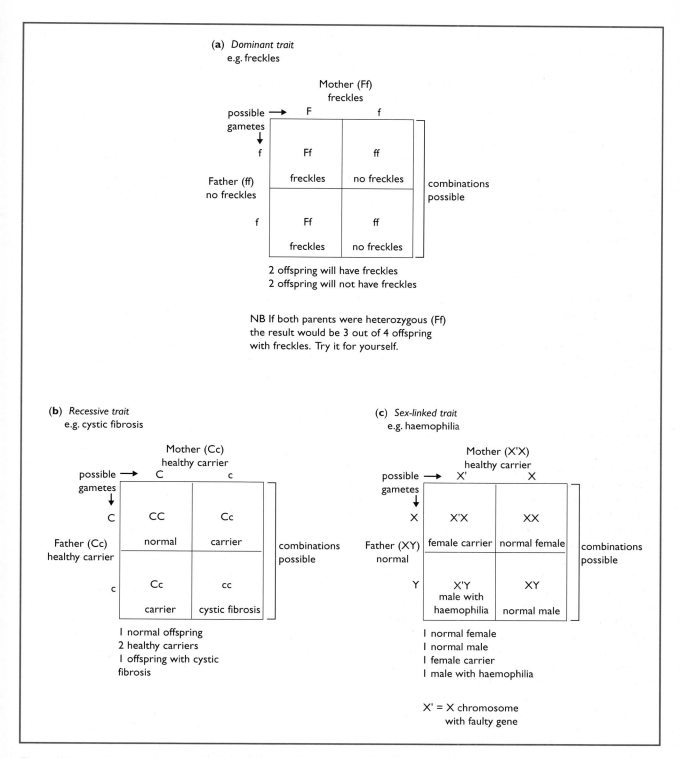

Figure 21.2 Punnett squares showing types of inheritance. **(a)** Dominant trait; **(b)** recessive trait; **(c)** sex-linked trait.

Table 21.1 Dominant and recessive traits and diseases
Dominant traits and diseases (expressed in homozygous and heterozygous states)
A. Autosomal Freckles Polydactyly (extra digits) Abnormal vision – long sight, astigmatism Normal pigments – skin, hair, etc. Achondroplasia (fetal death in homozygous state) Huntington's disease Brachydactyly (short fingers) Normal phenylalanine metabolism Normal production of mucus Normal brain lipid metabolism
B. Sex-linked (X chromosome) Normal blood clotting Normal colour vision Normal muscle metabolism
Recessive traits and diseases (expressed in homozygous state)
A. Autosomal No freckles Normal number of digits Normal vision Abnormal pigmentation – Albinism Normal growth of bone/cartilage Normal basal nuclei (no Huntington's disease) Fingers of normal length Phenylketonuria Cystic fibrosis Tay–Sachs disease
B. Sex-linked (X chromosome) Haemophilia Red–green colour blindness Duchenne-type muscular dystrophy   These X-linked diseases are expressed in the male because there is no normal X chromosome to counter the faulty gene. A female would need two faulty genes to have the disease.

Table 21.1 Dominant and recessive traits and diseases.

depends on whether the chromosome is paternal or maternal. This inheritance is called genetic imprinting and results in two distinct conditions that arise from the same mutation; for example, chromosome 15 change can result in Prader–Willi syndrome (learning disability, short stature and obesity) if inherited via paternal chromosomes and Angleman syndrome (severe learning disability, poor muscle tone and ataxia) when the chromosome is maternal.

Early Days

Life before birth involves three stages: pre-embryonic (see Chapter 20); embryonic, which starts 2 weeks after fertilization up to the end of the eighth week; and fetal, from the ninth week to birth.

Overview of embryonic development

The 2 week embryo has three primary germ layers (the ectoderm, mesoderm and endoderm, which form all tissues – see *Table 21.2*) and soon organogenesis (organ formation) will commence as the disc-like embryonic plate/disc elongates and curves, and the notochord (axial stiffener) forms from mesoderm (see *Figure 21.3*). It is during these early days/weeks that the embryo is vulnerable to agents, e.g. viruses and drugs, that cause malformations.

Soon the neural plate and crests will form the neural tube and nervous system development moves ahead (see Chapter 4). The body cavities are forming, as are the primitive organ systems, which soon start to function, e.g. the heart by the fourth week (see Chapter 10). The skin, skeletal muscle, ribs and vertebrae form from paired mesodermal segments called somites, which develop either side of the neural tube.

Special Focus **Screening for genetic problems and prenatal abnormalities**

Genetic screening (blood test or pedigree) for carrier status for some conditions is now possible, e.g. cystic fibrosis. This knowledge allows couples to make choices about reproduction, but can cause anxiety and depression. It is essential that adequate counselling accompanies any genetic testing. Readers requiring more information are directed to Further Reading, e.g. Skirton (1995a, b, c).

Investigations during pregnancy can detect some, but not all, prenatal abnormalities. Termination of pregnancy may be an option for couples when serious embryonic/fetal abnormality is diagnosed. Again couples should be offered genetic counselling, where the risk of subsequent pregnancies being similarly affected can be assessed, allowing people to make informed decisions about planning future pregnancies.

Some of the tests

A blood test that measures alpha-fetoprotein, unconjugated oestriol and total human chorionic gonadotrophin (hCG) – the 'Triple test' – in maternal serum is used early in pregnancy to predict the estimated risk of conditions such as Down syndrome and neural tube defects. For example, a reduced alpha-fetoprotein and oestriol with an elevated hCG would indicate an increased risk for Down syndrome. This test is a crude screening of risk which is calculated in conjunction with age, gestation and weight; where the risk prediction is 1 in 250 the couple are offered more specific tests (see below). A word of caution – the test for Down syndrome does produce false positives and negatives, and Gilbert *et al.* (1996) found that women of Asian origin had a significantly higher risk for false positive results (possibly because age is not always known).

A technique called chorionic villus sampling (CVS) is available [see *Figure 21.4(a)*] where samples of fetal tissue are obtained via the cervix for the detection of genetic abnormalities during early pregnancy (around 11 weeks). This has the great advantage of early and rapid diagnosis, and if necessary a less traumatic early termination. However, an evaluation of CVS (MRC, 1991) showed it to be less safe than amniocentesis (where the miscarriage risk is 1–2%) and its decreased accuracy means that retesting may be required. Another major problem was identified when babies with malformed limbs started to arrive – this was soon linked to CVS timing. Limb reduction was most severe when CVS took place between days 49 and 65, which corresponds to the times of limb development (Firth *et al.* 1994).

Many single gene and chromosome abnormalities can be diagnosed from testing amniotic fluid and fetal cells shed into the amniotic fluid surrounding the fetus. The sample is obtained by amniocentesis, whereby a wide-bore needle is passed into the amniotic sac via the abdominal wall (suitably anaesthetized) [see *Figure 21.4(b)*]. Fetal cells obtained from the fluid are grown and examined for chromosomal abnormalities such as Down syndrome. The amniotic fluid may contain chemical markers for a particular abnormality; for example, the presence of alpha-fetoproteins may indicate neural tube defects (see Chapter 4).

The major disadvantage of amniocentesis is that it is best performed at 16–18 weeks gestation and a further wait for the chromosome tests means that the couple are faced with the possibility of a very late termination. Earlier amniocentesis at 10–14 weeks may be developed as an alternative to CVS (MRC, 1991).

Chromosomal examination can also reveal the sex of the fetus – which is relevant where a history exists of sex-linked genetic conditions such as haemophilia.

Both CVS and amniocentesis are invasive and carry an increased risk of spontaneous miscarriage; this should be explained to the couple. These tests are not routine and are normally offered only to: women in their late 30s; couples with a history of previous fetal abnormality; or couples with a family history of genetic disorders.

Ultrasound scan (USS), a non-invasive technique, is used routinely to check the progress of normal pregnancies and assist in the diagnosis of fetal (Down syndrome and neural tube defects) and placental abnormalities.

By the end of the eighth week the embryo, which originally was only 2 mm long, has grown to 3 cm and the head is huge compared with the body. The organs are in place, the eyes and ears are forming, the limbs and digits are present, bone ossification has started and skeletal muscles are contracting – and all in 6 weeks.

Overview of fetal development

The fetal stage is dominated by spectacular growth and further development and differentiation of the structures formed as an embryo (see *Figure 21.5*). Considerable growth takes place between weeks 9 and 20, and fetal crown to rump (CR) length doubles by week 12 to around 8.5 cm. However, the head, which is very large, grows more slowly and allows the body to 'catch up'.

During the fourth month fine lanugo hair develops to cover the body by week 20 and fatty vernix forms to protect the skin. By week 16 the **fetus** is some 14 cm in length, increasing to 18.5–20 cm at week 20.

During the next 10 weeks the fetus 'plumps out' as fat is deposited under the skin and organ systems mature to the point at which the fetus becomes viable (capable of independent existence). However, those born very early require sophisticated support, with oxygenation (lack of surfactant see Chapter 12), and nutrition and temperature control (see Chapter 19). Fetal CR length continues to increase during this period – to 22–23 cm at week 24 and 28 cm by week 30.

The final 10 weeks sees considerable growth and weight gain, and babies born at 40 weeks, or term (remember it is really 38 weeks because conception occurs 2 weeks after

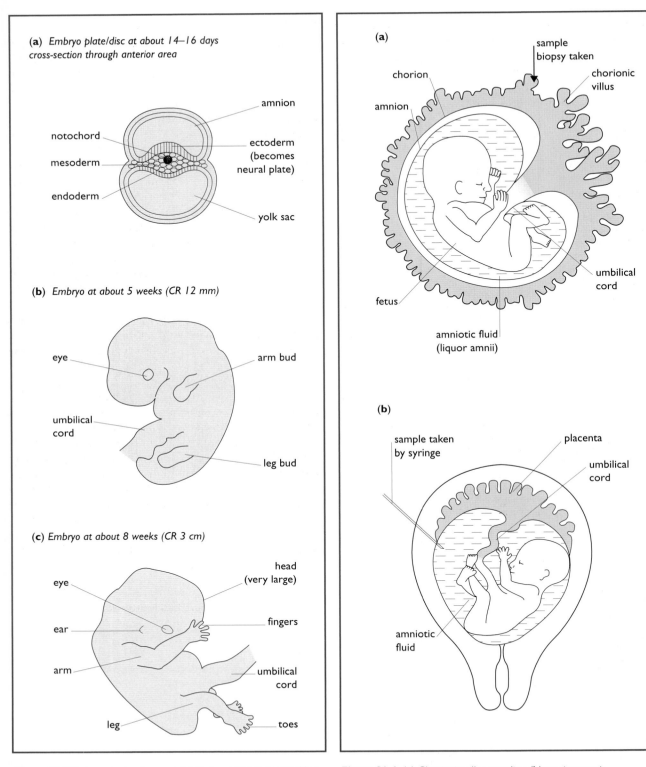

(a) *Embryo plate/disc at about 14–16 days cross-section through anterior area*

amnion

notochord

mesoderm

endoderm

ectoderm (becomes neural plate)

yolk sac

(b) *Embryo at about 5 weeks (CR 12 mm)*

eye

arm bud

umbilical cord

leg bud

(c) *Embryo at about 8 weeks (CR 3 cm)*

eye

ear

arm

leg

head (very large)

fingers

umbilical cord

toes

(a)

chorion

amnion

sample biopsy taken

chorionic villus

umbilical cord

fetus

amniotic fluid (liquor amnii)

(b)

sample taken by syringe

placenta

umbilical cord

amniotic fluid

Figure 21.3 Embryonic development. (a) Early – embryonic plate/disc (cross-section); (b) at 5 weeks; (c) at 8 weeks.

Figure 21.4 (a) Chorionic villus sampling; (b) amniocentesis.

menstruation), weigh between 2500 and 4500 g, with a CR length of 35–40 cm (total length is around 50 cm). The testes descend into the scrotum in male fetuses. Most lanugo disappears and vernix is usually only found in the skin creases of mature newborns.

<table>
<tr><td colspan="2" align="center">Table 21.2 Primary germ layers</td></tr>
<tr><td colspan="2" align="center">Primary germ layer derivatives</td></tr>
</table>

A. Ectoderm
(I)   Surface
      Skin – epidermis, nails, sebaceous glands and hair
      Eye – lens
      Ear – inner ear
      Tooth enamel
      Anterior pituitary gland
      Mammary glands
(II)   Neuroectoderm
      Neural tube – CNS, posterior pituitary, pineal gland, retina
      Neural crest – cranial & spinal nerves, autonomic nerves, melanocytes, adrenal medulla and mesoderm for head

B. Endoderm
Epithelial part of – tonsil, pharynx, thyroid, parathyroids, middle ear, trachea, bronchi and lungs
Epithelium of gastrointestinal tract, liver, pancreas and bladder

C. Mesoderm
Bone, muscles and connective tissues
Skin – dermis. Teeth – dentine
Urogenital tract – gonads, ducts and glands
Cardiovascular system and blood
Lymphatic system – spleen and cells
Adrenal cortex
Visceral muscle, serous membranes, visceral connective tissue

Adapted from England MA (1983) A Colour Atlas of Life Before Birth . Wolfe Medical Publications

Table 21.2 Primary germ layers.

Fetal circulation

During embryonic/fetal development the cardiovascular system is adapted for intrauterine life, where metabolic needs are met via the placenta. There are extra blood vessels and shunts that are converted at or soon after birth to an adult circulation pattern (see Chapter 10), which includes the pulmonary circulation.

By week 4 the embryonic heart is beating and blood vessels are developing at a rapid rate. Soon the embryo is connected to the placenta by umbilical vessels, which remain the vital 'lifeline' until birth and the infant's first breath (see Chapter 20).

Fetal blood, at 80% oxygen saturation, returns from the placenta within a large single umbilical vein to the liver (see *Figure 21.6*). Most of the blood bypasses the liver and goes directly into the inferior vena cava via a shunt called the ductus venosus. The inferior vena cava takes blood, now mixed with poorly oxygenated blood from the cells, to the right atrium.

From the right atrium some blood is shunted through the foramen ovale (opening in the septum) into the left atrium. This blood enters the left ventricle and leaves via the aorta to supply the head and upper limbs.

Blood returning via the superior vena cava to the right side of the heart and reaching the pulmonary artery is redirected to the aorta via the ductus arteriosus, a shunt between the pulmonary trunk and the aorta.

The foramen ovale and ductus arteriosus are shunts that enable most blood to bypass the non-functional lungs and pulmonary circulation. Blood flows through the shunts in the correct direction because pressure differentials are created by the minimal venous return from the lungs and blood flows from high to low pressure areas.

Poorly oxygenated blood with waste flows through the distal aorta to leave the fetus via the internal iliac arteries and the two umbilical arteries that carry the blood back

Figure 21.5 Fetal development.

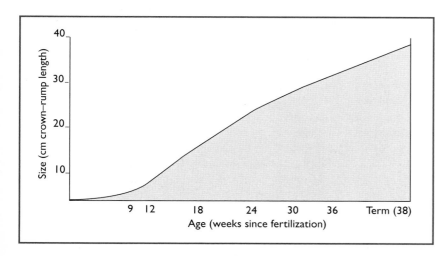

Figure 21.6 Fetal circulation.

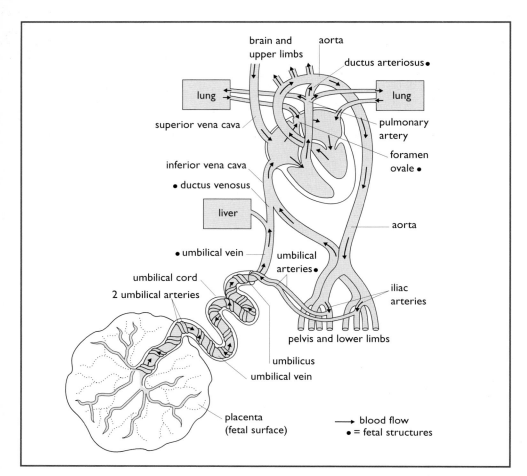

brain and upper limbs

aorta

ductus arteriosus •

lung

lung

superior vena cava

pulmonary artery

inferior vena cava

foramen ovale •

• ductus venosus

liver

aorta

• umbilical vein

umbilical arteries •

umbilical cord

2 umbilical arteries

iliac arteries

pelvis and lower limbs

umbilicus

umbilical vein

placenta (fetal surface)

→ blood flow
• = fetal structures

to the placenta. Here fetal blood passes through the capillary network to exchange substances with maternal blood prior to returning via the umbilical vein.

It is important to note that the liver, lungs and gastrointestinal tract are mostly bypassed because their functions are covered by maternal systems; they do, however, receive sufficient blood for their development.

Early Years–Growth and Development

The emphasis here will be the first year after birth, with only a brief mention of growth occurring during childhood. For the first 28 days after birth the baby is a neonate (newly born) and up to the first birthday it is classified as an infant.

Circulatory adaptations to extrauterine life

Several changes occurring at birth ensure that the infant adjusts to extrauterine life, but the most immediate is the establishment of respiration. The newborn usually gasps and starts breathing in response to the sudden exit from its cosy uterine surroundings.

The first breath, which inflates the lungs, causes enormous circulatory changes (*Figure 21.7*). Blood flowing through the pulmonary circulation decreases pulmonary artery pressure and increases that in the left heart and aorta. This reversal of pressure has two effects:
- The ductus arteriosus constricts and eventually becomes a fibrous cord.
- A flap occludes the foramen ovale, although closure will take some months to complete.

The umbilical vessels constrict and the ductus venosus empties. Eventually they become fibrosed, but persist as ligaments, e.g. the umbilical vein becomes the ligamentum teres of the liver (see Chapter 14).

Congenital heart defects may be due to continued patency of the foramen ovale or ductus arteriosus, which, as you can imagine, can cause considerable problems for the infant. Defects causing problems are usually treated surgically, soon after birth.

Nursing Practice Application **Apgar score**

At birth, and again after 5 min, the infant's physical condition is assessed using the five physical signs of the Apgar rating (designed for Caucasian new-borns). The infant is scored on a scale of 0–2 for heart rate, respiratory effort, colour (not always used), reflexes and muscle tone, which gives a maximum score of 10 (see *Figure 21.8*). Most healthy infants, such as Harvey (see Chapter 20), would be expected to score 8 or above.

Figure 21.7 Changes to circulation at birth.

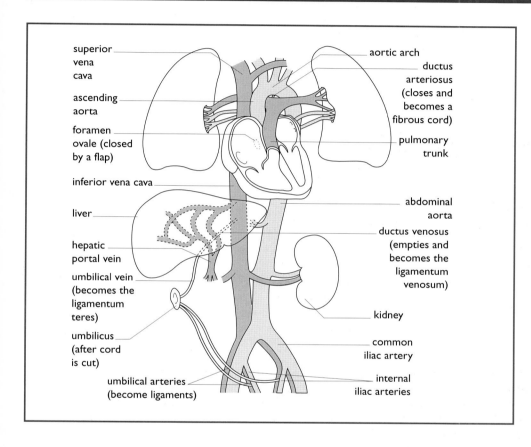

Labels: superior vena cava; ascending aorta; foramen ovale (closed by a flap); inferior vena cava; liver; hepatic portal vein; umbilical vein (becomes the ligamentum teres); umbilicus (after cord is cut); umbilical arteries (become ligaments); aortic arch; ductus arteriosus (closes and becomes a fibrous cord); pulmonary trunk; abdominal aorta; ductus venosus (empties and becomes the ligamentum venosum); kidney; common iliac artery; internal iliac arteries

The newborn

The usual weight for babies born at term, in the UK, is around 3400–3500 g, with boys slightly heavier than girls. Birth weight at term can vary between 2500 and 4500 g, and depends upon genetic inheritance, ethnic origin and the quality of the intrauterine environment; for example, multiple pregnancies and maternal smoking tend to produce smaller babies. A baby weighing around 3500 g usually has a total length of about 50 cm and a head circumference of 33–34 cm. A large and increasing head circumference may indicate hydrocephaly (see Chapters 4 and 18).

All newborns are assessed at birth (see Apgar score), weighed, measured, examined for abnormalities, e.g. spina bifida (see Chapter 4), and later have screening blood tests for phenylketonuria (see Chapter 13), thyroid function (see Chapter 8) and possibly cystic fibrosis (see Chapter 12).

Abilities and characteristics

Mature newborns can hear and respond reflexly to loud noises (Moro or startle reflex), see objects at about 25 cm, smell and taste, and usually waste no time in letting everyone know if they are hungry. Other primitive reflexes present at birth include: 'rooting', where the head turns, searching for a nipple, when the cheek is stroked; and the 'grasp' reflex, where the infant holds an adult finger. The reflexes disappear at different times and are used to assess maturity and development.

Newborns have poor temperature regulation, but deposits of brown fat offset this by providing a source of rapid release energy (see Chapter 19).

Now suddenly parted from its food supply, the infant's digestive tract must meet its needs from breast milk or formula, but most lose some weight in the early days whilst

Apgar score			
	Score		
Signs/Criteria	0	1	2
Heart rate	absent	slow, below 100/min	over 100/min
Respiratory effort	absent	slow, weak, irregular	good chest movements or crying
Muscle tone	limp	poor tone, some movement	active resistance, strong movement
Reflex irritability (response to stimulation such as sole flicks)	none	slight withdrawal	vigorous movement, cries
Colour (NB designed for Caucasian newborns)	pale or blue	extremities blue	completely normal colour

Figure 21.8 Apgar score.

Healthier Living Preventing sudden infant death syndrome

One of the commonest causes of death in infants aged between 1 month and 1 year is sudden infant death syndrome (SIDS), or 'cot death' (most deaths occur before age 6 months). Some factors are linked with an increased risk for SIDS, e.g. low birth weight and maternal smoking. Nurses have a role in identifying risk factors and working with parents to decrease these risks (Noyes et al. 1996). There are, however, several measures that reduce risk for all babies. Those caring for infants should be encouraged to:

- Put infants on their back or side to sleep.
- Avoid infant overheating.
- Ensure that people do not smoke anywhere near the infant.
- Consult the doctor at once if the infant appears unwell.

These points are detailed in the DoH leaflet 'Back to Sleep', issued as part of a campaign to reduce SIDS, during the early 1990s. An evaluation of the campaign (Hiley and Morley, 1994) found that deaths from SIDS had halved in 1 year.

Recently, further advice was added: use the bottom half of the cot to stop small babies slipping under their bedding.

Parents of bottle-fed infants may worry because most authorities suggest that there is a reduced incidence of SIDS with breast feeding. A study by Gilbert et al. (1995) found that bottle feeding was not a significant risk factor in isolation but that the increased risk associated with bottle feeding was linked to other factors, including preterm birth, parental employment and maternal smoking.

the digestive system 'gets its act together', e.g. acid and enzyme production, and feeding regimens, are established (see lactation, Chapter 20).

Dark green/black stools (meconium) are passed over the first few days and gradually change to the soft yellow/brown stools (4–6 daily) of milk-fed babies – the colour depends on whether breast or formula feeding is used.

Another problem for newborns is liver immaturity, which may lead to physiological jaundice (see Chapter 14). There may be a deficiency of the clotting factor prothrombin because of liver immaturity and low levels of vitamin K, which exist until the intestinal bacteria needed for its synthesis are in place. Prophylactic vitamin K injections (oral forms available) have been used in newborns for many years to counter the risk of haemorrhagic dis-

ease, which can cause intracranial bleeding. A recent study suggested a link between intramuscular vitamin K and cancers including leukaemia, but other studies found no link. Life-threatening haemorrhagic disease is preventable and Zipursky (1996) has suggested that all newborns should have vitamin K supplements.

Infancy – growth and development during the first year

The time from birth until the first birthday includes the breathtaking changes that convert the completely helpless newborn to a child able to communicate, control their posture, pick up small objects, crawl and possibly walk.

Much of this stunning development occurs concurrently with myelination (see Chapter 3). At the same time the

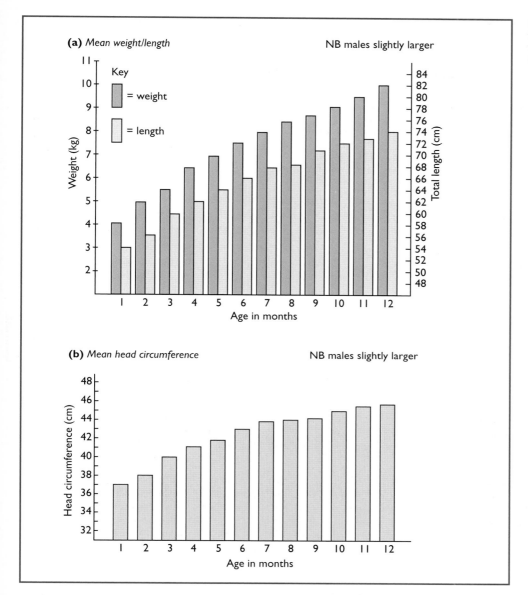

Figure 21.9 Growth in the first year (female). (**a**) Mean weight/length; (**b**) mean head circumference.

brain increases in size from around 400 to 1000 g. Babies smile and turn to look at a speaker's face by 6 weeks. By 3 months they kick vigorously and by 4 months they can laugh. Babies of 6 months communicate (babble and coo) and can bear weight on their legs. They sit unsupported by 8 months and some may crawl. At one year they are able to sit, pull themselves up and walk using furniture, and some may walk independently.

Physical growth occurs rapidly during the first year – babies weighing 3500 g at birth can be expected to weigh at least double this at 6 months (7 kg) and approximately treble the weight at 1 year (10–10.5 kg). More detail of mean weight, length and head circumference is provided in *Figure 21.9*.

The timing of developmental milestones, e.g. sitting up, and growth is used by health visitors and doctors to assess a child's progress and the early detection of unsatisfactory development, which allows for prompt investigation and the introduction of remedial measures.

Teeth

In Chapter 13 we mentioned the first dentition of 20 deciduous teeth and the second of 32 permanent teeth [see *Figure 13.6 (a), (b)*]. The eruption of the first teeth, at around 5–6 months, is another guide to developmental progress. Babies with conditions such as congenital hypothyroidism may have a delay in the eruption of teeth, as may those who are malnourished.

The first teeth to appear are usually the two lower central incisors followed by the two upper central incisors, two upper lateral incisors and two lower lateral incisors – some babies have these eight teeth at 1 year, but others may only have three or four. During the next 18 months the four first molars, four canines and four second molars will erupt to complete the first dentition at around 2 1/2 years.

The second dentition will start to replace the deciduous teeth between the ages of 5 and 6 years, and replacement is nearly complete by about 12 years of age; however, the third molars (wisdom teeth), if they erupt, will appear between age 18 and 25 years. As the permanent teeth erupt, the jaw enlarges to accommodate the increase in both size and numbers, and this eventually produces the adult facial proportions.

Bone changes and spinal curves

The bones are well ossified at birth (see Chapter 16) and secondary ossification centres form in the epiphyses during early childhood in a set order, resulting in further bone formation until only the epiphyseal growth plates remain as cartilage. Bone growth after birth, which continues throughout childhood and adolescence, is usually complete by the late teens (females) or early 20s (males). As infants becomes physically active the rather plain bones are subjected to stresses, which cause the development of the adult 'bony landmarks', e.g. tubercles (see Chapter 18).

During the first year the C-shaped fetal spine alters as two secondary curves are formed – the first in the cervical region when the infant lifts its head and the second in the lumbar region when the infant sits up and then stands (see Figure 18.14).

Growth and development during childhood

After infancy, growth and development continue more slowly through several stages – toddler, preschool and older child – until **puberty** occurs. Boys tend to be taller and heavier than girls until the earlier puberty in girls reverses this trend for a while. A guide to average weight and height for children aged between 2 and 11 years is provided in Table 21.3, but readers requiring more information are directed to Further Reading, e.g. Illingworth (1991).

Influences on growth

Earlier we mentioned some influences on prenatal growth and birth weight. Many factors continue to influence growth after birth and include:
- Genetics (genes determine maximum adult height).
- Health status; for example, children with cystic fibrosis may not achieve full adult height because of nutritional problems and recurrent chest infections. Interestingly, a study of 11-year-olds (sample $n = 554$) by Patel et al. (1994) found that the 11% who were positive for *Helicobacter pylori* (see Chapter 13) showed growth retardation (mean 1.1 cm) between 7 and 11 years of age.
- Proper nutrition is vital for growth, and children whose diet is deficient (quantity or quality) are likely to be below average weight and height for their age.
- The levels of growth hormone, thyroid hormones and sex hormones all affect growth; for example, a deficiency in growth hormone leads (untreated) to poor growth and short stature (see Chapters 8, 16 and 20).
- Security, stability and a loving environment all appear to influence the physiological processes required for normal growth; for example, growth may slow in children who experience bereavement.

Table 21.3 Childhood growth (2–11 years).

Age (years)	Male		Female	
	Weight (kg)	Height (cm)	Weight (kg)	Height (cm)
2	12.5	87.4	12.2	86.5
3	14.5	96	14.2	95.5
5	19.2	111	18.5	109.5
7	24.4	124	23.5	122
9	30	135.3	29	133
11	35	144	35.5	144.5

Table 21.3 Childhood growth (2–11 years)

NB Average weights and heights.

Adolescence and Puberty

Adolescence is the developmental stage starting with the onset of puberty and ending with adulthood. It lasts for several years between the ages of 9 and 20, with considerable individual variations.

The development of functional reproductive structures and secondary sexual characteristics, which occurs during the first few years of adolescence, is called puberty.

During childhood small amounts of adrenal sex hormones inhibit gonadotrophin-releasing hormone (GnRH) release but, as puberty nears, the hypothalamus becomes less sensitive and GnRH is released. This in turn stimulates follicle stimulating hormone (FSH), luteinizing hormone (LH) and the gonadal sex hormones – the male testosterone and the female oestrogens and progesterone (see Chapter 20). At puberty the secretion of sex hormones activates the individual's reproductive potential; gametogenesis is stimulated, the secondary sexual characteristics develop and general growth occurs (see *Figure 21.10*).

Puberty in the male

Timing varies, but it usually starts between age 10 and 14 years, with some changes continuing into the 20s, e.g. body hair development.

As already discussed, it is testosterone that initiates the changes of puberty. These include:
- Enlargement of the testes, penis and accessory glands.
- Growth of the seminiferous tubules and spermatogenesis.
- Laryngeal enlargement (see Chapter 12) and deepening of the voice; this 'breaking' of the voice curtails the singing life of a 'boy soprano'.
- Growth of facial, pubic, axillary and chest hair.
- Increased sebaceous gland activity, which is linked to acne (see Chapter 19).
- Formation of the male physique, 'growth spurts' and increase in muscle mass (see Chapters 16–18), all of which are linked to anabolic testosterone. Bone growth may continue into the late teens/early 20s.
- Development of libido, spontaneous erection and nocturnal emissions of semen.
- Possible influences on behaviour and mood, but many sociocultural factors contribute to this aspect of pubertal change.

Puberty in the female

Puberty in the female may start any time between the age of 9 and 13, but for most girls breast development and the growth of pubic/axillary hair occur at around 11 years of age. The **menarche** (commencement of menstruation) usually occurs between age 11 and 17, but the mean age in developed countries is 12–13 years – around 2 years after breast development starts. The actual timing of the menarche appears to be linked with achievement of a minimum body weight (fat) in relation to height and does not occur until the major growth spurt in height has taken place. This theory can be used to explain the fall in mean age of menarche over the last century in developed countries. It is probable that improved standards of health and nutrition have resulted in better growth rates which trigger an earlier puberty. Body weight (fat) influences are also demonstrated by the cessation of menstruation (amenorrhoea) following severe weight loss, e.g. with anorexia nervosa, 'crash diets' or excessive exercise.

Early menstrual cycles may be irregular and, as already mentioned in Chapter 20, the cycles are usually anovulatory. It comes as something of a surprise to a girl who has so far had pain-free periods to experience the dysmenorrhoea that starts when ovulation becomes a regular event.

The onset of puberty in the female is generally earlier than in the male and is of shorter duration. Oestrogen accounts for most of the physical changes, which include:
- Breast growth and development.
- Development of internal genitalia.
- Restarting oogenesis, commenced in fetal life, and follicle development.
- Vaginal mucosal changes with the production of an acid environment.
- Body hair – axillary and pubic.
- Development of female physique, e.g. pelvic shape (see Chapter 18), fat deposition and 'growth spurts', which are usually complete by age 15–17 years.

Young Adulthood and Mid-life

Young adulthood covers the years from 20 to 39, which for most of us represents the time when all systems are functioning well. It is a quiet time from the developmental viewpoint, but some occurrences are significant, e.g. reproductive function reaches its zenith, the percentage of fat as part of the total body weight increases from age 20 years and has more than doubled by late mid-life, and achieving peak bone mass between age 35 and 40 years (see Chapter 16). Mid-life has several definitions, but most include age 40–65 years. From the fifth decade people become aware of changes; for example, near vision deteriorates, necessitating reading glasses, and skin wrinkles, which announce the normal ageing process yet to come. For women, however, mid-life also includes the **climacteric** (see pages 522–523) – a tangible sign of ageing.

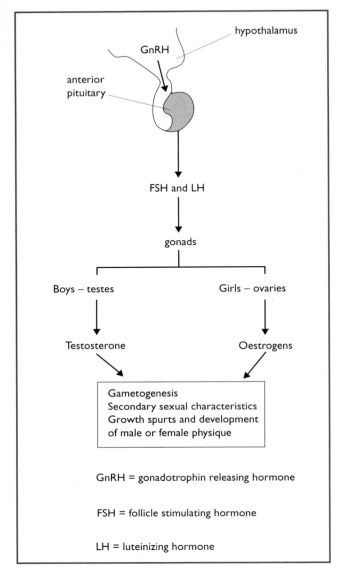

GnRH = gonadotrophin releasing hormone

FSH = follicle stimulating hormone

LH = luteinizing hormone

Figure 21.10 Hormones and the changes of puberty.

Climacteric and menopause

Female reproductive function and hormone production decline over a period of time known as the climacteric; this generally occurs between age 46 and 55 years, but may take place earlier or later. The cessation of menstruation, known as the **menopause**, is a distinct episode occurring during the climacteric; the mean age for the menopause is 50.8 years in the UK. The menopause can only be recognized retrospectively and most authorities accept a year without periods as evidence that the menopause has occurred. (NB ovulation may occur in the months after the menopause, but pregnancy is unlikely.) Often the term menopause is used, quite erroneously, to describe the climacteric.

Premenopausal women are often anxious that hysterectomy (removal of the uterus) will cause the climacteric to occur. If their ovaries are left intact they will not experience the climacteric until the naturally determined time, because ovarian hormone production continues as normal. They will, however, stop menstruating and become infertile.

Obviously the climacteric and menopause bring to an end a woman's fertility, but the reduction in oestrogens also produces metabolic effects ranging from short-term problems such as 'hot flushes' to lasting changes, e.g. raised serum cholesterol.

The menopause occurs because the ovaries fail to respond to the gonadotrophins; there are still plenty of follicles, but they no longer develop. Some women stop menstruating suddenly, but for most the cycles become anovulatory and erratic, and blood loss decreases. Eventually ovulation and menstruation cease and levels of oestrogen and progesterone decline. In response to this reduction in ovarian hormones the hypothalamus stimulates the pituitary to secrete more and more FSH and LH. The physical and psychosocial effects of the climacteric are due either to declining oestrogen or elevated FSH and LH, and include:

- Atrophy of internal genitalia.
- Weakening of the pelvic floor, which in some women will eventually cause stress incontinence (see Chapter 15) and uterovaginal prolapse (see Chapters 18 and 20).
- Labial atrophy and thinning of pubic hair.
- Breast atrophy.
- Vaginal mucosa thinning and becoming dry. The loss of the acid environment increases the vulnerability to infection. These changes of atrophic (senile) vaginitis can make intercourse painful/difficult (dyspareunia).
- 'Hot flushes' and night sweats caused by sudden vasodilation of skin vessels. LH surges and declining oestrogen levels appear to cause this vasomotor instability occurring in some women.
- Mood changes, e.g. depression, irritability and loss of confidence. These may be linked with negative attitudes to the climacteric which many women call the 'change of life' and to major life events occurring concurrently, e.g. children leaving home. Some women fear the effects of the climacteric on their sexuality and relationships.
- Later bone changes increasing the incidence of osteoporosis in postmenopausal women (see Chapter 16).
- Loss of oestrogenic influence on serum cholesterol, which, with triglyceride levels, rise after the menopause. Postmenopausal women will eventually develop the same risks for coronary heart disease (CHD) as men of similar age (see Chapter 10).

Bleeding occurring a year after the menopause (postmenopausal bleeding, or PMB); this is considered abnormal and should always be investigated to exclude uterine

---

Nursing Practice Application **Coping with the climacteric**

For some women, hormone replacement therapy (HRT) – low-dose oestrogen and progesterone (with intact uterus) on a cyclical basis – will help to alleviate some distressing effects of the climacteric, e.g. 'hot flushes'. The addition of progesterone prevents endometrial overstimulation. Testosterone may be given with oestrogens to treat osteoporosis, and other steroids that have androgenic effects, e.g. tibolone, can be taken by postmenopausal women and require no additional progesterone.

Women need information regarding the monitoring required during HRT to detect problems, which may include hypertension, and endometrial and breast malignancies (incidence of breast cancer increases statistically with long-term therapy). Also on the minus side, HRT will not prevent ageing or restore youth, in spite of many anecdotal accounts to the contrary appearing in the popular press. Another effect of HRT that might not be appreciated by women is that vaginal bleeding occurs with some types of treatment. HRT does, however, help many

women cope with the climacteric and it has obvious benefits in preventing osteoporosis and protecting against coronary heart disease (CHD), but progesterone partially negates this oestrogenic effect. Providing information about the climacteric and the options open to women is an important role for nurses. Hughes (1992) describes the development of information meetings at a GP surgery and discusses the results. Many women will derive benefit from self-help, e.g. vaginal lubricants, counselling and complementary therapies such as aromatherapy.

---

malignancy. The bleeding may be due to vaginitis, which can be remedied with topical oestrogen preparations.

Mid-life and male reproductive function

Male reproductive function, unlike that in the female, continues well into old age. Men have no physiological equivalent of the climacteric, and, although there is a decline in reproductive capacity, are capable of fathering children into their 80s and beyond. Testosterone levels decrease gradually from the fourth decade, but receptor sites in target tissues become more sensitive to reduced levels and spermatogenesis continues unabated throughout life. Ageing, however, will affect sexual response (see Chapter 20); the latent period lengthens and the ability to achieve erection and ejaculation may be affected by other factors, e.g. antihypertensive drugs.

Later Life and Ageing

The changes of normal ageing, occurring in older adults (aged 65 and over), mark the last episode of our developmental story that unfolds across the continuum of life. Ageing and death may not seem like a very good idea for individuals, but the very existence of the species depends upon a 'turnover' of people and genes as babies are born, develop, mature, reproduce, age and die. Biologically there is no point wasting energy in maintaining organisms once they have produced and reared offspring; besides, if we lived too long there would be no room.

A point to consider is the rate at which people age – there are huge individual variations. Some people enjoy 'good health' and remain independent until dying at a

'ripe old age', whereas others are frail and dependent for many years before death. It is also important to distinguish between the normal changes in physiological processes associated with ageing and the altered function and pathology that disrupts homeostatic balance in older adults.

During the 20th century the percentage of older adults in the population of developed countries has grown as life expectancy has increased. What is interesting is the steady rise in those aged 75–84 years and the big increase in those over 85 years, who as a group use disproportionate amounts of health and social care resources.

Most people in developed countries can expect to live longer than their forebears with the positive effects of improved social conditions and advances in medical science. Certainly, as health professionals, more and more of your energies will be devoted to the needs of older adults – in health promotion, acute care and planning longer-term initiatives in conjunction with social services.

Theories of ageing

Put simply, we grow old because molecules and cells 'wear out' and are no longer repaired or replaced. Not only do people age at different times, but individual cells/tissues have their own ageing timetable. Additionally, we tend to inherit longevity (or not) along with other genetic characteristics – some people have genes that initiate early ageing and in extreme cases, e.g. the progeria syndromes, the person ages during childhood.

In Chapter 1 there is more detail about cell ageing and you may care to refresh your memory. A summary of current theories of ageing, which may all operate to some degree, include:

- Genes that determine when cellular repair and replication will fail as DNA runs out or is no longer synthesized.
- Repeated cell injuries by free radicals, toxins, chemicals, radiation or lack of oxygen and nutrients.
- A breakdown in immunological responses that normally prevent cell damage by micro-organisms, malignant changes or autoimmunity (see Chapter 19).
- Decline in pituitary hormones, e.g. growth hormone, which may increase vulnerability to physiological stress, plus thymosine and melatonin (see Chapter 8).
- Lack of energy for DNA maintenance and cell repair (disposable soma theory).

Physiological effects of ageing

All cells, tissues, organs and functional systems undergo changes as part of normal ageing. These changes will inevitably affect the efficiency of body processes and will lead to a reduction in functional reserves, which diminishes our ability to maintain homeostasis in the face of physiological stress. Imagine for a moment an older person having 'forty winks' in a chair when the telephone rings – they wake suddenly, get up too quickly, feel giddy and flop back into the chair. They miss the call because their 80-year-old cardiovascular system has no reserves and cannot adjust blood pressure to cope with sudden changes in posture as quickly as 40

Table 21.4 Physiological effects of normal ageing	
1. Cell growth and repair	• reduced ability to replace or repair cells damaged by toxins etc.
2. Regulation, communication and control (nervous system, sense organs and endocrine system)	• loss of cells in cerebral cortex, changes to proprioception as cerebellum and vestibular nuclei deteriorate. Memory changes. • visual acuity declines, e.g. presbyopia, lens clouding occurs. • taste and smell decline, appetite affected. • high frequency hearing loss (presbycusis). • decline in hormone levels (see theories of ageing). • decreased sensitivity to insulin results in a decline in glucose tolerance. • thirst centre does not function so well; dehydration can occur.
3. Body transport systems (blood, cardiovascular and lymphatic systems)	• erythrocyte sedimentation rate increases, blood becomes more viscous. • stroke volume decreases, large arteries become less elastic – leads to increase in systolic blood pressure and postural hypotension. • thymus gland consists of connective tissue.
4. Obtaining and using raw material for metabolism and excreting waste (respiratory, gastrointestinal, biliary and urinary systems)	• lungs become less elastic with a decrease in FEV_1, increase in dead space. Exercise tolerance declines unless regular activity continues. • appetite declines and capacity smaller. Digestion less efficient. Constipation. • loss of hepatocytes, impaired drug/toxin metabolism. • GFR declines, drug excretion less efficient. Renal tubules work less efficiently and ability to concentrate urine decreases. Nocturia and risk for dehydration.
5. Movement and stability (bones, joints and muscles)	• loss of bone mass without bone deposition increases risk for osteoporosis. • loss of muscle tissue (lean body mass) and loss of strength. • joint stiffness especially with immobility (may progress to osteoarthritis).
6. Defence and survival strategies (skin, body defences)	• skin thins, becomes less elastic and is more easily damaged. • healing takes longer (inflammatory response decreased and vascular system brings less blood). • hair thins. • temperature regulation less efficient, less body fat, failure to feel cold or shiver, all increase risk for hypothermia. • skin has less fat and water to act as reserve store. • inflammatory response declines, increasing risk for infection. • immune response (humoral and cell mediated) declines, which increases risk for infection, cancers and autoimmunity.
7. Ensuring continuity (reproductive systems)	• female reproductive function ceases in mid-life during the climacteric, but sexual responses continue. • male reproductive function and sexual response continues throughout life (NB poor health may alter sexual response).

Table 21.4 Physiological effects of normal ageing.

Healthier Living **Staying healthy in later life**

We cannot halt the biological ageing process, but we can be proactive in helping to ensure that later life is as healthy as possible. Nurses can provide health promotion for older adults which assists in maintaining function, independence and enjoyment. Relevant areas for consideration include:

* Nutrition (see Chapter 13).
* Suitable exercise (see Chapter 17).
* Mental stimulation – courses, interests and hobbies.
* Health screening, e.g. for cancer. In an article by Faithfull (1994) epidemiological data indicates that, in the UK, 70% of cancers are diagnosed in people aged over 60 years.
* Sensible alcohol intake improves appetite and protects against CHD; however, alcohol misuse may increase falls and the likelihood of malnutrition in older adults (see Chapter 14).
* Stopping or reducing smoking (see Chapter 12).
* Stress management (see Chapter 6).
* Maintaining dental/oral care (see Chapter 13).
* Immunizations against influenza (especially those in long-term care) and tetanus.
* Sleep/rest (see Chapter 4).
* Keeping warm (see Chapter 19).
* Checks for sensory impairment – vision and hearing loss (see Chapter 7).
* Home safety/security, e.g. smoke and carbon monoxide detectors (see Chapter 12).
* Using medication safely (prescribed and nonprescribed).

Lastly, but vitally important, is enabling people to adopt a positive attitude and to 'get on with' what might be 25–30 years of post-retirement life. You will certainly think of other areas in the light of your own practice and experiences.

years previously (see Chapter 10), but at least they can check who called once homeostatic balance returns.

The physiological changes occurring in individual functional systems are covered in *Table 21.4*. Some age changes are also covered in appropriate chapters, e.g. inability to concentrate urine (see Chapter 15). As physiological processes change so does the way in which drugs are detoxified and excreted by the liver and kidneys (see Chapter 14).

Ageing, however, is much more than biology – it also has social and cultural components. For example, how society values older adults and makes financial provision for them will influence ageing. If you have negative perceptions of ageing and expect to be old at 65 you probably will be.

Dying and death

Until the second half of the 20th century the definition of death was straightforward – no breathing and heart beat. These criteria are still used, but are now extended to irreversible cessation of heart beat and breathing, because the development of cardiopulmonary resuscitation has resulted in the recovery of hundreds of thousands of people previously classified as dead.

The use of life-support systems means that those who would otherwise die may be maintained indefinitely on mechanical ventilation. Where life is being preserved by life-support systems and a heart beat is present it is necessary to use different criteria for the definition of death;

namely, lack of brainstem activity, which is ascertained by testing reflexes, e.g. pupillary and gag (see Chapter 4). A diagnosis of brain death can only be made in the absence of factors that may depress brainstem activity, e.g. narcotic drugs or abnormal blood chemistry.

The blood can be oxygenated outside the body (extracorporeal), e.g. via bypass during cardiac surgery where the heart has been stopped to facilitate surgery, and dialysis can substitute for kidney function (see Chapter 15).

Persistent vegetative state

The totally dependent persistent vegetative state occurs when the cerebral cortex is irreparably injured but the brainstem, which controls vital functions, continues to work. The individual, who is apparently conscious but unresponsive, may live for years with care and feeding. In the UK recent court rulings have allowed that feeding be withdrawn in specific cases and the person be allowed to die. These are obviously very difficult decisions for loved ones and health professionals to make. Diagnosis of a vegetative state is not always easy and because the possibility of error exists it is necessary to proceed with extreme caution where the discontinuation of feeding is being considered.

Death – causes and types

In developed countries the leading causes of death are cardiovascular disease and cancers, followed by accidents/violence and suicide (commonest causes in younger people), respiratory illness and infections. The causes of death in developing countries reflect differences in standards of living that result in poor nutrition and infection, e.g. gastroenteritis in infants.

Sometimes death occurs suddenly – usually from stroke (see Chapter 4) or heart attack (see Chapter 10). It may occur some hours or days after the acute episode, e.g. the heart attack victim who survives the first attack only to die of irreversible ventricular fibrillation some hours later.

Other people may die gradually as their functional systems decline to a point where they cannot maintain homeostatic balance, e.g. the person with chronic obstructive pulmonary disease (COPD) (see Chapter 12) who is unable to regulate blood pH as carbon dioxide is retained.

The terminal stages of any illness, e.g. cancer or muscular dystrophy, can be made much easier for the individual and those who love and care for them if pain and other symptoms are controlled (see Family-centred Study).

After a death those left behind will need help and support while they grieve and cope with their loss. This includes health professionals, who need the opportunity to talk about feelings, e.g. anger and helplessness, perhaps in staff support groups or in counselling. Lloyd-Richards and Rees (1996) have stated that hospital nurses feel unprepared to support bereaved relatives and that they too need support.

Family-centred Study **Last days at home**

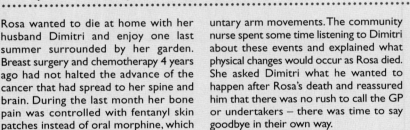

Rosa wanted to die at home with her husband Dimitri and enjoy one last summer surrounded by her garden. Breast surgery and chemotherapy 4 years ago had not halted the advance of the cancer that had spread to her spine and brain. During the last month her bone pain was controlled with fentanyl skin patches instead of oral morphine, which had caused constipation.

The couple were supported by their family, the community nurses, the GP and the local hospice, who provided night nursing.

During the days before her death Rosa gradually lost consciousness, but Dimitri was upset by her facial grimaces and invol-untary arm movements. The community nurse spent some time listening to Dimitri about these events and explained what physical changes would occur as Rosa died. She asked Dimitri what he wanted to happen after Rosa's death and reassured him that there was no rush to call the GP or undertakers – there was time to say goodbye in their own way.

When Rosa died she was painfree and her constipation had resolved; other signs/symptoms that might affect the terminal stages of an illness depend upon the underlying condition and include:
- Anxiety, agitation and confusion.
- Nausea, vomiting and hiccups.
- Diarrhoea.

- Dyspnoea and cough.
- Extreme weakness.
- Dry mouth.
- Bronchial secretions producing noisy breathing ('death rattle'), which distresses family and friends.

There is considerable debate about whether the terminally ill should be rehydrated to relieve a dry mouth as any benefits must be balanced against a possible increase in bronchial secretions and the distress of having an intravenous infusion. Readers are directed to Further Reading, e.g. Fox (1996) and Regnard and Tempest (1992).

Summary/Check List

Introduction
Genetics – chromosomes, problems, Nursing Practice Application – Down syndrome. Genes, alleles, inheritance – dominant, recessive and sex-linked.

Early days – embryonic development. Special Focus – screening for genetic problems and prenatal abnormalities; fetal development, fetal circulation.

Early years-growth and development – adaptations to extrauterine life. Nursing Practice Application – Apgar score, the newborn, infancy. Healthier Living – preventing sudden infant death syndrome; childhood; influences on growth.

Adolescence and puberty
Young adulthood and mid-life – climacteric and menopause. Nursing Practice Application – coping with the climacteric.

Mid-life and male reproductive function.

Later life and ageing – theories and effects of ageing. Healthier Living – staying healthy in later life; dying and death. Family-centred Study – last days at home.

Self Test

1 Explain: heterozygous, homozygous, dominant and recessive.
2 You are asked about risks associated with CVS. What would you say?
3 Why are drugs and viruses more dangerous to the embryo before week 8?
4 Explain how the fetal circulation is adapted for intrauterine life.
5 What information would you give to new parents about preventing SIDS?

6 Put the following in their correct pairs:
(a) FSH and LH
(b) menarche
(c) puberty
(d) first menstruation
(e) adolescence
(f) gonadotrophins.
7 Describe the physical changes associated with the climacteric.
8 What would you include in a health promotion programme for older adults?

Answers

1 See pages 509–510.
2 Decreased accuracy, miscarriage, limb damage.
3 Organogenesis is occurring.
4 See pages 515–516.

5 See page 518.
6 a–f, b–d and c–e.
7 See page 522.
8 See page 525.

References

DoH (undated) *Back to Sleep. Reducing the Risk of Cot Death.* London: HMSO.

Faithfull S (1994) Negative perceptions. *Nurs Times* **90** (1): 62–64.

Firth H, Boyd P, Chamberlain P *et al.* (1994) Analysis of limb reduction defects in babies exposed to chorionic villus sampling. *Lancet* **343**:1069–1071.

Gilbert L, Nicholl J, Alex S *et al.* (1996) Ethnic differences in the outcome of serum screening for Down's syndrome. *BMJ* **312**:94–95.

Gilbert RE, Wigfield R, Fleming P *et al.* (1995) Bottle feeding and the sudden infant death syndrome. *BMJ* **310**, 88–90.

Hiley CM, Morley CJ (1994) Evaluation of the government campaign to reduce risk of cot death. *BMJ* **309**:703–704.

Hughes Y (1992) Menopause – women of a certain age. *Nurs Times* **88** (12): 36–37.

Lloyd-Richards C, Rees C (1996) Hospital nurses' bereavement support for relatives: study report. *Int J Palliative Care* **2**(2): 108–110.

MRC Working Party on the Evaluation of Chorionic Villus Sampling (1991) MRC European Trial of Chorionic Villus Sampling. *Lancet* i:1491–1499.

Noyes J, Stebben V, Sobhan G *et al.*(1996) Home monitoring of infants at increased risk of sudden death. *J Clin Nurs* **5**(5): 297–306.

Patel P, Mendall MA, Khulusi S *et al.* (1994) *Helicobacter pylori* infection in childhood: risk factors and effect on growth. *BMJ* **309**:1119–1123.

Zipursky A (1996) Editorial – Vitamin K at birth. *BMJ* **313**: 179–180.

Further Reading

Belchetz P (1994) Hormonal treatment of postmenopausal women. *New Eng J Med* **330**(15):1062–1071.

Coni N, Davison W, Webster S (1992) *Ageing: the Facts.* Oxford: Oxford University Press.

England MA (1983) *A Colour Atlas of Life Before Birth – Normal Fetal Development.* London: Wolfe Medical Publications Limited.

Fox ET (1996) IV hydration in the terminally ill: ritual or therapy? *Bri J Nurs* **5**1:41–45.

Illingworth R (1991) *The Normal Child*, 10th edn. Edinburgh: Churchill Livingstone.

Mueller RF, Young I (1995) *Emery's Elements of Medical Genetics*, 9th edn. Edinburgh: Churchill Livingstone.

Redfern SJ, ed (1991) *Nursing Elderly People*, 2nd edn. Edinburgh: Churchill Livingstone.

Regnard C, Tempest S (1992) *A Guide to Symptoms Relief in Advanced Cancer.* Manchester: Haigh & Hochland.

Skirton H (1995a) Psychological implications of advances in genetics – 1. Carrier testing. *Prof Nurs* **10**(8): 496–498.

Skirton H (1995b) Psychological implications of advances in genetics – 2. Prenatal diagnosis. *Prof Nurs* **10**(9): 597–598.

Skirton H (1995c) Psychological implications of advances in genetics – 3. Predictive testing. *Prof Nurs* **10**(10): 644–646.

International System of Units (SI)

Introduction

The International System of Units (SI) or (Systeme Internationale) is a system of measurement used for medical, scientific, and technical purposes throughout most of the world. In the United Kingdom, SI units have replaced those of the Imperial System, e.g. the kilogram is used for mass instead of the pound (NB in everyday situations, both mass and weight are measured in kilograms although weight, which varies with gravity, is really a measure of force).

There are seven base units and several derived units within the International System of Units. Each measurement unit has its own symbol and can be expressed as a decimal multiple or sub-multiple of the base unit by the use of prefixes (see Appendix B).

Writing Large Numbers and Decimals

Before we look at the details of SI, it would be helpful to establish the ground rules for writing large numbers and decimals. These have particular relevance for practice, e.g. prescriptions for medication and laboratory results, where it is essential to be clear and accurate so as to avoid confusion and error.

Large numbers should be written in groups of three digits (from right to left) with spaces, but without commas (which are used in some countries as a decimal point).

For example:

ten thousand	should be written as	10 000
one hundred thousand	should be written as	100 000

NB Numbers with four digits are written without the space, e.g. one thousand – 1000.

Decimals should always have a zero (0) before the decimal point, which should be positioned near the line, e.g. 0.25 and 0.005. Decimals with more than four digits should be written in groups of three digits (from left to right) with spaces, e.g. 0.000 25.

Base Units and Symbols

Measurement	SI Base Unit and Symbol
Mass	kilogram (kg)
Length	metre (m)
Temperature	kelvin (K)
Time	second (s)
Amount of substance	mole (mol)
Luminous intensity	candela (cd)
Electric current	ampere (A)

Derived Units (with nursing practice application)

Measurement	SI Derived Unit and Symbol
Celsius temperature	degree Celsius (°C)
Frequency	hertz (Hz)
Energy/quantity of heat/work	joule (J)
Absorbed dose of radiation	gray (Gy)
Radioactivity (radionuclide)	becquerel (Bq)
Dose equivalent	sievert (Sv)
Pressure	pascal (Pa)
Force	newton (N)
Electrical potential / Potential difference / Electromotive force	volt (V)
Power	watt (W)

Factors, Symbols and Prefixes for Decimal Multiples and Submultiples

Factor	Prefix	Symbol
10^9	giga	G
10^6	mega	M
10^3	kilo	k
10^2	hecto	h
10^1	deca	da
10^{-1}	deci	d
10^{-2}	centi	c
10^{-3}	milli	m
10^{-6}	micro	μ
10^{-9}	nano	n
10^{-12}	pico	p
10^{-15}	femto	f

NB As kilogram already contains a prefix, the convention is to use the prefixes with gram (g), e.g. milligram (mg).

Anomalies (encountered in clinical nursing practice)

Temperature – Celsius (°C) temperature is used in clinical practice for measuring temperature, rather than kelvin (K).

Time – although the second (s) is the SI base unit for time, it is acceptable to use minute (min), hour (h) and day (d), e.g. GFR = 125 ml/min.

Volume – the litre (l/L) is used clinically to measure volume of fluids and gases. The litre is based on the volume of a cube (10 cm × 10 cm × 10 cm). A smaller unit, the millilitre (ml), which forms one thousandth part of a litre, has numerous clinical practice applications, e.g. recording fluid balance.

Pressure – the SI unit for pressure is the pascal (Pa), but in some areas, e.g. recording blood pressure, the old unit – millimetres of mercury pressure (mmHg) – is still widely used. The kilopascal (kPa) is increasingly used to measure blood gases and would replace mmHg pressure for blood pressure. Other clinical applications where the pascal is not used include: central venous pressure (CVP), which is measured in centimetres of water pressure (cm/H_2O); and the pressure of cerebrospinal fluid (CSF), which is measured in millimetres of water pressure (mm/H_2O).

Energy – the SI unit for energy is the joule (J) and for calculating energy composition or requirements the SI unit, kilojoule (kJ), is used. An old unit of measurement, the Calorie or kilocalorie (kcal), is however, still used (NB 1 kcal = 4.2 kJ).

Amount of Substance – the SI base unit for amount of substance is the mole (mol), but some substances, e.g. enzymes in the serum, are measured in International Units (*IU* or *iu*).

The Components of Medical Words and Terms

The Components of Medical Words and Terms
Prefixes, Suffixes, Word Roots and Combining Forms

Medical words or terms are usually compound words which contain more than one component part. They are formed from the addition of a prefix or a suffix to a word root or combining form. An understanding of medical terms will be achieved more easily if you become familiar with the main prefixes, suffixes and combining forms. Once you learn the 'code', it will often be possible for you to work out the meaning of new words when you enounter them.

Component	Meaning	Example
a/an -	without, lack of, not	*A*nuria (lack of urine)
ab -	away from	*Ab*duction (move a limb away from the body)
- able	capable of	Vi*able* (capable of living or surviving)
acro -	extremity	*Acro*megaly (enlarged extremities – jaw, hands and feet)
ad -	towards	*Ad*duction (move a limb towards the body)
adeno -	glandular	*Adeno*ma (benign tumour arising in glandular tissue)
- aemia	blood	An*aemia* (lack of blood – reduction in red cell numbers or haemoglobin)
aer -	air	*Aer*obic (requiring oxygen)
- aesthesia	sensation	Par*aesthesia* (disordered sensation – 'pins and needles')
- algia	pain	Proct*algia* (pain in the rectum)
ambi -	both	*Ambi*dextrous (equally skilled with both hands)

Component	Meaning	Example
andro -	male	*Andro*gens (male hormones)
angio -	blood vessel	*Angio*graphy (X-ray picture taken after injection of opaque fluid into the vessel)
aniso -	unequal	*Aniso*cytosis (inequality in red blood cell size)
ante/antero -	before, in front	*Ante*natal (before birth)
anti -	against	*Anti*coagulant (substance which delays or prevents blood coagulation)
arthro -	joint	*Arthro*scopy (endoscopic joint examination)
- ary	associated, connected	Urin*ary* (associated with urine)
- asis/esis	state of	Cy*esis* (state of being pregnant)
- ase	enzyme	Lip*ase* (enzyme concerned with fat digestion)
auto -	self	*Auto*graft (graft taken from a person's own body)
bi/bis -	two	*Bi*cuspid (having two cusps)
bili -	bile	*Bili*rubin (a bile pigment)
bio -	life	*Bio*chemistry (the chemistry of cell life)
- blast -	germ, bud	Haemocyto*blast* (an immature stem cell which can develop into any blood cell)
bleph -	eyelid	*Bleph*aritis (inflammation of the eyelid)
brachi -	arm	*Brachi*al artery (an artery of the arm)
brachy -	short	*Brachy*cephaly (short skull)
brady -	slow	*Brady*cardia (abnormally slow heart rate)
broncho -	bronchi	*Broncho*spasm (constriction of the bronchial muscle which narrows the air passages)
bucc -	cheek	*Bucc*inator (a cheek muscle)
carcino -	cancer	*Carcino*genic (agent which causes or predisposes to cancer)
cardio -	heart	*Cardio*myopathy (disease of heart muscle)

Component	Meaning	Example
carpo -	wrist	*Carpo*metacarpal joints (joints between the wrist and hand bones)
cata -	down	*Cata*bolism (part of metabolism when substances are broken down)
- cele	swelling/hollow	Hydro*cele* (fluid filled swelling associated with a testis)
cent -	hundred	*Cent*imetre (unit of length, 100th part of a metre)
- centesis	puncture	Amnio*centesis* (aspiration of amniotic fluid for diagnostic purposes)
cephal -	head	*Cepha*lometry (measurement of the head)
cerebro -	brain	*Cerebro*spinal fluid (fluid which surrounds the brain and spinal cord)
cervic -	cervix/neck	*Cervic*itis (inflammation of the uterine cervix)
cheil/cheilo -	lip	*Cheilo*plasty (plastic operation on the lips)
chemo -	chemical	*Chemo*receptor (receptors able to respond to chemical stimuli, e.g. oxygen levels in the blood)
chol/chole -	bile	*Chol*ecystokinin (hormone which stimulates gallbladder contraction and bile release)
cholecyst-	gallbladder	*Cholecyst*ectomy (removal of the gall-bladder)
choledocho -	bile ducts	*Choledocho*lithotomy (opening the bile duct to remove gallstones)
chondro -	cartilage	*Chondro*blast (an embryonic cartilage-producing cell)
chrom -	colour	Haemo*chrom*atosis (a condition where abnormal deposition of iron gives rise to skin pigmentation)
- cide	killing	Sui*cide* (self-destruction)
circum -	around	*Circum*duction (circular movement where the limb traces a cone in space, e.g. arm at the shoulder)

Component	Meaning	Example
- cle/cule	small	Fasicle /fasicule (small bundle of fibres, e.g. of muscle)
co/con	together with	Coenzyme (substances, e.g. some vitamins, required for certain metabolic processes)
coli -	bowel	Coliform bacteria (organisms normally found in the bowel)
colpo -	vagina	Colporrhaphy (repair of the vagina)
contra -	against	Contraceptive (device or drug which prevents conception)
cost -	rib	Intercostal muscles (muscles between the ribs)
cox -	hip	Coxalgia (pain in the hip)
crani -	skull	Cranium (part of the skull enclosing the brain)
cryo -	cold	Cryosurgery (surgical technique which utilizes intense cold)
crypt -	hidden	Cryptomenorrhoea (apparent amenorrhoea where menstrual blood is retained due to an imperforate hymen)
cyan -	blue	Cyanosis (blue discoloration of the skin and mucous membranes caused by poor oxygenation)
cysto -	bladder	Cystoscopy (endoscopic examination of the urinary bladder)
- cyte	cell	Leucocyte (white blood cell)
cyto -	cell	Cytotoxic (substance which is toxic to cells)
dacry -	tear	Dacryadenitis [inflammation of the tear (lacrimal) gland]
dactyl -	digit (usually fingers)	Polydactyly (presence of supernumerary digits)
de -	away	Decalcification (loss of calcium salts from bone)
deci -	tenth	Decilitre (one tenth of a litre – 100 ml)

Component	Meaning	Example
demi , hemi-	half	*Hemi*paraesis (weakness affecting one side of the body)
dent -	tooth	*Dent*ine (substance forming the bulk of a tooth)
derma -	skin	*Derma*titis (inflammation of the skin)
- desis	bind or fix together	Arthro*desis* (operation to fix a joint)
dextro -	right	*Dextro*cardia (congenital transposition of the heart to the right side)
di/diplo -	twos, double	*Di*saccharide (a sugar formed from two monosaccharide units, e.g. sucrose)
dia -	through	*Dia*pedesis (passage of white blood cells through blood vessel walls)
dis -	separation	*Dis*location (displacement of the articular surfaces of the bones forming a joint)
dors -	back	*Dors*al (relating to the back or the posterior part of an organ)
- dynia	pain	Pleuro*dynia* (pain felt in the intercostal muscles)
dys-	difficult, painful	*Dys*menorrhoea (difficult or painful menstruation)
ec-	out from	*Ec*topic (outside the normal place, e.g. a gestation where an embryo develops outside the uterus)
- ectasis	dilation	Bronchi*ectasis* (a condition where the bronchi are abnormally dilated)
ecto -	outside	*Ecto*derm (outer germ layer of primitive embryonic tissue)
- ectomy	removal	Gastr*ectomy* (removal of the stomach)
electro -	electrical	*Electro*lyte (substance which dissociates in water to form electrically charged ions)
em -	in	*Em*pyema (collection of pus in a cavity)
- emesis	vomiting	Hyper*emesis* (excessive vomiting)

Component	Meaning	Example
en/end/endo -	in, into, within	Endometrium (inner layer of the uterus)
entero -	intestine	Enterokinase (intestinal enzyme which activates trypsinogen)
epi -	above, on, upon	Epicondyle (bony eminence above or upon a condyle)
erythr -	red	Erythrocyte (red blood cell)
eu -	well, normal	Euthyroid (having normal thyroid function)
ex/exo -	away from, out of	Exophthalmos (abnormal protrusion of the eyeball out of the orbit)
extra -	outside	Extrapyramidal (outside the pyramidal tracts)
faci -	face	Facial (relating to the face)
- facient	making	Abortifacient (a drug which induces abortion)
- ferent	carry	Afferent (carry towards the centre)
ferri/ferro -	iron	Ferritin (a storage form of iron)
feto -	fetus	Alpha-fetoprotein (a protein produced by the fetus)
fibro -	fibrous, fibre	Fibrosis (formation of fibrous tissue in areas of tissue damage)
flav/flavo -	yellow	Flavoproteins (coenzyme substances involved in metabolic processes)
fore -	before, in front of	Forebrain (front part of the brain)
- form	having the form of	Filiform (resembling a thread)
galact -	milk	Galactose (a monosaccharide which combines with glucose to form lactose – milk sugar)
gastr/gastro -	stomach	Gastrin (local hormone produced by the stomach)
- genesis/genetic	formation	Gluconeogenesis (formation of glucose from non-carbohydrate sources)

Component	Meaning	Example
- *genic*	capable of causing	Pyro*genic* (causing fever)
genito -	genitals	*Genito*urinary (relating to the genital and urinary structures)
ger -	old age	*Ger*ontology (study of ageing)
gloss/glosso -	tongue	*Gloss*al (relating to the tongue)
glyco -	sugar	*Glyco*lysis (series of reactions which break down sugar)
gnath -	jaw	Micro*gnath*ia (abnormally small jaw)
- *gogue*	increasing flow	Galacta*gogue* (agent which increases the flow of milk)
- *gram*	a tracing or drawing	Electroencephalo*gram* (tracing of brain-wave patterns)
- *graph*	instrument for recording	Electroencephalo*graph* (instrument for recording brain wave patterns)
gynae -	female	*Gynae*comastia (male breast enlargement)
haem/haemo/haemato	blood	*Haem*opoiesis (formation of blood cells)
hemi -	half	*Hemi*anopia (loss of sight in half the visual field)
hepat/hepato -	liver	*Hepat*ocytes (parenchymal cells of the liver)
hetero -	different	*Hetero*zygous (where the paired genes for a particular characteristic are different)
hexa -	six	*Hexa*gonal (having six sides, e.g. a liver lobule)
hist -	tissue	*Hist*iocytes (macrophages – phagocytic tissue cells)
homeo -	same, like, unchanging	*Homeo*thermic (warm-blooded; an animal which maintains the same core temperature range)
homo -	same	*Homo*zygous (where the paired genes for a particular characteristic are the same)
hydro -	water	*Hydro*lysis (breakdown of complex substances by the addition of water)

Component	Meaning	Example
hygro -	moisture	*Hygro*scopic (having the ability to absorb moisture)
hyper -	above, excessive	*Hyper*capnia (excess carbon dioxide in the blood)
hypno -	sleep	*Hypno*tic (drug which induces sleep)
hypo-	below, deficient	*Hypo*thalamus (area of the brain below the thalamus)
hyster -	uterus	*Hyster*ectomy (removal of the uterus)
- ia, iasis -	state of, condition	Myop*ia* (condition of shortsightedness)
- iatric(s)/iatry -	healing, medical specialty	Geri*atrics* (medical specialty which deals with the disorders of later life)
iatro -	physician	*Iatro*genic (condition caused by the physician)
- ician	person skilled in a particular field	Paediatr*ician* (person skilled in the treatment of children)
idio -	peculiar to an individual, self	*Idio*pathic (condition with no apparent cause)
ileo -	ileum	*Ileo*caecal valve (valve between the ileum and caecum)
ilio -	ilium	*Ilio*femoral (relating to the ilium and femur, e.g. iliofemoral ligament)
im, in	not, in, within	*Im*potent (not potent)
immuno -	immunity	*Immuno*globulins (protein antibodies concerned with immunity)
inter -	between	*Inter*vertebral (between the vertebrae)
intra -	within	*Intra*uterine (within the uterus)
intro -	inward	*Intro*vert (an inward looking person)
ischio -	ischium	*Ischio*rectal (relating to the ischium and rectum, e.g. ischiorectal abscess)
- ism	condition/state	Hyperthyroid*ism* (condition where the thyroid gland is overactive)

Component	Meaning	Example
iso -	same, equal	*Iso*topes (forms of the same element where atoms have a different number of neutrons)
- itis	inflammation	Cys*itis* (inflammation of the bladder)
kerato -	keratin, horn, cornea	*Kera*titis (inflammation of the cornea)
- kin -	movement	*Kin*etics (study of movement or change)
kypho -	rounded	*Kypho*sis (deformity of the thoracic spine with the formation of a rounded hump)
lacri -	tears	*Lacri*mal (relating to tears, e.g. lacrimal gland)
lact -	milk	*Lact*ation (process of milk production)
laparo -	abdomen	*Laparo*tomy (opening the abdomen)
laryngo -	larynx	*Laryngo*spasm (spasm of the larynx)
later -	side	*Later*al (on the side, away from the midline)
leuco/leuko -	white	*Leuco*cyte (white blood cell)
lingua -	tongue	*Lingua*l (relating to the tongue, e.g. lingual artery)
lip/lipo -	fat	*Lip*ids (large group of fatty substances)
- lith/litho -	stones	*Litho*tripter (device which uses shock waves to disintegrate stones, e.g. kidney stones)
- lithiasis	presence of stones	Chole*lithiasis* (stones in the gallbladder)
- logy	science or study of	Cyto*logy* (study of cells)
- lysis	breakdown	Hydro*lysis* (breakdown of complex substances by the addition of water)
macul-	spot	*Macul*a lutea (yellow spot of the retina)
mal -	bad	*Mal*absorption (inability to absorb nutrients in sufficient quantities from the small intestine)

Component	Meaning	Example
- *malacia*	softening	Osteo*malacia* (softening of the bones – adult rickets)
mamm/mast -	breast	*Mamm*ogram (radiographic examination of the breast)
medi/meso -	middle	*Medi*an (in the middle, e.g. the median line an imaginary longtitudinal line which divides the body down the centre)
mega/megalo -	large	*Megalo*blastic (a type of anaemia characterized by abnormally large red cells)
- *megaly*	enlargement	Hepato*megaly* (enlarged liver)
melano -	black	*Melano*cytes (skin cells which produce the black pigment melanin)
meta -	after, beyond, between	*Meta*physis (the part of a long bone between the diaphysis and epiphysis)
- *meter*	measure	Thermo*meter* (device for measuring temperature)
metro -	uterus	*Metro*ptosis (prolapse of the uterus)
micro -	small	*Micro*cyte (abnormally small red blood cell)
milli -	thousand	*Milli*litre (thousandth part of a litre)
mio -	smaller	*Mio*sis (pupil constriction)
mono -	single, one	*Mono*nuclear (having a single nucleus)
- *morph* -/*morpho* -	shape, form	Poly*morph*ous (having several forms)
muco -	mucus	*Muco*lytic (substance which reduces the viscosity of mucus)
multi -	many	*Multi*cellular (having many cells)
myel-	marrow, spinal cord	*Myel*oblast (primitive bone marrow cell)
myo -	muscle	*Myo*metrium (uterine muscle)
narco -	stupor	*Narco*tic (drug which produces stupor and is used to relieve pain)
necr -	dead	*Necr*osis (death of tissue)

Component	Meaning	Example
neo -	new	Neoplasm (new growth)
nephr/nephro -	kidney	Nephron (functional unit of the kidney)
neuro -	nerves, nervous system	Neuroglia (non-excitable supporting cells of the nervous system)
noct/nyct -	night	Nocturia (passing urine at night)
normo -	normal	Normocyte (a red blood cell of the correct size)
null/nulli -	none	Nulliparous (never had a child)
oculo -	eye	Oculomotor (concerned with eye movement, e.g. oculomotor nerve)
odonto -	tooth	Odontoid (tooth-like, e.g. odontoid peg of the second cervical vertebra)
- ogen	precursor	Angiotensinogen (the inactive precursor of angiotensin)
- oid	likeness	Sigmoid (shaped like the Greek letter sigma, e.g. sigmoid colon)
oligo -	diminished	Oligomenorrhoea (infrequent or sparse menstruation)
- ology	science or study of	Gynaecology (study of disorders affecting the female reproductive structures)
- oma	tumour	Sarcoma (a malignant tumour of connective tissue)
onco -	tumour, mass	Oncogenic (an agent or substance which causes a tumour)
oo -	egg	Oogenesis (production of the egg or oocyte – the female gamete)
oophor -	ovary	Oophoritis (inflammation of the ovary)
ophthalmo -	eye	Ophthalmoscope (instrument used to examine the inside of the eye)
- opia	defect of vision or eye	Hypermetropia (long sight)
orchido -	testis	Orchidectomy (removal of the testis)

Component	Meaning	Example
oro -	mouth	*Oro*pharynx (part of the pharynx behind the mouth – between the soft palate and the hyoid bone)
orth -	normal, straight	*Orth*optics (straightening or correction of visual problems such as strabismus)
os -	mouth, bone	*Os* calcis (bone of the heel also called the calcaneus)
- osis	condition	Otoscler*osis* (condition of chronic thickening of middle ear ossicles with progressive hearing impairment)
oss, osteo -	bone	*Osteo*cyte (a bone cell)
- ostomy/stomy	opening	Trache*ostomy* (an opening into the trachea)
ot/oto -	ear	*Oto*liths [tiny calcium deposits (ear stones) found in the utricle and saccule of the inner ear]
- otomy/tomy	incision	Osteo*tomy* (incision into bone)
ovari -	ovary	*Ovari*an (relating to the ovary, e.g. ovarian artery)
ovi -	ovum, egg	*Ovi*duct (tube conveying ovum from ovary to uterus; also called uterine or Fallopian tube)
oxy -	oxygen	*Oxy*haemoglobin (haemoglobin which is combined with oxygen)
pachy-	thick	*Pachy*dermia (thickening of the skin)
paed -	child	*Paed*iatrics (medical specialty dealing with the disorders of childhood)
pan -	all	*Pan*cytopenia (a reduction in the numbers of all blood cells)
para -	beside, near	*Para*median (close or near to the middle)
part -	birth	*Part*urition (the act of giving birth to a child)
path -	disease	*Path*ogenicity (capacity to cause disease)
- pathy	disease	Nephro*pathy* (kidney disease)

Component	Meaning	Example
- *penia*	lack of	Leuco*penia* (lack of white blood cells)
pent -	five	*Pent*ose (a five carbon sugar)
peps -	digest	*Peps*in (an enzyme which starts to digest protein)
per -	through	*Per*fusion (flow of fluid such as blood through an organ)
peri -	around	*Peri*natal (relating to the time around birth)
perineo -	perineum	*Perineo*rrhaphy (repair of the perineum)
- *pexy*	fixation	Orchido*pexy* (the operation to bring down an undescended testis and its fixation in the scrotum)
- *phag -*	ingest, swallow	Macro*phage* (a tissue cell which ingests particles by phagocytosis)
- *phagia*	eating, swallowing	Dys*phagia* (difficulty in swallowing)
pharmac -	drug	*Pharmac*ology (science dealing with drugs and their effects)
pharyngo -	pharynx	*Pharyngo*tympanic tube (tube between the pharynx and middle ear)
- *phasia*	speech	Dys*phasia* (difficulty in speaking)
- *phil -/ philo/philic*	affinity for	Neutro*phil* (white blood cell which has an affinity for a neutral stain)
phlebo -	vein	Thrombo*phleb*itis (inflammation of a vein with thrombosis)
- *phobia/phobe*	fear of	Claustro*phobia* (fear of enclosed spaces)
phono -	voice, sound	*Phono*cardiography (recording of heart sounds and murmurs using a phonocardiograph)
photo -	light	*Photo*therapy (treatment using light, e.g. for physiological jaundice in the newborn)
phren -	diaphragm, mind	*Phren*ic (relating to the diaphragm, e.g. phrenic nerves)

Component	Meaning	Example
- *phylaxis*	protection	Pro*phylaxis* (measure taken for protection, e.g. immunization)
pilo -	hair	Arrector *pili* (muscle fibres around the hair follicle)
- *plas* -	form, grow	Hyper*plas*ia (grow larger by new cell production)
- *plasty*	reconstruct, plastic surgery	Rhino*plasty* (operation to reconstruct the nose)
- *plegia*	paralysis	Hemi*plegia* (paralysis down one side of the body)
pleur/pleuro -	pleura	*Pleur*isy (inflammation of the pleura)
pneumo -	air, lung	*Pneum*onia (inflammation of the lungs)
- *pnoea*	breathing	A*pnoea* (no breathing)
- *poiesis*	making	Erythro*poiesis* (making red blood cells)
poly -	many	*Poly*morphonuclear (many-shaped nucleus)
post -	after	*Post*ganglionic (relating to the nerve fibre after or distal to a ganglion)
pre/pro -	in front, before	*Pre*ganglionic (relating to the nerve fibre before or proximal to a ganglion)
proct -	rectum, anus	*Proct*ology (study of disorders affecting the rectum and anus)
pseudo -	false	*Pseudo*cyesis (false pregnancy)
psycho -	mind	*Psycho*genic (originating in the mind)
pulmon -	lung	*Pulmon*ary (relating to the lungs, e.g. pulmonary artery)
pyelo -	renal pelvis	*Pyelo*lithotomy (operation to remove stone(s) from the renal pelvis)
pyloro -	pylorus	*Pyloro*myotomy (operation to cut the muscle of the pylorus)
pyo -	pus	*Pyo*metra (pus in the uterus)
pyr -	fever, fire	*Pyr*ogen (substance causing fever)

Component	Meaning	Example
quadri -	four	*Quadri*ceps (large four-part muscle of the anterior thigh)
radio -	radiation	*Radio*isotope (an unstable isotope which emits radiation)
re -	back, again	*Re*flux (flowing back, e.g. of stomach contents into the oesophagus)
ren -	kidney	*Ren*in (proteolytic enzyme produced by the kidney)
retro -	backwards	*Retro*version (turned backwards, a displacement of the uterus)
rhin -	nose	*Rhin*opathy (disease affecting the nose)
- rhythmia	rhythm	Ar*rhythmia* (without rhythm, usually applied to a disturbance of cardiac rhythm)
- rrhage/rrhagia	to burst, pour, excessive flow	Meno*rrhagia* (excessive menstrual flow)
- rrhaphy	to repair	Hernio*rrhaphy* (operation to repair a hernia)
- rrhoea	flow, discharge	Leuco*rrhoea* (white vaginal discharge)
rub -	red	*Rub*or (redness, a sign of inflammation)
sacro -	sacrum	*Sacro*iliac (relating to the sacrum and ilium, e.g. sacroiliac joints)
salpingo -	uterine/ Fallopian tube	*Salpingo*graphy (radiographic investigation to ascertain uterine tube patency)
sarco -	muscle, flesh	*Sarco*lemma (cell membrane enclosing a muscle fibre)
sclero -	hard	*Sclero*sis (hardening, e.g atherosclerosis)
- scope	instrument for examining	Gastro*scope* (instrument used to examine the interior of the stomach)
- scopy	to examine, looking	Gastro*scopy* (endoscopic examination of the stomach)
semi -	half	*Semi*lunar (shaped like a half moon, e.g. semilunar cartilages or menisci of the knee)

Component	Meaning	Example
sero -	serum	*Sero*us (containing serum)
- soma/somat -	body	*Somat*ic (relating to the body, e.g. somatic nerves)
somni -	sleep	In*somni*a (not able to sleep)
- sonic	sound	Ultra*sonic* (high frequency sound beyond the range of the human ear)
sphygm -	pulse	*Sphygm*omanometer (instrument for measuring arterial blood pressure)
splen/spleno -	spleen	*Splen*omegaly (enlargement of the spleen)
spondyl/spondylo -	vertebra	*Spondyl*itis (inflammation of the intervertebral joints)
- stasis	stand still, lack of movement	Haemo*stasis* (no bleeding - the arrest of haemorrhage)
steato -	fat	*Steato*rrhoea (passing undigested fat in the faeces)
steno -	narrow	*Steno*sis (abnormal narrowing, e.g. mitral valve stenosis)
stern/sterno -	sternum	*Stern*ocleidomastoid (relating to the sternum and mastoid, e.g. sternocleidomastoid muscle)
sub -	below	*Sub*arachnoid (below the arachnoid mater)
super/supra -	above	*Supra*condylar (above the condyles, e.g. fracture of the elbow)
sym/syn -	together, union, with	*Syn*ergist (a muscle which works with other muscle groups
tachy -	fast	*Tachy*cardia (fast heart rate)
tars/tarso -	foot, eyelid	*Tars*als (bones of the ankle)
teno -	tendon	*Teno*synovitis (inflammation of tendon sheath)
tetra -	four	Fallot's *tetra*logy (congenital heart condition consisting of four defects)

Component	Meaning	Example
thermo -	heat, temperature	*Thermo*graphy (investigation which measures and records heat production in different parts of an organ or the body)
thorac/thoraco-	chest	*Thorac*ic (relating to the chest or thorax, e.g. thoracic vertebrae)
throm/thrombo -	clot	*Thrombo*plastin (clotting factor)
thyro -	thyroid	*Thyro*xine (a hormone produced by the thyroid)
tox -	poison	*Tox*ic (poisonous, e.g. toxic shock syndrome)
trache/tracheo-	trachea	*Tracheo*-oesophageal (relating to the trachea and oesophagus, e.g. tracheo-oesophageal fistula)
trans -	across, through	*Trans*urethral (through the urethra, e.g. resection of prostate gland)
tri -	three	*Tri*cuspid (valve with three cusps)
trich -	hair	*Trich*omycosis (fungal disease of hair)
- tripsy	crushing	Litho*tripsy* (crushing stones, e.g. in the bladder)
- troph/trophy-	growth, nourishment	*Troph*oblast (cells covering the blastocyst; they invade the decidua and are concerned with the nutrition of the early embryo)
- trophic	changing, influencing	Adrenocortico*trophic* hormone (the hormone which influences the adrenal cortex)
ultra -	beyond, extreme	*Ultra*microscopic (particles too small to be viewed with a light microscope)
uni-	one	*Uni*lateral (on one side)
uretero-	ureter	*Uretero*vesical (relating to the ureter and bladder)
urethr/urethro-	urethra	*Urethr*itis (inflammation of the urethra)
uri/uro -	urine	*Uro*bilinogen (pigment excreted in the urine)
- uria	urine	Dys*uria* (pain or difficulty passing urine)

Component	Meaning	Example
uter/utero -	uterus	*Uter*ine (relating to the uterus, e.g. uterine tubes)
vas/vaso -	vessel, duct	*Vaso*constriction (contraction of blood vessels)
vene -	vein	*Vene*puncture (inserting a needle into a vein)
vesico -	bladder	*Vesico*vaginal (relating to the bladder and vagina)
viscer -	organs	*Viscer*al (relating to the internal organs, especially those of the abdominal cavity)
xero -	dry	*Xero*derma (dry skin)
zoo -	animal	*Zoo*nosis (disease transmitted from animals to humans)